S0-BNW-073

Fundamentals of Nursing

Fourth Edition

Fundamentals of Nursing

The Humanities and The Sciences in Nursing

Elinor V. Fuerst, R.N., M.A.

Formerly Educational Consultant, Muhlenberg Hospital School of Nursing, Plainfield, N. J.; Assistant Professor of Nursing, Cornell University—New York Hospital School of Nursing, New York; Test Editor, Department of Measurement and Guidance of National League of Nursing Education; Educational Director, Christ Hospital School of Nursing, Jersey City, N. J.

LuVerne Wolff, R.N., M.A.

Consultant, College of Nursing, Arizona State University; Formerly Research Associate, Institute of Research and Service in Nursing Education, Teachers College, Columbia University, New York; Supervisor in Nursing, State Education Department, Albany, N. Y.; Assistant Director of Nursing Service and the School of Nursing, American University of Beirut

J.B. Lippincott Company

PHILADELPHIA ● TORONTO

Fourth Edition

Distributed in Great Britain by
Blackwell Scientific Publications.
Oxford, London, and Edinburgh

ISBN-0-397-54078-7

Library of Congress Catalog Card No. 70-77964

Printed in the United States of America

7 9 8

Fondly dedicated to

Mrs. Jennie Fuerst

and

Mr. and Mrs. Edward H. Wolff

Preface

This edition has been expanded to include nursing measures which are now considered fundamental to the care of all patients. It also has undergone an extensive revision in the arrangement of content. The focus of the text is on the three principles that guide nursing action, namely, maintaining the individuality of man, maintaining physiologic functioning, and maintaining a safe environment.

Matters concerned with nursing as a practice are considered in Unit One. This includes the status of current health problems, nursing's place in the health field, and technics related to practice, such as problem solving, teaching, and communicating by means of both the written and spoken word.

Nursing measures that are most directly related to man as a person have been organized in Unit Two. This includes consideration of the role of the patient, and the anxiety, stress and fear that may accompany that role.

Nursing measures concerned with environmental factors and with controlling the spread of infection have been organized in Unit Three. This content was placed before Unit Four—Man as an Organism—because the concepts of medical and surgical asepsis are essential to the care considered in Unit Four.

It will be noted that Unit Four considers the basic needs of man, i.e., hygiene, nutrition, rest, fluid and electrolyte balance, elimination, respiratory integrity, and so forth. The latter part of the Unit is concerned with some common problems of illness, such as pain, vomiting, and impaired elimination from the gastrointestinal or genitourinary tracts. Care of the terminally ill patient was placed at the end of this Unit.

Unit Five considers the many therapeutic measures which are commonly prescribed for the care of patients, and are essential to supporting the three preceding Units—man as a person, his environment, and his physical well-being.

Some common therapeutic and diagnostic measures are considered in Unit Six.

The format of this revision is not designed to constitute a particular sequence in teaching. It is hoped, however, that its arrangement is more flexible than heretofore, so that instructors can use it to select content to fit into their individual teaching patterns. It is also hoped that students and others using the text may find it easier to locate what they wish under this arrangement.

It is not the intent of the authors to fractionalize the patient, but rather to help the reader become increasingly aware of the fact that nursing is not just "treating" a patient.

Some procedures were deleted because they are so seldom used, or have been replaced by other measures, or in some instances depend too much upon local practice to be helpful in a text; for instance, charting and nursing care plan examples, which tend to follow the practice of the agency.

The patient study at the end of the text is offered as an example of teamwork as it can operate in the home. With the kind cooperation of the patient's family, it was possible to present this situation in the hope that it may help others. Nurses are often in a position to suggest to families means by which they can cope with many nursing care problems and still have their loved ones at home.

Acknowledgments

If we were to acknowledge our gratitude to all who have in some measure contributed to this book, we would need to omit the contents and write only of our past experiences and those associates, patients, and students who have helped to mold our philosophies and convictions. We deeply appreciate the assistance that we have received, directly or indirectly, from so many of our friends in nursing.

We wish to express our thanks to J. B. Lippincott Company, especially to Mr. Walter Kahoe, Medical Director, and Mr. Barton H. Lippincott, Vice-President, who were responsible for involving us in this adventure; and special thanks go to Mr. David T. Miller, Editorial Manager, Nursing Department, who offered valuable assistance and guidance during the preparation of both the previous edition and this new one.

We also wish to acknowledge our thanks to the following: Miss Mary T. Bielski, Associate Professor of Medical Nursing, Cornell University–New York Hospital School of Nursing, New York, N. Y.; Mrs. Dorothy F. Corona, Associate Professor of Nursing, College of Nursing, Arizona State University, Tempe, Arizona; the Rt. Rev. Msgr. James G. Wilders, Director, Hospital Apostolate, Archdiocese of New York, New York, N.Y.; Rabbi Albert Plotkin, Temple Beth Israel, Phoenix, Arizona; the Rev. Julian Alexander, Jr., Scotch Plains, New Jersey; William G. Burke, D.D.S., Phoenix, Arizona; Mr. Paul R. Messinger; and to Mrs. Louise J. Giuffre, for her valuable assistance in the preparation of the manuscript.

We have used three J. B. Lippincott Company publications generously, because their content fitted our format and purposes so well. We wish to thank Madelyn Titus Nordmark and Anne W. Rohweder, authors of *Scientific Foundations of Nursing*, J. Trygve Jensen, Author of *Introduction to Medical Physics*, and Norma M. Metheny and William D. Snively, authors of *Nurses' Handbook of Fluid Balance*.

Table of Contents

UNIT ONE: THE PRACTICE OF NURSING

UNIT THREE: NURSING IMPLEMENTATION—MAN AND HIS ENVIRONMENT

UNIT FIVE: NURSING RESPONSIBILITIES IN RELATION TO OTHER COMMONLY PRESCRIBED THERAPEUTIC AGENTS AND MEASURES

UNIT SIX: NURSING RESPONSIBILITIES IN RELATION TO ASSISTING THE PHYSICIAN WITH DIAGNOSTIC AND THERAPEUTIC MEASURES

UNIT SEVEN: NURSING IN A HOME SITUATION: A PATIENT STUDY

The Practice of Nursing

Unit 1

CHAPTER 1

Nursing and Its Responsibilities: Prevention—Care—Rehabilitation

When modern nursing began in the United States shortly before the turn of the century, it was primarily concerned with the physical care of the ill in hospitals. Nursing was task-oriented and much of nursing education was devoted to learning procedures and hospital routines. In keeping with the changes occurring in the world today, nursing is in transition. It is becoming indispensable in helping to provide society with comprehensive health care.

Nurses recognize that there are important social and psychological, as well as physical, aspects of patient care. They note too that nursing is rightly concerned with preventing illness, promoting health, and assisting with rehabilitation. This broader concept of nursing results from the application of principles rather than of empirical knowledge only. It implies that nursing is concerned with helping persons in need of health care, no matter where such care is given—at home, in a clinic, in a hospital, in a nursing home, or at other types of health agencies. In addition, nursing is concerned with these persons as individuals and with the way their personal requirements may affect their health problems. This approach places primary emphasis on the person being served rather than on the mechanics of procedures and routines.

Defining Nursing

Because nursing is in a state of transition, and has been for many years, the literature abounds with attempts to keep abreast of its changing status and the role of the nurse. Other health professions are also in transition and many new types of health personnel are being prepared. No profession can remain stationary. All are affected by forces both from within and without, scientific and social. These factors make it seem certain that nursing will continue to undergo re-definition.

The authors of this text define nursing as an art in the ministering of health services. It is based on scientific principles and is rendered by persons who have a sincere concern for the welfare and well-being of others. Nursing provides certain services to society that are therapeutic, in that they help people to stay well, help prevent illness or injury, help people regain their best health potential, and give care and comfort to the dying.

Circumstances in the related health professions with which the nurse is associated require that nursing assume some coordination responsibilities in addition to its care and cure functions. There is no question but that the services rendered to patients by different health team members overlap somewhat. For example, a physician, a dietitian, or a social worker can answer some questions a patient may have. Physicians, technicians, nurses and even family members can bathe a patient. What, where, when and how is nursing's contribution to the health services unique? Hopefully the answer will be made evident throughout the text.

In defining nursing, it must be remembered that it is the physician (except in certain emergency situations) who plans and prescribes a course of therapy. Nurses carry it out as directed. For example, if a physician believes that one of his patients needs a drug, he prescribes the exact medication, the time it is to be given, the dosage and the route of administration. A nurse is then responsible for giving the medication according to these orders, modifying the procedure, if necessary, to meet the patient's needs, and observing the results.

But nurses also initiate and control nursing care that augments and complements the physician's plan of care. Consider this example. An ill patient in a hospital needs a bath and oral hygiene. The nurse will either give (or assign an assistant [aide, volunteer or practical nurse] to give) the patient a bath and mouth care. She does not need a phy-

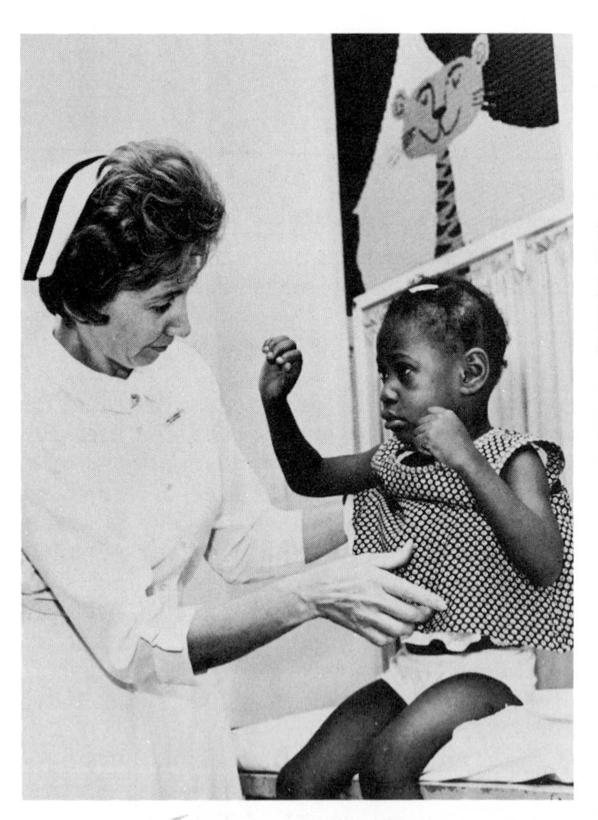

Fig. 1-1. Nursing is assisting in preventive care: Helping a pre-school child get ready for her physical check-up is a common experience for the nurse, but it is not so for a patient. In this instance, the nurse also needs to reduce some doubts and prevent some tears from forming. (Photo by Warren R. Vroom)

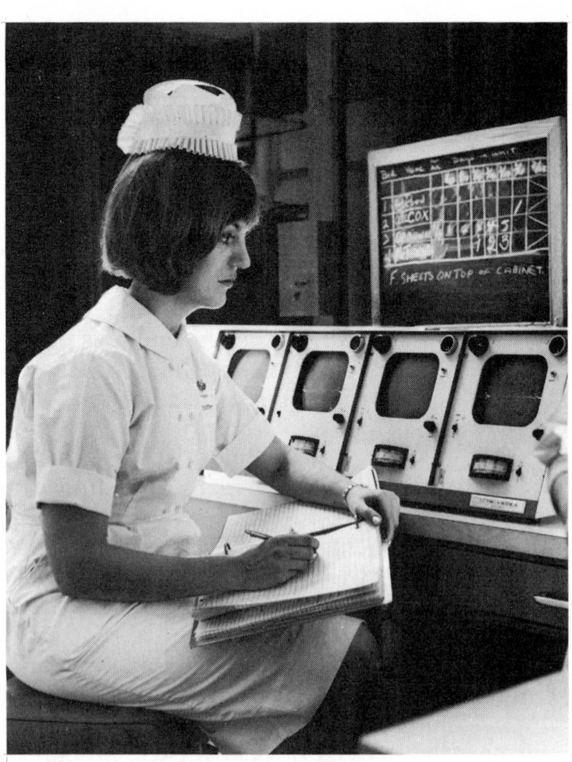

Fig. 1-2. Nursing is administering care to the sick: In addition to direct care of the patient, nurses must be knowledgeable about modern therapy. This nurse is at a monitoring station of the coronary care unit. (Courtesy of New York Hospital—Cornell Medical Center)

sician's order in order to provide this service; rather she recognizes the patient's nursing requirements and takes action on her own. When it is necessary to provide for individual variations the nurse develops a plan of care and modifies it as changes occur.

There is no single approach to nursing action. Each patient is a person having characteristics that make his situation unlike that of other persons. Therefore, there is variation in nursing care as applied to several individuals or even to one individual at different times.

The goal of the nurse's plan of care is not different from that of the physician or other health workers. All aim to help a person to conserve his health, to prevent or to cure illness and to sustain life. However, the contributions of each differ.

In many places where nurses practice, persons other than physicians and nurses are involved in carrying out the plan of therapy prescribed by the physician. For example, a physician may order a patient to have certain physiotherapy and a special diet. In this case, a physiotherapist and a dietitian also play an important role in the care of the patient. Nursing becomes involved in coordination, seeing that there is continuity of care for this patient, as well as working cooperatively with the other health workers. If, in this example, the physiotherapist had ordered

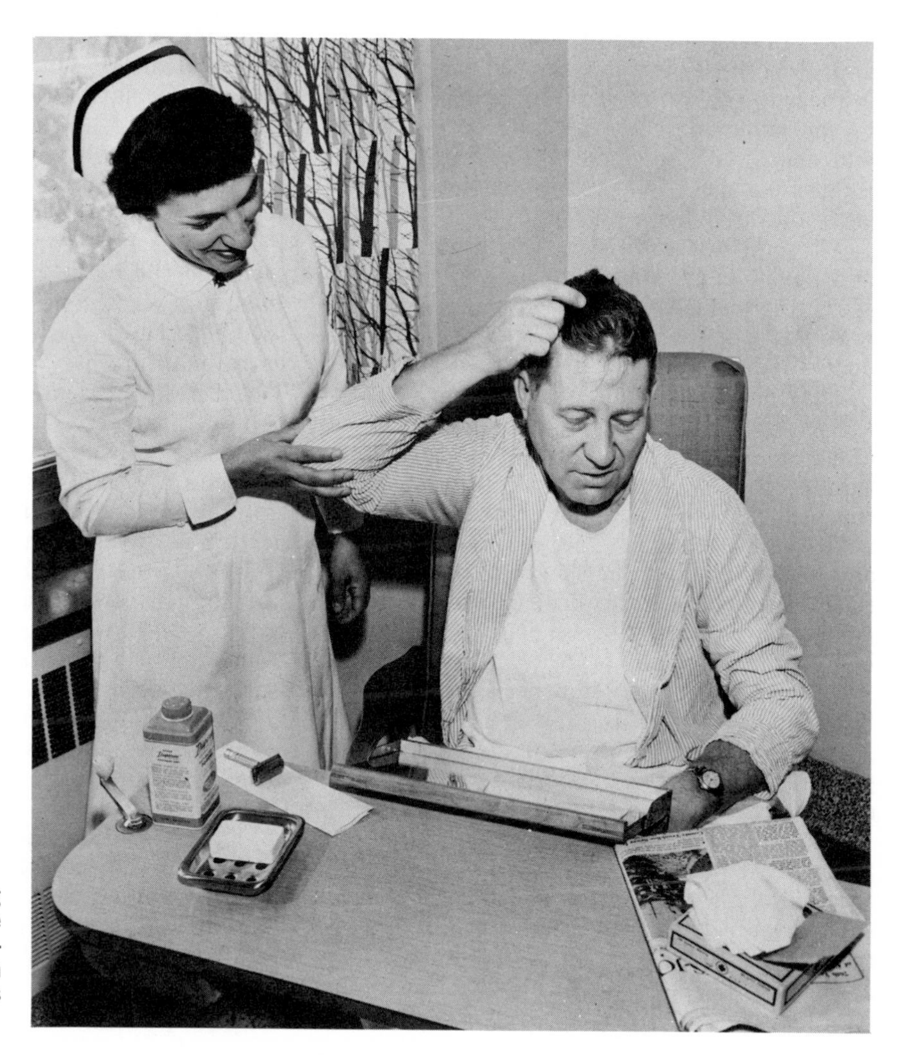

Fig. 1-3. Nursing is assisting in rehabilitation: Here the nurse is encouraging a patient to regain range of motion in his arm by encouraging him to comb his hair.

the patient to have periodic exercises for an extremity, in most agencies the nursing staff would be responsible for carrying out that order. Assume that the patient will continue with the special diet after leaving the hospital. The nurse, in cooperation with the dietitian, will see to it that the patient is given instructions concerning the diet.

The Role of the Nurse

There are certain abilities and qualities associated with the role of the nurse. The nurse should be sensitive to social needs and have a sincere desire and willingness to help others. She has the desire and the ability to master the knowledge and the skills required for practicing nursing. She possesses a creative imagination and develops an analytical and objective point of view. She has a willingness to grow intellectually, a desire to add to the body of knowledge of her profession and the ability to make adaptations as she judges her practice in light of new experience and knowledge.

Through her knowledge of human growth and development and interpersonal relationships, the nurse tries to "know" herself. She tries to work cooperatively and harmoniously with others and uses sound judgment in sharing responsibility with them.

She sincerely believes in the promotion and the restoration of health and the prevention of disease, and she reflects her beliefs through her own personal habits and daily activities. Therefore, she is a teacher by example, and through her own activities helps to instill in others the desire for health.

The nurse recognizes her obligations to her community, her state and her country. As a member of a democracy, she accepts her responsibilities as a citizen and upholds the tenet of equal rights for all persons, regardless of race, color, creed or social or economic status.

One writer illuminates the nurse's role as follows: "I believe that the true virtue, the true calling of the nurse, consists neither in following doctor's orders nor in administering prescribed treatments (although she ought to do both conscientiously) but in the true aspects contained in the very name of the profession: to nurse and to nurture, to feed the body and to nurture the soul."[2] The author acknowledges the necessity of carrying out the physician's plan of care but recognizes that the utmost value of nursing is what a nurse can do for an individual when she comes to know him as a person.

Nursing and the Law

In the last decade or two there has been a considerable increase in the number of legal actions in the United States involving nurses. At regular intervals the American Nurses' Association collects and reports information concerning court actions involving nurses to help keep nurses informed of their legal responsibilities. The American Journal of Nursing carries a bimonthly article written by an attorney who describes various laws and their relationship to nursing. The purchase of professional liability insurance is on the increase, including policies recommended by the American Nurses' Association. Nursing is so intertwined with the law that it behooves every nurse, students included, to examine the ways in which the law protects those for whom she is caring and the agency in which she is learning or working, as well as to examine her own legal status.

A detailed discussion of the legal aspects of nursing generally is included in curricula of schools of nursing near the time when students are graduating. Hence, the discussion here will be brief. However, because certain aspects of the law involve nurses from the time they begin their education in nursing, it seems appropriate to give an early over-view. As you read on in this text, there will be repeated mention of the legal implications of many of the nurse's responsibilities. Examples include legal implications involved in making entries on patients' records, in taking orders from a physician, in caring for patients' personal clothing and valuables and in reporting a medication error. New and experimental equipment may present dangers that could result in lawsuits. In addition, as nursing changes, so often do nursing responsibilities. Certain practices, intravenous therapy being an example, once were administered by physicians only. More and more nurses are assuming some of these responsibilities, with legal implications not yet clearly defined by either statutory or common law. The legal implications in the use of monitors and computers have not been defined.

Legal responsibilities inherent in nursing will continue to be described throughout your educational program. Losing sight of them could lead to serious results.

Sources of Laws. There are four main sources of laws or rules of conduct in our country. These sources are the constitutions, the legislatures, the judiciary system and administrative regulations.

Constitutions. In any society there must be an authoritative body if chaos is to be prevented. Although authority comes from the people, each individual relinquishes certain rights in order that a form of government can be established and given the authority to govern. The government is charged with the responsibility of maintaining order and protecting the general welfare of its people.

The constitution of the federal government and of each state indicates how its government is created and given authority. These constitutions state the principles and provisions for establishment of specific laws. Although they themselves contain relatively few laws (called constitutional laws), they are constant guides to legislative bodies. In our country each state constitution directs the governing of a specific geographic area, but it can in no way violate principles set down in the federal constitution.

Although individuals relinquish certain rights in order that a government can be created, the constitutions are not without their limits. For example, the first ten amendments of the federal constitution are referred to as the Bill of Rights. These amendments restrict the passage of laws that infringe on certain basic liberties; for example, freedom of worship, freedom of speech, freedom from unwarranted search and seizure of our homes and persons, and the like. Each state constitution sets similar limitations.

The Nurse Practice Acts in our country are based on constitutional laws and principles. These acts will be further discussed later in this Chapter.

The Legislatures. Our government under the constitution has created legislative bodies that are responsible for enacting laws. These bodies are called the Congress at the federal level and legislatures at the state level. Certain legislative bodies at the local level (county, municipalities, and the like) may be established also. A law enacted by a legislative body is referred to as *statutory law.* These laws must be in keeping with the federal constitution and, within each state, with that state's constitution as well. The Nurse Practice Acts are statutory laws.

The Judiciary System. Our government provides for a judiciary system which enforces the laws of the land. When conflicts arise, courts in the judiciary system make decisions in relation to the laws involved in the conflict. This multitude of decisions is called *common law.*

Common law is based on the principle known as *stare decisis,* or "Let the decision stand." In other words, once a decision has been made in a court of law, that decision becomes the rule to follow when other cases involving similar circumstances and facts arise. Court decisions can be changed but only when strong justification exists. Common law helps prevent one set of rules being used to judge one person, and another set to judge another person in similar circumstances.

Common law that is directly concerned with nursing exists. Under common law, for example, students in hospital-controlled schools of nursing have been considered as employees of the hospital. In the absence of legal action, there is question as to whether students in programs independent of hospital control (such as university and college programs) would be considered as employees.

Administrative Regulations. When a law is passed, the executive branch of our government (the President or a governor) or an administrative agency frequently is given the power to make certain regulations in relation to the law. These administrative regulations act as laws themselves and are enforceable just as any law in the country.

The state boards of nursing are administrative agencies which are granted power to make regulations in relation to state nurse practice acts.

Laws applicable to nurses and nursing practice are derived from all of the sources just described. Nurses, whether they are considered employees or independent contractors (as private duty nurses) are responsible for their actions in the course of their practice and can be held liable when a wrong has been committed. Torts and crimes and a few common examples will be described briefly.

Torts and Crimes. Torts and crimes are wrongs. A tort is a wrong committed by a person against another person or his property. In most instances, the court in a civil case (that is, a case involving a tort) will settle damages in terms of money, rarely in terms of imprisonment.

A crime also is a wrong against a person or his property but the act is considered to be primarily against the public. In a criminal case, the government (referred to as The People) prosecutes the offender. A crime is punished either by fines or imprisonment or both. Certain crimes carry the death penalty in some states.

A wrong may be prosecuted either as a tort or a crime or both. For example, crimes are torts by their very nature, and a person committing a crime may be tried in both a civil and a criminal action. But a wrong tried as a crime (and hence, a wrong against the public) usually implies a more serious offense with more legal implications than a tort.

Negligence. A negligent act occurs when a person performs an act that a reasonable person under similar circumstances would not do—or, conversely, fails to do what reasonably should be done. Malpractice also is negligence. To quote one authority, "Malpractice is only a term of limited nomenclature. Negligence is all-inclusive. In other words, malpractice and negligence are not two separate torts, but one and the same. What is necessary to constitute an act of negligence is essential to constitute an act of malpractice." (Lesnik: 235.)

One investigation found that nurses have been held liable for negligent acts such as these: burns, as caused by hot water bottles and electrical equipment; injuries, as a result of falling and improper treatment; losses, as sponges used in surgical procedures; and errors, as in diets and medications.

Assault and Battery. Assault is a threat to, or an attempt to, make bodily contact with another person without that person's consent. A battery is an assault that is carried out. Every person is granted freedom from bodily contact by another unless consent has been granted. In the field of health, a person operated upon without his consent can sue the surgeon and/or the health agency involved. Hospital personnel cannot force patients to do things against their will, unless consent has been granted, without fear of legal suit. Certain consent forms are discussed later in this text and others will be discussed in other parts of your educational program.

Slander and Libel. Slander is an untruthful oral statement about a person that subjects him to ridicule or contempt. Libel is the same, except that the statement is in writing, signs, pictures, or the like. False statements, for example, that indicate someone is unfit for the practice of his profession can be held as slander or libel. Falsely accusing someone of committing a crime constitutes slander or libel. Nurses who make false statements about their patients or their co-workers, for example, run the risk of being sued for slander or libel.

False Imprisonment. Preventing the movement of another person without proper consent can constitute false imprisonment. Such a wrong would be committed if any person were forcibly held in a health agency unless the proper consent had been granted. The indiscriminate and thoughtless use of restraints is another example of an act that can constitute false imprisonment.

Invasion of Privacy. Everyone is free to withhold himself from public exposure. If a person is exposed to the public, either personally or through pictures, the person responsible for such exposure can be held liable. As in other cases, this is not true if the patient has granted permission for the exposure.

Torts in relation to autopsies are discussed later in this text.

Examples of Crimes. A definition of crime was given earlier. Examples of crimes include murder, manslaughter and the illegal possession of narcotics. Murder is killing a person with malice aforethought. Manslaughter is killing without malice aforethought. Any person who is practicing nursing (or medicine) unlawfully and whose patient dies as a result of the illegal practice can be tried for the crime of manslaughter.

In our country, narcotic control is governed by the Harrison Narcotic Law. Persons found violating this law or any of the regulations issued to aid enforcement of the law are guilty of committing a crime.

Defenses for Torts and Crimes. The person or government bringing suit against another is called the *plaintiff*. The one being accused of a tort or crime is called the *defendant*. The defendant has every opportunity in our courts of law to defend himself; philosophically, he is presumed innocent unless proven guilty. Recent Supreme Court decisions, some of which gained considerable publicity, were predicated on the tenet that in our country every effort shall be directed toward justice for the accused. Hence, being *accused* of a tort or crime does not imply guilt.

The law also provides in certain instances for what is referred to as a privilege. When privilege is present, grounds for a suit may be absent. One privilege has already been mentioned, namely consent. For example, if a rational patient has signed a proper consent for surgery, he is in no position to sue the surgeon for having performed the operation for which he consented.

Emergency situations also give persons certain privilege. For example, if an unconscious patient is in need of a surgical procedure which in the opinion of a physician constitutes a lifesaving measure, and if no one is available who can legally give consent for the patient, the emergency justifies the operation without consent.

Everyone is granted the privilege of defending himself from harm. Hence, within reason and depending on circumstances, a person can perform acts of defense without being held liable for them. In the case of libel and slander, if the defendant can prove that the statement he made about another person is true, no case exists. For the interested reader, additional examples of privilege are cited in references at the end of this chapter.

Nurse Practice Acts. It has been pointed out that the federal and state constitutions provide for governments that we as individuals charge with the responsibility of securing the public welfare. Legislative bodies have used this principle to enact laws that control certain occupational and professional groups. In other words, to secure public welfare, laws governing these groups are designed to prevent incompetent persons from practicing. In general the goal of these laws is accomplished through two channels: (1) schools preparing practitioners must maintain certain minimum standards of education; and (2) graduates of the educational programs may be licensed only after satisfactory completion of an examination.

Nursing is one group operating under state statutory laws that were designed in keeping with federal and state constitutional principles to promote the general welfare. The first law in the United States dealing with the practice of nursing was enacted in 1903 in North Carolina. At the present time there are nurse practice acts in the 50 States, the District of Columbia, Puerto Rico and the Virgin Islands.

The laws vary considerably from State to State. Some laws define nursing, while others describe what a nurse may or may not do in the practice of nursing. In some States the law requires that a nurse be licensed in order to practice; such a law usually is referred to as a mandatory nurse practice act. In other States, the law merely allows the licensed nurse to refer to herself as a Registered Nurse or an R.N.; such a law usually is referred to as a permissive nurse practice act, since a license is not required in order to practice.

The administrative agency in each state that has power to make regulations in relation to nurse practice acts is the state board of nursing. The regulations made by these boards become laws in themselves, as previously described. Some typical responsibilities of these state boards include determining minimum standards for education for nursing, setting requirements for licensure, and deciding when a nurse's license may be suspended or revoked.

Study Situations

Criteria of a profession include requirements for its members to seek improvement in the services they render by continued study, self-evaluation, identification of problems and research. Throughout this text there are Study Situations such as the ones below. Consider them carefully. They are intended to help you recognize that there is more information available on the topics presented in each chapter, and they will refer you to other opinions on some topics. They also are intended to help you recognize problems needing further investigation, and to help you gain additional knowledge of principles that can guide nursing practice.

1. Nursing, as other careers, is influenced by social forces. As society changes, so must nursing change as it assumes its responsibilities for meeting health needs most efficiently. What social forces are likely to influence nursing practice during the next decade or two? The following references will assist in preparing answers to these questions:

- Hassenplug, L. W.: The world of nursing . . . 2000 A.D.
  AMER. J. NURS. *62*:100-102, August, 1962.
- Lambertsen, E. C.: Changes in practice require changes in education.
  AMER. J. NURS., *66*:1784-87, August, 1966.
- Mullane, M. K.: Has nursing changed?
  NURS. OUTLOOK *6*:323, June, 1958.
- Nahm, H.: A decade of change.
  AMER. J. NURS., *59*:1588-1590, November, 1959.
- Webb, M. W.: The nurse and the challenge of the sixties.
  AMER. J. NURS. *61*:48-50, August, 1961.
- Wheeler, D. V.: Who determines nursing's destiny?
  AMER. J. NURS., *63*:65-66, December, 1963.

2. In the following article, note the author's emphasis on the role of the nurse as coordinator of patient care. What other responsibilities does this author see as important in nursing?

- Wolford, H.: The nurse of the future.
  NURS. OUTLOOK, *14*:41-42, April, 1966.

3. Read the following article:

- Macdonald, B. D.: Nursing's many meanings.
  NURS. OUTLOOK, *14*:56-57, July, 1966.

In this author's description of her philosophy of nursing, what seven elements does she discuss as essential to nursing? How does the author elaborate on the statement, "Nursing is a reciprocal situation."?

4. For those readers interested in nursing's constant struggle for definition, the following historical articles would be of interest:

- Worcester, A.: Is nursing really a profession?
  AMER. J. NURS., *2*:908, 1901.
- Stewart, I. M.: Professional school or trade school?
  AMER. J. NURS., pp. 1105, *29*:1105-1110, September, 1929.
- Cabot, R. C.: What's worth while in nursing?
  AMER. J. NURS., p. 277, March, 1931.
- Bixler, G., and Bixler, R.: The professional status of nursing.
  AMER. J. NURS., p. 730, *45*:730-735, September, 1945.

5. A typical comment made by the prospective student in nursing is that she wants to "help people," and it is common for her to see herself helping the helpless. Consider the following references concerning man's drive to assert personal worth and his motivation to regain independence.

- Self-help, self-esteem, and self-determination. Editorial.
  AMER. J. NURS., *62*:57, September, 1962.
- Heckman, M. K.: What if it were I?
  AMER. J. NURS., *66*:768-769, April, 1966.

6. In considering the role of the nurse and the patient's expectations of the nurse, we must not overlook the child's image of the nurse and some of his expectations. See the following:

- Goodman, J.: A nurse is a heck of a nice thing.
  AMER. J. NURS., *67*:550-551, March, 1967.

7. The following article describes how the legal doctrine of *res ipsa loquitur* has been applied in several court cases:

- Hersey, N.: The doctrine that helps the plaintiff.
  AMER. J. NURS., *68*:120-121, January, 1968.

What was the primary purpose of using *res ipsa loquitur* in the case of the injured patient described in this article?

References

1. Baziak, A. T.: Prospects for change in nursing.
   NURS. FORUM, *6*:134-154. #2, 1967.
2. Bettelheim, B.: To nurse and to nuture.
   NURS. FORUM, *1*:60-76, Summer, 1962.
3. Donahue, J. C. (Guest Editor): Symposium on the nurse and the law.
   NURS. CLIN. N.A., *2*:115-197, March, 1967.
4. Fagin, C. M.: Psychotherapeutic nursing.
   AMER. J. NURS., *67*:298-304, February, 1967.
5. Heckman, M. K.: What if it were I?
   AMER. J. NURS., *66*:768-769, April, 1966.
6. Hersey, N.: The law and the nurse.
   AMER. J. NURS., see author's series of articles appearing bimonthly.
7. Lesnik, M. J., and Anderson, B. E.: Nursing Practice and the Law, 400 p.
   ed. 2 rev. Philadelphia, Lippincott, 1962.
8. Olszewski, L.: Is scientism destroying nursing?
   AMER. J. NURS., *67*:1052, May, 1967.
9. Palmer, D. A.: The nurse as a whole person.
   R.N., *27*:55-57, March, 1964.
10. Regan, W. A.: You, doctor, and hospital: Equals before the law.
    R.N., *28*:86-98, October, 1965.
11. Reiter, F.: The nurse-clinician.
    AMER. J. NURS., *66*:274-280, February, 1966.
12. Sarner, H.: The Nurse and the Law. 219 p. Philadelphia, W. B. Saunders, 1968.
13. Schlotfeldt, R.: A mandate for nurses and physicians.
    AMER. J. NURS., *65*:102-105, December, 1965.
14. Schutt, B. G.: The promise in practice. (Editorial)
    AMER. J. NURS., *67*:2515, December, 1967.
15. Silverburg, R.: We are swimming against the tide.
    NURS. FORUM, *6*:363-367, #4, 1967.
16. Stokes, J., III: Physicians' assistants.
    AM. J. NURS., *67*:1441-1443, July, 1967.

CHAPTER 2

Health and Its Implications for Nursing

The United States is pledged to promote the general welfare of its people. Implicit in this pledge is the belief that health belongs to everyone as one of the fundamental rights of mankind. No longer is health a privilege of only a few. Rather, it is a just claim to which everyone is entitled.

Health for its citizens is a concern of all nations. It has been recognized as a potent force in world leadership and has been used as an instrument of international relations. It has been employed constructively as a part of our foreign policy. In fact, nations throughout the world are recognizing that the health of their citizens is one of their most valuable assets.

A concept that embraces health for all has numerous implications. Persons engaged in the health fields have an obligation to promote the best kind of health services for everyone. In addition, this concept implies a need for a variety of health services, including nursing services, that can adapt continuously to the ever-changing demands and requirements of society.

Definition of Health

Many definitions of health can be found in both professional and lay literature, all of which in general are based on the premise that health represents physical fitness, emotional and mental stability and social usefulness.

The U. S. President's Commission on the Health Needs of the Nation reported that health means ". . . optimum physical, mental, and social efficiency and well-being." The Commission went on to state that the first requisite for leading a full life is health, which makes possible maximum self-expression and self-development of man.

The World Health Organization, one of the specialized agencies of the United Nations, defined health in the preamble to its constitution as ". . . a state of complete physical, mental and social well-being and not merely the absence of disease or infirmity." It goes on to state that health is ". . . one of the fundamental rights of every human being without distinction of race, religion, political belief, economic or social condition."

These definitions of health indicate that what constitutes health is not necessarily constant in nature. Health and illness may be considered to be on a continuum. In other words, there is no exact point at which poor health ends and good health begins. It is accepted commonly that health is relative in nature, and that for each individual there is a considerable range or latitude in which he may function and enjoy good health.

Comprehensive Health Services

What services are necessary to attain and maintain health? It is generally agreed that a comprehensive health program consists of two main parts: personal health services and environmental health services.

Personal Health Services. The National Commission on Community Health Services described the necessary components of comprehensive personal health services this way:

". . . These services should embrace those directed toward promotion of positive good health, application of established preventive measures, early detection of disease, prompt and effective treatment, and physical, social, and vocational rehabilitation of those with residual disabilities." (Health Is A Community Affair. 5:17)

To list and describe these services does not imply that any one of them is an entity unto itself and unrelated to the others. In fact, it is difficult to define exactly where one service ends and another begins, since all are related in many ways. For example, in certain instances good rehabilitation practices promote health and thereby prevent disease and disability. Practices that promote health often prevent disease. Technics that promote health and prevent disease have often improved as a result of improved methods for diagnosing and treating disease.

Nor should it be assumed that health personnel usually are concerned with only a part of these services. Many professional groups concerned with health contribute to all areas, and nursing is one of those groups. Each of the services is of major concern to nurses, and the various ways in which nurses contribute to them will be discussed throughout this text.

Although the promotion of health, the prevention of disease, the detection and the treatment of disease and rehabilitation are interrelated, a brief description of each service is presented in order that the student may visualize what constitutes a comprehensive personal health program.

Promotion of Health. Within recent years, science has made great progress in describing what good health is and how it can be promoted. It has been recognized that promoting good health includes supporting and developing mental as well as physical health programs. Psychologists and psychiatrists in particular have studied individual responses to stress and strain. From such studies, programs that help the individual to cope with the demands of everyday living are enabling more persons to enjoy better mental and social well-being. The numerous counseling programs are examples of a service that aims to promote good mental health.

An example of promotion in the area of physical health may be cited from the field of nutrition. Basic food requirements of the body have been well established. Animal experimentation as well as scientific observations of the dietary customs of humans have illustrated the effects of both poor and good eating habits. Through intensive educational programs, nutritionists and their allied coworkers have contributed immeasurably to health promotion by helping people to learn how to select proper foods.

Just as the services of personal health programs are interrelated, so also are mental and physical health. The medical profession has made great strides in illustrating the close relationship of mental and physical health, and various studies have pointed out how rarely they can be considered independently of each other.

Prevention of Disease. It has been pointed out that promoting health helps to prevent disease. However, despite good health promotion, disease still attacks man, and science is constantly at work in order to find measures that will prevent disease. In numerous instances, fortunately, the challenge of disease prevention has been well met. Certain communicable diseases that harassed this country as recently as a half century ago are now almost nonexistent, due primarily to a nation-wide development of immunization programs. Examples are smallpox and diphtheria. Certain other diseases such as typhoid fever, once common, have been reduced to a minimum by means of improved sanitation.

While energy continues to be directed toward prevention of disease, at least three trends are apparent in preventive medicine. Many acute illnesses have been largely conquered as mentioned above, but many chronic diseases have not. There is a trend now to attempt to identify signs of chronic illness long before it occurs. Increased publicity is devoted to the advisability of regular physical examinations for all ages.

A second trend is an increased interest in health problems related to a change in our population structure. The number of persons over 65 years of age has increased considerably in the United States during the last few decades. Practitioners in preventive medicine have become increasingly concerned with preparing people for those years when it may be necessary to adapt to a new way of life with different but still challenging interests.

A third trend is an interest in environmental factors that may cause certain illness. For example, people working under stress are urged to take regular vacations and rest periods (such as coffee breaks) in order to help prevent stress diseases. In fact, vacations and rest periods are recognized as important in all industrial programs today. The promotion of safe working conditions is another example of concern for environmental factors affecting the health of employees.

Detection and Treatment of Disease. Although great progress has been made in promoting health and preventing disease, illness will persist; and the detection and the treatment of disease remain an essential responsibility of the professions concerned. The nurse's role in detection and treating disease traditionally has been one of assisting the physician with treatments and caring for the ill. Although this role is largely unchanged, the nurse's responsibilities have increased. Through her observations, reporting and skills in carrying out many complicated treatments, she aids the physician who is responsible for diagnosing the disease and prescribing the treatment. Often the nurse is called on to assist with medical research, and through her contributions it has been possible in many instances for medical research to move forward more rapidly.

Rehabilitation. Although rehabilitation has been concerned particularly with restoring a disabled person to his best possible health, a much broader concept is accepted today—that rehabilitation is an important aspect of all health care. It is concerned with emotional and intellectual disability as well as physical disability. It encompasses all age and occupational groups. It is not limited to that period of time when, for example, a patient may be helped with muscle reeducation in order that he may learn new skills to enable him to regain economic and social usefulness.

Rehabilitation begins with the earliest contact with any person receiving health care. It encompasses all elements of care and continues throughout the period of illness and thereafter until the patient is restored to the best state of health possible for him.

Rehabilitation begins with helping the patient to understand his illness and to make the necessary emotional and physical adjustments. Time was when it was believed that nurses as well as other health personnel should provide complete personal care for the patient, even though his physical condition did not necessarily warrant such care. It is still important that health personnel provide care, but it is important, too, to think in terms of rehabilitation. Rehabilitation is in progress when the patient is taught or assisted to help himself so that he loses neither the desire for self-sufficiency nor the abilities required in day-to-day living and eventually will be able to care for himself. Participation in a program of self-help provides the physical and the mental stimulation that contribute to the restoration of health. Self-care also improves patient morale and dignity. Most patients experience great satisfaction and a sense of personal worth as they gradually regain their ability to care for themselves and to make whatever adjustments in living that their illnesses or disabilities necessitate.

Environmental Health Services. The National Commission on Health Services described comprehensive environmental health services thusly:

"Optimum health can be fostered by prospective planning and management of comprehensive environmental health services. This means going far beyond assuring pure water, clean air, and safe food. It means assuring hygienic housing to provide space for adequate privacy and family sociability, for places of rest and quiet and places for activity and recreation. It means assuring an external milieu for man designated to stimulate his greatest growth potential."[5]

The Commission goes on to state that

"The American environment is being contaminated at a rate rapidly approaching saturation and the health of the people is in jeopardy as a consequence. . . . Moreover, people are using physical, biological, and chemical products indiscriminately, unaware, for the most part of their hazards."[5]

Accidents may be considered an environmental hazard. Approximately 52 million people are injured annually; of these, about two million require hospitalization, while 45 million require some kind of medical attention. About 65,000 hospital beds are used annually for the treatment of accidents; and it is estimated that 88,000 hospital personnel are needed to care for the injured. It is easy to see that accidents increase the load on our health facilities and personnel markedly. Certainly nurses, as health personnel—as well as individuals—can play a positive role in helping to attack the accident health problem.

Providing society with these elements of health care requires the services of many. No one professional group works alone or independently of others; rather, many groups work together to render the services described. Nurses today assume responsibility in many areas; in addition to caring for the ill in hospitals and homes, they rec-

Table 1. Average remaining lifetime in years at specified ages: 1900-1902 to 1965

[For 1900-1902, data are for 10 States and the District of Columbia; for 1919-21, for 34 States and the District of Columbia. Beginning with 1939-41, data are for the United States]

Age	1900–1902	1919–21	1939–41	1949–51	1959–61	1965
0	49.24	56.40	63.62	68.07	69.9	70.2
1	55.20	59.94	65.76	69.16	70.7	70.9
5	54.98	57.99	62.49	65.54	67.0	67.2
10	51.14	53.79	57.82	60.74	62.2	62.3
15	46.81	49.37	53.10	55.91	57.3	57.4
20	42.79	45.30	48.54	51.20	52.6	52.7
25	39.12	41.47	44.09	46.56	47.9	48.0
30	35.51	37.68	39.67	41.91	43.2	43.3
35	31.92	33.89	35.30	37.31	38.5	38.7
40	28.34	30.08	31.03	32.81	33.9	34.1
45	24.77	26.25	26.90	28.49	29.5	29.7
50	21.26	22.50	22.98	24.40	25.3	25.5
55	17.88	18.90	19.31	20.57	21.4	21.6
60	14.76	15.54	15.91	17.04	17.7	17.9
65	11.86	12.47	12.80	13.83	14.4	14.6
70	9.30	9.74	10.00	10.92	11.4	11.7
75	7.08	7.49	7.62	8.40	8.7	9.0
80	5.30	——	5.73	6.34	6.4	6.7
85	3.96	——	4.31	4.69	4.6	4.7

U.S. Department of Health, Education and Welfare, *Facts of Life and Death*, 1967.

ognize their responsibility to society by contributing to comprehensive personal and environmental health programs.

Figure 2-1 illustrates comprehensive health services as just discussed. In addition to the basic resources, as the figure indicates, action of the entire community is essential if we are to attain the goal of the best possible health for everyone.

Accomplishments in the Field of Health

Health does not lend itself easily to measurement. To establish the absence of disease is often not a particularly difficult task, but to measure personal well-being is another matter. However, available statistics do reflect (at least in an indirect manner) the status of health in this nation. They also illustrate some of the advances made in the field of health as well as some of the problems concerning health that are still largely unsolved. Although health personnel recognize the limitations of such statistics, they have offered guidance in planning health programs. A few of these statistics will be described to illustrate accomplishments in the health field.

Many of the accomplishments made in the

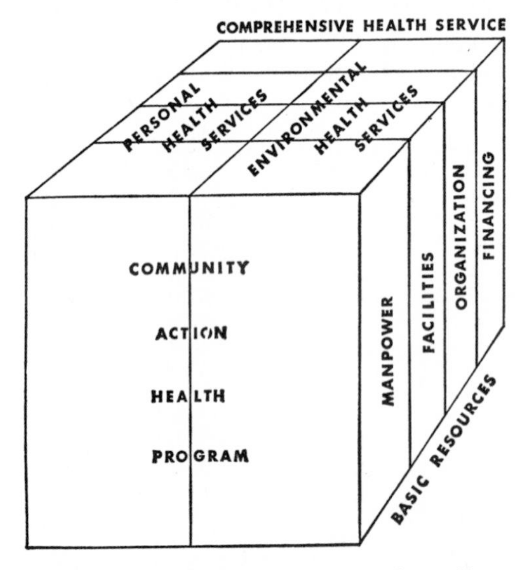

FIG. 2-1. Comprehensive health services. (from Health Is a Community Affair, Report of the National Commission on Community Health Services, p. 126. Cambridge, Mass., Harvard University Press, 1966.)

field of health are reflected in statistics which illustrate a lower premature death rate and an increased life expectancy. For example, infant mortality in the United States has continued to decrease in general since 1930, with a less dramatic decline since 1960. Figure 2-2 illustrates this finding.

Death rates, including all causes of death, have decreased also in the United States, as Figure 2-3 illustrates. Advances in health care are primarily responsible for this decline. Decreases in the mortality rates, especially among the young and middle-aged population, account for an increase in the population of people over 60 years of age.

Table 1 illustrates the average remaining lifetime at specific ages. Note that for each age, life expectancy has increased since 1900 and even since 1961.

Improved methods for promoting and restoring health, for preventing disease and for diagnosing and treating disease have all helped to increase the average life span in this country. Safe food and water supplies have practically eliminated in some areas, and greatly reduced in others, such diseases as typhoid fever, vitamin deficiencies and certain infant diarrheas. Vaccination and immunization programs and the use of antibiotics have aided in controlling most of the communicable diseases. Early disease detection programs have been important factors in the control of such diseases as tuberculosis. Improved equipment and laboratory technics have been important diagnostic aids for the physician. The rehabilitation movement has worked miracles in many instances to prevent individuals from becoming socially and physically disabled. Modern drugs, appliances and technics to prevent and cure disease are impressive in scope and quality.

Having passed legislation that provided for Medicare and Medicaid, our nation took great strides toward providing health services for the older citizens in our population. Now all persons over 65 are granted some health services at a minimum of cost. Persons otherwise unable to pay for medical, hospital and extended care now can receive substantial assistance. Also, Old-Age, Survivors and Disability Insurance (OASDI or

Social Security) has assisted many persons to live a more comfortable life. In 1966, payments from OASDI amounted to 20 billion dollars.

Dramatic surgical developments indicate that a new health horizon is upon us. For example, it has been demonstrated that in selected cases, diseased organs can be replaced by transplanting well-functioning substitutes for them. Although human transplantation might well be considered in its infancy, the implications are that great accomplishments in the field of health are in view.

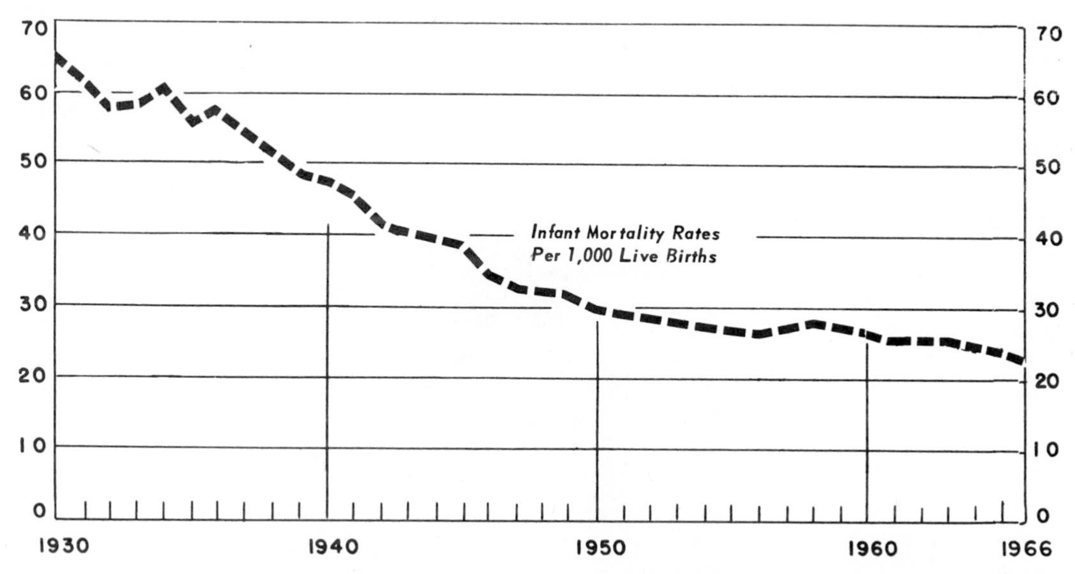

FIG. 2-2. Infant mortality rates: 1930-1966. U.S. Department of Health Education and Welfare, **Facts of Life and Death,** 1967.

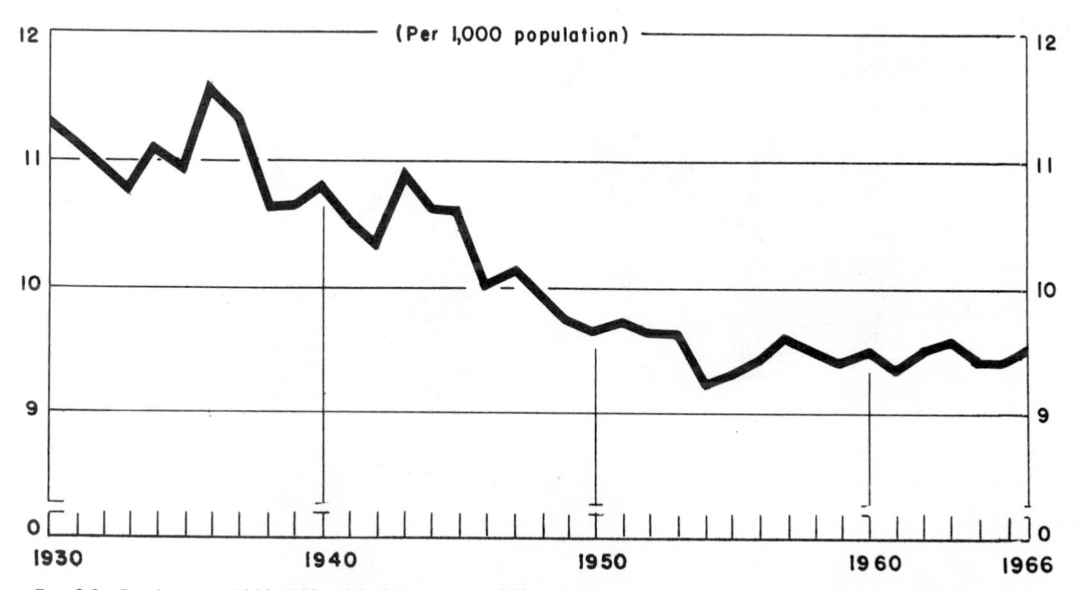

FIG. 2-3. Death rates: 1930-1966. U.S. Department of Health, Education and Welfare, **Facts of Life and Death,** 1967.

Current Health Problems

Accomplishments are encouraging indeed, and health personnel may well look at past accomplishments with pride. However, there is still much to be done in order that even more people may enjoy good health. In a message to Congress in 1963, the President of the United States stated:

"This Nation has built an impressive health record.

But each improvement raises our horizons; each success enable us to concentrate more on the remaining dangers, and on new challenges and threats to health. Some of these new challenges result from our changing environment, some from new habits and activities. More people than ever before are in those vulnerable age groups—the very young and the very old—which need the greatest amount of health services. More people are living in huge metropolitan and industrial complexes, where they face a host of new problems in achieving safety even in the common environmental elements of food, water, land, and air. The hazards of modern living also raise new problems of psychological stability."

The decrease in untimely deaths and the increase in life expectancy have resulted in this nation's having more elders in the population. Table 2 illustrates. Note that there

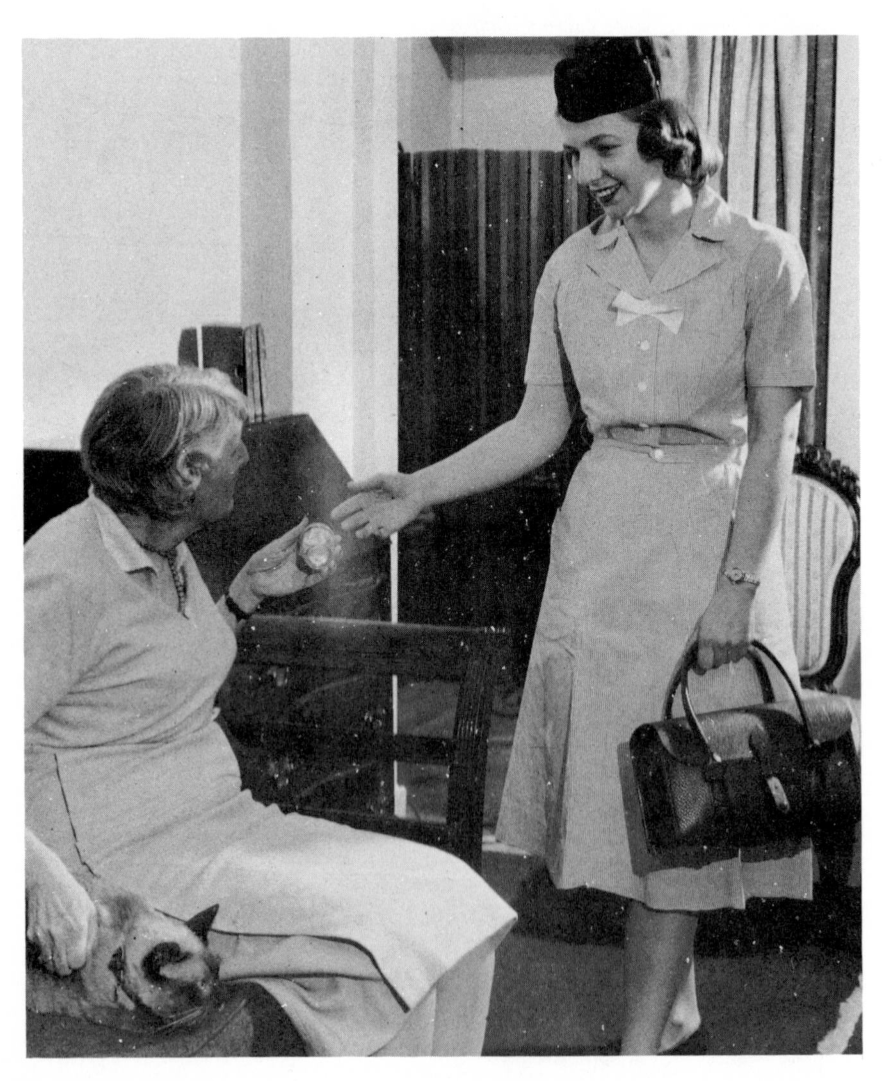

FIG. 2-4. The increase in the number of older persons in our population has created a demand for services outside health agencies; e.g., home care, out-patient care, and increased use of visiting nurse services.

Table 2. Population residing in the United States, by age, and per cent of total population in each age group: 1940, 1960, and 1965

[Enumerated as of April 1 for 1940 and 1960 and estimated as of July 1 for 1965]

Age	Population in millions			Per cent of total population in age group		
	1940	1960	1965	1940	1960	1965
All ages	131.7	179.3	193.8	100.0	100.0	100.0
Under 5 years	10.5	20.3	20.4	8.0	11.3	10.5
5–9 years	10.7	18.7	20.5	8.1	10.4	10.6
10–14 years	11.7	16.8	19.0	8.9	9.4	9.8
15–19 years	12.3	13.2	17.0	9.3	7.4	8.7
20–24 years	11.6	10.8	13.3	8.8	6.0	6.9
25–29 years	11.1	10.9	11.2	8.4	6.1	5.8
30–34 years	10.2	11.9	10.9	7.7	6.6	5.6
35–39 years	9.5	12.5	11.9	7.2	7.0	6.2
40–44 years	8.8	11.6	12.4	6.7	6.5	6.4
45–49 years	8.3	10.9	11.4	6.3	6.1	5.9
50–54 years	7.3	9.6	10.6	5.5	5.4	5.5
55–59 years	5.9	8.4	9.2	4.5	4.7	4.7
60–64 years	4.8	7.1	7.8	3.6	4.0	4.0
65–69 years	3.8	6.3	6.3	2.9	3.5	3.2
70–74 years	2.6	4.7	5.2	2.0	2.6	2.7
75 years and over	2.6	5.6	6.7	2.0	3.1	3.4

U.S. Department of Health, Education and Welfare, *Facts of Life and Death*, 1967.

were about 18 million persons over age 65 in 1965. This figure is expected to reach 21 million by 1975 and 25 million by 1980. One of the primary health problems of the aged is that of chronic disease. Although chronic diseases affect all age groups, invalidism and dependency due to chronic illness are particularly prevalent in the older age groups.

Some of the more common causes of chronic illness in this country are arthritis and rheumatism, blindness, cancer, cardiovascular diseases, cerebral palsy, deafness, diabetes mellitus, epilepsy and mental diseases. Although the seriousness of chronic illness has long been recognized, the public now is becoming increasingly active in supporting programs to aid in the solution of problems associated with them.

One chronic disorder that, despite public attention, still presents a particularly acute health problem is mental illness. More than one half of all hospital beds in the United States are for the mentally ill, and many more people who are not hospitalized or attending clinics are in need of care. There have been concerted efforts in recent years to establish programs that will promote mental health and prevent mental diseases, but the magnitude of the problem of mental illnesses remains.

In a message to Congress, President Kennedy summarized the problem of mental illness and mental retardation in the following statement:

"Mental illness and mental retardation are among our most critical health problems. They occur more frequently, affect more people, require more prolonged treatment, cause more suffering by the families of the afflicted, waste more of our human resources, and constitute more financial drain upon both the Public Treasury and the personal finances of the individual families than any other single condition."

In his 1965 health message to Congress, President Johnson said:

"Forty-eight million people now living will become victims of cancer. Nearly 15 million people suffer from heart disease and this, together with strokes, accounts for more than half the deaths in the United States each year. . . . Today we are challenged to meet and master the three killers which alone account for seven out of 10 deaths in the United States each year—heart diseases, cancer and stroke."

Figure 2-6 illustrates these statistics graphically.

Coronary heart disease has reached what might be called epidemic proportions. In 1965, about one-third of the deaths from this disease claimed persons under age 65, a serious problem of premature death in this country. In general this problem has made the country coronary-conscious. But reducing the toll of coronary deaths, especially among persons in the prime of life, remains a big challenge.

Upper respiratory infections are the most frequent cause of absence from work and school for all age groups. Alcoholism, careless use of insecticides, air pollution, and indiscriminate use of drugs are considered by many health workers as primary health problems today. Accidents are the first cause of death from ages one to 36, and fourth for all ages. Motor vehicle fatalities are of special concern and on a general increase annually. In any year it is estimated that 60 per cent of the population do not receive dental care. It is estimated that about 25 per cent of our children have facial disfigurement or are unable to chew properly because of poorly aligned teeth and jaws. The preceding statements point up additional health problems in need of concerted efforts to overcome.

It is ironic that the application of knowledge in the health services lags considerably behind knowledge on hand. The toll of the diseases most responsible for illness and for death in the United States could be reduced markedly if we but used available skill and knowledge. What good is knowledge if the person needing it is unaware of its existence? Or is unable to pay for the services he needs? Or refuses for one reason or another to observe health practices known to prevent certain illnesses? Or cannot have certain services for the lack of personnel to provide them? As these questions indicate, certain health problems are intertwined with social, psychologic, environmental and economic issues. Hence, their solution will require effort from our entire population. But health personnel in particular should play a dominant role in identifying problems and in seeking the support of the general population to help solve them.

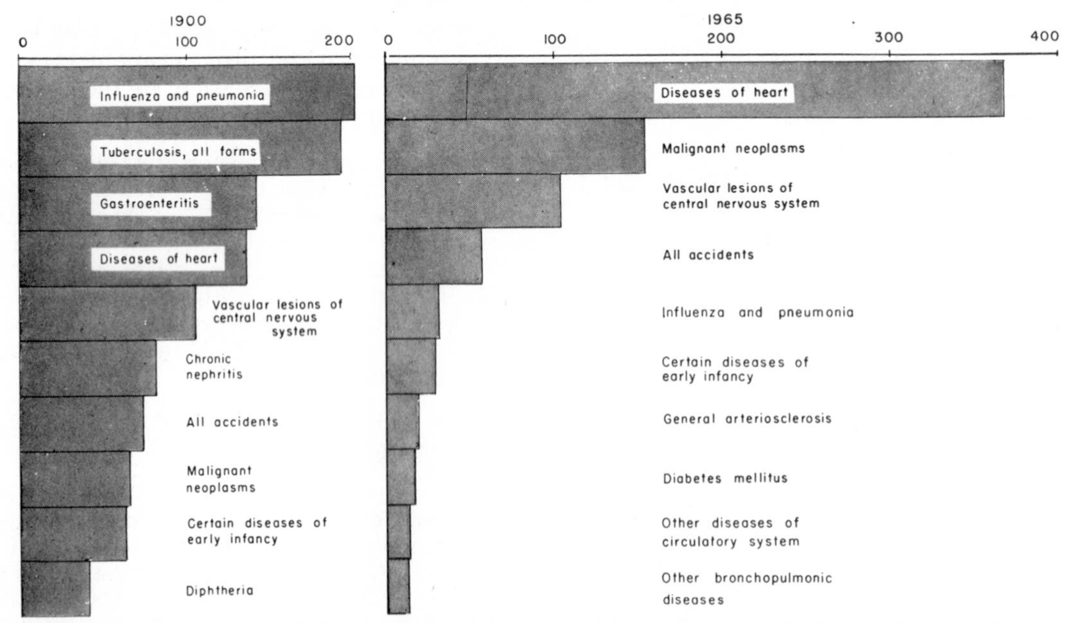

Fig. 2-5. Death rates per 100,000 population for the ten leading causes of death, 1900 and 1965. (From U.S. Department of Health, Education and Welfare, **Facts of Life and Death,** 1967.

There are some health problems for which solutions become global in nature. Two examples are the eradication of malaria and of smallpox. Considerable work has been done in this area, especially through agencies of the United Nations. But much more needs to be done in the future.

No one group of persons can be held responsible for the solution of health problems. The cooperation of all personnel engaged in the field of health, either directly or indirectly, as well as the support of the public, are required. Nurses must share in this responsibility; they have an obligation to society which is not limited to on-the-job performance. Rather, their obligations continue constantly, and their contributions can be invaluable through teaching the public and winning public support and interest in programs that help to solve the nation's health problems.

Study Situations

1. Mention has been made of the increased number of elders in the population and of the fact that health problems are intertwined with factors other than illness per se. The following excerpts were taken from a letter by Virginia T. Holcombe, R.N., to the editor of Nursing Outlook, 13:22, March, 1965.* In this letter, what factors does the author stress as problem areas for senior citizens, other than health problems?

". . . In looking forward to senior citizenship, there are a few points which cause anxiety. Why not consider the possibility of society developing patterns of living which will help young and old adjust together? Does the future have meaning for the senior citizen or is he slowly being pushed into clean, neat, quiet, nutritious nothingness?

What chance has individualism against batteries of consultants? . . . Is there any hope for geriatric nursing gypsies or slower bohemians? Who decides what is 'useful'? While looking at the present aged, why not look at the middle aged and young? What are they doing to establish solid values and simple pleasures . . .?

Take one man for example. Edward was up in his eighties when he spent his last days in a modern hospital with all the comforts. Probably he seemed a 'difficult' patient, always wanting to go home. What a wonderful life he had had, living close to nature, enjoying sun or rain, spring or fall, hunting, fishing, or planting. One day the neighbor's cat killed a rabbit in the field and brought it to Edward. When the neighbor asked, 'Did you eat it, Edward?', the answer was, 'No. I just skinned it.' It was *his*.

Edward was nearly eighty when his horse died. The neighbor asked, 'Why do you want a horse? You don't need one. As it is you have to plow and raise corn to feed him.' Edward said, 'A man has to have a horse.' Would it have been a greater service to give what little care was available at home?

Who is to say that a man's life is to be shorter, living in his way — or longer, living it according to a pattern considered reasonable by his family or consultants? It is not surprising at all that old people become taciturn. Is it going to distress society that I leave the windows open to let in the birds to share my peanut butter sandwich? Will it upset the smooth running of society that I prefer a shack, where I can sit in the rocking chair with the cat in my lap and watch the sun and shadows on the green gold filigree of leaves?

Of course I am saving up now so as not to be a financial burden to society and am going on record to state that if I endanger public safety, it is society's job to protect others. Having made a reasonable allowance for others in this rapidly changing world, even if my heart is bad and my head fuzzy, let me go to the Army-Navy game or the International Congress of Nurses 30 years from now.

In our studies to lengthen life, let us not forget to look for the meaning of life and freedom. Sometimes a man has to have a horse."

2. The following editorial points up several problems in relation to present day health care:

- Schutt, B. B.: Crisis in health care. AMER. J. NURS., *66*:1281, June, 1966.

In what areas has nursing already aided in taking positive action to assist in meeting certain health problems? Where does the author believe nurses must take even more action in helping people attain better health care standards?

3. In the first two pages of the following article, note the statistics concerning loss of lives due to heart disease, cancer and stroke:

* Reprinted, with permission, from Nursing Outlook, March, 1965.

- Leone, L. P.: The attack on heart disease, cancer, and stroke: Is nursing ready? AMER. J. NURS., *65*:68-72, May, 1965.

In the section entitled, "Slow Follow-through," what statistics aid to confirm the statement that the application of knowledge lags far behind knowledge on hand?

References

1. Ashenburg, N. J.: The effects of air pollution on health.
NURS. OUTLOOK, *16*:22-25, February, 1968.
2. Bettelheim, B.: To nurse and to nurture.
NURS. FORUM, *1*:60-76, Summer, 1962.
3. Challenges to nursing in medicare.
AMER. J. NURS., *65*:68-75, November, 1965.
4. Gregg, M. B.: Communicable disease trends in the United States.
AMER. J. NURS., *68*:88-93, January, 1968.
5. Health Is A Community Affair, Report of the National Commission on Community Health Services. 252 p.
Cambridge, Mass., Harvard University Press, 1966.
6. Nahm, H.: Nursing dimensions and realities.
AMER. J. NURS., *65*:96-99, June, 1965.
7. Potter, H. R.: Public health and social trends.
NURS. OUTLOOK, *13*:53-55, September, 1965.
8. Sheahan, M. W.: Through community action: A health commission reports.
AMER. J. NURS., *66*:1298-1302, June, 1966.
9. Snyder, J. D.: New era dawns for health planning.
HOSP. MANAGE., *105*:45-46, February, 1968.

CHAPTER

3

Using Problem Solving in Nursing Practice

Introduction

In Chapter 1, it was stated that nursing has a role in helping to provide society with comprehensive health care—preventive, curative and rehabilitative. Such a broad spectrum of services cannot be spelled out entirely in routines and technics. It is obvious that in nursing certain skills are important. For example, a nurse unable to master the skill of assembling a syringe would be useless in many situations. However, much more than manual skill is required of the nurse. Individuals and groups of individuals present myriad nursing problems that require independent analysis and action.

In other words, the effective nurse needs the ability to recognize when a patient, his family or a group of patients is in a state of need and provide care that is of benefit to those concerned. Such nursing practice depends on the ability of the nurse to use the problem solving process.

Problem solving is systematic investigation. It involves the *objective* collection and analysis of facts, which should result in a course of action that will resolve or alleviate the problem. Problem solving is akin to the more sophisticated technics of research. This text is not designed to include technics of research but it does give information useful in the process. The organization of content around three broad principles, hopefully, should guide the nurse in meeting problems.

Although problem solving aids in finding the logical solution to a problem, one must remember that not every problem confronted in life has an available answer. Also, some problems may have no one right answer. Depending on circumstances, there may be several correct courses of action. However, the person who approaches a problem with logic is far ahead of the one who faces problems with frustration and anxiety, secure only when someone is there to tell him what to do; or worse, yet, simply avoids it.

Problem solving also is a means to improve practice by finding better ways of doing things. Change for the sake of change has little value, but change with the intent to improve practice is a responsibility of professional practitioners. Consider just a few discoveries and changes that have occurred in recent years, which have already had, and will continue to have, marked influence on everyday living: space exploration, automation, the population boom, increasing numbers of aged persons in our population, and the constant discovery of new drugs and new medical therapy. As society changes, so must the practice of nursing. If this practice is to be of high caliber it must keep up with the increased demands upon it. A practitioner functioning at a professional level needs a sound background in scientific principles, an ability to identify problems, and the knowledge of how to solve them.

The Problem Solving Process

There are five essential steps in the problem solving process. Some authors may describe more—or fewer—inasmuch as one step is sometimes broken into several parts or combined with others.

Statement of the Problem. A statement of the problem is an essential step in careful investigation. Unless the person knows exactly what question he wishes answered, he cannot collect and analyze the findings with any precision. Sometimes a problem may have several facets, in which case each part of the problem should be stated clearly. It helps to determine which facet should be investigated first. Sometimes a problem is well on its way to being answered once it has been clearly stated and examined.

Collection of Data That Will Assist in Answering Questions Posed by the Problem. How much data does one need to study a question? This cannot be stated categorically, except to say one needs enough to answer the question accurately and without bias. Often only a few items of data are really necessary.

On the other hand, some problems require a great deal of data. In that case, an instrument for the collection of data usually is needed. Sometimes one must obtain a sampling of data, because it would not be practical, convenient or necessary to use all the data available. Procedures for the preparation and use of instruments for data collection can be found in references at the end of this chapter.

Analysis of the Data in Relation to the Problem. The analysis of data usually requires tabulation so that the data can be examined and studied. For some problems, an objective arrangement of findings may be simply all that is needed. When a problem involves a great deal of data, statistical analysis may be necessary.

Preparing the Answer to the Problem on the Basis of the Data Collected. Once the data are analyzed, possible answers to the problem under investigation can be stated. Great care must be exercised here. The best investigation of a problem is of no use if the data are not analyzed correctly and objectively. Deleting information or giving less attention to some aspects of the data nullifies the whole procedure of problem solving. It is similar to thinking that if we do not like certain aspects of a situation, ignoring them will make them go away. If we try to sway the answer to our liking by juggling the data, the answers are not objective and, in all likelihood, will not solve the problem.

Testing the Course of Action Selected. Once a a course of action has been selected and tried, it carries with it a concurrent aspect of evaluation. It *is* or *is not* answering the problem. If not, a reappraisal is needed. An incorrect course of action could be the result of an error in any of the phases of the process.

The following illustration shows how basic the use of problem solving can be to the practice of nursing.

A patient is not eating the food served on his tray. On one occasion he pushed the tray away so briskly that some of the liquids spilled on the bed linen.

The problem in this example is that the patient is not eating. From psychology, one knows that behavior is purposeful—the patient is not eating for a reason. From a knowledge of nutrition and its relationship to maintaining physiologic function, the nurse knows that it is important that the patient have adequate nourishment. The approach to this problem becomes one of attempting to learn why the patient is not eating; then to take a course of action, based on the probable cause, that hopefully will result in his eating.

Several things have occurred when a problem is identified as just described. First, there is recognition that a problem exists. The patient's refusal to eat has not been ignored. Second, the problem has been identified as a patient problem. The problem does not "belong" to the nurse (although she may be the one who will have to change the soiled linen). Nor does the problem "belong" to the diet department.

Collecting data on the problem of the patient's not eating involves a compilation of all of the possible reasons why this patient refused food. The nurse might start by asking the patient. He may state that he would eat if the "soup wasn't always cold." This may be the real problem and would be relatively easy to solve. But, he may say no more than a defiant "I don't want it!" Then additional data must be collected. The nurse recalls what she knows concerning patients' reactions to illness and hospitalization. One could ask: is the patient refusing food that his faith prohibits? does the patient, because of his cultural background, consider the particular food served him inappropriate for an ill person? Collecting data also may involve asking the patient's family or physician about his behavior.

As was stated earlier, it is impossible to state categorically how much data one needs. In this particular example, it is possible that sufficient data have been collected to work out a satisfactory course of action after the patient indicated that cold food annoyed him sufficiently to cause him to reject all food. On the other hand, no amount of data might point to the real cause of the patient's behavior.

When the nurse collects data on the patient's problem, she needs to look at it objectively and analyze its appropriateness to the problem. No statistical analysis is involved with a case like this, but each piece of data should be weighed carefully, considering all of the pros and cons. Nearly everyone is familiar with some of the tricks (or errors) in handling information that can result in very inappropriate or wrong conclusions. Even in this example of the patient's not eating, subjective thinking or careless weighing of all of the factors involved could lead to ineffective action.

If an analysis of the findings indicated that the patient simply did not like the particular food served, then a logical course of action is to see to it that he is served food that he enjoys but which is still appropriate when considering his illness.

Assume in this case that the analysis of the data did not lead to a relatively easy course of action. Possibly the patient reacted as he did because of bitter resentment of illness and the resulting dependency. In this case, there may be little the nurse can do except to offer help if there is anything the patient would like. The physician may find it necessary to give this patient nourishment intravenously.

Once a course of action is taken, the nurse studies the success or failure of her attempt at solution. If giving the patient food that he likes results in his eating, one can assume that a satisfactory course of action has been taken. If all nursing action fails and the patient's refusal to eat is creating a hazard to him, the physician, as previously stated, must act on the medical problem.

Why did the nurse consider the patient's not eating a problem? Many persons might simply say, "Leave him alone. When he gets good and ready, he will eat." But the nurse's background helps her to recognize that she is confronted with a problem that cannot be ignored.

The nurse's action in pursuing the matter is guided by a knowledge of principles. She understands that inadequate nutrition has implications for the production of energy for the body, for tissue building and repair, for fluid and electrolyte balance, and the like. The nursing goal is to make certain the patient has an adequate nutritional intake. Therefore, it becomes necessary to seek a solution when the patient has refused to eat.

Throughout this text, there are principles that can aid in identifying and solving nursing care problems. No one principle from any one scientific area is unique to nursing alone. It is a combination of principles as used by nurses that is a key factor in helping identify nursing as having a body of activities, responsibilities, and technics unique from those of other health fields.

Definition of a Principle

There is difference of opinion as to the meaning of the word "principle" and also as to what is credited with being a principle. The term as it is used in this text is defined as follows:

A proved fact, or a group of facts so interrelated that they formulate a law, or a generally accepted theory, or a moral doctrine generally accepted by a society, may be considered to be a *principle*.

Principles serve as guides to action, especially in problem solving. They do not specify what must be done. However, depending upon the results desired or the problem being acted on, they help to determine the action that is necessary.

The following examples may clarify further the role of principles as guides to action:

A *proved fact* from the science of bacteriology is: *microorganisms in the nose and the throat can be transmitted to other persons via droplets dispersed by coughing, sneezing or talking, or by direct contact.* Knowing this fact, we are taught to cover the nose and the mouth when sneezing or coughing and to refrain from breathing directly on other persons. When an infectious organism is known to be present, as in the case of a person having pulmonary tuberculosis with positive sputum, more drastic action often is indicated. In this case the patient and health workers and visitors may be asked to wear masks to help to prevent the spread of the organism by droplets.

A *law* from the science of physics is Archimedes' Principle: *any body submerged or floating in a fluid is buoyed up by a force equal to the weight of the fluid displaced.* This principle is in operation when a boat remains afloat on a body of water. It is also

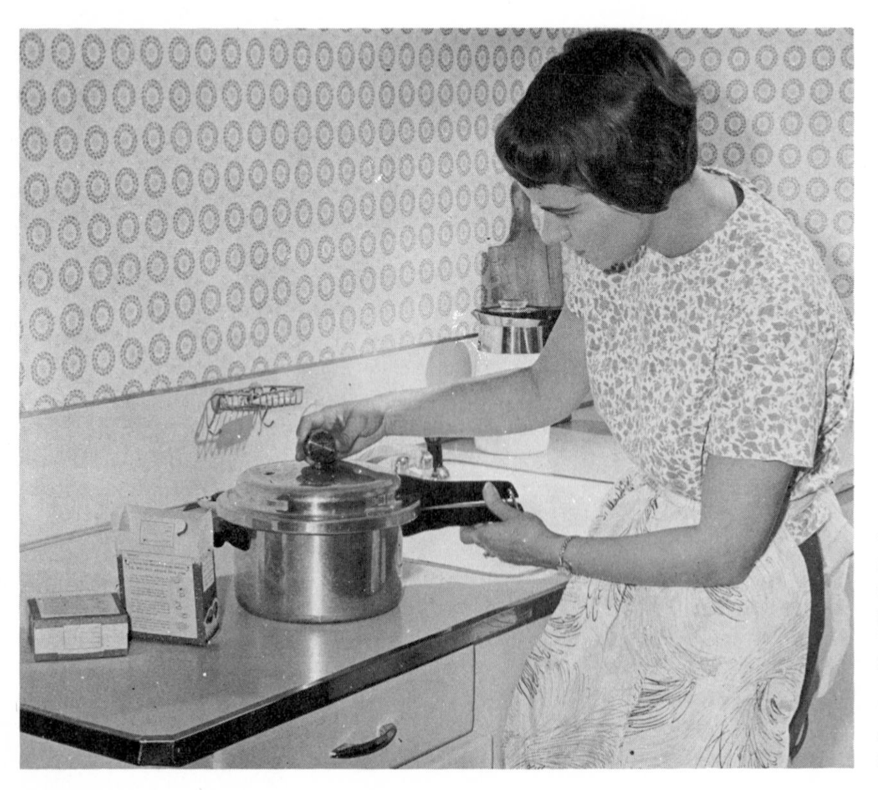

Fig. 3-1. Principles guide action. Many different actions can stem from the same set of principles. Water is vaporized under pressure, and therefore a higher temperature is achieved. The autoclave is used for sterilizing items in the hospital, and the homemaker uses a pressure cooker to prepare foods more quickly.

in effect when paralyzed or arthritic patients are placed in a pool of water in order that their extremities may be manipulated easily because the water buoys them up.

A *theory* is a hypothesis or a scientific conjecture. In the field of health maintenance there are still many unproved phenomena in illness. Aspects of some illnesses have been studied and are understood up to a point. Beyond that point there are tentative conclusions which, in a way, form a theory that guides health workers. For example, the ability of antibiotics to combat many illnesses and infections is unquestioned. However, laboratory studies and case histories have raised the question of their ability to be effective repeatedly for the same patient. There is evidence that not all infections can be controlled by antibiotics. Also, there are some strains of bacteria that have become resistant to antibiotics presently available. Therefore, until such time as the entire phenomenon of bacterial invasion and control in the human is understood, health workers must accept the conjecture that strict adherence to precautionary measures, personal cleanliness, rest and good nutrition are the best means of preventing illness and infections caused by many disease-producing organisms elusive to known chemotherapeutic agents.

Another example is seen in the present controversy over the relationship of smoking to cancer of the lungs. There is evidence that persons developing cancer of the lungs have also been smokers. However, there are many persons—some heavy smokers—who do not develop cancer. Until such time as more evidence of cause and effect are forthcoming, it seems best to go on the theory that the reduction of irritation to the lungs caused by smoking is an aid toward prevention of cancer in that area.

A moral doctrine is concerned with the teaching or advocation of behavior which is considered good and right. As members of society, we arrive at standards of conduct from a variety of sources, such as our family, religion, education and social and cultural groups. These standards we hold as truths, and they affect our beliefs and behavior. We can learn what is normal from a physical and physiologic standpoint and predict what may occur to a person under a given set of circumstances. However, we cannot predict how another person will behave or react if we do not have an awareness of his own moral code.

An example of a moral doctrine accepted by our society is: *every effort is made to save the life of another person.* A lay person at the scene of an accident will give whatever aid he can until help arrives. Physicians and nurses continue to care for a terminally ill patient until death occurs, even though death has been imminent for days. However, in our civil defense plan in the event of a nuclear attack, the reverse holds true; those with medical authority would separate persons who are injured beyond help of recovery from those who have a chance of surviving and give preference to the latter. While the logic of this system of priorities in the civil defense program is understood, nevertheless it could create extreme mental conflict because it is inimical to a fundamental ingrained attitude.

Standards of conduct and moral doctrines change, as is evident throughout the world today. Whereas once there was little change from one generation to another, now there is change even within each generation. These changes are reflected in health services—not only in care and cure, but in interpersonal relationships as well.

Principles as Guides to Nursing Practice and Problem Solving

In succeeding Units in this text, certain procedures are described under titles beginning with "Principles Guiding Action etc." Principles and the suggested action are given. Not given are the details of the procedure. Such details would not be principles. Hospitals and other agencies design their own methods and specify details for carrying out procedures. A point of clarification is being made here because it is possible that details of a certain activity can be stressed to such a degree that they cloud the principles. Various methods may work equally well if principles are not violated. For example, the way bread is baked commercially now bears no resemblance to the home-baking process of 75 years ago. But the principles underlying bread-baking are the same.

When making a hospital bed it is customary to anchor the sheet by making a square or mitered corner. Both are effective if properly done. However, a contour sheet is certainly an improvement over both of these methods, especially if there is a plasticized mattress cover. The contour sheet is designed to "hook" over the mattress—something a flat sheet cannot do.

When a straight sheet is used to make a corner on a plasticized mattress cover there is a tendency for the corners to pull out—a mighty discouraging sight for the effort expended. Herein lies a principle: friction is the resistance present whenever two surfaces slide on each other. When both sheet and mattress covering have nap there is more resistance (friction) and consequently the sheet will not loosen readily. A plasticized covering does not offer much friction; hence, a sheet slips upon it with ease.

Consider an example from the text. On page 395, there is a section with the heading, "Principles Guiding Action in Applying Hot Moist Applications to a Body Area." In the text the reader is given those aspects of the treatment which should not be violated if it is to be effective and safe. In other words, the principles hold true no matter where or how the treatment is given. Examples in-

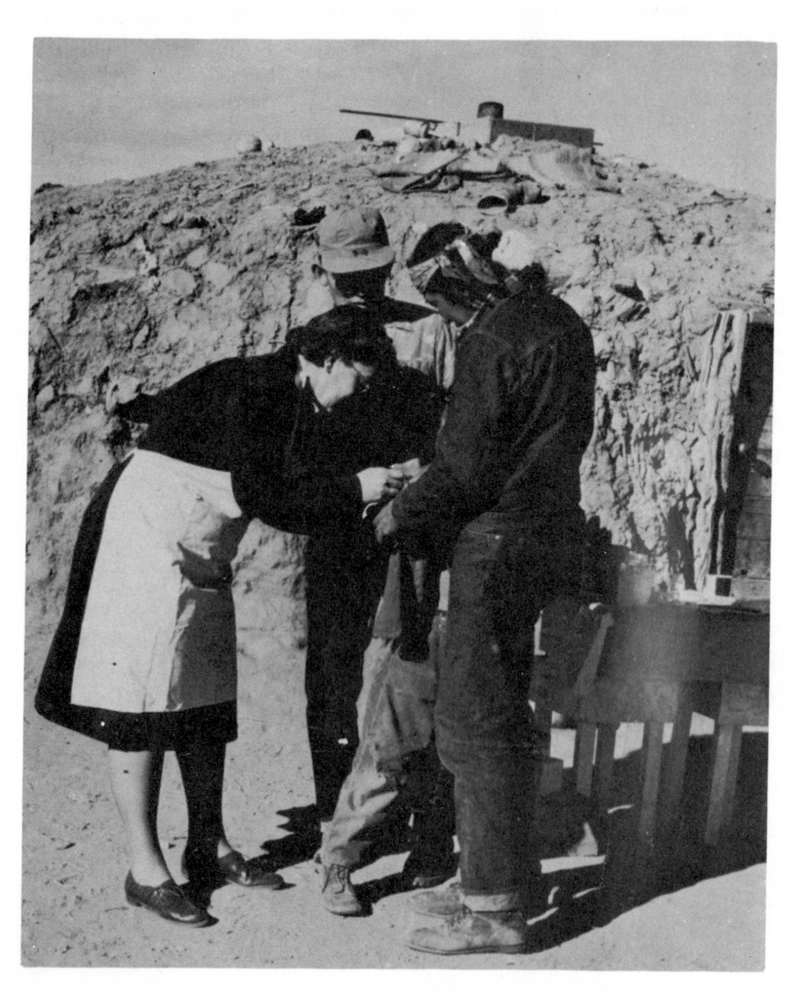

FIG. 3-2. Sound understanding of principles in both nursing technics and human relationships makes it possible for this nurse to function effectively on the Navajo reservation. Her work area for administering immunization injections is in front of a native dwelling. (U.S. Government photograph)

clude: the basis for selecting a certain type of cloth, for using lubricant on the skin and for using waterproof material to cover the wet pack. Most health agencies in which the procedure of applying applications might be carried out would have a detailed method for doing it written in their procedure manual. It would specify where flannels could be obtained, what kind of container is used for the water and the flannels, what method is used to keep the water hot, what type of waterproof material is used, and what device is used to wring water from the packs. A nurse going from one agency to another would want and need this information no matter how well she understood the principles of applying heat; it is a matter of knowing what there is to work with and where it may be obtained. In carrying out the suggested method the nurse does have the freedom to make adjustments if they are in the best interests of the patient and as long as principles are not violated.

Agencies prefer to have written procedures so that there is as much uniformity in practice as possible, and it is economically unsound to allow for personal preferences. Suppose that one nurse wanted an electrically heated container with a wringer on it, another preferred a basin on an electric stove with a canvas wringer, and a third nurse wanted a press wringer. The cost would be prohibitive to the agency. Also, having each nurse use a different method may not be adding to the patient's feeling of security.

In the search for principles—the *why* of all actions—it becomes possible to separate the details of the *how*. For instance, this same procedure of applying hot applications might have to be done at home. A nurse teaching a patient would stress the principles and then seek a way of doing it. What is available in the home? It may be that a bath towel would need to be used. A pot on the stove may have to suffice for heating the material; wax paper may be the waterproof material, etc. Methods can vary with the place and the circumstances and be effective as long as principles are not violated.

In addition to procedures, there is also the matter of *policies* with which the nurse must be concerned. In some instances agencies find it necessary to insist that all personnel carry out an activity in a specific manner. No one is permitted to make variations on his own. Students in the situation also are obliged to observe this order, which is referred to as a *policy*. A policy may eventually be changed or modified, but while in force it leaves no room for individual action upon it.

A policy very often is a safety measure for the agency, or the patient, or his possessions. Policies are written by administrative personnel and kept on file so that they may be referred to as necessary. It is possible for persons to become so accustomed to following a policy in one agency that they consider it to be universal practice. For example, in Hospital A there is a policy stating that all patients having artificial dentures are to be given denture cups and instructed to use them. The hospital will not be responsible for loss if patients do not use the containers. It is the nurse's responsibility to see to it that the policy is made known to the patient. Failure to do so could mean her paying for dentures in the event that they are damaged or lost. The hospital takes this precaution to ensure safety for the patient's possession. A nurse who has lived with this policy for a long time would feel uncomfortable if she were to go to Hospital B where there is no such policy. This nurse might feel so strongly the need for safeguarding the dentures that she continues to observe the precaution even though it is not expected of her.

Another example of policy is frequently seen in connection with visiting hours: which hours visitors may see the patient, how many may visit at one time or in one day, who the visitors may be (i.e., husband–wife–mother–father), where they receive permits and how long they may visit. Policies for visiting patients vary from one agency to another and even from one clinical unit to another.

Now consider an example that illustrates both method and policy as well as problem solving. A nurse has two patients who are to have their baths given to them in bed. One is not permitted to bathe herself because of the possibility of heart strain. She is able to move about easily and is not receiving any treatments at this time. The other patient, who is elderly, has severe limitations to the extent that she cannot move, and in addition requires several treatments. Guided by principles, the nurse will make variations in the way she bathes these two patients. For the patient who has heart impairment, the nurse would give the bath and make the bed so that as few movements as possible, such as turning or sitting upright, are required of the patient. (Increased effort increases heart action.) For the helpless patient it would be beneficial to bé turned more than the other patient. (Decreased activity causes stasis, pressure on areas, decreased respirations, and so on.) Also, for the second patient the nurse would want to do the treatments which could soil the bed linen, such as irrigating the catheter and changing the dressing before the bath rather than at the completion of it and making the bed.

In this same hospital there is a policy which states that all patients over 65 years of age must have bed siderails up at all times. The nurse must comply even though her elderly patient is incapable of turning or moving herself. Her other patient is not 65 years of age but must remain in the sitting position at all times and receives medications that make her feel drowsy. The nurse decided to keep this patient's bed siderails up also. The nurse identified a problem and took action.

What are some of the principles underlying the action of the nurse in placing siderails up for the patient who is not 65 years of age? One could say that it is just common sense. However, there are principles underlying the action, and the nurse was aware of them. First, a person is incapable of maintaining a position which requires conscious effort when dozing or sleeping. Secondly, the body will move in the direction of greatest gravitational pull. If this pull should be toward the edge of the bed, the patient could fall out of bed if the line of gravity goes out of her base of support. Thirdly, with the bed as high as it is, a fall from that distance to a hard surface could result in injury.

Neither clearly written procedures or policies are sufficient to sustain a lack of awareness of principles. A sound background of knowledge will help nursing personnel identify problems and give the best possible care to patients.

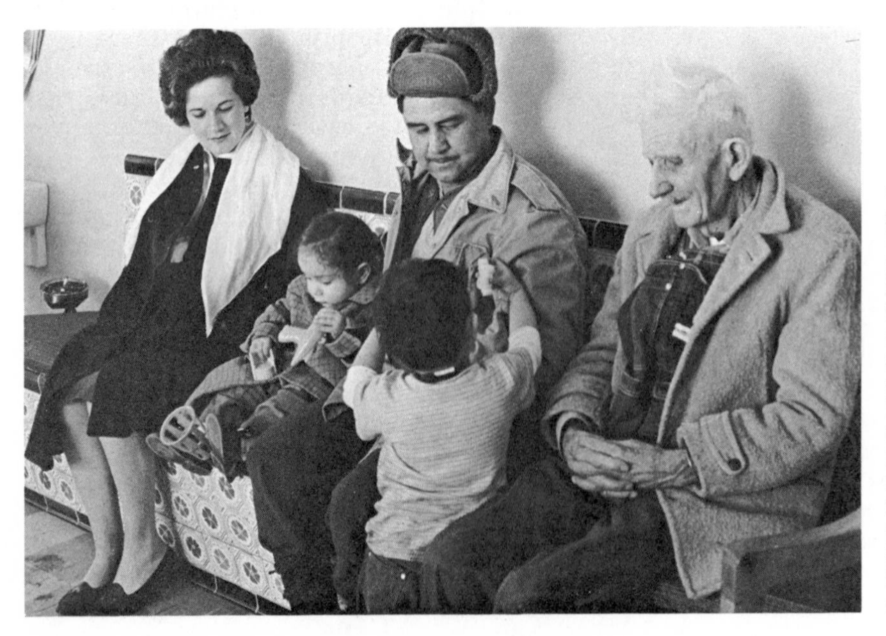

FIG. 3-3. Scene: the waiting room of a clinic. As the nurse greets each patient and brings him to the physician, her approach should be appropriate to the age of the person and his health problem, if she knows about it. Each one is not another case. In her appraisal of each person in the picture, what could be some of the things the nurse should consider about each as an individual—such as, What do I need to know? How do I assess this information? What approaches or actions should be attempted?—then, Did it work? (Photograph by Mary Ann Gehres of Presbyterian Life)

Study Situation

Many helpful suggestions concerning the solving of problems are found in the following article. It concerns sampling, reliability of sources of information, interpretation and other facts to be kept in mind when collecting and analyzing data.

- Means, R. K.: Interpreting statistics: An art.
  NURS. OUTLOOK, *13*:34-37, May, 1965.

Study Situations in succeeding chapters of this text will call attention to nursing situations in which the problem solving process was applied.

References

1. Abdellah, F. G., and Levine, E.: Better Patient Care Through Nursing Research. pp. 11-29.
   New York, Macmillan, 1965.
2. Fox, D. J.: Fundamentals of Research in Nursing. 285 p.
   New York, Appleton-Century-Crofts, 1966.
3. Meyer, B., and Heidgerken, L. E.: Introduction to Research In Nursing. pp. 14-20.
   Philadelphia, Lippincott, 1962.
4. Research—how will nursing define it? (Symposium Report).
   NURS. RES., *16*:108-129, Spring, 1967.
5. Spalding, E. K., and Notter, L. E.: Professional Nursing, ed. 7, pp. 512-518.
   Philadelphia, Lippincott, 1965.
6. Stevens, L. F.: Look at your own practice.
   AMER. J. NURS., *65*:106-107, June, 1965.

CHAPTER

4

Three Principles Guiding Nursing Practice

Introduction

The previous chapter indicated that principles are often the means by which problems are recognized. They may also be used as the source of information by means of which problems are solved. There are three principles that can guide the nurse in giving care to any person. They are broad in their scope because each represents a total of many principles from several sciences. These principles are concerned with maintaining the individuality of man, maintaining physiologic functioning in man, and protecting man from external causes of illness.

There is no nursing care situation in which one, two or all three cannot be used to guide practice. To the extent that the nurse's fund of knowledge increases, the actions inherent in the three principles will increase also. These principles are stated as follows:

MAN AS A PERSON

Each person is an individual member of society who has rights, privileges and immunities which should be respected, regardless of race, creed, social or economic status, and has personal fears and needs which usually are exaggerated when there is a threat to his well-being.

MAN AS AN ORGANISM

The human body requires that certain physiologic activities be maintained if the body is to function effectively.

MAN AND HIS ENVIRONMENT

Appropriate precautionary measures will help to reduce or eliminate physical, chemical or biologic factors in the environment which cause illness or injury to man.

Understanding the significance of each will require time. None of these principles can be developed fully in the short space of this chapter, nor even of this text. However, it is hoped that introducing them at this time will help to develop their full meaning through increased understanding in other areas of learning and practice in the care of patients. As each nursing care activity is encountered, it will be helpful if the nurse questions the degree to which each of the three principles functions. In this way, it becomes possible to recognize rather soon that each principle is not involved to an equal extent in every situation. Each one will guide actions according to the needs of the specific situation.

It will also be helpful to the student to relate areas of learning in the curriculum to these three guides. For example, where does the course in microbiology fit among this trio? Communication skills? Anthropology? Chemistry? Public health? It can be noted that all areas of learning in the curriculum are the sources of knowledge which are the "woof" and the "warp" of these three principles.

To explain further, consider a nurse who knows how to keep a patient clean, free from bedsores and free from infections by the use of good technic in handling dressings and is skilled in giving injections. She is not really giving total or even good nursing care if she has paid no attention to the emotional, the spiritual or the cultural needs of her patient. For example, if the nurse fails to understand that he is an Orthodox Jew who observes his Sabbath on Saturday and would appreciate the opportunity to do this, or that he is worried about his invalid wife at home who must depend on neighbors for care, the quality of her nursing leaves something to be desired.

On the other hand, if a nurse is concerned primarily with the emotional aspects of a patient's care, protects him from harmful factors in the environment but is not concerned with certain aspects of his physical care, his recovery may be delayed because of altered bodily functions, such as loss of muscle tonus, nutritional deficiency or unsatisfactory fluid balance. This, too, is neither good nor total nursing care.

As another example, consider the nurse who attempts to meet adequately the psychological and the physical needs of a patient but who is not too aware or concerned with the protective factors in his care, and as a result the patient falls out of bed, develops an infection or is burned. This also falls far short of total or good nursing care.

All three principles are involved in the care of every patient. The extent to which one has the priority role in the patient's care is dependent on the needs of the patient, and even then there will be variation from day to day and in some instances from hour to hour. They represent a foundation on which the practice of nursing can be developed. They are broad and firm. They are designed to accommodate a broad and high-level type of performance if that performance is guided by scientific knowledge and sound judgment.

Principle Relating to Man as a Person

> *Each person is an individual member of society who has rights, privileges and immunities which should be respected, regardless of race, creed or social or economic status, and has personal fears and needs which usually are exaggerated when there is a threat to his well-being.*

This statement is accepted as truth by many other professions besides that of nursing. It emphasizes that patients are individuals and that the effectiveness of ministrations to them is, to a very large extent, dependent on an understanding of human development and behavior. It implies that the nurse, too, must try to understand herself if she is to develop optimum relationships with others.

Probably, the whole concept of this principle could be expressed in the phrase, *nursing is caring*. Sometimes, mentally or physically handicapped children or older disabled persons are placed in institutions for what is described as good care, the connotation being that at least they will be fed, clothed, kept clean and given protection. But *caring* is more than that. It is having sincere concern for and interest in the patient, as well. If one really cares for a person, then one has thought and regard for him. Nursing is not really nursing unless it is caring.

To those who have had little experience with illness or the care of the ill, there may be some question as to why it is even necessary to belabor this statement any further. It is so obvious. Unfortunately, it is still a common occurrence for patients to be shorn of personal identity and personality during an illness and to be treated only in terms of the diseased areas or organs. The pressure of circumstances makes it easy for this to happen unless the nursing personnel are deeply concerned with the *person* as well as with the care he requires.

When a person assumes the role of a patient and requires care from members of the health team, whether in a hospital, a home, a clinic or a doctor's office, he does not suddenly become a "coronary" or a "diabetic." He is still the same individual he was before the onset of his illness, dynamic in his own way, who has need of care because of impaired cardiac or pancreatic function. But all too often attention is focused on the affected body organ or part and not the person.

One of the basic arts in the practice of nursing is a sound understanding of and skill in the use of interpersonal relationship technics. This ability to create pleasant relationships with people, as pointed out earlier, is an important asset. Without it, little of what the nurse will do in actual practice will attain effectiveness. The relationship of the nurse to the patient should be one of *mutual planning and consent*. It is disastrous for the nurse to assume an authoritarian role and place the patient in the position of a recipient of care which he may neither understand nor want, nor have an opportunity to explain his own needs or to ask questions.

A person who recognizes the need for therapy and takes the initiative to seek help has acknowledged that he needs the assistance

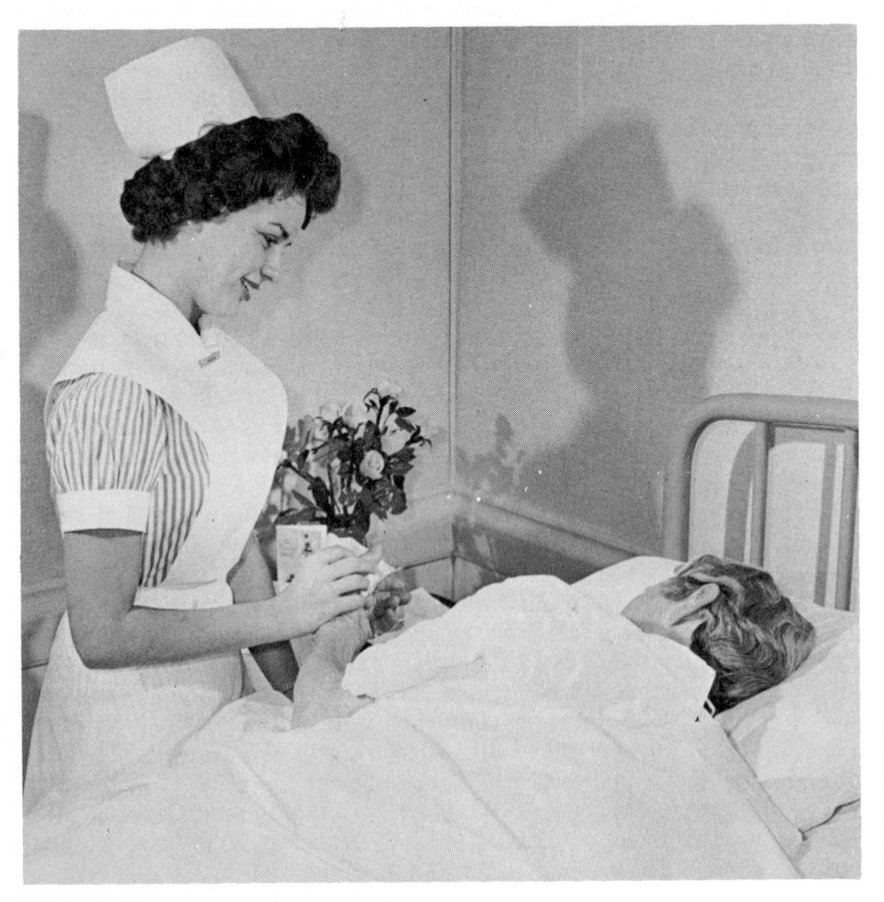

FIG. 4-1. Nursing is caring . . . feeling for the persons we serve. Having just turned this patient on her side and made her comfortable, this student nurse touches the patient's outstretched hand and smiles at her before leaving.

of others in order to achieve relief from the fears associated with his problem. Seeking assistance suggests an initially mutual act, and this mutuality should not be lost once the course of assistance has begun. The individual does not surrender all his rights in the agreement nor does he give *carte blanche* to those caring for him. The goal is more likely to be achieved and the experience is more likely to be a mutually pleasant one if the patient is always considered, to some degree, to be a member of the health team. This is based on the accepted belief that the amount of effort that an individual makes in his own behalf has a direct bearing on the outcome.

When the situation is complex and includes a large number of health workers, such as in an outpatient clinic, a nursing home or a hospital, it is not easy to keep a relationship in which the patient contributes to his own plan of care. Usually, this is put into operation more easily in more individualized situations, as in public health nursing, small industrial health programs and physicians' offices. This is due primarily to the fact that the numbers of patients and workers and the vast number of activities in hospitals require routines—and rightly so. Without organization, routines and planning, patients would be at an even greater disadvantage and inconvenience in the resulting confusion. It is this pattern of routines for expediency in work performance, and also the presence of a large number of workers contributing to patients' care, that very easily can cause the patient to be lost. Things are being done to him and for him rather than with him because it is easier that way.

Understanding the impact of illness on any individual is important to the nurse for another reason. In recent years, auxiliary personnel have come to be recognized as assistants in the nursing care of patients. They enter upon this work after relatively little preparation and orientation. These auxiliary workers, for the most part, are taught how to do certain phases of care which authorities in nursing and medical practice believe they can do safely. Little, if any, detail can be devoted to teaching them the psychosocial aspects of patient care. Therefore, the nurse, as a leader of these auxiliary workers, must assume responsibility for imparting by word and by deed that illness usually produces anxiety and fears in the one affected. Anyone who is the recipient of or "consumer" of nursing services is usually one who has *concern* for his total welfare as well as *need* for specific treatment. The personal needs of any patient are as important as his physical needs. The former may not always be in evidence to others, but it cannot be assumed that therefore they do not exist.

All too often, a patient may be typed on the basis of a superficial characteristic of behavior, with no effort made toward further understanding. For instance, there was an occasion when an aide commented that a 16-year-old Japanese boy "was a good kid. He's not full of nonsense like American teenagers. He does everything he is told to do and doesn't give you a hard time." If conforming was being good, then he was. But further conversation with this boy, whose father was a diplomat, revealed that his behavior was the result of personal convictions and upbringing and not merely a desire to keep peace with the nursing staff. He talked about the sports he played and enjoyed at school in Japan, namely, judo and karate. One could not help understanding, if one really listened, that the philosophy of young Japanese men was not the importance of winning or losing but of obedience. Self-discipline, politeness, dignity and self-control were stressed as much as physical fitness. Once the label of "good kid" was removed and his behavior understood on the basis of a philosophy of life and of this cultural group, the staff saw him in a different and much more interesting light. Judo became a major topic of interest among the nursing staff; and in other ways, when given the opportunity, the patient contributed to a better understanding of another culture group with which this staff had had little contact. Most important of all, they acquired a much deeper understanding of the patient as an individual.

While auxiliary personnel are being oriented to the activities related to patient care, it is a function of the nurses who supervise them to develop further their awareness of the patient as a person. Planning sessions, conferences and other joint activities are means by which the nurse helps her assistants in patient care to see and feel that their acts are services to others. Personnel should be cautioned against imparting an air of being overworked or too busy to be bothered by questions or any other form of interruption. Nurses, and others, may sometimes feel overwhelmed by the work that must be done and the orders that must be carried out, but they should not reveal this to patients by either word or act.

Consideration should always be shown for the patient by offering explanations for treatments and providing opportunity to ask questions. Few, if any, forms of therapy should be administered without the nurse's explaining and discussing them with the patient, insofar as it is possible under the circumstances and according to the physician's wishes. In this way, the patient has the opportunity to convey anxieties and to shed some of his fears; however, equally important, he comes to feel that he, too, is participating in the plan, that others see him as a person, not just as a "case."

The nurse should expect that some patients will be resistant and that some apprehensions which patients have cannot be dispelled by explanations and attempts at interpretations. But it is in learning how to approach resistance, and how to allay anxiety, and how far and for how long one must take over the lives of others, that the nurse finds one of the most challenging and never-ending fields of learning.

There is no rule of thumb or set of rules in interpersonal relationships which can be learned and then practiced until perfected. The student's understanding of others is the product of experience supplemented by constant learning. But this understanding cannot be acquired without a basic respect for the individuality of man.

A full discussion of this one principle alone would require several volumes. Each patient contact, each experience with other members of the health team and all new learning in the psychosocial sciences will aid in developing interpersonal relationships further. Unit Two is concerned with the development of this principle.

However, as a beginning, consider the following examples of actions based on the principle that each person is an individual member of society who has rights, privileges and immunities which should be respected, regardless of his race, creed or social or economic status and whose fears and needs are exaggerated when there is a threat to his well-being.

Understand that for most persons, on being removed from their usual environment and receiving treatment for illness or injury, fears and anxieties are created. The nurse can reveal an awareness of this state of mind by the manner of approach and the consideration shown to the patient.

Consider the patient's understanding of his plan of care before ministering to him. In circumstances where it is determined that the patient does not understand his care, or his illness makes it difficult for him to understand, make every effort to explain and interpret all activities (both prescribed and routine) before initiating the care. No matter how simple or routine a measure may seem to the nurse, it may still be unfamiliar and awesome to the patient.

Make every effort to gain an understanding of the common interests, needs and problems of various age groups so that they may be taken into consideration in establishing relationships.

Respect and try to understand the religious beliefs of others. Recognize that, during periods of illness, spiritual support is often of vital importance in the patient's recovery and his acceptance of his problems. Make every effort to help the patient continue or establish habits of prayer and devotion if he shows an inclination to do so.

Respect differences of opinion and beliefs which others may have. Avoid discussions which may be disturbing to the patient.

Respect and try to understand different culture patterns. Consider cultural and religious patterns which may be interfering with therapy as factors that require serious and careful handling. Avoid discussing them with the patient until a satisfactory plan can be worked out with the cooperation of the physician and a family member and/or a religious counselor.

Remember that a patient is not an isolated individual. He is a part of a family unit, a community member, and his illness may be creating anxiety reactions in the lives of many others.

Listen to the patient and his family members. The patient's ability to talk to someone is therapeutic as well as a valuable asset in the nurse's understanding of him.

Try to provide an atmosphere that helps the patient to feel comfortable in spite of the strangeness of his new surroundings.

Principle Relating to Man as an Organism

> *The human body requires that certain physiologic activities be maintained if it is to function effectively.*

Another aspect of the nurse's ability to give the best kind of care is to have a sound understanding of the body's needs and what may be expected if these are not met.

Most people have some understanding of physiologic needs through education, experience or hearsay. They come to realize, for instance, that loss of rest and sleep produces fatigue; poor eating habits may produce gastric distress, constipation, diarrhea and weight gain or loss; excessive perspiration produces thirst; cutting off oxygen supply can quickly produce suffocation, and so on. It is obvious that the nurse's responsibilities in patient care require her to have a superior understanding of the details of the body's functions and the needs relating to them.

Before proceeding further, it should be pointed out that this principle cannot be isolated from the one discussed previously relating to man as a person, nor the one that follows, man and his environment. Our way of life can help our bodies to run smoothly or keep them in constant need of repair. Practices that are within voluntary control affect our bodies—such as habits of eating and sleeping, patterns of dress, types of work and recreational activities and uses of tobacco, alcohol and medications. It follows, then, that the more one understands about a person and his individual characteristics, the easier it will be to try to help him maintain effective functioning of his body processes.

The human body is complicated beyond belief. It takes a great deal of study to understand even the smallest part of it. Research is swelling the already overwhelming sources of knowledge pertaining to the body and its discrete functions. No lay person following the events of the trips into space can avoid learning about some of the functions of the body and the changes that may occur under varied circumstances. Nor would anyone escape the fact that research in space medicine has been established. The news media abound in information related to health, and nurses can be prepared for patients to be quite knowledgeable about many physiologic activities. Suffice it to say that the nurse needs to continue to expand her knowledge in the area. One course in anatomy and physiology cannot sustain the nurse in her practice for life. It is only the beginning. A background in other related fields such as chemistry, physics, microbiology and pathology is equally essential in understanding how the body functions.

Knowledge of the normal state is the basis for understanding the abnormal and its requisite therapy. It is also essential in helping the person to attain or retain his best state of health. Although signs and symptoms produced by various physical conditions can be memorized, a much more valuable approach is to understand the reasons for their appearance. The next step is to try to understand the relationship of these signs and symptoms to the normal functioning of a particular person.

When the nurse is carrying out measures prescribed by the physician, her responsibilities include understanding the therapy prescribed, the desired results and the difficulties that might occur. Furthermore, the nurse should be capable of observing signs that could be considered as abnormal whether or not they are related to the present illness or therapy. For instance, a patient may be hospitalized with a tumor of the mouth. In the course of caring for him, the nurse notices that the patient's urinary output is below what she knows to be normal. Although this condition is seemingly unrelated to the patient's tumor, the nurse immediately recognizes its physiologic importance and reports it to the physician. Such an observation is rarely possible by the physician; he depends on nurses to bring these observations into the total picture. Therefore, it is obvious that nurses' observations can be responsible for effecting change in therapy for a patient and, in some instances, for saving a life.

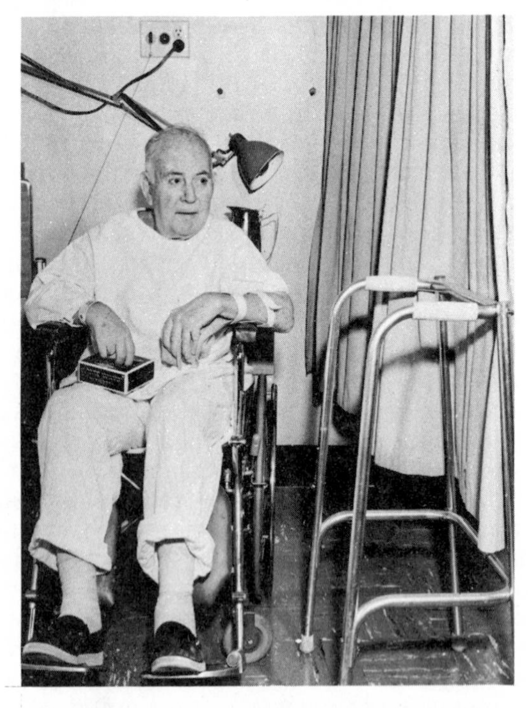

FIG. 4-2. Helping the patient to maintain physiologic functioning and to maintain a safe environment for him requires a good deal of mutual planning between the patient and the nurse. This gentleman has an adjustable bed, his wheelchair, a walker, elastic bandages on his feet and legs, a protective hand and wrist splint, which is adjusted periodically during the day for repositioning his wrist; and, not seen in the picture, a suction machine on his bedside table. He allows as how he is a busy man between his trips to physiotherapy and "all this getting around."

Often, a nurse is the one who can help a patient to accept a plan of therapy. It is one thing for a physician to prescribe, but it may be another matter to put a plan of therapy into effect. This may be due to the fact that the patient does not understand the therapy that the physician has prescribed or the need or the value of it. Rather than omit the therapy until the physician can be consulted or carry it out in spite of the patient's objections, attempts should be initiated to find a way of making the therapy acceptable to the patient.

Consider the following example of action initiated by a nurse who was understanding of the rationale of the therapy, the physiologic state of the patient and the patient's feelings concerning her physical condition. An elderly patient was in the hospital for diagnosis of pains in the left side of her chest with the possibility of its being of cardiac origin. A nurse came in to give her the second dose of medication since admission. The previous nurse had explained that the drug was for her heart. The patient insisted that her heart was fine. She did not wish to take the pills. She said that her trouble was from a gallbladder operation about 60 years ago and explained how sick she had been because in those days the "doctors didn't know very much." She seemed to feel that she had been suffering ever since from this episode, and stated emphatically, "And I told the doctor that!"

The nurse listened to the patient's emphasis on the previous surgery. She had a hunch that the patient would be pleased if she were to receive a drug for what she considered to be her real problem. She was also determined that the patient accept the medication because it was for the patient's benefit. Therefore, the nurse replied by telling the patient that the drug had more than one action. It was to improve the total blood circulation; and since she may have had changes in circulation due to the surgery, this drug was good. The patient accepted the pills after this explanation. The easy way out of the situation would have been to concede to the patient's refusal and to report it to the doctor. However, the nurse realized that the patient needed the medication; she permitted her to explain why she did not wish to take the pills; she guessed that the patient wanted something for her long-standing ailment and therefore capitalized on this fact. She made the explanation more general and yet did not tell an untruth.

Consider another example. A 38-year-old mother of three children who was under the care of a gynecologist in an outpatient department expressed the hope that she would not have any more children. She said, "I get fatter after each one. Some women are like that and I'm one of them." The nurse asked if she really believed that. Her response indicated that she did indeed. Following the nurse's report, much time and effort were devoted to helping this woman. The medical and nursing personnel worked together to convince her that food, especially the kind she fancied and in the quantities she ate, was responsible for her weighing 210 pounds. She broke several appointments because, as she later admitted, she was afraid her eating habits would be discussed. Eventually she began to accept the fact that she was setting the stage for serious physical problems for herself, as well as the psychological ones she now had. She was referred to another clinic for a planned program for weight loss. After losing weight and adjusting to her new eating pattern, she had the courage to joke and tell the nurse who started her on the right path, "I don't hide custard doughnuts in an empty soap box any more."

In the role of coordinator, the nurse also is able to implement plans of other members of the health team. Diet therapy, physical therapy, radiation therapy, hydrotherapy and speech therapy may be other aspects of a patient's over-all plan. The nurse, by virtue of her understanding of the interrelatedness of body functions, is in a key position to encourage the patient to follow through on courses of action by these other therapists. In the next chapter, nursing care plans are discussed. They reflect both immediate and long range nursing problems in maintaining physiologic functioning. These plans may result from the recognition that the patient will have some physical limitations for a period of time and may also need to have some treatments continued at home. The patient and his family are assisted so that the necessary measures can be continued and the persons involved in carrying them out can understand them. The way has been prepared for smoothing the transition from the hospital to the home. In many instances, it may include plans for visiting nurse services as well. To permit the patient to go home without such assistance may result ultimately in harm. Hence, the nurse as a coordinator has directed her attention toward helping a patient to continued improvement in his health.

Principle Relating to Man and His Environment

Appropriate precautionary measures will help to reduce or eliminate physical, chemical or microbiologic factors in the environment which causes illness or injury to man.

As mentioned previously in the discussions on health and the role of the nurse, prevention of illness is a responsibility of all members of the various health fields. Prevention implies that, through an ever-increasing knowledge of illness and injury, there will develop a corresponding awareness of potential dangers to health and of ways to protect persons from these dangers.

This principle cannot be isolated from the two previous ones. All safety measures carried out on any person's behalf are intended to keep him in the best state of well-being. In many instances, knowing much about the person as an individual can be a guide to initiating safety measures that might not be indicated for other persons.

Action based on this principle ranges from what might be considered plain common sense to that which is guided by technical knowledge. For example, in getting a patient out of bed for the first time after a prolonged illness, the nurse will anticipate the possibility of his becoming faint; she provides protection, as support when the patient stands, and a chair close by. This may very well be considered as just good sense.

The nurse is concerned with additional areas of safety. Factors in the environment must also be considered: room temperature, ventilation; the possibility of the patient's slipping if he has new footwear and the floor is hard and smooth; wires or other items that might be in the way or fall on him if he reaches out suddenly or pushes the table or chair. There is also the matter of knowing how to lower the patient into the chair or support him if he begins to faint. This requires an understanding of body mechanics, which is the correct use of the body guided by principles of physics.

There are other sources of potential danger to patients which are not quite so obvious. They require special understanding. Getting a patient out of bed for the first time may involve much more than providing a means for support and a chair close by. If the patient has a drainage tube attached in a body site, there is need for protecting such a tube from dislodgment; there is also the possibility that the tube must be kept in such a position that drainage is not disrupted; that

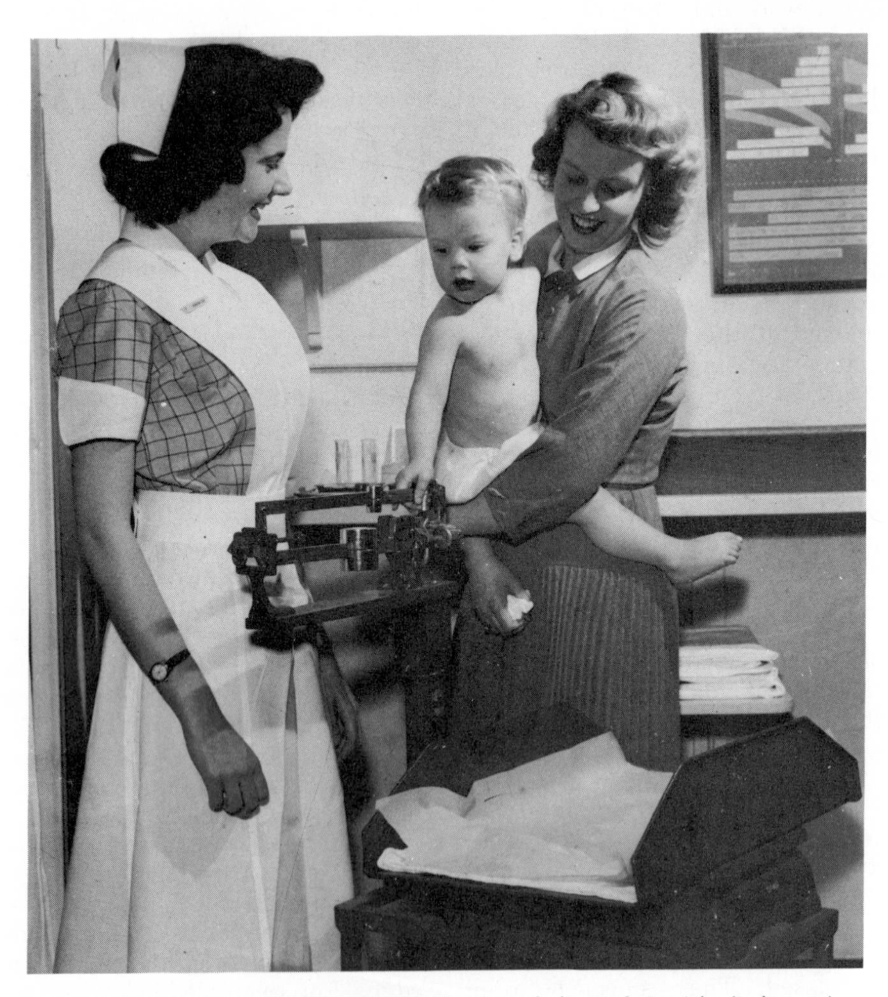

Fig. 4-3. What surrounds a child prompts his curiosity—unfortunately, it does not always last. Most adults do not question many things that may be in their environment, some of which are potentially dangerous. A part of nursing is the prevention of accidents to patients before they happen.

the tube must be protected from contamination by harmful agents; that the patient should understand how to manage the drainage tube so that he is not afraid of it.

Some persons might ask, "What is there to giving pills? Anyone can buy pills, read the label and take them." While this is true, it must be recalled from discussion of the principle of maintaining physiologic functioning that a nurse has many responsibilities when administering therapy. It is not only a question of reading the labels and the dosages correctly; the nurse must know the action of the drug, why it is being given, what it should do that is desired and what it might do that is undesired, etc. From the standpoint of safety, the nurse understands that any drug might be harmful. Some persons may have a low tolerance for a drug, others may have allergic reactions of various kinds, and still others might have side-effects that could be harmful if the drug is continued. Any activity in nursing, performed skillfully, might be made to look easy. But it might be likened to an iceberg: there is more beneath the surface than above it.

Another area of nursing requiring special understanding is the control of microbiologic agents in the environment in order to prevent the transmission of disease. Practices in this area may range from simple daily activities related to personal care to the management of a unit for patients who have communicable diseases. The nurse's actions in innumerable situations are based on scientific principles by which she must be guided. Here, again, is an area in which the nurse has unlimited opportunities to serve as a health teacher, both by example and by more direct methods.

The activities directly related to protecting the environment from microbiologic factors—namely, medical and surgical asepsis and communicable disease control—are discussed in more detail in Unit Three.

In addition to exercising every precaution possible when carrying out the physician's orders or other acts of nursing care, the nurse also must be aware of hazards that exist in the environment. While maintenance of equipment is not a nursing activity, all personnel in health agencies should observe the same precautions that they would at home. Wet or slippery floors, frayed electrical cords, objects on the floor, broken furniture—all are potential hazards. So are the objects that the nurse uses, such as needles, glassware and the variety of electrical appliances. When potentially harmful factors are recognized, handled properly and kept in good working order, the safer the environment will be.

It seems to be appropriate to mention at this time that the nurse is a registered practitioner. Registration by a state certifies that the nurse can practice safely. Safety in the practice of nursing is not brought about by brief exposures to certain information. It requires continuous study, keeping abreast of the latest literature and a constant increase of scientific knowledge. If a nurse is involved in an act which results in harm to a patient, a suit for malpractice may well result. Misapplication of any activity generally understood to be within the nurse's scope of responsibility, or failure to carry out such a duty when needed, could be classified as negligence. Illness occurring from uncontrollable circumstances is always regrettable; when it is a consequence of carelessness, it is tragic.

As Chapter 2 indicated, environmental health service personnel are concerned with hazards affecting all of us. Air and water pollution are major health problems in many countries. Chemicals used to control pests and drugs used in animal experimentation may be hazards to man. Protecting the public in regard to these problems requires the efforts and cooperation of scientists, industrialists and legislators, as well as health personnel.

Study Situation

In the American Journal of Nursing, *66*: 1747-1761, August, 1966, there is a group of articles under the title, "Syndrome of Poverty." Read the articles and look for implications in relation to this chapter. Consider how problems of the "have nots" can be viewed in terms of man as a person, man as an organism, and man and his environment.

CHAPTER

5

Communicating the Patient's Health Status And Need for Care

Introduction

The practice of nursing requires skill in the use of many different types of written communication. Without effectively recording the reporting among the various members of the health team, there would be utter chaos, with the patient the loser. This chapter is concerned with the kinds of written communications nurses use in their practice. Some report on the care given to the patient as directed by the physician's orders—charting. Others are related to planning the individualized care for patients—nursing care plans. Others, referrals, provide for extended care for patients if they use the services of other agencies—home care services, for instance.

Records can occupy a great deal of the nurse's time, so much so that nurses have been criticized for spending all of their time at desks. The use of personnel other than nurses, such as ward clerks, and newer technics for reporting and recording are helping to ease this situation.

The Patient's Chart

A record is an integral part of planning for the patient's care in almost all health agencies. In his office, the physician keeps a history of the patient's past health and a detailed summary of all therapy. In health stations and clinics, there are similar records. Visiting nurses are guided by records which give the physician's orders and an account of what was accomplished during each visit.

When a patient is admitted to the hospital, a record, the chart, either accompanies him or is sent to the unit as soon as possible after his admission. This record is used by all professional personnel contributing to his care. When it is completed at the termination of his stay in the hospital, it is a complete history of the patient's therapy, reaction to his illness, and progress while in the hospital, with possibly a recommendation for future care if necessary.

The recording that is done on the chart is referred to as *charting*. Each health agency has its own forms and specific details for charting: for example, some require using blue ink for recording during day hours and red ink for evening and night hours and the sequence of forms. For many years it was considered essential for the nurse to print all entries on a patient's chart. Since there is no legal justification for this practice, in many health agencies notations may be written.

Records are less bulky, more nearly accurate, more presentable in appearance and far easier to use if typewritten. In many agencies, provisions are made for typing medical, laboratory and x-ray reports, and addressographs (or a similar machine) are used on all chart and request forms.

While there is variation in detail, charts of most hospitals and other health agencies include certain similar information. Generally, charts include the following forms: a face sheet which gives general information about the patient, such as his name, address, age, sex, marital status, religion, name of next of kin, etc.; a release which when signed by the patient or responsible person gives consent to therapy; a graphic form for recording temperature and pulse and respiratory rates, days postoperative, days postadmission, fluid intake and output, height and weight; a form for recording the patient's past medical history, the physical examination and the physician's diagnosis; a form to guide the physician in recording details of the patient's progress; a form to aid the laboratory in recording the results of tests; and a form on which the nurse records all medications administered to the patient as well as observations about him. Other forms may be used, depending on the nature of the clinical service to which the patient is admitted—for example, anesthesia and operative records in surgery; behavior records in psychiatry; labor and delivery records in obstetrics. In addition, special forms are used by various departments if a patient utilizes their services, such as physical therapy and x-ray therapy.

The Physician's Orders

Once a patient has been admitted to the hospital and the routine aspects have been completed, there is little that can be done until the physician sets a plan into action. In some situations, even fluids and food are withheld until there is an order for the patient to have them. The physician's orders are the basis of the patient's plan of care.

The physician's orders are directed toward specific therapy for the patient. They include the type of diet the patient should receive, the medications, the treatments and the amount of activity he is permitted, and requests for consultation with other physicians or health workers, if necessary. It is the nurse's responsibility to see that the physician's plan is put into action.

The method of posting orders can be managed in a number of ways. Once written by the physician, orders may be transferred to a treatment book, a treatment sheet, a Kardex or the like; or they are transferred onto a record which includes both the physician's orders and information about the patient which reflects his immediate or future needs.

The Nurses' Notes

The patient's chart is one of the basic tools used by the nurse both in helping to plan care and in recording care. Therefore, it is important that the entries made by the nurse be significant and helpful to others.

Legal Aspects. There is considerable difference of opinion as to the legal status of the chart, especially in relation to the nurses' notes. The variation on this point exists because state laws differ on the admissibility of a patient's record as evidence in a court of law.

In some instances, the nurses' entries are removed from the chart and filed separately after the chart has been forwarded to the record department; in other instances, they remain as a part of the chart. There also are variations from state to state as to whether or not the nurses' entries must be kept as a permanent part of the record. The length of time that certain parts of a patient's chart are kept depends on the statute of limitations within the state, usually 6 to 7 years. However, the vital parts of the chart, such as the physician's diagnosis, a record of treatment, a discharge diagnosis and a summary, are rarely destroyed.

There have been a number of court actions involving patients' records, and all have been judged on an individual basis, depending on the laws existing in the state and the type of hospital involved. From these cases, many of which are cited in texts dealing with legal aspects of medical practice, one point is clear—namely, that all who record on a chart must do so with great accuracy. It is best for the recorder to be well prepared in technics of charting. Such technics include the formulation of concise and objective statements, aimed at avoiding loose reporting such as hearsay. Statements made on a patient's chart which legally are termed as hearsay are those made by the recorder after he has been told something by someone else. In effect, he heard something and then repeated it; he was not involved directly in either the incident or the observation.

There is no universal practice among either nurses or health agencies regarding the kind of recording that should be done. A variety of practices exist. Some are as simple as checking off certain phases of patient care and behavior on printed forms or making one summary-type entry on a patient's record every 24 hours. Other practices could be described as pertinent progress notes reflecting all prescribed care, the patient's emotional adjustment, health teaching in progress and other related patient-care information. Since both types of entries are acceptable, depending on the situation and the program of care in effect, the nurse should be prepared to do both.

The Nurse's Charting. A common criticism of the nurses' entries on charts is that they report little else but routine care, such as the fact that orders for medications and treatments have been carried out. It takes practice to develop skill in writing nurses' records that objectively and concisely describe the nursing problems encountered and the progress made in relation to them.

Many details governing nurses' entries on patients' records are a matter of individual method and policy of an agency. There is no universal procedure for keeping nurses' records, and the nurse will have to acquaint herself with the details wherever she practices. For example, there are such details as: how frequently entries are to be made; if routine nursing care is recorded; if the signature must appear in full or if initials are permitted; if identifying letters such as P.N. for practical nurse, S.N. for student nurse and R.N. for registered nurse must be used; if abbreviations such as OOB for out of bed may be used; how errors are corrected; if lines can be skipped; if physicians' visits are recorded, etc.

Because the recording is time-consuming, it is no wonder that details, accuracy in spelling and legibility suffer; and this is unfortunate for the impression that it creates of nurses. Some agencies are now using recording machines. The nurses dictate their comments into a recording machine, and in turn the comments are entered on the patients' chart by a secretary. In terms of time saved, improvement in the quality of entries and the appearance of the records, the results are worth it. Dictation also is a skill and requires practice. It is expected that the practice of using machines and other automatic equipment will become increasingly widespread.

Nursing Orders and Nursing Care Plans

In almost all health agencies there are routines that guide nursing personnel and ensure some uniform quality of care for all patients. These routines are the result of joint administrative investigation and planning and consideration of personnel available. In hospitals they include such details as how much linen should be changed per day, when meals will be served and by whom, how many visitors may be permitted to see the patient and at what times, and the hours for routine admission and discharge of patients. There is little that a nurse can do to change these.

Within the nursing department additional routines are established such as when patients are bathed and when other hygienic measures shall be performed. Nurses make modifications in routines if they are acceptable to the patient, make him more comfortable and contribute to his plan of care. These modifications may be written into a nursing care plan which is apart from the patient's chart.

A nursing care plan as part of effective nursing service to the patient has several objectives: to aid in the patient's return to his best state of health; to help him to maintain his individuality and his way of life, as far as possible; to save time by having information about a patient's plan of care readily available; and to effect a smooth transition between the patient's discharge from the hospital and his care at home. Good planning includes preparing for the patient's discharge, even if the discharge date is unknown or possibly several weeks away.

There are any number of nursing care forms in use; no one form could serve the purposes of all nurses in all situations. The form used by any group of nurses is based on the philosophy of care accepted by the institution, its medical staff and its nursing service. In some services, the nurse has more authority than in others, and this is reflected in the kind of form used. For example, in some hospital services, the nurse is expected to evaluate the activity needs of patients and to encourage certain types of bed exercises. This may not be possible in other situations. When the nurse is expected to make such judgments, the form of nursing care plan used will usually take this into consideration.

Without a written plan, a nurse caring for a patient for the first time is unable to continue with the plan developed by other nurses without having to ask the patient the details of his routine care. Is it necessary for the patient to be denied the routine that he helped

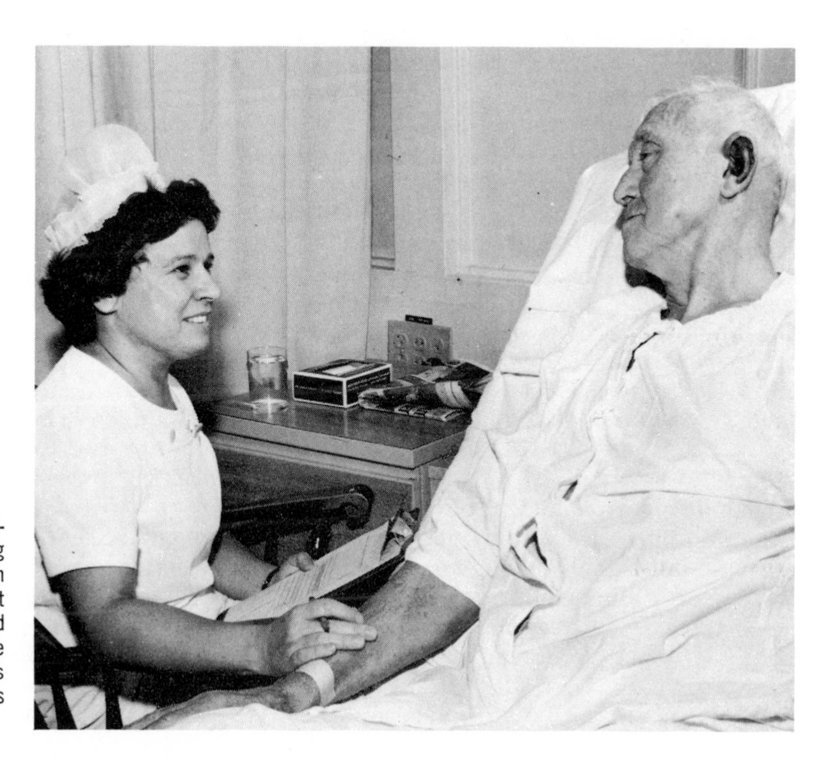

FIG. 5-1. Interviewing the newly admitted patient for the purpose of gaining information to initiate a nursing care plan can do much to help the patient feel at ease. The elderly person who is confused and concerned about himself cannot be rushed into fast answers. In spite of his many physical problems, this gentleman's sense of humor had not been affected.

to establish with the cooperation of his previous nurses?

With a written plan, the nurse can see immediately how a bath is managed, whether a feeding problem must be considered, whether there is a problem related to elimination, or whether the patient prefers his dressing or irrigation done in a certain manner. In addition, the nurse is able to continue with any special teaching that the patient may have been receiving without the risk of boring the patient with repetitious or confusing information.

For chronically ill patients, nursing care plans are invaluable. Such patients have definite routines that are the result of much investigation and planning on their part as well as on the part of physicians and nurses and possibly other health workers. It is often disturbing to patients if they must explain to each newcomer on the nursing staff why a certain thing must be done a certain way.

A comment about recording on the nurses' notes form on the patient's chart and on a nursing care plan is needed to clarify the difference in purpose of the two. The patient's chart should contain those notations which have a direct bearing on the patient's health problem. They stem from the nurse's observation of the patient. To guide the nurse in deciding upon entries on the chart, the question might be asked, "What does the physician want and need to know?" The physician reads the chart and he is concerned with finding out (1) whether the prescribed therapy was carried out and if not, why not; (2) the reaction of the patient to the therapy; (3) any observations possibly not related to the therapy but which should be investigated and (4) the progress or the status of the patient in matters related to the health problem but not necessarily a part of the written orders.

Numbers one and two above are definitely akin to fulfilling the nurse's responsibility for carrying out the physician's orders. Number three is fulfilling the responsibility to the physician by assisting in observing the patient. Number four can reveal what the nurse's own part in the patient's care has been. It should not be a duplication of what is on a nursing care plan but rather a comment or a progress notation from it.

The nursing care plan is for the use of the nursing personnel and contains information pertinent to the nursing care of a particular patient. For example, if there was a nursing care plan for a patient who had a leg amputation and also had many other physical limitations and is learning to crutch-walk, it could be quite detailed. There might be a routine for helping him out of bed and supporting him, exercises for strengthening his arms and evaluating his progres in learning to use the crutches. All this detail does not belong on the chart. However, a progress comment would be helpful to the physician.

Consider another example of a patient who is confined to bed and asks for a glass of hot water every morning before breakfast, stating that he does this at home "to keep my bowels regular." This is a minor request considering all that can result if it is denied. The patient may become emotionally upset, he may develop feelings of resentment against the nursing personnel or he may feel that hospitalization is prisonlike and that nothing may be requested. It may interrupt his regularity of elimination and, as a result, he may require enemas or cathartics. If he receives the latter, they may cause distress, and he may be even more upset. If he receives enemas, it is creating more work for the nursing personnel which would have been unnecessary had they given him the glass of hot water in the first place. If enough disruption is caused by the whole process, the patient may need to spend several weeks at home becoming readjusted, both emotionally and physically.

Such modifications in a patient's care should be written either on a nursing care plan or the Kardex by the nurse responsible for the patient's care. In a sense, they are *nursing orders.* All other nurses observe them. A reason for the order is often helpful when it is not obvious. In the above example, the nurse would record, "Give glass of hot water before breakfast." Anyone caring for the patient would do so. Other examples of nursing orders might be as follows: keep turned on either side except for meals; do not serve lunch on Mondays or Thursdays since patient has nausea after cobalt therapy; allow to walk only when nursing personnel or family are present; use lotion on feet daily; give him dentures for meals and remove after eating.

Patients often make requests of auxiliary personnel. If a close team relationship exists between the nurse and auxiliary personnel, such requests are channeled and then investigated. As mentioned earlier in Unit One, one of the roles of the nurse is to guide and help the auxiliary members in nursing service who are contributing to patient care. Through reporting sessions and conferences on patient care, the auxiliary personnel can be helped to understand the type of information that should be relayed so that it can be incorporated in nursing care plans.

Nursing orders, then, are those modifications in the patient's care which the nurse, by virtue of her understanding of the patient's illness and the physician's plan of care and wishes, can make for the patient's comfort and safety. In succeeding Units, there will be discussion of modifications frequently seen in various situations. Many of these can be recognized by the nurse and acted on without the physician's writing an order for them.

Nursing Care Plans and the Patient's Future Needs

Estimating the Patient's Future Needs. A logical approach to planning for the patient's care is to include him in the planning from the outset. In many instances the nurse will know that a patient will need to have assistance with dressings, irrigations, injections, medications, exercises or diet changes, even before the patient is aware of this. On the other hand, the patient may have many questions going through his mind, unanticipated by the nurse, about what is to become of him after hospitalization. A purpose of mutual planning is to avoid having a concentrated confused period of preparation for discharge take place minutes before the patient is to leave the hospital.

To understand if a patient has any concern about the future, the nurse should provide him with the opportunity to express his feelings about his care after discharge and to encourage him to ask questions. Many patients have the feeling that what happens to them after they go home is of no concern to the personnel in the hospital. When this occurs, is it because no one took the time to find out what was to become of the patient after he did leave?

Sometimes, the concern that patients have over their illness or their care after discharge is not expressed verbally but may be manifested in their attitudes or behavior. They may feel reluctant to talk about certain problems either out of embarrassment or because they themselves may not know that the nurse can assist them. Examples of such problems include lack of funds to buy equipment which

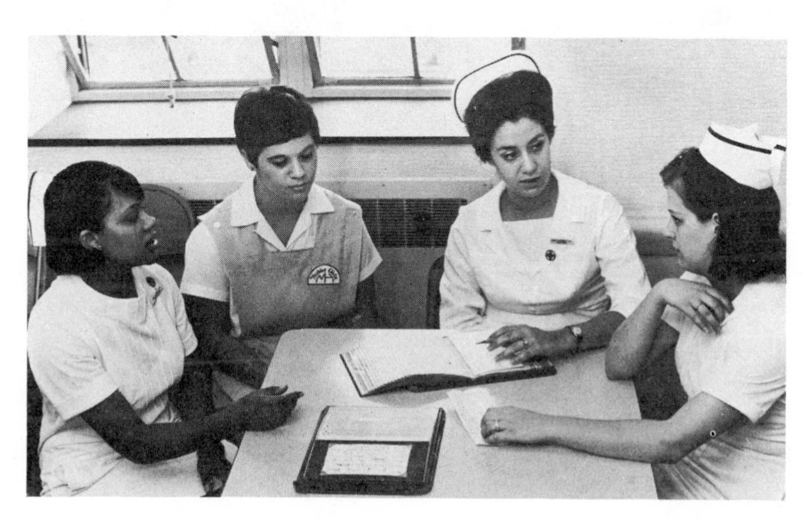

Fig. 5-2. A part of preparing nursing care plans and keeping them up to date is the use of team conferences. Here the team is meeting following the care of a group of patients. They are pooling their information and adjusting each patient's care plan according to his current needs. (Photo by Warren R. Vroom)

they may need; not knowing where and how to purchase special foods; fear of harming themselves when they give themselves injections at home; uncertainty about measuring drugs accurately; misgivings over the way their new way of life is going to affect others; worry over being a burden to others or causing so much expense. One of the unique contributions that the nurse can make is to help the patient to see that as a health worker she has an understanding of such problems and that if she is unable to help directly, there are others she may call on for assistance with the problem while he is still in the hospital. The problem stated by the patient and the action taken by the nursing staff is recorded on the nursing care plan.

Planning With the Family and the Patient. Some patients are able to get all the information that they need and to share it with the family members concerned, while others will need family members to assist in the planning. The latter is especially true for the patient who is dependent on someone else for a part of his care, or has a language handicap, or whose mental state is such that it is best if others are also aware of the details of his care. Planning with family members should also begin early, for the sooner they know what to expect, the sooner they are able to make their own adjustments, as necessary. How family members are being used in preparing a patient to go home should be recorded on the nursing care plan.

In some instances, the nurse will need to channel problems through other persons, such as the social worker or the public health nurse. Agencies differ in the amount of latitude granted the nurse in planning without the collaboration of the physician; but in almost all instances, problems which require referrals to other departments or outside agencies will need the physician's endorsement. However, physicians are grateful to nurses who are able to help to prepare the patient and his family adequately for his dis-

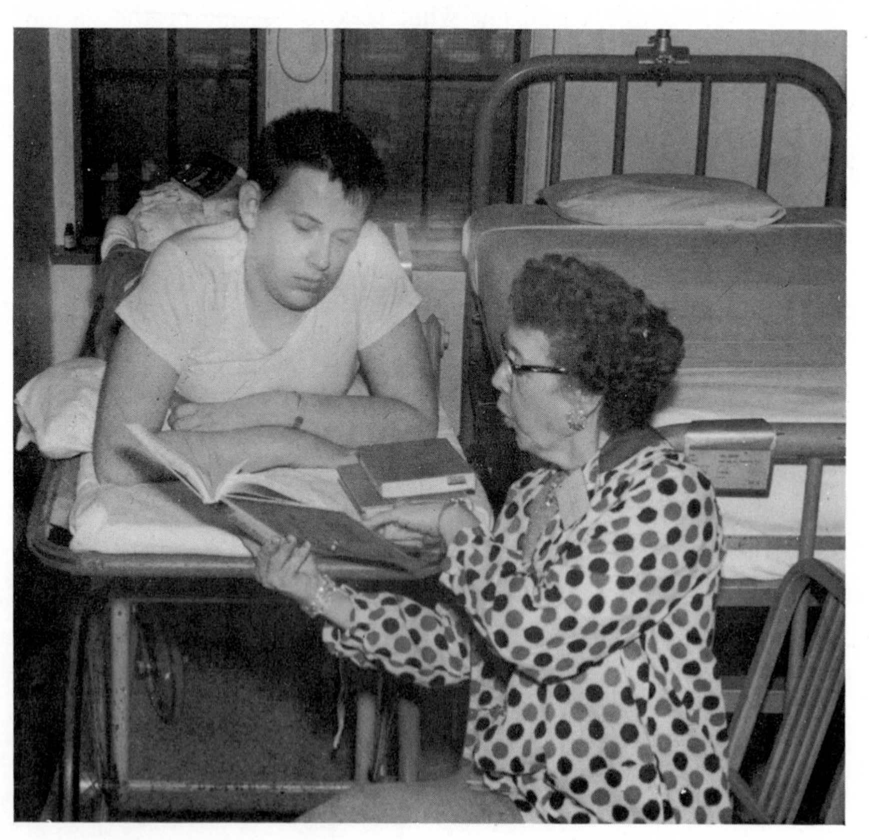

FIG. 5-3. This boy is continuing his studies while in the hospital. A nursing care plan for him should include the days and the hours that his teacher is with him so that he is ready for her and her time is not wasted. It should also include plans for uninterrupted study periods for him. This is another example of the nurse's part in coordinating the various phases of a patient's care during illness and convalescence. (University of Illinois Research and Educational Hospital.)

charge, since failure to do so may create other problems. For instance, if a patient were hurriedly instructed about medications to take at home and then through a misunderstanding failed to take them properly, it could impair his progress, causing concern to the patient and his family and possibly resulting in a middle-of-the-night call to the physician. It may also require a period of time to get the patient "straightened out" again.

Instructions for Home Care Should Be Written. In addition to verbal presentation, all instructions that involve procedures, diets, etc., should be made available in written form. Although written instructions require time to prepare, their value in the months that follow cannot be overestimated. It is a great relief to both the patient and his family to know that they have this material to refer to at home. It is a further assurance that the instructions are likely to be carried out more accurately. A mistake that the nurse can make in preparing the patient and the family members for the discharge is to assume that every word which she has told them is understood clearly and remembered perfectly. Instructions needed by a patient and given to him in written form should also be indicated on the nursing care plan.

Referrals to Other Departments and Agencies

The means by which information about a patient is transferred to another group of health workers who will help to provide continuity in the patient's care is another form of reporting and recording and is called a *referral*. However, it is common practice for most persons to associate the term "referral" with a public health agency. The referral is the physician's request to the public health agency to accept the patient and to give the care prescribed. Referrals also may be made to social agencies, rehabilitation centers, nursing homes and sometimes to other hospitals.

While the request for continued care is made by the physician, it is the nurse's responsibility to prepare a summary of the patient's present nursing care plan and other pertinent comments. The public health nurse who is to continue the plan of care initiated in the hospital will find this helpful. This saves her time but what is more important is that the transition is comfortable for the patient.

In some agencies there are intramural referrals which provide a means for sharing information about a patient which is not likely to be found on the patient's chart. For example, the outpatient department may have been caring for a patient for many months, and it is decided that he needs hospitalization. The key points in his care which the outpatient department personnel may consider important to communicate to the succeeding group of health workers are entered on a referral and passed along. Or, a patient may be discharged from the hospital needing follow-up care in the outpatient department, and the nursing and medical staff may wish to send a referral to the outpatient department.

If a nursing care plan has been kept on a patient, it will be relatively easy for any member of the nursing staff to complete the nursing portion of a referral. However, a meager and uninformative report as to what has been done for the patient and family, will help no one. In preparation of a referral, the nurse can be guided by this thought: "What would I want to know about this patient if I were the person who had to continue his care at this point?"

Study Situations

1. Read the following article and identify some of the points made previously in this text concerning the role of the nurse in initiating individualized care. Also, note the stress on using principles to guide action, observing, using effective written and oral communication, continued study to improve patient care and having concern for the patient's total health problem, not merely a segment of it. Does it strengthen the concept that the practice of nursing is not procedure-oriented but rather the result of being able to use knowledge to aid another individual in a way that is not provided for by other health workers, by routines or by the physician's plan of care?

- Chambers, W.: Nursing diagnosis.
  AMER. J. NURS., *62*:102-104, November, 1962.

2. If you were to be a patient in a hospital where you were unknown, what are some of the things that you might wish the nursing staff to know about you? Do you have any patterns of eating, sleeping, grooming or hygiene that you would not like to have disturbed? Suppose you were rather helpless and had to be bathed, and each morning when a new person arrived to care for you, you had to tell her not to use soap on your face, not to use mouthwash on your toothbrush, and so forth.

3. The following article lists some of the more common "sins of omission and commission" in relation to the patient's chart, especially the nurses' notes, and why an audit is helpful:

- Estes, M. D.: Introducing the nursing audit.
  AMER. J. NURS., *64*:91-92, September, 1964.

4. Read the following article for a description of how notes relative to a patient's behavior can be automated. Note that the authors believe the proper use of automative technics can result in ". . . a more flexible type of treatment program for the optimum care of the patient."

- Rosenberg, M., and Carriker, D.: Automating nurses' notes.
  AMER. J. NURS., *66*:1021-1023, May, 1966.

5. Nurses often feel deluged with paper work beyond the scope of communicating the patient's health status and needs, as the following article illustrates:

- DeMarco, J. P.: Automating nursing's paper work.
  AMER. J. NURS., *65*:74-77, September, 1965.

When systems as the one described in this article become common in health agencies, nurses will be freed of much desk work.

6. That nurses' notes leave much to be desired in many instances is a problem that nurses must face. The following article describes how one agency, using a problem solving approach, attempted to gain information as a means for further study and action:

- Healy, E. E., and McGurk, W.: Effectiveness and acceptance of nurses' notes.
  NURS. OUTLOOK, *14*:32-34, March, 1966.

Note that nurses and physicians did not always agree as to what belonged on charts. Can you see a relationship between these areas of differences and the philosophy of nursing care plans?

7. Although the content of this chapter is primarily concerned with written communication, it does not mean to exclude the fact that oral communications are often essential also. Note how the author of the following article used the problem solving approach to resolve an oral communication problem she and others faced:

- Schwartz, D. R.: Planning the telephone call.
  NURS. OUTLOOK, *13*:44-45, January, 1965.

References

1. Banks, A. W. *et al*: Tape-recorded nurses' notes.
   NURS. OUTLOOK, *14*:42-44, October, 1966.
2. Farrell, M. B.: Health service records at a glance.
   AMER. J. NURS., *66*:312-313, February, 1966.
3. Jamison, E. F.: Physician's order books—revised.
   NURS. OUTLOOK, *16*:39, March, 1968.
4. Kelly, N. C.: Nursing care plans.
   NURS. OUTLOOK, *14*:61-64, May, 1966.
5. Little, D., and Carnevali, D.: Nursing care plans: Let's be practical about them.
   NURS. FORUM, *6*:61-76, #1, 1967.
6. Mansfield, E.: Use of patient care plans by aides.
   NURS. OUTLOOK, *15*:72-74, April, 1967.
7. McCain, F. R.: Nursing by assessment—not intuition.
   AMER. J. NURS., *65*:82-84, April, 1965.
8. McPhetridge, M. L.: Nursing history: One means to personalize care.
   AMER. J. NURS., *68*:68-75, January, 1968.
9. Melody, M., and Clark, G.: Walking-planning rounds.
   AMER. J. NURS., *67*:771-773, April, 1967.
10. Morgan, E. M.: New chart forms solve old problems.
   AMER. J. NURS., *65*:93-96, March, 1965.
11. Park, W. E.: Patient transfer form.
   AMER. J. NURS., *67*:1665-1668, August, 1967.
12. Rosenberg, M. *et al*: Attitudes of nursing students toward computers.
   NURS. OUTLOOK, *15*:44-46, July, 1967.

13. Schwartz, D. R.: Toward more precise evaluation of patients' needs.
NURS. OUTLOOK, *13*:42-44, May, 1955.
14. Tenney, D. A.: Patients' progress—one step forward.
NURS. OUTLOOK, *15*:30-33, November, 1967.
15. Turner, C., and Mahoney, R. F.: After hospitalization.
AMER. J. NURS., *64*:137-139, September, 1964.
16. Wahlstrom, E. D.: Initiating referrals. A hospital-based system.
AMER. J. NURS., *67*:332-335, February, 1967.
17. Walker, V. H. *et al*: A care plan for ailing nurses' notes.
AMER. J. NURS., *65*:74-76, August, 1965.
18. Walker, V. H., and Selmonoff, E. D.: A study of the nature and uses of nurses' notes.
NURS. RES., *13*:113-121, Spring, 1964.
19. Weil, T. P., and Weil, J. W.: The use of computer systems in patient care.
NURS. FORUM, *6*:206-217, Spring, 1967.
20. Woods, M. F.: Measuring a patient's needs and progress.
NURS. OUTLOOK, *14*:38-41, October, 1966.

CHAPTER

6

Using Teaching Skills in Nursing Practice

Introduction

In the practice of nursing, there are innumerable opportunities for teaching others. Often, the nurse's teaching is done concurrently with nursing care activities. However, there are instances when the nurse plans and participates in formal scheduled teaching of specific groups of patients. Such groups might be mothers learning to care for their newborn infants or diabetic patients learning about their diets and the ways in which their diets may be worked into family meals.

With greater emphasis being placed on patients assuming self-care activities as soon as their physical state permits, the nurse's role as a health teacher has increased steadily. At one time, patients had almost everything done for them by the nurse during their stay in the hospital. Now nurses are helping patients to learn to do as much as possible for themselves. As the values of increased activity and decreased bed rest have been noted, some authorities in physical medicine and rehabilitation concluded that the old approach of too much "tender loving care" was actually harmful. While there may be some loss of function through the illness mechanism itself, undue loss may result from keeping the patient inactive longer than is necessary and by not involving him in his own care and recovery. To help the patient understand why he is being asked to walk soon after surgery, or that he is being encouraged to try to tie the strings on the back of his gown because his shoulder muscles need exercise, is an important part of nursing care. It involves teaching the patient about his own body needs, which will be of value to him long after he has recovered from his present illness.

Since teaching is often a very important aspect of a patient's care, there is need for recording the progress made just as there is need for recording that an order for a treatment has been carried out. If this is not done, there is the possibility that the teaching started by one nurse may never be completed, or that the patient may be taught the same thing by a succession of different personnel—both possibilities irritating to the patient.

In each Unit in this text, there is information that the nurse may wish or need to share with others. The nurse who uses teaching skills as an integral part of her nursing practice is likely to give more effective care. Several Study Situations in this text show that patients respond well to teaching as part of their care.

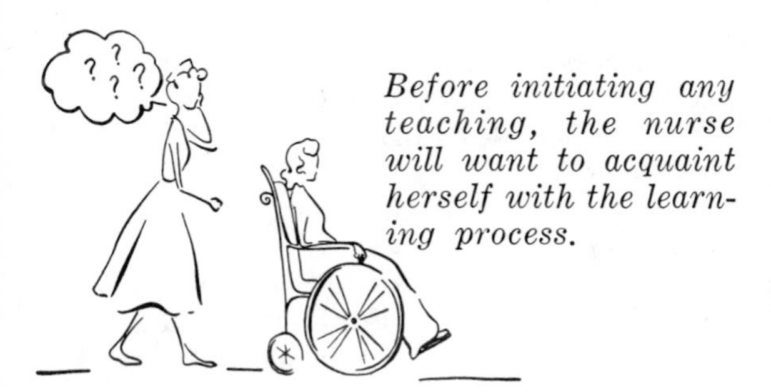

Before initiating any teaching, the nurse will want to acquaint herself with the learning process.

The Learning Process

A person has learned when a teaching activity results in a change in his behavior. This change may be in knowledge, attitudes, appreciation or skills. How does the learner become involved, and how does one know when changes in behavior have been effected? The following aspects of learning should help the nurse understand some effective teaching technics.

Individual Needs. When learning is in progress, the learner is attempting to satisfy a need. Psychologists often use the term "goal" as the target for which the learner is striving. The individual wants to master something in order to attain his goal. For example, a child may wish a cookie that is in a jar outside his reach; therefore, he needs to learn how to reach the jar. A college football star can remain on the team if his scholastic average is above a certain rating; therefore, to attain his goal he must do well in classes. A bride wishes to please her husband by serving delicious meals, therefore, she learns to cook to attain her goal.

Assume that a nurse wishes to teach a mother the care of her newborn baby. Most new mothers are excited about caring for their babies, and, although they may be somewhat apprehensive, they have and recognize the need to learn how. The patient's need to learn this care is one that a nurse can usually discern with ease.

Often, an individual's goals cannot be defined clearly, and in some cases the person may even attempt to conceal them. For example, a patient may not seem to be interested in doing certain things for himself or in learning self-care activities. Although he may never admit it, his real goal could be to remain dependent if he has learned to find satisfaction in having things done for him, or continuing in a state of "ill health" helps him remain away from an unsatisfactory work situation.

Interest in Learning or Desire to Learn. The interest in learning or the desire to learn—often referred to as motivation—is closely associated with an individual's goals. Unless there is an interest or a reason for attaining a particular goal, learning will proceed slowly if at all.

An example will illustrate how teaching may fail when the nurse does not recognize a patient's feelings about a certain learning situation. Most authorities feel that breast feeding, when it is possible, is the method of choice for feeding newborns. Assume that a particular physician advocates this strongly, but his patient does not want to breast feed her baby. It can be predicted that the nurse's effort to teach this mother to breast feed her baby may fall on deaf ears if the nurse has failed to consider that the patient at this point needs not technics but gentle suggestion. The patient's interest will govern her learning—not the desire of the nurse or the physician.

When motivation is lacking, the nurse may stimulate a patient's interest. Possibly, the mother just described does not know or understand why her physician recommends breast feeding, and she may think that breast feeding means that she can never skip feeding her baby by substituting an occasional bottle. It is possible that with explanations the nurse may stimulate in the patient an interest which did not exist formerly, and then teaching can proceed with greater ease. However, the nurse must understand her own feelings and be certain that she neither furthers nor imposes her own interests on a patient without the patient's accepting them, in which case learning will not occur.

Readiness to Learn. This depends on the capabilities a person has that influence his ability to learn. Readiness involves several factors, three of which are intellectual capacity, physical and emotional maturity and previous educational experiences.

Intellectual Capacity. An individual's intellectual capacity will affect his ability to learn. If he is well endowed and if he puts his inheritance to good use, the learner can assimilate much in little time. The person who is limited may never learn as much and often needs to spend considerable time in achieving what he does learn.

Physical and Emotional Maturity. The degree to which an individual has matured physically and emotionally will influence learning. For example, most children learn to walk at some time between the ages of 12 to 16 months; prior to this period, most children's musculoneurologic maturity is insufficient to permit them to learn to walk, and attempts to teach them to do so result in failure.

Physical maturity is easier to determine than emotional maturity, since the former can be judged, to a large extent, in relation to the individual's chronologic age. Estimating emotional maturity is a different matter; and simply judging it on the basis of chronologic age sometimes leads to false conclusions. For example, a young adult presently dependent on a wheel chair may have sufficient physical maturity to have learned the skills of a mechanic, but he may not demonstrate sufficient emotional maturity to see why he should bother with the rehabilitation that eventually will afford him the ability to earn his own living.

Physical maturity should not be confused with physical ability. For example, a patient may have reached physical maturity, but be-

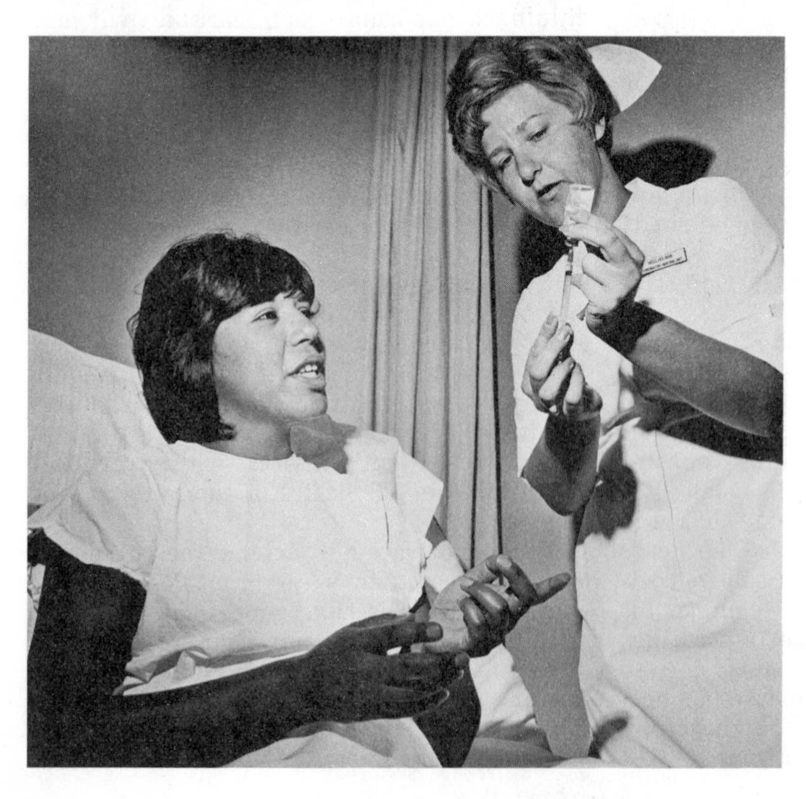

Fig. 6-1. Teaching is often given to the patient who must manage a problem, such as injections at home. (Good Samaritan Hospital, Phoenix, Arizona)

cause of a handicap, say a paralysis of an arm following an injury, he cannot be taught to give himself a subcutaneous injection. This patient may never be physically ready to learn a technic such as giving himself an injection.

Consider another example that illustrates how emotions may influence learning. A young woman has had a breast removed, and to ensure retaining the best possible function of the arm and the shoulder, exercises are essential. The teaching of the exercise may be ineffective if the patient is still in a period of depression over the loss of this body part. Emotionally, she is almost in a state of mourning, and until she is able to adjust to this change and accept it, the exercises might be carried out better without too much emphasis on teaching. As soon as the patient sees how the exercises are helping her, she usually will want to learn and to practice them.

Previous Learning. An individual's previous cultural and educational experiences will affect the learning process. For example, certain cultures believe that a person is not ill unless he feels and looks ill. Assume that it has been found on a routine examination that a person reared in such a culture has pulmonary tuberculosis and positive sputum but that the disease has not progressed to the point that the patient feels and looks sick. Unless a nurse knows and understands what this patient has learned from his culture, it may be difficult or even impossible to teach him to care for himself in order that he regain health and refrain from exposing his family and friends to the disease.

A person's previous educational experiences play a vital role in his learning. For example, a patient who is a college graduate with a major in human physiology is ready for information that a patient who is also a college graduate but has a major in English literature is in no position to understand. Or, consider teaching two patients how to irrigate their wounds; one is a college graduate, the other has reached only the 10th grade. Despite the difference in their educational experiences (and other things being equal), the nurse may teach both in a very similar manner. The amount of formal education that an individual has does not necessarily indicate his ability to learn; some

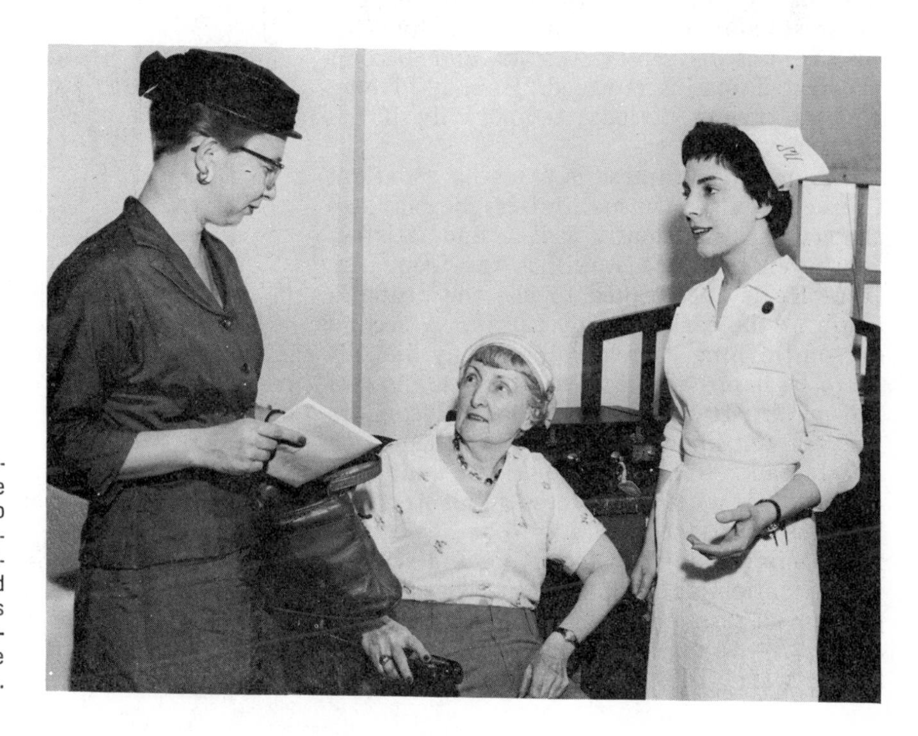

Fig. 6-2. Teaching may also involve the family, so that those who must help the patient also understand the care. Verbal instructions are not sufficient. Written instructions should be offered as reminders. Usually patients and family members are not emotionally "free" to concentrate when given verbal instructions.

very intelligent people have not had educational opportunities. But the *nature* of either a formal education or self-teaching to which an individual has been exposed usually influences his readiness for learning.

Response to a Learning Situation. When an individual is learning, he will make a response to the learning situation. The response may be in physical movements or spoken words; or it may be an internal reaction, such as a feeling of pleasure, that cannot be observed except possibly indirectly.

After responding to a learning situation, the learner evaluates the results of his response. If the response is one of satisfaction, he will be motivated to learn more.

Evaluation of the response usually is an unconscious experience, i.e., the learner rarely expresses this response nor is he consciously aware of it. For example, the student in nursing usually feels satisfaction and pleasure after being taught to give a patient an injection. However, she may be quite unaware of having evaluated her response.

If the learner decides that his new response is unsatisfactory, one of two things is likely to occur. The learner either will try again and modify his response until he experiences satisfaction, or he may feel thwarted by the unsatisfactory results and become frustrated and discouraged. He may give up further trying, at least temporarily if not permanently.

Assume that a nurse is teaching a patient to use crutches. On his first try he may use the crutches sufficiently well to find satisfaction, even though his skill is far from perfect. He is encouraged to use the crutches again at the earliest opportunity. A second person learning crutch-walking may find little to be happy about in his early trials and become frustrated, but he eagerly attempts it again, until he does learn to use them with satisfaction. But a third patient, unable to use crutches with any success on his first try, becomes frustrated, stating that he is perfectly happy using a wheel chair and refuses further attempts to practice. These three persons all responded to a learning situation, and each evaluated his response in a different way. The first patient experienced sufficient satisfaction to be stimulated to further learning; the second was dissatisfied, but the dissatisfaction became a challenge to try again; and the third was dissatisfied, frustrated and willing to give up.

Adjustment in teaching methods sometimes is helpful when a patient seems dissatisfied or frustrated. Perhaps too much is being taught too fast, and the learner is not experiencing satisfaction by having mastered one thing at a time. Perhaps the nurse's or the patient's goals were unrealistic.

Sometimes, pointing out small degrees of success and giving the patient praise and encouragement help to stimulate him to further learning. It is always safer to begin with small segments of relatively easy teaching so that the learner may enjoy satisfaction. Then, the amount and the speed can be geared to the learner's ability and interest.

The nurse evaluates her teaching on the basis of how well the patient is responding and showing signs of changes in behavior. She asks, "How well is the patient assimilating and using his new knowledge?"

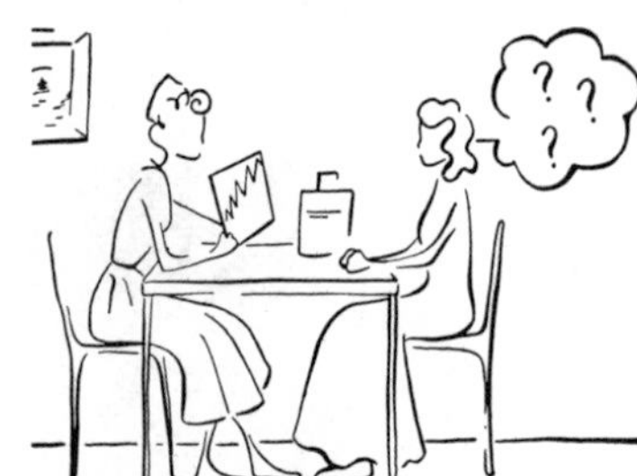

While the teaching goes forward, there is need to determine whether the patient is making progress and then proceed accordingly.

The Learning-Teaching Environment

Learning can occur any time and any place. While learning can occur under the most adverse conditions, every effort should be made to provide a comfortable environment.

An environment conducive to learning usually takes at least the following factors into consideration:

Give and Take. There still exists a stereotype in nursing that can be detrimental to a good teaching-learning situation, and nurses should be aware of it. The public has an impression that nurses are too busy and also that their word is law. If a patient has this feeling, his ability to learn is impaired by fear or unwillingness to be a nuisance. A give-and-take atmosphere should be established. The feeling, the tone and the attitude of the person teaching are more important than many other environmental considerations. If the learner senses that the other person is interested in him and trying to help him, he will be more receptive and stimulated. But if he senses urgency or a superior attitude, the nurse's teaching will have little or no effect.

Comfort for the Learner and the Teachers. Ideally, the patient as well as the nurse should be comfortable. Suitable chairs, adequate lighting and good ventilation add to the comfort. Privacy also is desired.

Teaching Aids. It is helpful to have teaching aids available. For example, if the nurse wishes to teach the procedure for giving a baby a bath, she will wish to have equipment such as a mother may use at home so that she may demonstrate the procedure. Also, audio-visual aids are helpful, such as a film, a filmstrip, or slides. The nurse may choose to use these in conjunction with her teaching.

Books, pamphlets and printed sheets can be helpful teaching aids. Often, the nurse will find that the patient appreciates them, and the learning process is improved by a review of the material. Printed materials make it possible for the patient to study on his own and ask questions, besides serving as future references.

Being Free of Distractions. A person distracted with miscellaneous thoughts rarely is able to utilize learning opportunities to a maximum. Therefore, the nurse should plan to teach the patient when he is least likely to be distracted. Teaching planned to be given during visiting hours, for example, can hardly be expected to be beneficial, since the patient perhaps will have visitors waiting for him. The same is true if he knows that he is to be called to the x-ray department at any moment.

Selection of the Teaching Method. The nurse who uses stimulating and motivating methods of teaching usually accomplishes more than the one who tells what is to be learned. The stimulating teacher captures the patient's desire to learn when she utilizes appropriate methods interestingly and with skill. For example, the nurse might ask a patient how she cared for her leg ulcers before hospitalization and then concentrate the teaching on areas that need adjustment.

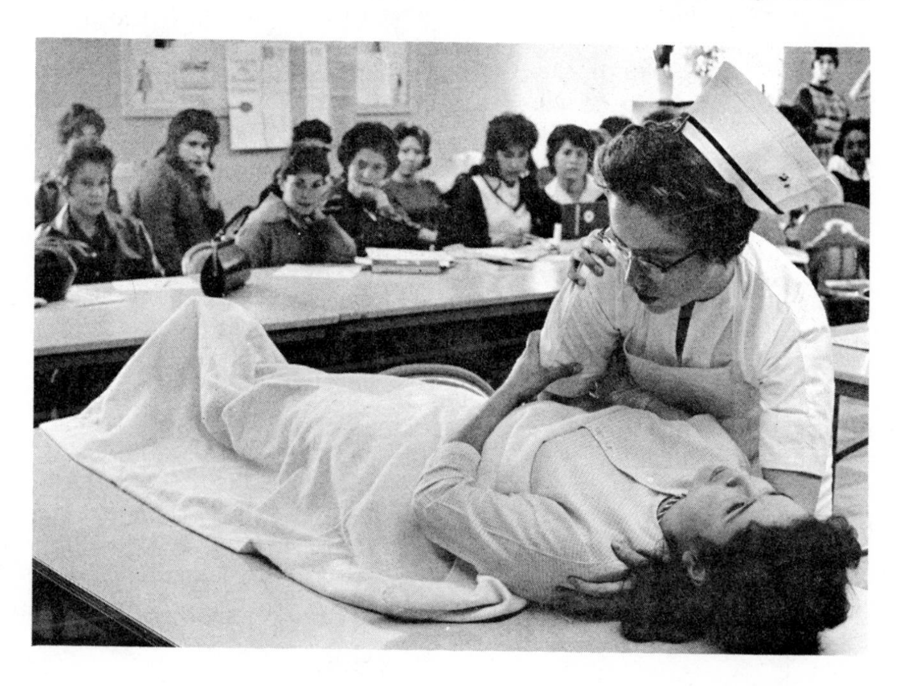

Fig. 6-3. When incomes are low and hospitals miles away, the seriously ill must often be cared for at home. Here, a nurse is teaching a group of girls how to move a patient and to avoid strain on themselves. (Photo by Mary Ann Gehres of Presbyterian Life)

Most persons will agree readily that whatever teaching method is used, the teacher should have her instruction organized. It has been said that learning and bewilderment may differ only in terms of organization. However, organization does not mean rigidity. Flexibility in teaching methods to capture the enthusiasm of the learner is as essential as organization.

The Nurse as a Teacher

We have discussed the learning process and an environment conducive to learning. A third facet in a discussion of teaching and learning concerns the teacher.

There is no dearth in the literature of education describing the characteristics of a good teacher. However, making generalizations concerning these characteristics is difficult, because teaching is a highly individualistic and creative matter. When we recall teachers we had who were outstandingly fine, we see that they were often very different from one another, both in their personalities and in their teaching methods. However, experienced teachers in general agree on at least two characteristics that seem essential for success in teaching.

Good Teaching Requires Good Scholarship. It may seem obvious that a person must be familiar with a field of knowledge before he can teach it. But in addition, the good teacher is a scholar, one who constantly seeks out new knowledge in his field and constantly seeks to increase his intellectual growth. While the nursing student is a beginner in the area of intellectual growth and knowledge in her field, an attitude of scholarliness with a sincere interest in her professional development will help her take the first steps toward becoming an effective teacher of her patients.

Good Teaching Requires the Ability to Communicate Excitement. This is not the excitement we feel when filled with great joy, although elements of it can occur in teaching. More typically, we are communicating enthusiasm, interest in what we are doing, and an interest in helping the learner. The important person in the teaching-learning situation is the learner. But the person who is enthusiastic about his teaching and keeps the learner's need foremost generally experiences more teaching success.

As indicated, technics and methods of teaching are innumerable. The nurse making early attempts at teaching patients may feel awkward and ill at ease. Experience, coupled with a sincere interest in wanting to help her patients and with enthusiasm for what she is doing, rarely results in failure.

Study Situations

1. The three articles listed below illustrate a variety of teaching mehods. See if you can identify some of them.

- Krysan, G. S.: How do we teach four million diabetics?

  AMER. J. NURS., *65*:105-107, November, 1965.

What aspects of a teaching program for diabetics does the author indicate need evaluation? Could her suggestions for evaluation be used in other patient teaching situations?

- Barnard, K.: Teaching the retarded child is a family affair.

  AMER. J. NURS., *68*:305-311, February, 1968.

Note how the process of learning applies to Stevie's situation.

- Healy, K. M.: Does preoperative instruction make a difference?

  AMER. J. NURS., *68*:62-67, January, 1968.

Describe how patients reacted when they felt responsible for some of their own recovery after being taught self-care procedures.

2. The following article reports findings when an investigation was made concerning questions to which patients wanted answers:

- Linehan, D. T.: What does the patient want to know?

  AMER. J. NURS., *66*:1066-1070, May, 1966.

Note the emphasis the author places on establishing what the patient wants to know, rather than on what health personnel feel the patient should know. Which principle in the learning process does this concern for the patient illustrate?

References

1. Amend, E. L.: A parent education program in a children's hospital.
   NURS. OUTLOOK, *14*:53-56, April, 1966.
2. Bailey, T. F.: Puppets teach young patients.
   NURS. OUTLOOK, *15*:36-37, August, 1967.
3. Cronbach, L. J.: Educational Psychology, ed. 2, 706 p.
   New York, Harcourt, Brace and World, 1963.
4. Hogan, A.: Launching programs for expectant patients.
   AMER. J. NURS., *66*:2227-2230, October, 1966.
5. Kornblueh, M.: The cafeteria food game.
   NURS. OUTLOOK, *15*:41, February, 1967.
6. Varvaro, F. F.: Teaching the patient about open heart surgery.
   AMER. J. NURS., *65*:111-115, October, 1965.

Nursing Implementation: Man as a Person

Unit 2

CHAPTER 7

Concept of a Therapeutic Relationship

This Unit is concerned primarily with the principle discussed in Chapter 4, Man as a Person. As previously stated, human beings are not made of a separated psychosocial entity and physical entity; rather, the two form a unity and function together as one. What affects a person from a psychosocial viewpoint influences his physical status, and vice versa. However, for the sake of trying to clarify the various facets of comprehensive nursing, this Unit is concerned with the psychosocial aspects of patient care.

Definition of a Therapeutic Relationship

What is meant by a therapeutic relationship, or by a therapeutic climate in which a person is cared for? The terms can be defined in many ways and, somewhat like the weather, are affected by innumerable forces. In this discussion, therapeutic relationship is concerned with the patient's social and psychologic well-being. When a patient *feels* better as a result of his contacts with those serving him, a therapeutic relationship exists; a therapeutic climate has been developed. How the *patient* feels is the important thing, not how those who are caring for him happen to feel. The patient is assessed in terms of his own requirements, not the staff's.

The nurse must remember that she also is a unique individual, different from everyone else and is constantly trying to cope with her needs also. She should try to understand her own attitudes (emotions, prejudices and such) and realize that she cannot divorce herself from them when giving care. Nevertheless, she is obliged to suppress any reactions on her own part which could detract from the quality of her care, if a therapeutic climate is to be established.

Promoting therapeutic relationships with patients has a clear objective. Because of the interrelatedness of the psychosocial and physical make-up of people, a therapeutic climate tends to provide a maximum likelihood of success in the care prescribed for the patient. Simultaneously, it tends to aid the patient in adjusting to whatever handicaps he may have as a result of his illness status and promotes a feeling of well-being.

Factors Tending to Promote Therapeutic Relationships

Many social psychologists have come to the opinion that a relationship becomes therapeutic when people feel *secure.* Included in a sense of feeling secure is the person's need to maintain his self-identity, his dignity, his sense of worth, and his feeling of belonging. This theory results from the insights social scientists have developed through study and research.

Knowledge about feelings of security has been applied to many aspects of daily living. For example, mothers are taught the importance of conveying security to their newborn babies. Holding an infant firmly, rocking him, fondling him, singing and talking to him, all make him feel secure and wanted.

Another example concerns the children of separated parents. These children, be they right or wrong, tend to question their sense of worth and often waver in developing security and identity as a person when one parent is absent. Parents of these children generally are counseled to do whatever is possible to help them feel secure and wanted.

For years industry has applied psychosocial insights in human relations. Studies have shown that employees are not necessarily motivated to higher rates of production and quality work by reward systems. More critical are these two factors—a feeling of belonging within the organization, and a feeling of satisfaction when employees can express their talents and abilities. Closely allied to these factors is the employee's need for being able to make decisions in his work and for sensing he has not lost control of his fate.

Programs for the older members of our population have objectives related to security. Basic to the success of such programs, it is generally agreed, is planning for activities that promote a sense of well-being in the participants. These people, just as others, need to feel a sense of worth and belonging. Providing activities that amount to little more than "busy work," lowering their sense of

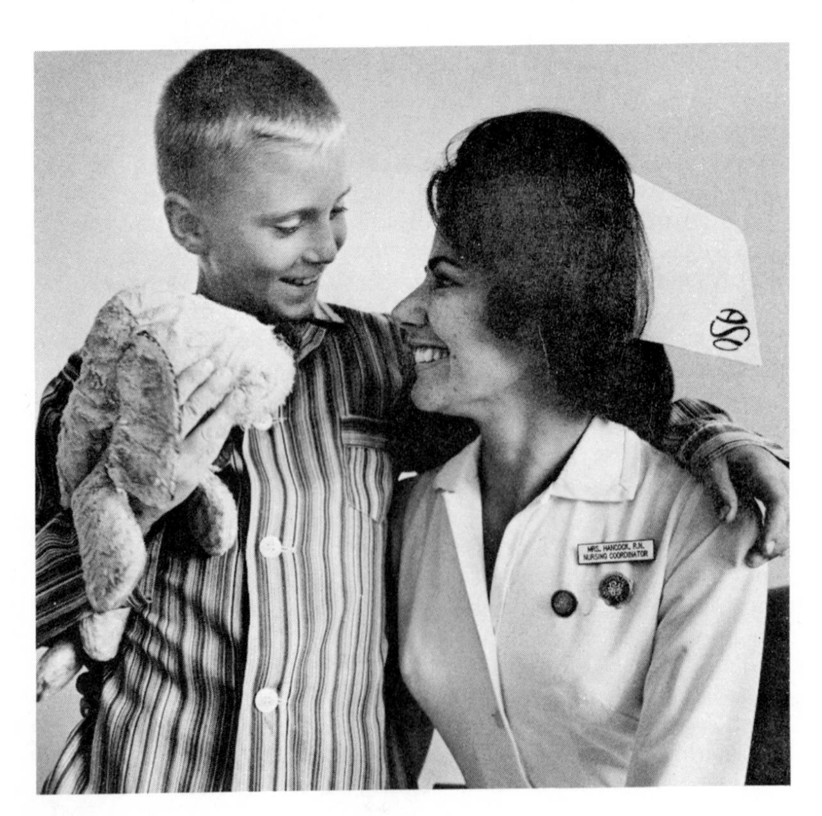

Fig. 7-1. To judge from the facial expression, this nurse appears to have established a warm and therapeutic relationship with her young patient. Note the child's favorite toy, which he was allowed to keep with him. (Good Samaritan Hospital, Phoenix, Arizona.)

dignity and taking decision-making from them, rarely succeed.

From these findings, it seems apparent that health workers too could employ knowledge that would promote a therapeutic climate for their patients. But the literature shows little evidence that such practices are in general use in our health agencies. There are many descriptions, in lay as well as professional literature, illustrating how little concern is shown for helping patients feel secure in the social setting of our health agencies.

Modern health agencies are planned with an eye for efficiency, orderliness and cleanliness, all certainly worthwhile objectives. But how many of these agencies have facilities to make the hospital seem more like a "home away from home"? How many have social rooms, cafeterias or dining rooms? Does the furniture have to be arranged in such a fashion that, as one patient stated it, "From my bed I could see only the midriff of a telephone pole through a window. I later learned that it overlooked a beautifully landscaped area"?

Patients are members of families and communities. Making decisions—from very simple ones often to very difficult ones—is an important part of daily life. Yet it is not uncommon for patients neither to be asked nor to be consulted concerning aspects of their care. Often they are not told what is happening to them or why something is being done to them. The privilege of making even simple decisions, it appears, is removed. In addition, they may no longer seem to have names and are referred to as a room number or by a diagnosis. Such practices can hardly contribute to a sense of well-being and security.

In this Unit, and throughout the text, factors that aid in promoting a therapeutic relationship with patients are discussed. Hopefully, the reader will find ways of helping patients to feel less bewildered and alone, and less bored, in what many patients refer to as an impersonal and cold setting.

Mr. Patza—Portrait of an "Uncooperative" Patient

While Mr. John Patza was driving his truck on a busy highway one rainy night, engine trouble developed. He managed to pull to the side, but not completely off the road, and was putting up flares when he was struck by an oncoming car. He was taken to the hospital with fractures of both legs and his right arm. There were other injuries, such as bruises and small lacerations. The accident occurred 400 miles from his home. That Mr. Patza was uncomfortable and distraught because of his situation was obvious. However, as days passed, he did not seem satisfied with the staff's efforts to care for him.

He had cigarettes in his bedside stand and would ask for one frequently. A nursing staff member would light the match for him and see that his ash tray was near. A comment was made that he could use a full-time person just to keep up with his smoking. It could have been this remark that started him off on trying to light the cigarettes by himself. With the use of only his left hand, the result was dropped matches and burnt bed clothes. He was cautioned about the hazard and told that he must have a nursing staff member light the cigarettes. This distressed him since he had already "gotten the message" that he wanted more cigarettes than nursing time

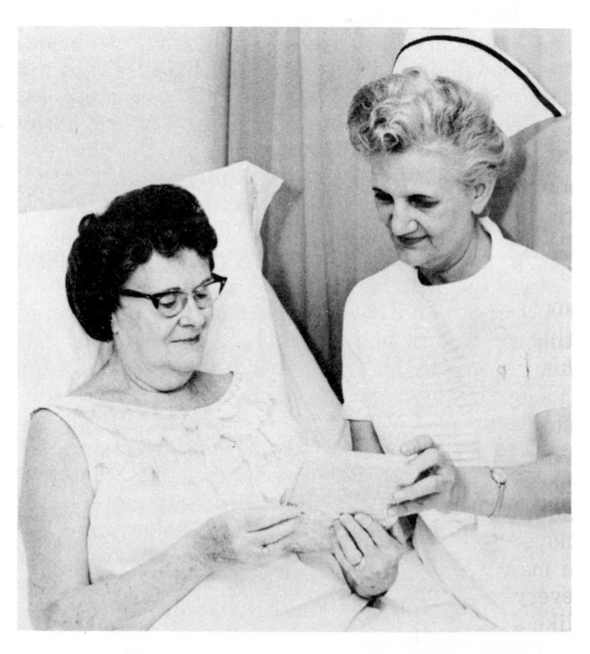

Fig. 7-2. Pictures of loved ones are often a real source of comfort to the patient. Sharing even brief moments with the patient helps the nurse to know the patient and her family better and to understand the patient's needs more adequately. (Photo: Warren R. Vroom)

could accommodate. So, he asked the other patient in the room, who was ambulatory, to light his cigarettes for him.

He also asked the patient's visitors to buy cigarettes for him. After another attempt at lighting a cigarette by himself was discovered, his cigarettes and matches were removed until the doctor could be consulted. This angered him to such a point that he responded with a tirade well sprinkled with profanity. He remained hyperactive, pulling at the top bed covers, shaking the bedside rail, then pushing his overbed table so forcefully that his tray almost slid off. He became demanding and expressed dissatisfaction with everything—his doctors, his nursing care, the food and the facilities.

Mr. Patza's behavior was such that none of the nursing staff felt comfortable being assigned to him. He was discussed at team conferences in an effort to resolve the situation. There was concern about the fact that he had received no mail or message from his wife. He had given her name as the family member to be notified. His employer had already sent a representative to see him.

The crisis came when one of the nursing aides was trying to clean his fingers and nails. His cast had been cut back a bit so that he could use the fingers of his right hand. While the aide was cleaning under his nails he snapped, "You're digging me." She did not believe that she was, but tried to cleanse more slowly. He pulled his arm away and shouted, "You're hurting me on purpose . . . get out and leave me alone." Things had reached a crucial point. The nursing staff members were aware beyond a doubt that he was not fond of them, nor could they feel kindly toward him. Something had to be done.

At this point, help came from an unexpected source. The other patient in the room was getting ready to go home, and, while waiting for his family, he came to the charge nurse. He confided that he felt sorry for Mr. Patza. "He is beside himself and in a tough spot. He is so far from home. He's got a wife he can't trust and her silence disturbs him more and more." He added that Mr. Patza, a heavy smoker, was annoyed by the smoking restrictions. He was also a man who had his " 'couple of shots of whiskey' every night and this has been stopped. He feels like a prisoner."

Thanks to the roommate, the picture of Mr. Patza's situation became clearer. The concern about his wife was not unfounded, and the effect of this nagging worry on his temper was understandable. The sudden denial of his "shots," the marked curtailment of his smoking, his immobility, his distance from home, all left him "shorn" and frustrated.

The care plan was promptly revised and implemented. The smoking situation was eased because Mr. Patza had better use of the fingers on his right hand. He was appreciative and said he did not want to be a bother. A social worker came to see him and, with the help of his employer, made arrangements to have him transferred to a hospital nearer home. This really pleased him; as he commented, "At least some of my buddies will come and visit me." He still made no mention of his wife to the nursing staff.

Perhaps the situation need not have reached the point of mutual distrust between patient and staff that it did. However, such situations do develop and this one is offered as an example. The more of them that can be avoided, the better for all concerned, especially for the one who is "down"—the patient. Behavior is purposeful; it always has meaning. If a patient turns hostile, there are always underlying reasons, and these must be sought out.

Study Situations

1. The following article describes a mother's reaction to her child's hospitalization. Although written some time ago, it illustrates poignantly how effectively health personnel helped to develop a therapeutic climate.

- Hemmendinger, M.: Rx: Admit patients at all times.

  CHILD STUDY, *34*:3-10, Winter, 1956-57.

This article also appears in the following book:

- Brown, E. L.: Newer Dimensions of Patient Care: Part 1: The Use of the Physical and Social Environment of the General Hospital for Therapeutic Purposes. pp. 143-154.

  New York, Russell Sage Foundation, 1961.

What did the nurses do in this situation that the mother felt contributed invaluably to her child's recovery?

2. Consider the following article in relation to developing a therapeutic relationship in a nursing home:

- McGinity, P., and Stotsky, B.: The patient in the nursing home.

  NURS. FORUM, *6*:238-261, #3, 1967.

Note the challenges facing the nursing staff in trying to maintain a person's individuality in this setting.

References

1. Dittmann, L. L.: A child's sense of trust. AMER. J. NURS., *66*:91-93, January, 1966.
2. Donohue, Sister M. A.: The I-thou relationship. NURS. OUTLOOK, *14*:59-61, August, 1966.
3. Hall, B. L.: Human relations in the hospital setting. NURS. OUTLOOK, *16*:43-45, March, 1968.
4. Johnson, J. E. *et al*: Interpersonal relations: The essence of nursing care. NURS. FORUM, *6*:324-334, #3, 1967.
5. Loder, E. R.: A gift for the nurse. (Editorial). NURS. OUTLOOK, *13*:21, December, 1965.
6. Nalls, S.: Developing a therapeutic relationship. AMER. J. NURS., *65*:114-118, December, 1965.
7. Streeter, S.: View from the inside. NURS. OUTLOOK, *15*:34-35, May, 1967.
8. Zorbo, N. R.: The professional bog. (Letters). AMER. J. NURS., *66*:252-255, February, 1966.

CHAPTER

8

Receiving a Patient in The Hospital

When a person needs to be hospitalized it is only one part of the total experience a patient has with his health problem. It is neither the end nor the beginning of it. This is an important point for the nurse in the hospital setting to bear in mind. A second point is that the estimated length of stay in the hospital in no way alters the nurse's responsibilities to the patient. Even if a person is admitted for so-called minor surgery or for a diagnostic or a therapeutic measure and remains in the hospital only overnight, the hospitalization period is still important to him. A patient having a short hospital stay may have as many and maybe more problems relating to his health than someone in for a longer period of time. Quite often, hospital personnel feel that there is nothing to be done with or for the patient who is in for a brief stay. However, understanding that hospitalization is only one part of the total experience will guide action in the way that a person is admitted, cared for during his stay and prepared for discharge.

Nursing Responsibilities in the Hospital Admission Procedure

Each health agency has a procedure for the admission of patients. These procedures vary from one agency to another. However, most include: the preparation of the patient's chart; the proper identification of the patient; the collection of data for billing purposes; the management of personal items and valuables; and then the determination of the patient's health status through such procedures as laboratory examinations, x-rays, obtaining the vital signs, and performing a physical examination. Personnel admitting the patient are expected to observe for bruises, insect bites or lesions and record their presence.

As far as the nurse is concerned she will have to perform those responsibilities assigned to the nursing department. For example, in hospitals with admitting suites, nurses are not concerned with many administrative details. Records are prepared and started, identification bands applied, blood and urine specimens collected and valuables checked. Some may have the patient put on hospital clothing. The patient's physician and the house staff may also be notified. In other hospitals, some or all of these details are performed by the nursing department. These details are a matter of hospital routine and may be changed from time to time to improve service or to make better use of personnel.

Maintaining the Individuality of the Person Being Admitted

Each person should be considered as an individual, in terms of both personality and extent of illness. All "gallbladders" are *not* the same, neither are all "tonsillectomies." Hospital, clinic or office routines very often are performed in a way that attempts to mold patients into a common pattern. Routines may appear to be logical, but the patient may feel that he is caught in a system which does not permit him freedom to participate.

Psychologists and psychiatrists have found that many children, for example, have had severe emotional reactions to the experience of having their tonsils removed. It is convenient for hospital personnel to separate the child from his parents almost immediately on admission. In this way, certain preparatory routines can be accomplished quickly with or without the child's cooperation. In rapid succession, the child is stripped of his own clothing, placed in unfamiliar garb in an unfamiliar bed and surrounded by unfamiliar children. He is examined; he may

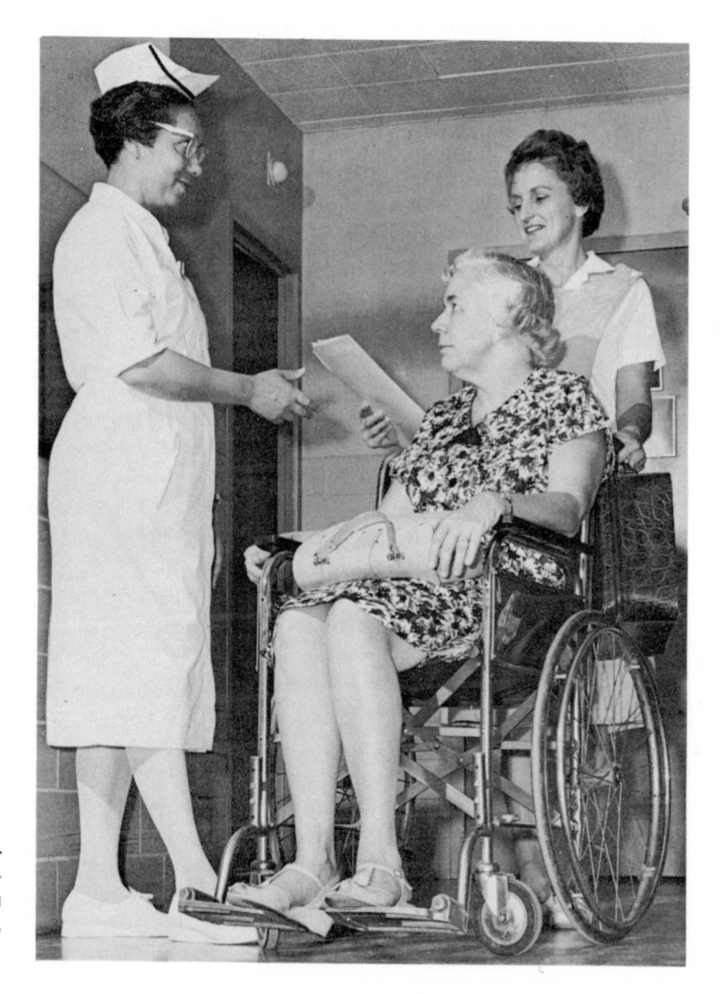

Fig. 8-1. The welcome that a patient receives on admission can do much to alleviate the feeling of tenseness that he may be experiencing. While the admission of a patient can become routine for the nursing staff, this is not the case with the person being admitted.

have laboratory work done, and then he is given preoperative medications. He may be carried away from his room on an object strange to him, brought to a strange place with furnishings unlike any he has ever seen, and, with little chance to get his bearings. Even if the method of transportation is made less frightening by the use of a "train" or a wagon, it is not of his choice in a place of his choice. He is surrounded by strange people who try to hold him down while another stranger tries to "smother" him, and screaming drifts off into oblivion. When he awakens, he feels sick. If he vomits, he may be frightened by the sight of the old blood he has swallowed. All of these events occurring in the span of a few hours can very well be a living nightmare not easily forgotten by the little "T and A."

While the preceding example may seem to be extreme, it can be repeated as easily with the adult. Patients find it comforting to be greeted pleasantly, as though they were being awaited. Patients like to be called by name and to learn to whom they are talking. It is helpful to the new patient if persons are identified by name pins. It is impossible to learn the names of many persons in a short span of time, and it means much to most patients to be able to connect names and faces.

The child is not alone in wanting someone to remain nearby when he is admitted to the hospital. Adults also find comfort in having a close family member or friend remain until they have the chance to become more adjusted to the new situation. As a matter of fact, talking for even a few minutes with the patient and his family will help the nurse considerably in understanding the patient and the patient in feeling more comfortable when left alone.

It is best for the patient not to be subjected to a routine which fits no one but is applied to everyone. For example, some patients may not wish to be dressed in hospital gowns and placed in bed immediately on admission. Sometimes, this is necessary but very often it is not. If there is no real urgency about the patient's admission, the comfort of wearing his own robe and bed clothing means much to him. If not acutely ill, he may wish to be out of bed to explore the place where he is to spend his time. He may want to know who his neighbors are if he is in a unit where there are other patients, for patients very often find companionship, consolation and reassurance in talking to each other. The new patient should be introduced to his roommates by whoever is admitting him to the unit. He should not be left to do his own socializing, since he may be so concerned for himself that it is not easy for him to approach others.

It is comforting for the patient to have some idea of what to expect concerning what will be done to complete his admission and to start his plan of care. Explanations are easy to give and do much to reduce apprehension. No matter how many details are included in a procedure for admitting a patient, they should be explained to him so that he may be helped to see that they are in his interest. In addition, the thoughtful nurse tells the patient about the call system, where the bathroom is, whether he has bathroom privileges, when he can expect meals to be served, what hours visitors may call, and the like.

Much has been said and written about making the transfer from a normal way of life to that of being a patient easier and more pleasant. A report of one study appears in the references at the end of this chapter.[1] Yet, the transition is not always easy. Health personnel who think only in terms of "getting the work done" rather than in terms of "getting to know the patients" are contributing little toward developing a therapeutic climate for the patient. Good nursing during the time that a patient is being admitted is largely dependent on the nurse's ability to put herself in another's place, and ask, "What would I like if I were the patient?" In most instances, the answer is easy to comply with and easy for all nursing personnel to offer—kindness, understanding and thoughtfulness.

Study Situations

1. In the following article, the process of "people stripping" is developed around the procedure for admission. The author has a

humorous way of bringing to light some of the many harmful acts committed when one succumbs to *procedure* and forgets that the patient is a person. Indicate which of the actions listed should be performed with this fact in mind and how this would affect the entire admission process.

- Taylor, C. D.: Sociological sheep-shearing. NURS. FORUM, *1*:79-89, Spring, 1962.

2. Read the following article, which so vividly analyzes 3 characteristics that differentiate people who are not "hospital sick" from those who are:

- Taylor, C. D.: The hospital patient's social dilemma.
  AMER. J. NURS., *65*:96-99, October, 1965.

3. Read the following article to learn how one hospital believed it accomplished a great deal in aiding new patients and their families in adjusting to the hospital environment:

- Dawson, M. J.: New patients dine with the nurse.
  AMER. J. NURS., *66*:287-289, February, 1966.

4. According to the following article, how did the nurse take steps to reduce tension with parents of children being admitted?

- Mahaffy, P. R. Jr.: Admission interviews with parents.
  AMER. J. NURS., *66*:506-508, March, 1966.

References

1. Elms, R. R.: Search or research? Nursing approaches to patients on admission to hospital.
   NURS. OUTLOOK, *13*:55, July, 1965.
2. Robinson, G.: From the hospital, where?
   NURS. OUTLOOK, *15*:47-49, July, 1967.
3. Tarnower, W.: Psychological needs of the hospitalized patient.
   NURS. OUTLOOK, *13*:28-30, July, 1965.

CHAPTER

9

Understanding the Role of the Patient

Definition of Patient

The dictionary defines the word "patient" as a person under medical or surgical treatment. Or, stated another way, a patient is one who is under the care or supervision of one of the health professions.

Generally speaking, it is assumed that a patient is ill. However, the illness or health of a person is not necessarily a criterion. For example, the obstetrician refers to women who seek out his professional care during pregnancy as his patients. The laboratory technician determining the hemoglobin count of someone's blood prior to that person's donating for a transfusion generally refers to him as a patient. In these two examples the persons may not necessarily be ill, although they are called patients. On the other hand, persons who are indeed ill are also called patients.

As has been pointed out, nursing offers services to people in good health as well as to those who are ill. However, this chapter is concerned primarily with patients whose health is not optimal and who are under the care of members of the health professions.

On Becoming a Patient

Persons who become patients continue to be just as different from one another as they were prior to the patient experience. Although the word "patient" is used to refer to many different kinds of people with many different kinds of problems, a patient is still an individual and different from all other patients.

For too long health personnel have expected a stereotyped performance from patients. Patients were expected to be "cooperative" at all times; they were not to question or suggest any change in procedure or routine; and they were expected to believe without query that all that was being done to them was for their own good. Especially, patients were not to complain. Behavior that was not in line with the expectations of the "good" patient was likely to be considered as "uncooperative."

When a person is ill, he assumes a role that is different from the one he had when his health problem was absent. From psychology we learn that behavior is adaptive and purposeful. In other words, all of living is to some degree a process of adapting to one's environment. Behavior is purposeful in that a person acts in a manner that to him has meaning, even when he may not be able to explain the reason for his behavior. Hence, in the process of adapting himself to the role of the patient, the person's behavior changes, because it is an attempt to adjust to something new.

Some people adjust to new settings with greater ease than others. For example, there are people who move about the country establishing new homes in markedly different surroundings with apparent ease. There are others who feel they cannot live happily except in a familiar environment. So too with patients. Some appear to adjust with ease, while others adjust with greater difficulty, to a hospital setting.

The degree or seriousness of an illness, from a medical viewpoint, may not necessarily be a useful indicator in predicting a person's attitude and reactions to his illness. Some patients whose illness may be considered minor in terms of complete recovery may view that illness with great alarm and concern. Other patients experiencing serious illness may appear to show little emotional reaction or concern. However, just as in other behavior, a person's reaction to his illness and hospitalization has meaning and is purposeful for each individual.

The transition from health to illness is an unpleasant experience for most people. It is a rare person who does not feel afraid and anxious, at least to some degree. Some may experience feelings of guilt and shame for being ill. Many ill people feel pessimistic and downcast. Men very often consider it an affront to be ill; women are less likely to feel this way. Breadwinners in the family generally view illness with apprehension if income is threatened. Women worry about the care of their families and homes. There is often dread of the invasion of privacy, with probing questions and detailed physical examinations. There may be fear of pain, which might indeed be a very realistic fear. Young adults may be concerned about interruptions in their education. Children may feel uneasy in strange surroundings as well as fearful of being deserted by their parents.

It is unrealistic to assume that patients' fears and anxieties could be eliminated. But there are means by which the nurse can take action that may ease mental and physical distress when a person becomes a patient. The philosophy of this text is founded on the belief that nursing can offer a unique health service to individuals when available knowledge is utilized to promote therapeutic relationships with patients.

Common Emotional Reactions to Illness: Fear—Anxiety—Stress

Physiology of Emotions. To understand the distress experienced by patients, one needs also to understand the physiology of emotions. This topic is considered in courses in psychology but a brief review will be presented here.

Most somatic responses to emotion operate through the nerve cells and fibers of the autonomic nervous system. This system consists of the sympathetic (thoracolumbar) and the parasympathetic (craniosacral) divisions. The parasympathetic impulses tend to control normal operation of the viscera, such as facilitating smooth muscle contraction, permitting salivation and slowing the heart rate. Sympathetic impulses increase heart action, inhibit salivation and gastrointestinal activity, raise blood pressure by constricting arterioles, dilate bronchioles, stimulate perspiration and increase the secretion of adrenalin, which tends to augment the effects of sympathetic innervation. Both the parasympathetic and sympathetic impulses act during emotion. However, the parasympathetic effects usually are masked by the stronger sympathetic effects.

The hypothalamus also plays a part in emotional responses, as does the cerebral cortex. Coordination of responses apparently occurs in part through activity of the hypothalamus, and the cerebral cortex appears to have a restraining or controlling effect on emotional responses.

Physiologic responses to emotion differ from person to person and, also, in the same person from time to time. Nor can one emotion be differentiated from another by physiologic reactions only. However, the physiologic responses to emotions are not disorganized. On the contrary, they are well organized, and even when emotion is strong the body responds harmoniously. What *may* be disorganized is behavior that results from an emotional experience. For example, a person experiencing extreme fear may be so consumed by his emotion that his behavior may become erratic, and, hence, less effective in eliminating or reducing the cause of his fear.

Fear. Fear usually is characterized by an expectation of harm or unpleasantness. Normally the body reacts by attempting to avoid or withdraw from the threat. When we are afraid, sympathetic innervation, as described earlier, places the body in a state of readiness for action to avoid or escape harm. The person who has fear usually is aware of the danger and has insight into the reasons for his fear. The causes in general are present and real.

Absence of the emotion of fear may seem ideal, but without it life would be infinitely more precarious. We have all experienced fear in our lives, and it might be doubted that we could have survived the many dangers had we not been fearful. For example, fear of accidents often results in safer automobile driving. Possibly one of the best life-saving "devices" for the non-swimmer is his fear of being in water over his head.

Patients with fears may express them rather freely. For example, a patient said he was afraid of receiving oxygen therapy because of the danger of an explosion. A few explanations from the nurse to the patient and to his visitors alleviated the fear readily.

On the other hand, some patients may be reluctant to express fears, believing that they may appear unintelligent and a nuisance if they ask questions. One patient, for example, eventually described having marked fear when he did not receive his breakfast when the other patients were served. Instead, a technician came to take a blood sample. The patient was sure his condition had worsened

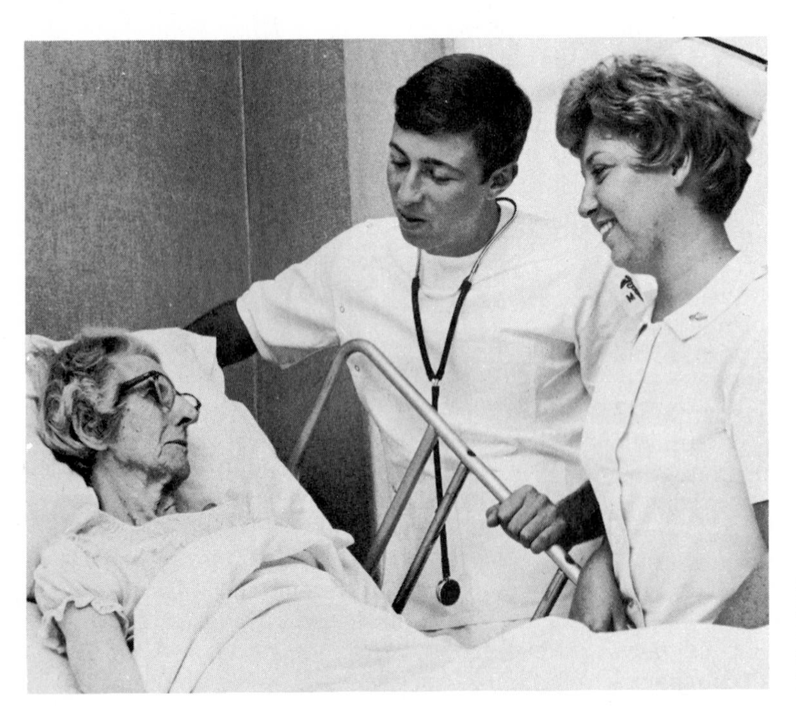

Fig. 9-1. The pattern should be one of planning with the patient, rather than for him, or doing things to him. Even brief visits should give the patient an opportunity to ask questions or discuss a matter that concerns him. (Photo by Warren R. Vroom)

and that he was about to receive some therapy. He was both fearful of what might be happening to him and fearful of asking anyone for an explanation. When one reads in the literature what patients have described as fearful experiences, it is easy to see that many of them could have been avoided or minimized, had someone just taken the time to give some explanations to these people.

Fears may be camouflaged by other behavior. For example, a patient, awakened postoperatively, saw that she was in a bed with siderails in place. She became very angry and told a family member that she "really told off that nurse who put up those railings." When asked why she was upset about having siderails on her bed, the patient said, most indignantly, "I came in here for a simple operation and I don't expect to be treated like someone who is insane. I've heard about how they treat insane people. They put them in beds and fix it so you can't get out. And I'm not crazy!" After the reason for the siderails was explained, the patient's anger quickly subsided.

Anxiety. The dictionary defines anxiety as uneasiness of mind caused by apprehension of danger or misfortune. It often is referred to as a persistent generalized fear of the unknown and is associated with some future event. Worry sometimes is called a mild form of anxiety, but the worried person usually is able to communicate the cause of the concern. Anxiety is characterized by a lack of awareness of the cause of fear. Although pervasive, it is vaguely organized in the mind of the person; hence, he feels helpless and uncertain concerning appropriate action to take.

Anxiety is more difficult to handle than fear. Should one be afraid of a dog, he can try to get away from the situation. But when anxiety is present, the person lacking insight as to its cause feels defeated and has dread of what will happen.

The physiologic reactions to anxiety result from sympathetic innervation. However, because of the nature of anxiety, the responses of the organs to stimulation are not usually as dramatic as when fear, for example, is present.

Because lack of insight is commonly present, an anxious person often directs his attention to the physiologic symptoms of anxiety. Common ones are fatigue, insomnia, diarrhea, urgency of voiding, nausea, anorexia and excessive perspiration. The so-called "nervous heart" is a common symptom of the anxious person. Or the patient may say he thinks his heart "stands still" at times. When anxiety becomes chronic and persistent, the services of a psychiatrist may be necessary.

Although anxiety can be destructive in nature, it also may be used constructively. This is especially true when the anxiety is not overwhelming. In fact, some persons believe that without anxiety, as well as some fear, the human race might not have survived in situations that made constructive action imperative. The anxiety associated with examination periods in school stimulates many students to carry out effective study programs. The anxiety of an elected official whose neglect of slum conditions may threaten his office can serve to stimulate constructive action.

Not only patients experience anxiety. This period in civilization has often been referred to as the Age of Anxiety. True, it is an age with great changes occurring rapidly. The threat of thermonuclear annihilation is almost ever present. Values have changed rapidly and tensions over appropriate behavior are increased. Civilization will have utilized anxiety wisely if action resulting from it can be put to constructive use.

Stress. Stress often is referred to as strain or tension. It occurs most often in circumstances necessitating an increased and often prolonged effort to adjust. Any factor that disturbs the physical, psychologic or physiologic equilibrium of the body may be stressful. As in the case of fear, the body strives to rid itself of the factor causing the stress.

Stress is a highly individualized experience. Some persons appear to be able to tolerate a great deal more than others. Or a situation that is stressful for one may not be for another person. The important thing is how each individual perceives and meets the situation that causes the stress. It is a rare person who does not experience stress as he assumes the patient role.

What the Patient Expects of the Nurse

When a patient submits to the care of members of the health professions, he has expectations concerning the behavior and abilities of those caring for him. Investigations have borne this out.

Patients expect the nurse to be *professionally competent.* This has been found to be especially true in relation to technical competencies. They are apt to doubt the competence of a nurse who seems unsure of equipment she is using. A casual spoken thought, like "I wonder how this works," or "I can't seem to get this to work," does little for a patient's confidence in the nurse. It is not surprising that a patient questioned his physician about his pulse rate after the nurse who came to take it kept shaking her watch and said she wondered if it was working correctly. But patients are quick to compliment the nurse who carries out a procedure with deftness and self-assurance. One frequently hears patients speak, for example, of the nurse who gives "good shots."

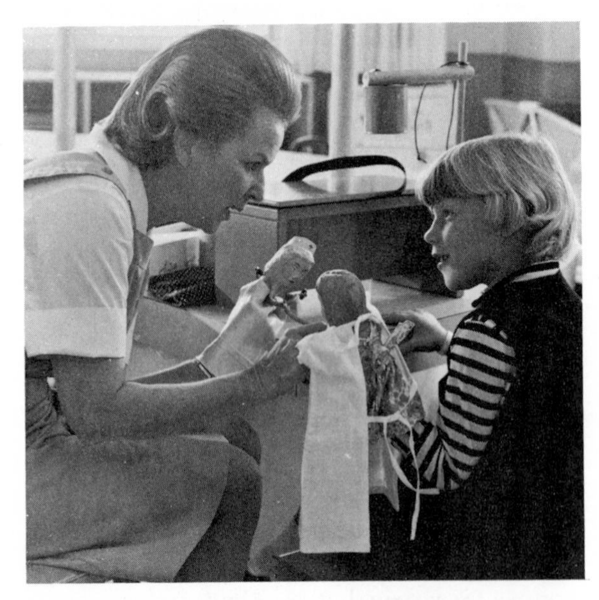

Fig. 9-2. By using puppets this volunteer is helping the little girl to feel more comfortable and at ease in a situation that could produce a great deal of anxiety. They are playing the role of the patient and the role of the nurse. (Courtesy of Good Samaritan Hospital, Phoenix, Arizona)

Patients expect nurses to be *serious about their work.* Human emotions can be contagious; hence, patients tend to enjoy having persons who are cheerful, but still obviously sincere, care for them. Patients often enjoy sharing a humorous experience with the nurse, but it is indeed a rare patient who accepts frivolity or casualness. Some patients may find it disturbing to see nurses in groups chatting and laughing. Families as well as patients also find it disconcerting when nursing personnel are laughing and talking outside a room in which someone is ill or deeply concerned with his health problem. In situations such as those just mentioned, the nurses might well be serious-minded about their work, but their behavior may cause the patient to be critical.

Patients expect nurses to be *understanding and accepting* of them. It is not that nurses are always expected to *do* something or *say* something. Just showing some consideration and remaining with the patient for a few minutes to listen to what he has to say is a great contribution to his comfort and well-being. Respect for the patient's worth and dignity are demonstrated by nurses who accept him as he is and make the effort to understand him and the way he perceives his situation.

When patients are unable to care for themselves, they expect the nurse to *assist them in meeting their hygienic needs.* Although the nurse may assign other members of the nursing team to this task, the patient still expects the nurse to know about them and what can be done about them. For example, they expect to be bathed when they feel unable to do so for themselves. Placing a basin of water in front of a one-day postoperative patient who has had major surgery and telling him that it is good to be active would be regarded as gross insensitivity, not therapy.

Patients can be made unhappy by having their hair left uncared for when they cannot care for it themselves. They do not like visitors to see them in a state that is embarrassing to them. Helping the patient to maintain normal bladder and bowel functions is appreciated, because neglect in these matters usually brings with it many disturbing physiologic problems as well as possible psychologic ones.

There may be times when there is too much dependence on the nurse. More will be said about this later in the text. But when a patient needs assistance, he expects the nurse to anticipate and to meet his needs.

Generally, patients expect nurses to *orient them to the hospital environment.* Nearly everyone is afraid of the unknown, and to be left in a hospital room without orientation can be a frightening experience. T. S. Eliot expressed the patient's point of view well in "The Cocktail Party," concerning an impersonal environment, when he wrote

All there is of you is your body
And the "you" is withdrawn.

Courtesies that help patients to feel that they are not just another person aid in developing a desirable therapeutic climate in which to care for them.

Implications for Nursing

There are several principles that the nurse will observe as she aids people to adjust to their roles as patients.

Emotional responses evoke widespread visceral changes affecting the circulatory, respiratory, digestive and glandular systems as well as the skeletal system.

This principle serves as an aid to the nurse in recognizing when a patient is, for example, anxious or fearful. Not many people admit readily to these emotional responses. This is especially true when patients believe that by so doing, they also are admitting to being unusual or strange. This principle, then, assists the nurse in observing patients for reactions that may have an emotional basis, such as excessive perspiration, frequency in urination and increased respiratory rates.

Emotional behavior is motivated behavior and there is cause for it.

By observing this principle, the nurse will realize that a patient's emotional behavior has reason or cause. Knowing that the behavior has reason guides the nurse in every approach to the patient. For example, a nurse notes that a patient is crying; the patient tells the nurse, "I'm crying, but for no reason." The nurse knows there is reason despite what the patient has stated. She stays with her, listening for her to express a possible reason. The nurse may feel personally disapproving of the patient's manner of handling the situation, but her behavior is that of supporting her.

When a stimulus for a particular kind of behavior is annoying, the body responds by attempting to avoid or reduce the stimulus.

Consider the example given previously of the patient found crying. Crying may be a last resort because she knows no way of avoiding an annoying stimulus. Assume this patient is fearful of a diagnosis that will require many subcutaneous injections which she will need to administer herself. Although no one enjoys administering injections to himself, by explanation the nurse might at least alleviate some of the patient's fears and thus diminish the annoying stimulus. Assume instead that this patient is fearful of a certain diagnosis, such as a malignancy, which she associates with death. Fear of death in that case becomes very real. Possibly the most the nurse can do is offer the patient support by listening to her and by being available when her fears become overwhelming. In this case the nearness of a nurse who offers support might at least reduce some of an annoying stimulus.

Study Situations

1. The following poem displays a sensitive and perceptive description of the meaning of life:

• Sanborn, J.: Quiet for one.
NURS. OUTLOOK, *13*:29, December, 1965.

How do you react to the thought that patients are more than human machines in need of mechanical repair?

2. The following article describes rest in its broadest sense—that is, freedom from the kinds of things that usually appear to cause stress, anxiety and fear for the hospitalized patient.

• Narrow, B. W.: Rx rest is . . .
AMER. J. NURS., *67*:1646-1649, August, 1967.

Describe with each example in the article how the perceptive nurse relieved or reduced fears or anxieties. Review the six characteristics of rest described on page 1649. Can you add others?

3. Read the following article:

- Field, W. E. Jr. *et al*: The senses taker. AMER. J. NURS., *66*:2654-2656, December, 1966.

What do the authors describe as the "indispensable means to patient care?" How do the authors describe emotional support? What kinds of people do these authors say are the least likely to adopt the "sick role"?

References

1. Anxiety, recognition and intervention. (Programmed Instruction). AMER. J. NURS., *65*:129-152, September, 1965.
2. Brooks, B. R.: Aggression. AMER. J. NURS., *67*:2519-2522, December, 1967.
3. Carnevali, D. L.: Preoperative anxiety. AMER. J. NURS., *66*:1536-1538, July, 1966.
4. Cockerill, E. E.: Reflections on my nursing care. AMER. J. NURS., *65*:83-85, May, 1965.
5. Erickson, F.: When 6- to 12-year-olds are ill. NURS. OUTLOOK, *13*:48-50, July, 1965.
6. Ishiyama, T. *et al*: Let's be patients. AMER. J. NURS., *67*:569-571, March, 1967.
7. Kilpatrick, H. M.: The frightened patient in the emergency room. AMER. J. NURS., *66*:1031-1032, May, 1966.
8. Nehren, J., and Gilliam, N. R.: Separation anxiety. AMER. J. NURS., *65*:109-112, January, 1965.
9. Perceptions of nursing care. Patients' views. AMER. J. NURS., *65*:127-129, May, 1965.
10. Selye, H.: The stress syndrome. AMER. J. NURS., *65*:97-99, March, 1965.
11. Tarnower, W.: Psychological needs of the hospitalized patient. NURS. OUTLOOK, *13*:28-30, July, 1965.
12. Webb, C.: Tactics to reduce a child's fear of pain. AMER. J. NURS., *66*:2698-2701, December, 1966.

CHAPTER

10

Using Communication Skills

Definition of Communication

Communication is the interchange of information. The information reaches us through hearing, seeing, tasting, smelling and touching. Everything one does or uses has communicative value—one's work, the house one lives in, the clothes one wears. All that impinges on our senses—a glance, a wink of the eye, a touch, the spoken word, a gesture, the odor of one's cologne—communicates something. In other words, we communicate in a variety of ways through talking, signaling, writing, gesturing, drawing, singing, and dancing.

Communications go on almost constantly in human activity. We hear the ring of an alarm clock, a signal to awaken from sleep. The smell of coffee tells us that breakfast is ready. The instruments on the dashboard of the car aid in indicating whether the car is in good order. Newspapers, magazines, radio and television convey innumerable messages that are used constantly in everyday living.

Communication is basic to all human relationships. Unless people communicate, no sort of relationship develops between them. The example of two strangers sitting next to each other in a theater demonstrates physical closeness without any type of relationship necessarily developing between them. However, if during the movie these two people exchange words or glances, that is, communicate, a relationship comes into existence. It matters not whether the communication is verbal (one makes a comment to the other) or nonverbal (one frowns at the other for eating popcorn loudly), hostile or friendly, a human relationship is there.

For communication to take place, there must be a sender with a message to convey and a receiver of the message being sent. The sending and the receiving of messages usually cannot be separated distinctly, since both often go on simultaneously. For example, assume that a nurse is talking with a patient who is describing his headache. While the patient talks, the nurse listens and receives the message. But at the same time, she may be sending messages to the patient by the expression on her face and her actions as the patient speaks (such as drumming her fingers impatiently). The patient, then, receives a message while transmitting one. Stop for a moment and consider any conversation with another person. One soon realizes that the interchange of messages is constant and simultaneous.

Kinds of Communication

Pictures. Prehistoric men communicated extensively through the use of pictures. Many found in caves are amazingly lifelike and communicate ideas concerning danger, superstition, religious beliefs, and the like.

Pictures are still used effectively in communicating today. Many cartoons found in newspapers and magazines carry vivid messages without the use of words. The patient in Fig. 7-2, p. 65, conveys information to the nurse through the picture she is showing. Illustrations of various sorts have been used with success in teaching programs designed to help patients. Illustrative material is used in many classrooms. Artists through the ages have shared information with observers through their pictures and sculpture. The preference we have for a certain kind of art also tells something about our own personalities. Pictures represent a common and often effective way of communicating, but they often are cumbersome and complicated to use in comparison with other symbols.

Symbols. Symbols are signs that represent an idea or object. Words are the commonest symbols in communication. They are names given to everything we know. It is not known when man first learned to talk, but words developed as man connected a particular sound (word) with a specific object or idea.

The use of words in communication often is called verbal communication. Reading, writing, speaking and listening use words and hence, are called verbal communications. Usually verbal communication is a voluntary act; one can speak or write or listen or read if one chooses.

There are numerous symbols other than words used in communication. For example, the national flag of a country is a well-known symbol. A dove connotes peace, while a hawk symbolizes war. A cross is one symbol of Christianity. The symbols of operation in mathematics (addition, subtraction, multiplication and division) are in constant use. H_2O is the chemical symbol for water. The symbol, ♀, means female while the symbol, ♂, means male. Doodling can have communicative value. An almost endless number of examples such as these illustrate the wealth of symbols used daily when sharing information.

Language and Writing. Language is a prescribed way of using words so that people can share information effectively. Language includes a common definition of words being used, as well as a method of arranging words in a certain order to convey the message. The development of language represented a great step forward in the history of communication, for now everyone using the same language could share information more readily.

Reading became a method of communicating with the development of writing. Writing probably began with record-keeping. At first writing used pictures, the hieroglyphics of Egypt being an example. But this was an awkward and time-consuming way to write. Eventually the alphabet was developed, with each letter having a certain sound. Information now could be exchanged in writing by grouping letters in a sequence to form words.

Signals. Signals are used to carry information from one place to another. For example, the drumbeat has been an important signal used in communicating in some parts of Africa. Whistles, horns, guns, sirens, and the like, are other audible signals used around the world in various ways to communicate messages.

Some signals depend on the use of sight. The American Indian used smoke signals to convey messages. Flags, flashing lights and beacons are effective communication media in some situations. Strips of cloth placed in a prescribed pattern to indicate distress often are used by persons stranded in remote areas to communicate with planes overhead.

Most hospitals use a light as a signal when the patient wishes a nurse. Flashing lights are used in some hospitals to signal personnel. These same lights, flashed in a particular manner, can be used to indicate that an emergency exists and additional personnel are needed to assist.

Gestures. Communication that does not necessarily depend upon words is called nonverbal communication. The sender of messages communicates by means of gestures—that is, by physical movements, facial expressions, tone of voice, personal appearance, and the like. Nonverbal communication is more likely to be involuntary and therefore less under the control of the person conveying the message. Hence, nonverbal communication is generally considered as being a more nearly accurate expression of true feelings. How many times have we asked or been asked, "What's wrong?" when obviously appearance and behavior showed that all was not well?

Nonverbal communication may be concurrent with verbal communication, and it can be of much greater significance. There is a proverb that states "What you do speaks so loud I cannot hear what you say." The tone of voice also can give different meanings to a word or phrase. The words "Hello" and "Goodbye" can be said in such a way that another's presence is either the best or the worst thing that could have happened. The way the nurse says "Good morning" to a patient often tells him much about how the nurse feels.

A common example of nonverbal communication can be seen when a child receives a gift. If he likes it, his whole appearance and his actions show it. If he is disappointed, he is equally demonstrative, not being sophisticated enough to cover this up with proper expressions of gratitude.

An important part of nursing is cultivating the art of observation, that is, to watch for and interpret nonverbal messages. For example, a patient may joke about his preoperative tests and be casual about his impending surgery, but his expressions do not fool the observant nurse who notes that he is in and out of bed, is unable to sit and read, smokes one cigarette after another, makes frequent trips to the telephone booth to call his wife and gets out of the corridor whenever he sees a stretcher coming along.

Common Problems of Communication

For effective communication there *must be a message delivered from one person to another.* A gesture indicating where a visitor may find a particular patient may not be seen. A letter may be lost in the mail. A child playing too far from home may not hear his mother's call. These illustrations demonstrate a breakdown in communication: a message was sent but not delivered to the intended receiver.

If one mumbles while talking, speaks too softly or to rapidly, if there are noises in the room, and so on—any of these may prevent what has been said being heard. Sometimes, patients have been reprimanded because they failed to follow instructions for taking medications at home when they probably did not clearly hear the instructions. For many people, especially the very ill or the elderly, it may be necessary to ask, "Did you hear me?" or "Was that clear?"

When a message is sent, it *must get the attention of the receiver.* A letter that has arrived at its destination must be read. Commercials on television and radio often are sent at a higher decibel level than the programs they interrupt. This device is intended to catch the attention of the audience. The patient's call light is a signal for a nurse, but the communication fails if the light does not catch the nurse's attention. Preoccupation with other thoughts may divert attention. For example, a patient may be so afraid of giving himself injections that his attention is diverted when the nurse attempts to teach him the procedure. Without an attentive receiver, effective communication is not possible.

Once a message has been sent and received,

it *must be interpreted.* Interpretation by the receiver is based on his past experience. If the sender and receiver have had different experiences in terms of the message being sent, a breakdown in communication can result. The sign language of the deaf cannot be interpreted by one inexperienced in this form of communication. A person listening to a message spoken in a language unfamiliar to him cannot interpret the sender's message. Pain means one thing to a person who has suffered a great deal, but it may mean something quite different to one who has experienced little. The grief of death may have relatively little meaning to a person who has not experienced the loss of a loved one.

Consider many of the adjectives used commonly in everyday conversations. What is a *big* car? A *small* child? A *good* meal? A *poor* movie? An *expensive* garment? A *high* temperature? A *rapid* pulse rate? Unless the sender's and receiver's past experiences are similar in relation to the manner in which these adjectives are used, effective communication is impossible.

It is of utmost importance for the nurse to use words that the patient can understand. A nurse speaking to a patient who is to have a blood test would not be of much help if she said, "You are fasting this A.M., since you'll have a V.P. for a B.U.N." She is more likely to convey a clearer message to the patient if she tells him that his breakfast will be delayed until after a blood sample has been taken, that the doctor wishes a study of his blood and that taking food may alter the blood findings. Often, nurses are accused of forgetting that most patients are not familiar with hospital jargon.

The message *must be stated in words having a common meaning to the sender and the receiver.* The study of the meaning of words is referred to as *semantics.* To persons speaking the same language, identical words may have entirely different meanings. For example, the word "democracy" means one thing to most people in the Western world but something quite different in the Eastern world, even when a common language is being used. Communication using such words as liberty, freedom, fraternity, love and hate will fail unless the sender and receiver attach common meanings to these words. A 45-year-old will be lost in a conversation with a teen-ager unless he knows current teen-ager jargon.

In the May, 1962, issue of The American Journal of Nursing, (p. 111), there is a section entitled "Euphemistically Speaking." Although this is presented as humor, it illustrates how phrases that generally are accepted to have one meaning can have a different one when used in certain situations. An example from this entry is a physician's progress note that states, "This patient is quiet and cooperative." The meaning given to this note is "It's a pleasure having him on the ward. We hardly know he's around."

For effective communication, a message *must be accepted and acted upon.* For example, a nurse may ignore a patient's call light. Until she accepts the signal as a call for her and acts to answer it, communication has not been established. When she answers the light, the patient complains of pain and asks for a medication. Communication still has failed if the nurse does not accept the patient's request as necessary and takes no action whatsoever.

A physician was of the opinion that one of his patients should lose weight. The excess weight was placing undue strain on his heart, already damaged by heart disease. Despite explanations, the patient ignored the physician's advice. Communication ceased when the patient failed to accept and act on the physician's message.

Possibly few people have missed hearing the repeated warnings issued by the American Cancer Society concerning the dangers of smoking. Yet, statistics illustrate that smoking has decreased little if at all. Presumably the Society's messages are not being accepted and acted on by any large number of people.

The following description illustrates certain gestures having a cultural basis. A communication problem resulted when the nurse failed to understand these gestures. The description also illustrates other problems of communication as discussed earlier. See if you can identify these problems.

A public health nurse visited Mrs. Martinez, wife of a Mexican migrant worker, and her new baby shortly after they were discharged from the hospital. The purpose of the visit was to establish rapport with Mrs. Martinez in order to learn why she had been hostile about participating in hospital routine concerning personal cleanliness. A language barrier existed to a certain extent, because the nurses in the hospital did not understand Spanish sufficiently well to know what the patient said when she spoke rapidly and angrily.

Upon entering the home the nurse was impressed with evidence of good care being given by Mrs. Martinez's mother. The baby, asleep in the arms of his grandmother, appeared well. The grandmother held the baby out slightly to the nurse, who thought the grandmother wanted her to see the baby more easily. The nurse did not touch the baby. The grandmother extended the baby out even further and while the nurse looked more attentively, she felt no need to touch and handle the baby. The hospital report indicated that the baby was normal and well and so it appeared. When the nurse spoke to the mother about her hospital stay, she quickly realized that she was making no progress. The mother barely answered the nurse's questions and often turned her face away. After a few minutes the nurse

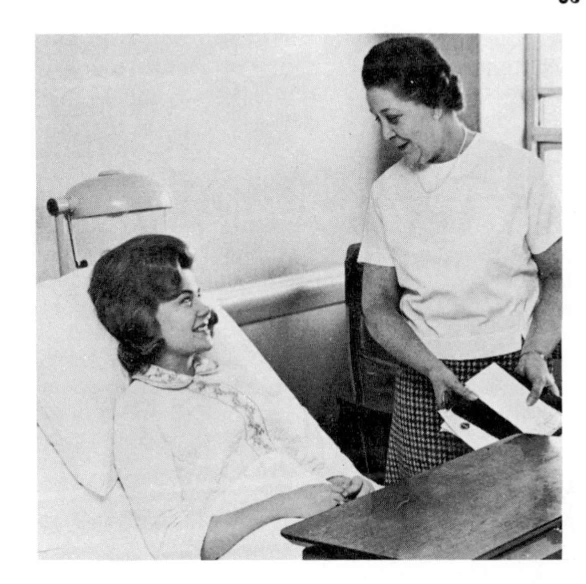

Fig. 10-2. Often the nurse understands that what the patient is asking for is something that she cannot handle. However, she can call upon other persons in a health agency to help meet the patient's needs; as for example, a "Patient Relations Representative," who can answer questions about costs of hospitalization and insurance, and other items that are of concern to the patient. (Courtesy of Muhlenberg Hospital, Plainfield, N. J.)

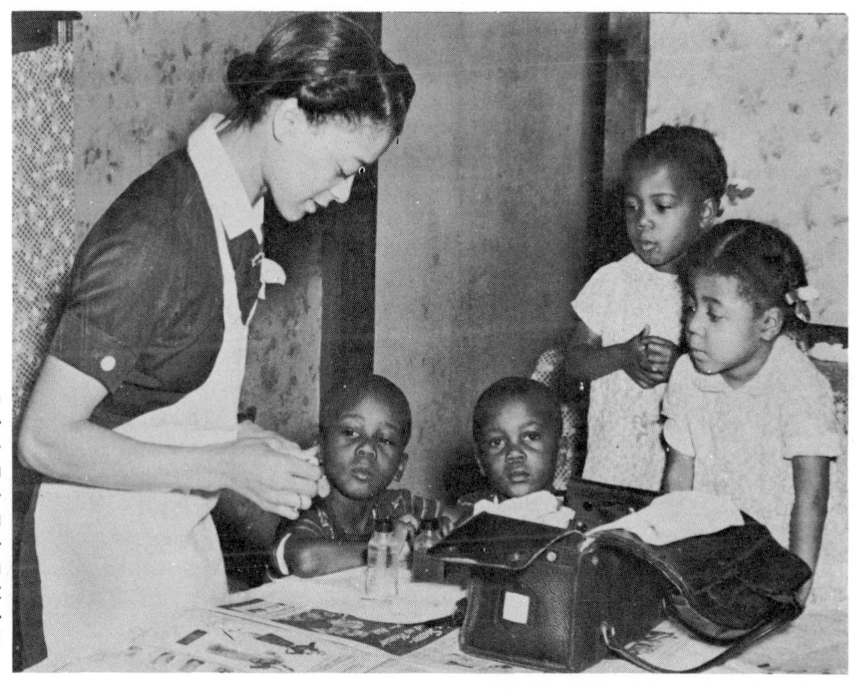

Fig. 10-1. The public health nurse has many challenges before her in relation to communication. Not only by her skill in giving care, but also in her relationship with the family and even with the neighbors. Her very attitude, gestures and bearing can do much to help others accept health care. (Department of Public Health Nursing, National League for Nursing.)

left, feeling frustrated for having failed in gaining rapport with Mrs. Martinez. When the nurse returned a few days later, the grandmother politely but firmly told the nurse her services were no longer needed.

The nurse discussed the calls with her supervisor, who was familiar with the culture of this family. Mrs. Martinez and her mother believed the nurse was possessed of an "evil eye" because she gazed at the baby but did not touch him. The nurse would then give *mal ojo*, or "evil eye sickness," to the baby. Had the nurse touched the baby, all would have been well.

When the nurse attempted to discuss personal cleanliness with the mother, the patient had said she was clean but became unclean in the hospital because she was forced to wash herself with water. This violated the prescription of *dieta*, a period after childbirth when mothers of this culture must not have water touch them because it makes them "unclean." The supervisor explained that when Mrs. Martinez left the hospital, she no doubt obtained a local remedy that would undo the harm done her in the hospital. In addition, the family would now seek the services of a *curando*, a woman in this culture with powers to cure the "evil eye sickness" the nurse transmitted to the baby.

Definition of Interviewing

Interviewing is a tool of communication. It is used purposefully for learning about people and for obtaining information. The person seeking information is referred to as the *interviewer*. The *interviewee* is the person being interviewed.

Interviews occur at various levels. Some are very casual and impersonal and might well be referred to simply as conversation. This type is useful when first getting to know a person. We use it in everyday living on numerous social occasions, and nurses too use casual conversation with patients. There is no reason why nurse-patient conversations should always be on a formal or structured basis. Much indirect benefit accrues to the patient if he finds his nurse to be a companionable person and an interesting human being. The nurse who is unable to speak on any subject but the health problem at hand may have a difficult time developing satisfactory relationships with at least some, if not most, patients. On the other hand, the nurse who seemingly avoids discussing the patient's health problem may place her competence under suspicion and possibly might cause the patient unnecessary fear.

Another level of interviewing is conversation of a more personal nature, which usually has more structure than the level just discussed. There usually is specific questioning involved—in nursing, the questions are directed toward eliciting information about the patient and/or health problems with which the nurse is attempting to help him.

A deeper level of interviewing involves attempts to learn about people's feelings. The conversation may or may not use questions directly related to feelings. It relies often on interpreting nonverbal communications, as gestures, facial expressions, tone of voice, and the like.

An even deeper level uses the technic of interviewing for assisting persons therapeutically. It is an essential tool in the care of psychiatric patients.

Successful interviewing depends on the skillful use of questioning, listening and observing.

Questioning. The purposes of using questions when interviewing include obtaining specific information we need and directing conversation to fruitful channels. Best results usually are obtained when the interviewer is sympathetic and supportive of the patient. In other words, it is best to avoid questions that "grill" the patient, that make him feel he is receiving the "third degree" or that are probing in nature. Also, questions that tend to make the patient feel his answers must fit the nurse's expectations are of little avail in helping to understand him.

Observing. Chapter 17 discusses observing the patient. This applies also to interviewing. If we are interested in learning about the patient, then the purposeful use of observation becomes essential. As has been pointed out earlier, it is primarily through observations that one becomes aware of nonverbal communication.

Listening. Listening is an active process in the art of interviewing. Good listening requires understanding of what is being said without adding personal interpretation. It requires the listener to be accepting of the other person so that responses can be made freely.

A common pitfall in interviewing is to assume that talking must be continuous. Sometimes, especially when the interviewee is expressing emotion, the beginning interviewer may feel uncomfortable when a silence occurs. Silence deserves respect also. It may be during a period of silence that the patient is exploring his feelings, and interruptions by the interviewer may disrupt the relationship.

Principles of Interviewing

There are several principles that nurses will wish to use as guides when interviewing patients.

Information essential to understanding a person and his problems can be obtained by the process of interviewing. To illustrate, if a nurse realizes that knowing something about a patient's usual daily activity pattern will aid her in planning his nursing care, she plans her interview accordingly. Unless an interview is used purposefully and constructively—that is, with a goal in mind—nurse-patient communications may become little more than a meaningless exchange of words.

Successful interviewing depends upon attitudes of acceptance, objectivity, kindness and warmth. This principle guides the nurse in her statement and selection of questions, her acceptance of the patient's behavior and her sincere effort to help and care for her patient.

A comfortable environment is conducive to successful interviewing. A comfortable environment is one in which both the patient and the nurse are at ease. Such items as comfortable furniture, proper lighting and provisions for privacy are essential. Also the atmosphere is conducive to effective relationships when it is relaxed and unhurried in nature. If the nurse seems preoccupied and "on the run," or if the patient is ill at ease for fear of missing visitors or an intra-agency appointment, interviewing is impaired.

Interviewing is more effective when geared to the interviewee's age and mental and physical capabilities. Interviewing a teen-ager is quite unlike interviewing a middle-aged person. Also, certain interviewing is fruitless if the patient is acutely ill.

Suggestions for Interviewing

There are many suggestions or tips that authorities list in relation to establishing therapeutic relationships between interviewer and interviewee. These are a few of the common ones.

In general, questions that can be answered by simply saying "Yes" or "No" are to be avoided. Such questions tend to cut off further conversation, even when the interviewee might well wish to go on.

The interviewee usually feels an attitude of acceptance when the interviewer's statements are noncommittal and nonjudgmental. Examples of such statements are "I understand" and "I see."

Placing events into a more meaningful sequence or order often occurs when the interviewer asks questions as "What led up to that?"

Broad openings or general leads are often helpful to encourage the interviewee to go on. Examples are "What are you thinking?"; "And then?"; or "You appear uncomfortable."

Statements that indicate no cause for anxiety or concern (such as "Everything will be all right," or "Don't worry. You will be all right.") and statements that indicate rejection (as, "We'd better not discuss that.") generally impair the therapeutic nature of an interview and tend to stop conversation.

Pretending to listen is a barrier to effective interviewing. It is a rare person who is insensitive to an attitude of apathy and boredom on the part of the interviewer.

Questions containing the words, *why* and *how*, generally elicit little information. For example, the question, "Why were you not tired enough to sleep?" might better be stated by asking "What were you doing while you were unable to sleep?" Questions using why and how tend to intimidate a patient such as, "Why didn't you see the doctor about that?"

Comments that indicate the interviewer might not have understood tend to encourage further explanations. An example of such a comment is "Are you saying that listening to music takes your mind off things?"

Listening selectively, or hearing only what one wants to hear limits the effectiveness of the interview. All of us, including patients, are guilty at times of hearing only what we want to hear. No one likes to hear bad news about himself; no one wants to hear that he must give up some of the pleasures of life; nor do we want to hear that there are difficult times ahead.

The nurse is aided in the interview if the following questions are kept in mind: What are the repeated themes in the patient's speech and behavior? What topics does the patient tend to avoid? What subjects tend to make the patient shift the conversation to other topics? What inconsistencies and gaps appear in the patient's conversation?

Beginning students probably will find that they will give nursing care slowly at first—perhaps too slowly—while also observing and listening to their patients. With practice, successful communication with patients can go on while a nurse is engaged in usual activities. If this important aspect of nursing is neglected in preference to manual skills, it robs the nurse of valuable knowledge of those under her care as well as many opportunities to bring satisfaction to both the patients and herself.

Study Situations

1. Look at the guide in the following article:

- Manthey, M. E.: A guide for interviewing. Amer. J. Nurs., *67*:2088-2090, October, 1967.

Study the guide in relation to the discussion on interviewing in this chapter. What was the purpose of the interview for which this guide was prepared? Consider how the guide might be adapted for other purposes.

2. Some of the standard phrases used by nurses and other hospital personnel can do more harm than good both to patients and their families, such as "He is doing as well as can be expected" or "He is resting comfortably." The following article is an interesting and informative one about patients' feelings when not being able to get information, especially in the hospital setting.

- Little, D. E.: The say-something tell-nothing concept of nursing. Nurs. Forum *2*, No. 1, 38-45, 1963.

3. In the following article, what does the author consider as the best way to establish communications with the deaf? Can you think of simple gestures in addition to the ones described that could assist a nurse in communicating with the deaf?

- Bender, R. E.: Communicating with the deaf. Amer. J. Nurs., *66*:757-760, April, 1966.

4. There are sketches of patients in the article listed below, on pages 2133 and 2134. Without reading the captions, describe messages you receive from the gestures these patients demonstrate.

- Understanding hostility (Programmed Instruction). Amer. J. Nurs., *67*:2131-2150, October, 1967.

5. The following article describes several kinds of communication between a patient and her nurse:

- Storlie, F. J.: Message from Marcia. Amer. J. Nurs., *67*:1682-1683, August, 1967.

Note the importance the author places on touch in communication. What was the message *to* Marcia from the nurse when their hands touched?

References

1. Bain, B., and Bailey, J.: How a communication tool led to the development of a nursing care plan. Nurs. Outlook, *15*:48-51, October, 1967.
2. Bermosk, L. C.: Interviewing: A key to therapeutic communication in nursing practice. Nurs. Clinics N. Amer., *1*:205-214, June, 1966.
3. Cohen, M. S.: Easy to listen to. Amer. J. Nurs., *66*:1999-2001, September, 1966.

4. Hays, J. S.: Analysis of nurse-patient communications.
NURS. OUTLOOK, *14*:32-35, September, 1966.
5. Johnson, B. S.: The meaning of touch in nursing.
NURS. OUTLOOK, *13*:59-60, February, 1965.
6. Juzwiak, M.: How skilled interviewing helps patients and nurses.
RN., *29*:33-40 and 76-80, August, 1966.
7. Kron, T.: Communication in Nursing, 244 p. Philadelphia, W. B. Saunders, 1967.
8. Lambertsen, E. C.: C. C. U. therapy must include support for patient's family.
MOD. HOSP., *110*:128, March, 1968.
9. Lewis, G. K.: Communication: A factor in meeting emotional crises.
NURS. OUTLOOK, *13*:36-39, August, 1965.
10. Paynich, M. L.: Cultural barriers to nurse communication.
AMER. J. NURS., *64*:87-90, February, 1964.
11. Peters, J. A.: On the patients' terms.
AMER. J. NURS., *65*:130-131, February, 1965.
12. Schutt, B. G.: Feeling safe. Editorial.
AMER. J. NURS., *65*:61, June, 1965.
13. Skipper, J. K.: Communication and the Hospitalized Patient. *In* Social Interaction and Patient Care, Skipper, J. K., and Leonard, R. C., (eds.), p. 61-82.
Philadelphia, Lippincott, 1965.

CHAPTER

11

Considering Cultural Influences on Behavior

In order to understand the patient as an individual and to maintain his individuality, it is necessary to see him in the context of his cultural background; therefore, some knowledge of cultural influences is basic to providing good nursing care. Our discussion here must necessarily be sketchy. Further principles and illustrations that can help to guide action are provided in other courses of study in the curriculum.

Definition of Culture

Culture represents the sum total of a way of life developed by groups of people and handed down to succeeding generations. This total includes language, art, morals, customs, laws and innumerable other factors which, when considered as a whole, constitute a cultural pattern. We are born into a culture that teaches us a system of values and beliefs necessary to the functioning of a group whose members are interdependent. We learn how to behave, what to eat, how and when to eat, what to wear, how to get along and communicate with others and how to care for ourselves. It includes such activities as using a language, running a government, rearing our children, getting married, making a living, and fighting a war.

The word "cultured" sometimes is applied to certain people who display appreciation of fine literature, art or music. Those not sharing this appreciation may be referred to as "uncultured" persons. But the word is not used in that connotation in this book. Nor is it so used by social scientists. When we speak of culture here, we are referring to man's behavior and to the ways in which human beings of all social levels carry out their activities of daily living.

Men live in clusters that social scientists refer to as *societies*. Members of each society share certain ways of behaving which constitute the society's culture. For example, a society of approximately 75,000 Navajo Indians lives on reservations in Arizona and New Mexico. The culture of the Navajo society includes the way these people dress, the language they share, the type of houses in which they live, rituals concerning the curing of illness, their religion, the manner in which they rear their children, and the like.

Cultures contain subcultures or "groups within groups." While sharing the broad traits of the larger culture, the members of a subculture also have certain special characteristics in common which establish that group's peculiar identity. American subcultures, for example, are almost infinitely divisible according to such factors as region, race, education, occupation, income, social class and so on. Moreover, each individual is the product of a number of subcultures, every one of which will affect his attitudes to some degree.

Subcultural points of view are most important for the nurse to keep in mind because they can be subtle and therefore deceiving. If a patient appears whose culture is sharply in variance with our own, e.g., a newly arrived East Indian, the usual tendency on the part of health personnel is to accept him as an exotic and thereby forgive his seeming oddities of speech, dress, diet and mannerisms as simply foreign. However, often our own nationals with differing but less obvious subcultural points of view may only invite prejudice because we believe that they ought to know better.

Cultures are Learned

All of mankind functions physiologically in much the same manner throughout the world. But even superficial observations illustrate that there is remarkable variation in mankind's patterns of behavior. This great diversity of man's behavior can be seen in any activity in which men engage. For example, the American teen-ager dresses very unlike the Saudi Arabian teen-ager. There is little resemblance between food customs in Samoa and Sweden. Although there may be elements of commonality, the Moslem religion is very different from Christianity. Examples such as these can be cited indefinitely.

Physical characteristics are genetically transmitted from one generation to another. This is not true of cultural characteristics. At birth man has no cultural ways of behaving. His manner of behaving is acquired through learning and over a period of years.

That we are influenced by the groups with which we are associated throughout life can be documented. There are many instances in which children in one family were separated in childhood and brought up under different circumstances. When they reunited in later life, the differences stood out by contrast. Let us take a hypothetical example.

If one child had been brought up in an apartment in a large city and the other on a farm, the city child probably would dress differently, have different ways of using his leisure time, find difficulty with such maintenance chores as painting a house, repairing machinery, installing electric fixtures and doing carpentry. He may even dislike manual labor if he is a "white collar" man. Differences in rural and in urban social life also could be reflected in their personalities. The one might feel lost and very uncomfortable in his unfamiliarity with the wide open spaces; the other might feel imprisoned in an apartment.

Other attitudes, beliefs and values can be as deeply ingrained. For example, if a woman has been taught and lived under the rule that "cleanliness is next to godliness" she may feel uncomfortable in a slovenly household. She might also be inclined to judge her relatives and friends solely on the basis of their housekeeping. The nurse also finds out that there are a goodly number of well-established attitudes and beliefs (superstitious and otherwise) relating to health. Many of these can interfere with care that is desirable or necessary. For instance, food prejudices may seriously hamper the maintenance of a therapeutic diet. A patient may refuse to have a blood transfusion because he has been taught that this should not be done. He is not necessarily being stubborn; he sincerely believes that this is wrong.

Cultures are Subject to Change

Cultures change primarily in two ways—by invention and by borrowing. An example of an early invention that changed culture was the invention of the wheel. When cultures meet, the borrowing of ideas and products is common. The impact of one culture on another through borrowing is called *acculturation.*

Consider the effect on American life, during the past half century, of such technologic innovations as electric lighting, mass-produced housing, television, automobiles, telephones, jets, super highways, atomic energy and automation. All have impinged on every aspect of our private lives to some degree. Think of the changes that continue to occur in our attitudes toward work and job opportunities, education, use of leisure time, langauge, modes of dress, concepts of morality, food patterns and countless other everyday considerations.

Paradoxically, although change is a law of life, nothing is more natural than the individual tendency—particularly on the part of those past middle life—to resist it consciously. It is always comforting to be able to preserve some vestiges of the "old ways" (many of which, of course, had been taken for granted and unappreciated until threatened with extinction). However, despite unwillingness to change, individuals undergo constant modifications of attitude throughout life—changes which may themselves be almost imperceptible until some circumstance brings them into dramatic relief. Consider the person who suddenly embraces a religion different from that which he always had practiced. Although his action may appear abrupt and arbitrary to others, it is likely to be the result of cumulative changes in attitude that have quietly taken place throughout the years. Thus, often we drastically modify our thinking despite ourselves.

If it is to our ultimate advantage to do so, we also can modify our attitudes by conscious effort: hence, the implication of the foregoing for the nurse. The word "barbarian," coined by the ancient Greeks, originally referred to all those who were not Greek. Most of us exhibit a tendency to think the same thing of anyone outside the pale of our own sociocultural world. For health personnel, this narrow outlook can be highly detrimental to the therapeutic relationship. If we feel comfortable only with individuals of our own nationality, religion, socioeconomic class, race and educational background, it becomes impossible to communicate beyond the most elemental level or to achieve any degree of understanding with patients and co-workers. It is wise to be aware that no one's cultural heritage is a static thing, that its horizons expand when a conscious effort is made to recognize other cultures. This implies not only passive tolerance but also an active desire to accept, learn and ultimately to understand.

Implications for Nursing

Anthropologists and sociologists have made tremendous contributions to the field of knowledge concerning cultures. Most, if not all, of them would agree that their findings are of great value when they can contribute to a better life for their fellow men. But the question arises—to what extent have we a right to change people's culture? Stated in another way, when we feel a cultural characteristic is undesirable for some reason, have we the right to persuade others to accept our culture "for their own good?"

These questions have produced much debate. Some scholars will say that just as we accept the right of a man to his own religious beliefs, we must also accept the right of a man to other aspects of his culture. They would add that no one has a right to deliberately change the culture of others.

Those who feel there is sometimes good reason for attempting to produce cultural change hold that it is justified *under certain circumstances.* They feel that individual rights are not violated when people are given sufficient knowledge concerning alternative behavior so that they can make an intelligent choice. This principle seems to be especially applicable in the field of health.

In a remote Mexican village health workers found that the only local beverage was an alcoholic drink made from the juice of a local plant. There was no safe source of water for drinking. But even when safe water was brought to these people, it was soon learned that they did not fare well. The local drink had been the only source of certain minerals and vitamins essential for health. This example illustrates that although it might well have been desirable for health reasons to change a cultural characteristic, the change became detrimental in another way until appropriate alternative behavior became available to these people.

In many instances, a patient's behavior differs so radically from that of the staff (and, for that matter, of most of the other patients) that his behavior and his beliefs seem to be hopelessly unacceptable. However, if the nurse applies the principle of cultural influence and change as just described, it may well be that she can transform the situation into a comfortable one for all concerned. Moreover, she might greatly benefit the patient by showing him possibilities of which he may not have been aware. In other words, she has given him knowledge so that he can make a choice. The following is an example:

Mike Ferrer was a young itinerant farm worker who lived in shacks when he worked and in his battered car the rest of the time. When he was brought into the hospital, he was placed in a small ward. Within a matter of a few hours the other patients were calling the nurses or coming to the nurses' station to voice complaints about him. Mike had voided in a wastepaper basket, he spat out the window from his bed; because he was warm, he threw the top bedcovers over the foot of the bed and lay semiexposed in only a short hospital gown. By the standards of the other patients and the nurses he was committing one social indiscretion after another. Considering what they knew of his background and circumstances, the nurses realized that this young man probably was not aware that he was doing anything "wrong." It took quite a bit of doing to explain the use of a urinal, the bathroom facilities, the wipes to expectorate in and their careful disposal and the inadvisability of letting himself be exposed. Some of the men recognized Mike's willingness to "do right" when he knew what to do and, out of kindness and in recognition of his potentialities, they did much to help him.

In this situation, notations were made on his nursing care plan which maintained consistency in the nursing approach to Mike. There was no need to ask the physician to "talk turkey" to him or to reprimand him (though nurses did inform the physician, who was pleased to see their results and to cooperate with them). Mike's illness, surgery and secondary chest problem kept him in the hospital for a while, during which time he expressed a desire to make some changes in his life for the better. With a nurse's help in obtaining a social worker to visit him, possibilities for the future were explored with him. After his discharge he visited the nurses when he came for his clinic appointments. He reported on his progress in learning to read and write, and then on his new job.

It must be obvious that verbal and nonverbal communication were equally important in this kind of situation. It is not only what we say to the other person but how we look and behave that tells him that we are trying to understand. This is not to say that the nurse necessarily subscribes to the patient's views, but that she can understand the *why* of the difference.

Cultural factors may influence a patient's reaction to illness. In our Anglo-American culture, health in general holds supreme value and illness is considered unpleasant and undesirable. In some other cultures, illness is sometimes accepted with less concern. For example, in India it is common knowledge that illness and lack of well-being are associated with protein starvation. Yet, because of cultural dietary habits, it has proven difficult to teach mothers to give their babies low-cost high-protein gruels that would aid in preventing malnutrition. Malnutrition is an accepted condition of life for many and is not viewed as a matter of concern.

Deep in the interior of South America, there are people who rarely give their children names until they are two years of age. So many babies die before this age that a child is not really considered an integral part of the family unless he survives the first two years. Hence, he is not named until then. In this South American culture, unlike our own, a high mortality rate is considered inevitable and part of life.

The following description illustrates how a cultural characteristic concerning *time* might well interfere with the development of a therapeutic relationship with certain patients.

The nurse lives in a world that exists in

carefully measured units on the clock. Not hours or even minutes are sufficient to serve as units of time; the second is pressed into service. The routines of health agencies start and end at specified times. The sweep-second hand on the wristwatch is ever-present. The clinic and the doctor's care are administered in little packages of time labeled "appointments." An appointment has a definite time for beginning and, by inference, a definite minute for termination. Drugs are given to the patient to be taken half an hour before meals, every four hours, once daily at 8 A.M., and so on. Time is an important denominator in the culture of most health workers.

To say the American Indian is not conscious of time is to do him an injustice. He has a wonderful time system that guides his life on the reservation. But it is a clockless world with events to separate time intervals: sunrise, the noonday sun, sunset, full moon. Until the nurse understands a culture in which the clock is a stranger, she is likely to criticize her patients as eternally tardy.

Other cultures may not use the American Indian's way of judging time, but they too may seem clockless. The nurse may encounter patients who ask, "What's the big rush?" A pill, for example, taken two hours late may pose no problem in their minds. The nurse will be frustrated unless she realizes that there may be a cultural difference in the patient's concept of time—his sense of "time" may be entirely different from hers.

Some cultural differences are seemingly slight, so much so that we may tend to disregard them in everyday life. However, in nursing we should take them seriously because such little things make a big difference to a sick person. For example, a person who drinks coffee with all meals and in between probably would serve coffee to her guests without offering a choice. If one of the guests were English, a cup of tea probably would be more enjoyable, but for such an occasion as this, it would not be important. However, if this guest were a patient and were given coffee with all his meals, he could become very distressed. A "good cup of tea" could be very important to his well-being, and a nurse should see that he received it.

Here are examples of other behavior, reflecting cultural differences, frequently seen in nursing: wanting to eat the main meal of the day in the evening rather than at noon; desiring highly spiced and seasoned foods; refusing to undress before a strange person; being upset because it is necessary to sleep in a room with a strange person; avoiding use of a bedpan as much as possible because someone else must care for the contents; keeping a religious object pinned to the bed at all times; refusing to take a shower or a bath each day; refusing to have a bath during the menstrual period; asking to have the windows shut at night because night air is "bad"; refusing to have a pelvic examination done by a male physician; moaning and crying loudly when in pain; unreservedly demonstrating grief when a relative dies. Because of the influences of her own cultural background, the nurse may find such behavior incomprehensible and type the patient as "odd," "ignorant" or "difficult." It is necessary for her to make the effort to understand that this is simply learned behavior, normal in many subcultures.

Study Situations

1. The following article, written by a Vietnamese, illustrates several points made in this chapter:

- Tao-Kim-Hai, A. M.: Orientals Are Stoic. *In* Social Interaction and Patient Care. Skipper, J. K., and Leonard, R. C., (eds.), p. 142-155.
  Philadelphia, Lippincott, 1965.

Note in the first paragraph the author's opinion concerning reasons for his problem while hospitalized as a result of cultural differences between the staff and himself. Point out instances that led the patient to believe that nurses have a "superiority complex" and were "without consideration or kindness." Can you identify reasons related to cultural differences that led the patient to feel he should ". . . enlighten the hospital staff about world tolerance . . ."? After he lost his temper, even though the staff may now have felt that the patient was very cooperative, how did the patient really feel?

2. The following article appears in the book listed in Study Situation 1:

- Jewell, D. P.: A Case of a "Psychotic" Navajo Indian Male. p. 184-195.

What did the author find that indicated the patient's behavior was a result of his cultural background rather than of a mental illness? Do you think we might sometimes label patients as "strange" or "ill" when their behavior is normal in terms of their cultural background?

3. The following articles describe nursing in different cultures. Select several of these articles to read. Direct your attention to the following questions: What customs of the people tended to interfere with introducing medical/nursing care as practiced in the United States? What behavior traits of the people described were different from behavioral traits that a nurse would expect to observe of patients from her home town?

- a. Cunningham, M. P. *et al*: We went to Mississippi.
  AMER. J. NURS., *67*:801-804, April, 1967.
- b. Devitt, H. E.: Nursing in a Vietnam village.
  NURS. OUTLOOK, *14*:46-49, December, 1966. (Note cultural characteristics that had to be taken into consideration when teaching assistants.)
- c. Jennings, C. R.: The stroke patient—his rehabilitation.
  AMER. J. NURS., *67*:118-121, January, 1967. (Note especially the cultural traits described on page 121.)
- d. Libbey, A.: Junior year in India.
  AMER. J. NURS., *66*:332-334, February, 1966.
- e. Loughlin, B. W.: Pregnancy in the Navajo culture.
  NURS. OUTLOOK, *13*:55-58, March, 1965. (Note that the author indicates a need to look at all cultural aspects of life before instigating a program of change. Note also the questions she posed as needing answers before health workers "suggest new methods" to peoples of cultures other than our own.)
- f. Lynn, F. H.: An American nurse visits two mental hospitals in Greece.
  NURS. OUTLOOK, *14*:50-53, December, 1966.
- g. Schneider, V.: Letter from Lambarene.
  AMER. J. NURS., *65*:128-130, October, 1965. (Note the author's description of Dr. Schweitzer's philosophy concerning the care of these patients, on page 130, "An Old-Fashioned Hospital.")
- h. Storlie, F.: Letter to Tommie's grandma.
  AMER. J. NURS., *67*:542-543, March, 1967.
- i. Weiss, M. O.: Nursing and nurses in Israel.
  NURS. OUTLOOK, *14*:58-60, October, 1966.
- j. Saba, V.: A nurse goes to Saudi Arabia.
  NURS. OUTLOOK, *14*:58-61, May, 1966.

References

1. Berry, E. J.: HOPE docks in Guinea.
   AMER. J. NURS., *66*:2238-2242, October, 1966.
2. Macgregor, F. C.: Uncooperative patients: Some cultural interpretations.
   AMER. J. NURS., *67*:88-91, January, 1967.
3. Smith, F. L., and Afek, L. B.: The Papagos teach our students.
   NURS. OUTLOOK, *16*:26-28, July, 1968.
4. Stallsmith, J. A.: Treat or tribulation?
   AMER. J. NURS., *66*:1782-1783, August, 1966.
5. Vogel, J. R.: Foreigner in Denmark.
   AMER. J. NURS., *65*:108-109, April, 1965.
6. Watts, W.: Social class, ethnic background, and patient care.
   NURS. FORUM, *6*:155-162, #2, Spring, 1967.

CHAPTER 12

Considering Religious Influences on Behavior

Anthropologists have found that some kind of religion is a part of every culture. Religion, in a general sense, may be considered as man's attempt to understand his relationship with the universe about him. It functions to provide orderly relations, more or less, between man and his surroundings. A religious faith often reduces anxiety for the believer.

There are almost countless varieties of religious practices, beliefs and rituals in the world. This chapter concerns itself primarily with Judaism and Christianity, the most commonly practiced religions in the United States.

Religion and Illness

It is common for most patients to seek support from their religious faith during times of stress. This support is often vital to the acceptance of an illness, especially if the illness brings with it a prolonged period of convalescence or indicates a questionable outcome. Prayer, devotional reading and other religious practices often do for the patient spiritually what protective exercises do for the body physically.

The values derived from religious faith cannot be enumerated or evaluated easily. However, the effects attributable to faith are in evidence to health workers constantly. Patients have been known to endure extreme physical distress because of strong faith. Patients' families have taken on almost unbelievable rehabilitative tasks because they had faith in the eventual positive results of their effort. Some of the greatest personal triumphs over disease and injury are recorded not in medical or nursing texts but in biographic literature. A health team composed of every type of expert in medicine can bring the patient only to a certain phase of recovery. The effort to take that which has been "repaired" and to develop it to its fullest must come from the patient. Even though not all patients are faced with major problems because of illness, all are in need of maintaining a constructive and hopeful attitude. Spiritual support often is the key to the hope and determination that helps them and it is a real comfort to many patients to be able to adhere closely to their religious practices during illness.

The presence of a Bible, a prayer book, rosary beads or other religious objects in the patient's unit is significant. It may well be that the patient spends a portion of each day in devotional reading and prayer. Although some patients may have no objection to do so in the presence of others, other patients may prefer privacy. Inasmuch as patients may feel that a request for privacy may not be understood, it is a thoughtful gesture if the suggestion is initiated by the nurse.

Many hospitals have chapels in which patients may worship, and in some instances regular services are held for various denominations. Where regular services are not held, patients are permitted to worship in the chapel at their convenience. Frequently, it is through the consideration of members of the nursing staff that patients are made aware of such facilities.

Although a person's religious faith frequently appears to speed recovery, there are instances in which a religious belief that conflicts with medical aims may hamper a person's adaptation to a health agency or his acceptance of therapy. For example, the doctrine of the Jehovah's Witnesses prohibits blood transfusions. In the Islamic religion, man is regarded as largely helpless in controlling his environment and illness is accepted as his fate rather than as something against which action might be taken. Some Navajo Indians still use a lengthy religious ceremony to "cure" certain diseases; tuberculosis is an example. For some people, illness is viewed as punishment for sin, and, therefore, inevitable. Even though concepts such as these may hamper the efforts of health personnel, every attempt should be made to understand them and what they mean to the patient. Only then can cooperation be obtained that may result in the patient's willingness to accept certain therapy. This may very well require the assistance of the patient's religious advisor.

It is important for the nurse to try to gain an understanding of what religion means to the patient. Even within the same faith, people interpret their religion differently. But the sensitive nurse treats the patient's belief with respect in any case. If a particular religious practice presents a problem in relation to the patient's medical regimen, the nurse can turn to the patient, to his family, or to the clergyman for assistance.

The Chaplain's Role in the Health Team

Because physical recovery is closely related to mental attitude and emotional stability, the patient's religious counselor plays a key role on the health team. There are instances when he serves as an associate to the physician and the nurse by interpreting therapy and its value to the plan of care. He may very well be the person who helps the patient to accept various phases of care.

While the chaplain serves a real purpose on the health team, usually he is not a member of the hospital staff. However, in many large hospitals, chaplains of various faiths are available at any time of the day or night. When the patient is in a hospital near his own community, the clergyman from his own church may also visit, and generally this is a satisfying experience for the patient.

The nurse can be helpful to a chaplain by greeting him and helping him to locate his parishioner. If the patient is in a single room with the door closed, the nurse should determine whether the patient is able to receive a call from the chaplain. Having him enter the unit at an inopportune moment is embarrassing to both chaplain and patient. In other instances, the patient may be located in a unit which has several patients in it. In this situation, too, the chaplain and the patient may be disturbed by a situation which exists in the unit. The patient usually identifies the chaplain as a personal visitor, not as a true member of the health team accustomed to hospital routine and hospital sights. The chaplain, too, recognizes that he does not have the freedom to enter units and be present in situations which a doctor or a nurse may take for granted.

Preparation of the Patient's Unit for the Chaplain's Visit. Preparation of the patient's unit for the chaplain's visit may vary with the purpose of the visit. If the occasion is one of a visit, the unit should be orderly and free from unnecessary equipment and items. There should be provision for the chaplain to be seated at the bedside or near the patient so that both can be comfortable during the visit. If a sacrament is to be administered, the top of the bedside table should be free of all items and covered with a clean white cover. A white paper tray cover is frequently more satisfactory than a towel. If the patient is located in a unit having several patients, he may appreciate having the bed curtains drawn partially so as to provide some degree of privacy. Almost always when a sacrament is to be administered, the entire unit is screened to provide privacy.

Judaism

Judaism teaches the unity of God, and God is considered the creator and source of all life. Each person is free to choose between good and evil. Man is considered as a child of God. Unlike Christianity and some religions of the Near East, Judaism does not hold resurrection and immortality as a central concept. One rabbi states that the aim of Judaism is salvation of humanity in history rather than salvation of the soul in the hereafter. Salvation is found by fulfilling social responsibilites. Death is considered part of the continuance of birth, growth and decay.

The spiritual adviser of the Jewish faith is the rabbi.

There are three forms of Judaism: Reform, Conservative and Orthodox. Reform Judaism is more liberal than the other two in its thinking, whereas Orthodox Judaism is the most conservative of the three. Conservative Judaism finds its place more or less between Reform and Orthodox Judaism.

The Jewish Sabbath and Holidays. The Sabbath begins on Friday at sundown and ends on Saturday at sundown. It is a day for rest and worship. For the patient who observes the Sabbath, treatments and procedures

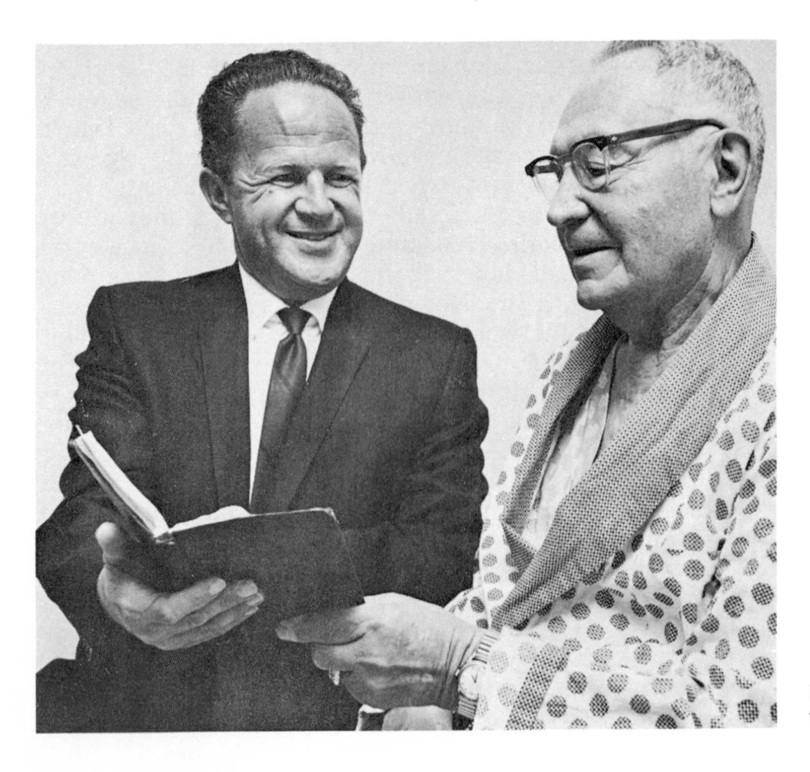

Fig. 12-1. The rabbi's visit and the reading of prayers together with him are comforting to the Jewish patient.

should be postponed if postponement will not cause harm to the patient.

In Judaism, New Year's Day is called Rosh Hashanah and usually occurs in September. Rosh Hashanah is the beginning of a ten day period for reflections and consideration of life and its problems. The period ends with the Day of Atonement or Yom Kippur.

Hanukkah usually occurs in December. It is a festival recalling ancient resistance to tyranny and is a time of rejoicing and giving of gifts.

Passover occurs in the spring and is observed for seven days. It is a festival of redemption that recalls the departure of the Jews from Egypt.

There are additional Jewish holidays but the ones just mentioned are observed most commonly by persons of Jewish faith.

Dietary Practices. Dietary practices are important for the nurse to understand, especially when she is caring for patients who observe Conservative or Orthodox Judaism. Reform Judaism does not hold these practices as relevant. Because dietary practices vary in Judaism and also occasionally among Jews practicing the same form of Judaism, the nurse should consult with the patient, a family member or a rabbi, if questions arise.

Dietary regulations permit the eating of meat of kosher animals and fowl. Animals are considered kosher if they are ruminants and have divided hooves, as cows, goats and sheep. Kosher fowl are primarily those that are not birds of prey, as chickens, ducks and geese. Fowl and animals are slaughtered, dressed and prepared in a prescribed manner in order to be considered kosher. Fish are considered kosher if they have both scales and fins, as salmon, tuna, sardines, carp, and the like. Shellfish, such as shrimp and lobster, are not acceptable. Fish do not have to be slaughtered and dressed in a prescribed manner.

Fish and meat products (such as oils and fats), milk and milk products and eggs are considered kosher if they are from the abovementioned animals. Plant or vegetable oils are acceptable.

Milk products may not be eaten with or immediately following meat products. An interval of six hours must elapse between eating meat and milk products. Meat products, on the other hand, may be eaten after milk products after an interval of only a few minutes. If a patient is having both meat and milk products during the same meal, serve the products separately, first the milk products and then the meat.

Fish may be eaten with dairy products if prepared with a nonmeat shortening or if broiled.

During the Passover period, leavened products, such as bread, cake, cookies, noodles or beverages containing grain alcohol, are not used.

Kosher foods may not be prepared in utensils used for the preparation of non-kosher foods unless they have been cleansed in a prescribed manner. Fruits and vegetables that have been steamed or cooked in non-kosher utensils are permissible if non-kosher sauce, gravy or shortening are omitted.

For the patient who is in the hospital and observing dietary practices, the following suggestions are helpful. Use paper dishes for the serving of food; substitute fresh vegetables and fruits for leavened products; if kosher meat or fish is unavailable, use an acceptable protein substitute, as milk products or eggs; suggest that the family bring matzos (unleavened bread product) for the patient.

If a Jewish patient's observance of dietary practices interferes with his medical regimen, Jewish law permits modifications. Before proceeding with modifications, the nurse should consult with the patient, a member of his family or a rabbi.

Circumcision. Male Jewish infants are required to be circumcised on the eighth day following their birth. However, the rite may be postponed for as long as necessary if the infant's health does not permit it at that time. The mohel (professional circumciser) may perform it or in some instances, it may be done by a surgeon of Jewish faith while a rabbi attends. A quorum of ten men attends the ceremony.

Death and Preparation for Burial. When possible, a service of confession and prayer is observed as death approaches. Preferably the rabbi is present for this—if not the patient's own rabbi, then one associated with the health agency.

A patient who has died may be washed and covered with a clean cloth. Should a Jewish patient who has no kin to claim the body die, a rabbi should be contacted.

Reform and Conservative Judaism do not object to post-mortem examination. An autopsy is considered by them to be a means by which medical knowledge learned from the dead can help the living. Either the patient gives consent for autopsy before death or the family grants such permission after death.

Christianity

Christianity teaches the trinity of God, that is, there are three Persons in one God: God the Father, God the Son, and God the Holy Ghost. God the Father is considered the creator and the source of life. The Son of God is Jesus Christ, who came into the world in human form, suffered and died for the salvation of all men. Christianity holds resurrection and immortality as a central concept. Although social responsibility is important in Christianity, salvation is found through faith in the triune God. However, the two go together—faith and good works.

In the United States, most Christians are Roman Catholics or Protestants. The spiritual adviser in the Roman Catholic faith is the priest. For Protestants the spiritual adviser is called a minister, pastor or preacher.

Sunday and Holidays. Most Christians observe Sunday as a day for worship. An example of an exception is the Seventh Day Adventists, who set aside Saturday for worship.

Although many holy days are observed in the various faiths in Christianity, two are held in common and are familiar to almost everyone.

Christmas is observed in most places in the world of Christianity on December 25. It is celebrated as the day on which Christ was born. The day is a joyous one and a time for giving of gifts in memory of Christ's birth.

In the spring, Christians observe Lent and the Easter season. Easter occurs in March or April. The six-week period prior to Easter is called Lent and the Friday before Easter is Good Friday.

Lent is a time for contemplation on the sufferings and death of Christ. Many Christians make personal sacrifices during Lent as a symbol of humility and in memory of Christ's suffering. These sacrifices often involve some kind of fasting, which may need to be taken into account during periods of illness, especially if it interferes with the medical regimen. Good Friday is a day of sorrow when the Christian recalls the agonizing death of Christ on the cross.

Easter marks the end of the Lenten period and is a day of great rejoicing. It commemorates the day when Christ arose from the dead. Belief in His resurrection confirms the Christian tenet that Christ is the Son of God.

Roman Catholicism

In the care of patients who are of the Catholic faith, the nurse will find it necessary to be acquainted with the following sacraments: baptism, communion and the sacrament of the anointing of the sick. Sacraments in the Catholic faith, by virtue of the fact that they are accepted as having been instituted by Christ, are believed to have the power to produce the effect that each signifies.

Baptism. Since a nurse is present during the delivery of a child or the miscarriage of a living fetus, it is imperative that she understand that, for a Catholic family, any child in danger of death must be baptized. At the time of death all Catholics must be in the state of grace, free from serious sin. It is mainly by means of the sacraments that sin is absolved and grace given. Baptism is the first sacrament and removes the first, or original, sin deriving from Adam and Eve. To the Catholic, this is absolutely necessary for salvation.

If a priest is not available, the nurse or the doctor should administer the sacrament of baptism. It is preferred that a Catholic nurse or doctor administer the sacrament, but if a Catholic is not available, anyone having the use of reason may do it. It is necessary that the person conferring the sacrament have the intention of doing what the Catholic

Church desires and use the proper form. The procedure is as follows: while pouring plain water over the forehead so that it flows upon the skin, say, "I baptize thee in the name of the Father, and of the Son, and of the Holy Ghost." In case of intra-uterine baptism, the water may flow on any exposed part of the infant's body.

Since baptism may be conferred when there is possible danger to the child's life, and since the family may not be aware of it, the fact that the sacrament of baptism was conferred should be recorded on the infant's chart. If a priest confers the baptism, he will notify the family that it has been done. If the child is baptized by someone other than a priest, the priest should be informed and then he can discuss it with the parents.

Holy Eucharist or Holy Communion. This is the most excellent of all the sacraments of the Catholic faith because, according to Catholic belief, it contains, under the appearance of bread and wine, the Body, Blood, Soul and Divinity of Jesus Christ. All Catholics in danger of death should receive communion if possible. Most Catholic patients wish to receive it frequently. Ordinarily, confession precedes communion. To receive communion, all Catholic patients, except those in danger of death, must fast; in the hospital, the patient is to fast only one hour from solid food. The patient is not required to fast from liquids and medications.

Prior to communion, the patient should be made comfortable, the unit prepared as described earlier, and the patient given privacy so that he may pray and prepare himself for the sacrament.

Sacrament of the Anointing of the Sick. When a patient is in serious danger of death, this sacrament is administered along with confession, communion and the last blessing (a special blessing of the Pope carrying with it a plenary indulgence which the priest is entitled to bestow on the dying person). However, apart from this, it is customary now to give the sacrament of the anointing of the sick to all persons who may be coming into danger of death from sickness, accident, old age or surgery. Therefore, the patient about to have heart, lung or other major surgery would ordinarily be given this sacrament. For as well as preparing one for death if it be God's will that the patient die,

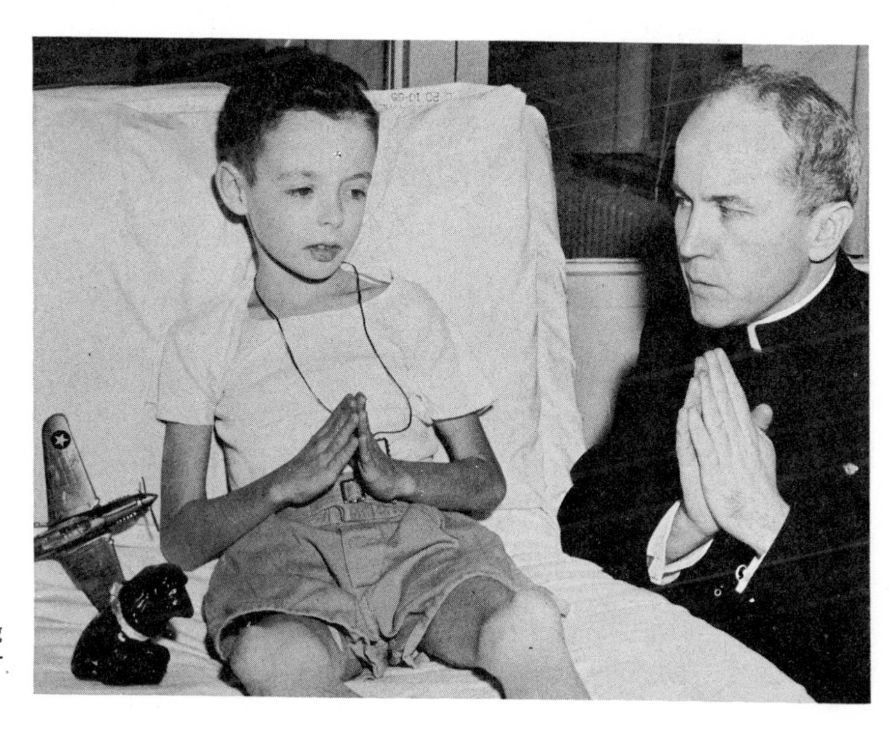

Fig. 12-2. The priest hearing the prayers of a child brings comfort to the child and his family.

this sacrament gives peace of mind and soul to the sick person and helps return him to bodily health if God so wills. In administering the sacrament of the anointing of the sick, the priest anoints the five senses in the form of a cross with holy oil and with beautiful accompanying prayers that beg for the peace of mind of the patient and return to bodily health.

These rites are very important to the Catholic patient, and it is imperative that the nurse notify the priest in time to administer them, no matter at what hour of the day or the night the patient's condition seems to warrant it.

If a patient dies very suddenly and has not had these rites, it is still possible for the priest to administer conditionally the sacraments of penance and anointing of the sick within hours following death. The sacraments are an important part of the Catholic faith.

Protestantism

The Protestant faith embraces a large number of denominations. Some of the religious groups that are active today originated before the Reformation, and others have developed since then apart from the Reformation influence. While certain doctrines are common to most of these denominations, there are individual practices and interpretations which give each a distinct pattern of its own.

While some denominations employ certain sacraments that are similar to those in the Catholic faith, others reject the concept of sacraments and observe baptism and communion as ordinances that are means of grace but not of salvation. Others, such as the Friends (Quakers), reject both ordinances and sacraments.

Baptism. Some Protestant faiths hold that baptism should be performed in infancy. The Baptists, the Disciples and some others hold that the ordinance of baptism should not be administered before the person reaches the age of accountability. If a child of Protestant parents is in danger of dying, the nurse should ask whether the parents wish to have the child baptized. If the parents wish it and a Protestant minister is not available, the child may be baptized as follows: a baptized nurse who has understanding and belief in the act that she is about to perform may baptize the baby by pouring water continuously over the baby's

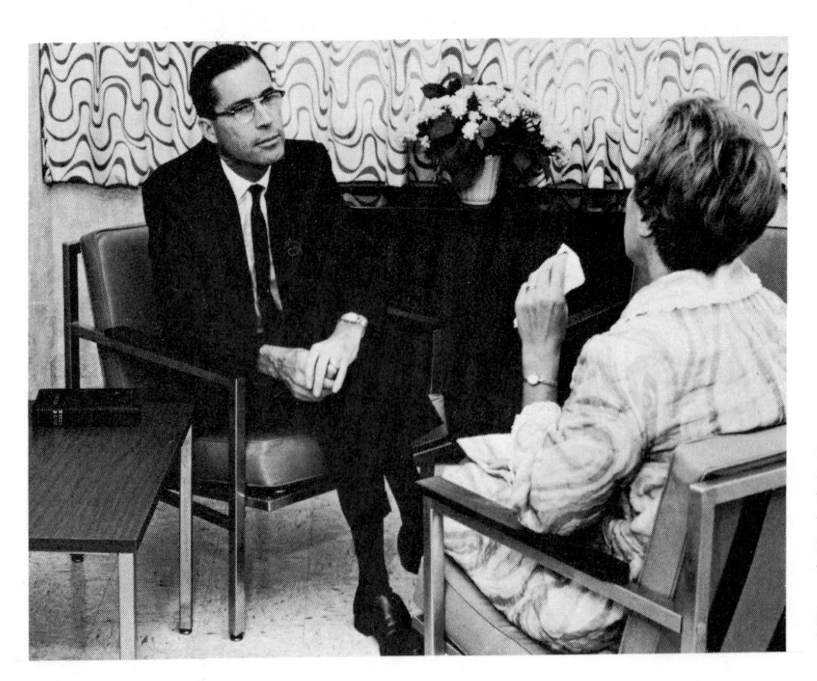

Fig. 12-3. It is understandable that we cannot reveal our fear or anxieties to just anyone. As much as nurses or doctors may try to help a patient, it is often the patient's minister who is needed on the health team. There is no question about the therapeutic value to the patient of being able to unburden a problem and being strengthened by prayer. (Photo: Warren R. Vroom)

forehead and saying the following words, "I baptize thee in the name of the Father, and of the Son and of the Holy Ghost. Amen." The baptism is recorded on the child's chart by the person performing it and the parents are informed as soon as convenient.

Communion. In most Protestant faiths, communion is administered less frequently than in the Catholic faith. However, many Protestant patients request it prior to surgery or during a period of illness. It represents the body and the blood of Christ which were sacrificed for the remission of sin. Before the arrival of the minister, the unit should be properly prepared and the patient given privacy so that he has an opportunity for prayer and self-examination.

Other Beliefs

In the course of her education and working career, the nurse can expect to care for persons holding beliefs less common than those just discussed. Examples include the Moslem, the Buddhist, the Coptic and the Confucian faiths. It is impractical to discuss all faiths in this text. However, the basic principle remains: in her attempt to understand each patient for whom she cares, the nurse should attempt to understand basic tenets of his faith and how these may influence his therapeutic regimen, his recovery and his adaptation to the hospital environment.

While sacraments, ordinances, forms of worship, doctrines and beliefs help distinguish one faith from another, all faiths provide the spiritual support which should and/or could help each man to face life constructively and to be of service to others. The nurse should never underestimate the power of religion as a part of the patient's recovery.

Some people do not accept any particular religious faith. Nevertheless, they deserve the same respect for what they choose to believe. They have as much a right to believe as they wish as those persons who accept a particular religious creed. Common courtesy demands respect for the beliefs of others.

Study Situations

1. Consider the following article:

- Berger, A. A.: Ethical implications of professional competency.
  J.A.M.A., *200*:200, June 12, 1967.

Although the article was prepared with the medical profession in mind, do you think that it is applicable to nursing?

2. The article given below is an excellent supplement to the section in this chapter describing Judaism. Note the magazine's foreword in italics, which emphasizes that the patient's religious beliefs can color his response to illness.

- Berkowitz, P., and Berkowitz, N. S.: The Jewish patient in the hospital.
  Amer. J. Nurs., *67*:2335-2337, November, 1967.

3. For examples of how clergymen have assisted the nursing team to meet patients' spiritual needs, you may wish to refer to the following article:

- Inman, K. *et al*: If you ask me: What specific assistance has a clergyman given you in helping a patient meet his problems?
  Amer. J. Nurs., *57*:737, June, 1957.

References

1. Barton, R. T.: Religious Doctrine and Medical Practice.
   Springfield, Illinois, Charles C Thomas, 1958.
2. Berkowitz, P., and Berkowitz, N. S.: The Jewish patient in the hospital.
   Amer. J. Nurs., *67*:2335-2337, November, 1967.
3. Peale, N. V., and Blanton, S.: Faith is the Answer. 280 pp.
   Carmel, New York, Guideposts Associates, Inc., 1955.
4. Piepgras, B.: The other dimension: Spiritual help.
   Amer. J. Nurs., *68*:2610-2613, December, 1968.
5. The National Association of Catholic Chaplains: The Apostolate to the Sick, A Guide for the Catholic Chaplain in Health Care Facilities. 128 p.
   The Catholic Hospital Association, 1967.
6. Sandmel, S.: We Jews and You Christians, 146 p.
   Philadelphia, Lippincott, 1967.

CHAPTER 13

Using Sources of Diversion as Therapy

Anyone who has been ill and confined at home or in a hospital knows how long the days can be and how slowly the hours seem to go by. Sometimes, these hours of idleness have a way of making the experience of being ill far more disagreeable than it need be. When one is busy, time has a way of passing quickly. (Hence, the saying, "If you want to kill time, try working it to death.")

In certain contexts a distinction is made between the words, "diversion" and "recreation." However, in this text the two are used synonymously.

Purposes of Diversional Activities

Diversional activities can serve a variety of purposes. Very often they are intended primarily to help a person to relax while doing things that are of interest to him. This is especially true of patients who are convalescing after acute illnesses but who can expect to return relatively soon to their usual leisure and work.

Diversional activity is credited with serving a therapeutic purpose in the prevention and the correction of some personal adjustment difficulties, and considerable investigation has been undertaken in this area. Findings of such investigations have benefited schools, colleges, homes for the aged and hospitals, as well as the home. It is now possible to purchase or to select games or projects on the basis of age, size of group and degree of difficulty of the activity, in relation to the desired purpose. For example, it is possible to assist quiet and withdrawn individuals to participate comfortably in a group situation or to select a diversion which will help to quiet and relax the more active individual.

When illness or incapacity is prolonged or chronic, recreation that a person enjoyed before his illness may not interest him, or certain activities may no longer be appropriate. Recreation then may be planned to find new and suitable means of spending leisure time. For example, a person with partial permanent paralysis following a cardiovascular accident may have to give up certain sports and find substitutes. He may lose all interest or retain some as a passive participant. In many health agencies for persons who are chronically ill or have prolonged illnesses, recreational therapy departments staffed with trained personnel are available. In such cases, the nurses' responsibility for helping to provide diversion is decreased. Some authorities now recommend that recreational therapy be included in the total rehabilitation program in hospitals, nursing homes and homes for the aged because it has great potential in the fulfillment of human needs.

Recreation is often a good way to keep a child contented in bed and relatively quiet during illness and convalescence. Although activity is restricted, imagination can travel far and wide through toys and games, making confinement seem less bridling. Robert Louis Stevenson's poem, "The Land of Counterpane," illustrates poignantly how toys can help the ill child roam far from his confining bed:

When I was sick and lay a-bed,
I had two pillows at my head,
And all my toys beside me lay
To keep me happy all the day.

And sometimes for an hour or so
I watched my leaden soldiers go
With different uniforms and drills,
Among the bed-clothes, through the hills.

And sometimes sent my ships in fleets
All up and down among the sheets;
Or brought my trees and houses out,
And planted cities all about.

I was the giant great and still
That sits upon the pillow-hill,
And sees before him, dale and plain,
The pleasant land of counterpane.

For older children allowed out of bed, group games offer both companionship and challenge for the participants.

Children's play often serves a useful purpose in aiding to evaluate physical and mental development. The observant nurse can use play as a tool for planning not only a youngster's recreation but many aspects of his care as well.

Diversional activities often are used in occupational therapy.

Occupational therapy is a prescribed and supervised rehabilitation procedure involving manual and/or creative activities. For instance, a patient may be referred by the physician to the occupational therapy department for an activity which will exercise certain muscle groups in the hand and the arm. There the patient may be required to do something that he never has done before, but in all instances the therapist will try to offer a choice of suitable activities so that the patient may thoroughly enjoy doing it. Some patients may be referred to the occupational therapy department to learn a new vocation so that they may seek employment after they are discharged from the hospital. Typical would be an amputee who used to be a bus driver. Or, some patients may be referred to the occupational therapy department to engage in an activity in which they already have some skill. For such a patient the immediate interest in a constructive activity is therapeutic because it gives him self-confidence from the beginning and occupies his time constructively. In still other situations, patients may wish to engage in activities which help merely to pass the time; such patients will return their finished products to the occupational therapy department.

Selection of Diversional Activities

The diversional needs of acutely ill patients may be little other than perhaps visits with family and friends and receiving and reading mail. When convalescence is short, patients may require very little assistance in finding diversional activities, since they usually begin to assume their usual way of life. Their ordinary interests appear, and these are pursued with little effort needed on the part of the nurse.

Diversions for the patient should be chosen according to several factors such as individual interests, age, sex, type of illness, physical capacity and duration of illness. Satisfaction for the patient should be uppermost. Giving a patient something to do just to keep him occupied is not sufficient.

In suggesting a diversional activity for a

patient, it is best to have some understanding of the patient's natural interests first. Diversions which a patient will take on because he wants to be like the others about him, or which he feels obligated to perform, may or may not be interesting. If the activity is the patient's choice, it stands a better chance of serving its purposes well.

Very often, the diversion is akin to a person's occupation, but it can also be the opposite. For example, it is not uncommon to see a person with excellent manual dexterity, such as a surgeon, paint or sculpt as a diversion, or a highway engineer building a model railroad layout at home. On the other hand, one with a confining occupation, such as a research chemist, may like gardening or golf or other outdoor hobbies. Helping a patient to feel more comfortable while ill very often requires the nurse's display of interest in his usual hobbies or diversions. It may be that he had not thought of them because he was confined. If it is not possible for him to enjoy the identical diversions, close substitutes perhaps can be found. Any diversion that can be provided or obtained from home which makes the patient more at ease contributes to a therapeutic climate.

Like adults, children are unsatisfied with activites that are of no interest to them. The diversion selected will have to be considered carefully from the standpoint of the child's interest in it, the amount of physical activity involved and the possible emotional reactions to it.

In certain instances, the patient may prefer group activity to solitary diversion, but here again his condition must be taken into account. Obviously, a patient in a full body cast cannot join in a game of ping pong, but probably he can play cards; a game of solitaire may suffice during times when other patients cannot come to join him in a group game.

Wherever group activites are concerned, like interests are involved. When organizing such events and inviting patients to join them, it should be remembered that recreation for one individual may not be such for another and that points of difference can cause stress and conflict for a patient. For example, if a nurse were to say to a group of patients on a sun porch, "I'll turn the television on so you can all watch the baseball game this afternoon," she may annoy those who have no interest in the game. In other words, the nurse should avoid making patients feel compelled to join in.

For persons confined for long periods of time, group activities usually are enjoyable. Just being in a group may be satisfying in itself. Some agencies have parties on patients' birthdays and on certain holidays, as well as planned events for other special occasions. If given the opportunity, some patients enjoy the challenge of organizing,

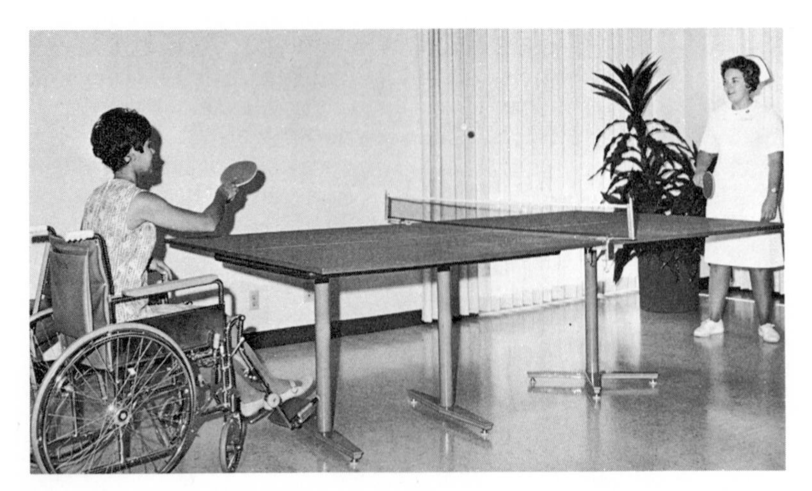

Fig. 13-1. In this agency's rehabilitation unit, nurses use recreation as a time when they can learn to know their patients better. Patients are encouraged to wear street clothes, if they so desire, as part of their preparation for returning to their homes and communities. (Institute of Rehabilitation Medicine of the Good Samaritan Hospital, Phoenix, Arizona.)

decorating and planning for group recreation, as for a party, a skit or a game.

When helping to select diversions, remember that most people need variety. Few care to pursue a single thing all day or day after day. Children and young adults are especially likely to succumb to boredom.

Common Diversions for Patients

Reading and Writing. Rare indeed is the patient who does not enjoy at least some reading when confined with illness. Books, magazines and newspapers are readily available in most health agencies. For those unable to visit the library, volunteers in many agencies bring reading materials to the patients. Many patients bring their own reading materials with them. In general, patients prefer "light" reading—something that is easy to read and understand.

Some persons enjoy writing while hospitalized. This is especially true with those who have long-term illness or are not acutely ill. Chronically ill persons often enjoy pen pals. New mothers usually plan to write birth announcements while hospitalized.

The arrival of mail generally is a pleasant experience for all patients. It is a way to keep in touch with family and friends, and many patients derive great pleasure in displaying the cards that they receive. Very ill patients, or those unable to open their mail, may appreciate help with this. The person bringing the patient his mail should offer to open the envelope and read the card or message to the patient if he so desires. It may be a comforting message from someone who is unable to visit the patient. If mail is not opened because the patient is unresponsive or does not wish someone else to do this, it should be carefully placed so that a family member or other responsible visitor can see it and assume responsibility for it.

Television and Radio. Most health agencies have provisions for patients to use television and radio sets. In most instances, agencies rent TV sets for a nominal fee. For those patients who are ambulatory, sets often are available in patient lounges and recreation rooms. Many people enjoy watching television or listening to a radio for at least part of every day; and except for the very ill and the very young, this usually is appropriate, not only for its entertainment value but also because of its associations with home. However, it should be remembered that television and radio programs may be a source of annoyance for other persons; therefore, the volume should be kept at a moderate level.

Arts and Crafts. Recreation involving any of the arts and the crafts can be especially rewarding in that something is created, and the end-products are useful and decorative. Frequently, arts and crafts are suggested to patients if the activity involved is also beneficial for a specific physical limitation.

Toys. Toys can be the source of much pleasure for the hospitalized child. They should be carefully selected on the basis of factors discussed earlier in this chapter. In addition, safety must be kept in mind when selecting toys. Those with small removable parts are to be avoided because of the danger of swallowing these parts. Also to be avoided are toys with sharp edges or points. Because of allergies, toys stuffed with feathers or wool are undesirable. Stuffed toys present a cleaning problem which limits their use in many situations.

Dining Rooms and Patient Lounges. Eating with others is a symbol of family life and is taken for granted in many cultures. Almost no one likes to eat alone, and efforts to bring patients together for meals usually are rewarding. Yet, facilities for patients to eat in groups are relatively rare in health agencies. Those having progressive patient care units may include dining rooms or cafeterias for ambulatory patients. Many of the chronic illness hospitals have patient dining rooms. Patients able to use them appear to enjoy being with others, and mealtime is a satisfying social experience.

Many pediatric services arrange to have children eat together. Often, children eat more willingly when with others, and the handicapped are stimulated to do their best in order to be more like their peers.

Patient lounges are seen commonly in psychiatric hospitals, rehabilitation centers and federal hospitals. In view of the many social activities that patients enjoy in such lounges, one would hope that more hospitals could provide them. Here, patients can enjoy games together, meet for chatting, watch television, and so forth. For persons who do not socialize readily, a patients' lounge with opportunities to meet or be near others often can make the difference between loneliness and the satisfaction of being one of a group.

Visitors. Most patients enjoy visits with family members and friends. At one time most health agencies observed very limited visiting privileges, the reason being that visitors often were thought to upset patients as well as the hospital routines. However, most hospitals are becoming increasingly lenient in the provision of visiting privileges, as health personnel are observing the therapeutic value for patients. On pediatric services, visiting privileges in the past often were extremely limited. But in those agencies where most barriers for visiting have been removed, the children have demonstrated a marked increase in morale, resulting in definite therapeutic benefit.

In addition to the pleasure the patient has when a relative or friend visits, some agencies permit the visitor to aid in the patient's care. Examples include assisting the patient with eating, with walking, and with caring for the nails and hair. Under some circumstances, it may even be helpful to the patient if a family member can aid in administering medications or convincing the patient to take them. This may seem in violation of the usual procedure relating to medications but circumstances may prove it to be acceptable. A concerned relative will certainly spend as much time and effort as is necessary to encourage a loved one to take a medication. This would be preferable to a busy nurse giving up after a few tries and reporting the dosage as "refused"; or to having the patient spit out the medication after the nurse departs from the bedside.

However, visiting can be overdone, and health personnel generally agree that some limitations still must be observed. For the very ill, a limitation on the length of time visitors may stay or on the number of visitors present at one time may be necessary. While visiting policies are necessary, good judgment still must be used on the basis of the individual situation. In certain instances, because of the danger of infection (such as following organ transplants) no visitors may be allowed.

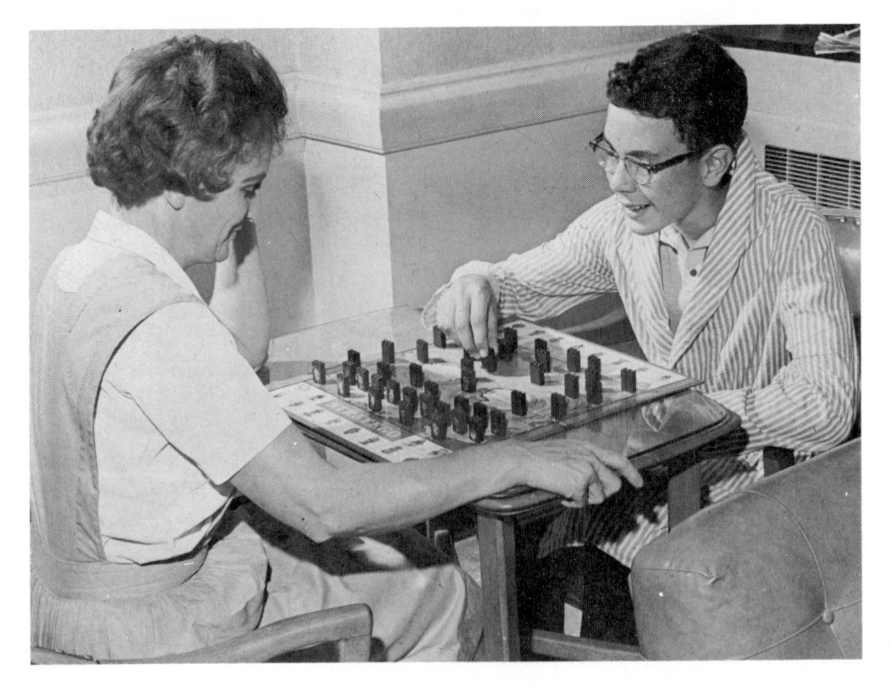

Fig. 13-2. The patient whose activities are limited usually appreciates some form of diversion to help pass the time. The teenage patient often is in an awkward situation, too old to be in pediatrics and too young to find companionship with his adult roommates. It is seldom that the nurse has enough time to play a game with him or to engage in some other pleasurable pastime. However, the nurse could plan for a volunteer or other assistant in nursing care to do this. Here, our young patient shows signs of having made a successful move.

Patients as Helpers. There was a time when patients were expected to help each other and to assist with work in health agencies when such work did not interfere with their recovery. However, using patients as helpers is uncommon today. In those agencies where this system has been used judiciously, the results have been impressive. For some patients, being able to help is gratifying and gives a feeling of personal accomplishment, besides relieving boredom. A few examples of things that patients can do to help are: acting as interpreter when language barriers occur, reading to patients who are unable to do so, making telephone calls for bedridden patients and writing letters for patients who are incapacitated.

Other Miscellaneous Diversions. Some agencies have facilities for swimming, movies, operating a radio station, canteens, auditoriums for social events, and the like. In general, it would seem that as facilities and opportunities for diversion increase, patients' attitudes toward health agencies would improve. Experiences in such places need not be as dreary and impersonal as was often the case in previous years.

It is true that not everyone wishes to keep himself occupied, even for a part of the time, with diversion or work. It is also true that nurses often cannot find the time to provide diversional activities for all patients. But there are times when nurses do have the opportunity to encourage patients in activities which they enjoy and in which they show an interest.

Study Situations

1. It was pointed out in this chapter that nurses may not always have sufficient time for providing activities for all patients. In the following article, note how volunteers working with nurses planned activities for homebound persons:

- Wilkiemeyer, D.: Unbinding the homebound.
  AMER. J. NURS., *66*:1803-1805, August, 1966.

How might volunteers or other nursing team personnel assist in a similar program when patients are still in a health agency?

2. The following article describes still another way in which volunteers were used to provide recreation for a group of mentally retarded children:

- Clark, J. W.: Volunteers in a new land.
  HOSP. J. AMER. HOSP. ASSOC., *40*:72-74, May 16, 1966.

Note that the agency held to the philosophy that retarded children were entitled to more than custodial care. How might a similar philosophy be applicable for agencies caring for the physically ill child?

3. Read the following article:

- Northrup, L.: Conferences mean better nursing.
  AMER. J. NURS., *66*:1342-1343, June, 1966.

Note in column three on page 1342 how diversion was planned for Mr. D. Indicate what purposes diversion served for this patient and what factors guided the selection of diversional activities.

4. For additional examples of how diversion was used purposefully to help patients, read the following article:

- Stevens, L. F.: Interventive nursing therapy.
  AMER. J. NURS., *64*:123-124, October, 1964.

Try to identify the cardinal aspects of nursing intervention for therapeutic purposes.

References

1. Asselmeier, D.: Pediatric unit *for* children. NURS. FORUM, *3*:81-95, #3, 1964.
2. Kurasik, S.: The need for recreational therapy in hospitals, nursing homes and homes for the aged. J. AMER. GERIAT. SOC., *13*:556-560, June, 1965.
3. Martin, S. E.: Party time in pediatrics. AMER. J. NURS., *66*:1770, August, 1966.
4. Nieters, S., and Forsyth, M.: Play is the business of children. AMER. J. NURS., *67*:2577, December, 1967.
5. Student nurses delight patients with "Fun in Fantasy." HOSP. TOPICS, *43*:65, November, 1965.
6. Toys at work. AMER. J. NURS., *65*:68-71, December, 1965.

Nursing Implementation: Man and His Environment

Unit 3

CHAPTER 14

Concept of a Safe Environment

Introduction

In Chapter 2, the discussion of environmental health indicated concern with everything about us—the air we breathe, our water and food supply, sewage disposal, and so forth. Although nursing is interested in, and concerned with, the environment of mankind and its effects on health, this Unit confines itself to the hospital environment.

The next chapter will consider maintaining a pleasant environment, the point being that a safe environment can also be an aesthetically pleasing one. The last chapter in this Unit discusses principles and practices that will aid in infection control.

Principles of infection control constitute a large part of this Unit. Other aspects of the environment affecting patient safety in the hospital are discussed later in the text. For example, restraints to prevent patients from hurting themselves are discussed in Unit Four. Safety in relation to administering medications is discussed in Unit Five. The safe use of various kinds of equipment is discussed along with the description of the equipment. The concept of protecting man from illness or injury is woven into the entire text. However, infection control underlies every nursing activity; therefore, it is presented early.

Hospital-Acquired Infections

Safe patient care in relation to infection control depends on the combined efforts of everyone. It has been estimated that the average cost of each hospital-acquired infection to all involved is approximately $400,000! Yet, investigations have shown that with the observance of basic sanitary practices, these infections could be substantially reduced or eliminated—a small price, it would seem, to prevent the costly result of what is often found to be carelessness and indifference.

Prior to approximately 1940, hospital personnel concerned themselves conscientiously with the dangers of infections communicated in hospitals and with methods to control and prevent their spread. When infections did occur, everyone scurried about with great dispatch to discover causes, and preventive and aseptic techniques were reviewed with scrutiny. The result was that infections communicated in hospitals were prevented with considerable success.

Then, the antibiotic era arrived. No one questions the value of chemotherapeutic agents, and since the discovery of antibiotics, many infections are treated effectively, quickly and easily. Hospital personnel did not necessarily assume that the discovery of chemotherapeutic agents was sufficient rationale for discarding all of the time-tested methods for preventing infections in hospitals. But changes did appear. Personnel in general tended to become somewhat careless about technic, and good technic, even though taught, was not carried out, because strict technics had been modified and replaced with more easygoing, less time-consuming methods.

There were sufficient early warnings that the repeated use of antibiotics could produce resistant strains of certain organisms, and everyone learned that these drugs were bacteriostatic, not bactericidal. But facts and warnings were often overlooked, and undue security based on the ability of antibiotics to take care of infections that were occurring, as well as to prevent them, was common. Widespread and often indiscriminate use of antibiotics occurred. The result was that antibiotic-resistant strains of at least one organism, staphylococcus, developed even faster than had been anticipated; and hospital-acquired infections came to constitute a world-wide problem.

Even though knowledge has advanced, there is still a lack of precision in controlling infections in the hospital environment. A single standard does not exist. In other words, there is no easy way to control hospital infections. To add to the complexity, people are among the weakest links in infection control. Medical science has developed fantastic weapons to fight many ills. But no one has found a cure for human indifference or carelessness.

Source and Spread of Infections. When hospital infections became more common, many persons asked whether these infections were communicated in the hospital; a common hunch was that patients had the infections before they were hospitalized and that after the patient was admitted the infections then reached clinical proportions, as a result of his being ill. In certain instances, this was no doubt the case. However, study findings also have indicated that it was doubtful indeed that many patients came to the hospital with subclinical infections. Furthermore, studies have illustrated that certain organisms are well adapted for creating cross-infections in the hospital environment. For example, one study reported that certain micrococci apparently are able to survive for months and even years in dust and bedding. Also, micrococci are sometimes present in the nasal passages of personnel and patients, without these persons necessarily always manifesting clinical signs of infection, and can be carried from person to person on blankets and mattresses, both of which are often cleansed in a haphazard fashion between patient uses. This same study found that the most vulnerable persons were debilitated patients, the newborn and those who had breaks in their skin, including even needle pricks received during the administration of intravenous therapy. Another study found that the hands of personnel most probably spread organisms among the newborn. Hospital floors also have been found to be a reservoir of infectious agents. Hospitals were finding that no clinical service and no age group was exempt from infections that were readily transmitted and often difficult to treat.

The Prevention and the Control of Infections. The increased prevalence of staphylococcal infections in hospitals has stimulated preventive efforts by all professional health workers. Professional periodicals as well as some of the popular lay magazines carry increasing amounts of information and suggestions concerning the dangers and the prevention of hospital infections. Uniformly, there is a plea for observing constant meticulous cleanliness, for a return to strict technics and for planned programs to aid in reducing infections.

Hospital Infection Committee. In 1958, the Joint Commission on Accreditation of Hospitals and the American Hospital Association jointly recommended that each hospital appoint a committee on infection control. It was also recommended that the committee have broad representation, including the nursing department. Since that time, many health agencies have followed the recommendation. These committees are charged with the responsibility of investigating all infections, establishing surveillance programs and providing leadership and guidance for the prevention and control of infections. They have worked well in many agencies to provide a safer hospital environment.

The importance of reporting infections in patients and in personnel to an infection committee cannot be over-emphasized. The nurse, as a member of the health team, has a responsibility for routine and prompt reporting in the manner established by the agency in which she is working or studying.

Hospital Population. No person in the hospital community can be exempt in a planned program to control the spread of infection. This includes patients, all hospital staff, students, visitors, auxiliary personnel and persons delivering items to patients. Thoughtful supervision and teaching become continuous processes to aid in attaining a safe environment for everyone. The role of the nurse as a teacher has already been pointed out in this text. In addition, by setting a good example in her own practice, the nurse transmits essential knowledge that helps to control hospital infections.

Environmental Sanitation. Most of the responsibility for environmental sanitation is delegated to departments other than nursing in a large percentage of health agencies. For example, the housekeeping department usually is responsible for cleaning the hospital building, including patients' rooms. The laundry cares for all linen and is responsible for its safe handling and care. Maintenance departments are charged with the responsibility of pest control. The dietary department takes care of sanitizing food service items. However, because the nurse understands the importance of sanitation, often she can assist in coordinating the efforts of many persons in making the hospital environment a safe one.

Study Situations

1. The American Journal of Nursing reported on an interview with the Matron of Groote Schuur Hospital in its April, 1968 issue, beginning on page 707. On pages 708 and 709, note the detailed precautions taken to prevent infection following heart transplantation. Why are patients having organ transplants especially susceptible to infection? Could you list additional reasons for high susceptibility?

2. The following article points up the seriousness of hospital-acquired infections:

- Hicks, J. T.: Hospital-acquired infections. Part 1—problems of environment.
  HOSP. MANAGE., *105*:27-31, January, 1968.

How was the cost of hospital-acquired infections arrived at? Which rooms, other than patient rooms, were found to harbor many organisms? How did the author account for the large number of organisms in these rooms?

3. Mention was made early in this chapter that a safe environment is concerned with more than infection control only. The following two articles describe factors, in addition to infection control, with which the nurse should be concerned in aiding to maintain a safe environment:

- Miller, R. R., and Johnson, S. R.: Poison control; now and in the future.
  AMER. J. NURS., *66*:1984-1987, September, 1966.
- Hymovich, D. P.: ABC's of pediatric safety.
  AMER. J. NURS., *66*:1768-1770, August, 1966.

References

1. Edgeworth, D.: Nursing and asepsis in the modern hospital.
   NURS. OUTLOOK, *13*:54-56, June, 1965.
2. Parisi, J. T.: Teaching infection control methods to ancillary service personnel.
   HOSP. J. AMER. HOSP. ASSOC., *42*:82-88, March 16, 1968.

CHAPTER 15

Maintaining a Safe and Pleasant Patient Unit

Although while we are constantly seeking for safety in the hospital environment, we also are interested in maintaining one which is as comfortable and as attractive as possible. Many factors in the hospital environment may not be within the nurse's control. Basic structures cannot be changed. However, occasionally nurses can make recommendations for desirable alterations, and frequently they are asked for suggestions when patients' units are being designed or furnished. Hence, there are times when nurses can aid in maintaining an aesthetic as well as a safe environment.

The Patient's Room

Walls and Floors. It is no longer considered necessary for a hospital room to be bare and "sterile-looking." White walls and white equipment are being replaced by more colorful furnishings and tastefully decorated walls. However, there is still need for careful planning in the use of color and design. It is best to use combinations that are attractive in an unobtrusive way, because unusual decor may appeal to relatively few people.

It has been found to be unsatisfactory to use wallpaper with a distinct design, such as large flowers, because during periods of illness some patients have been disturbed by designs, seeing faces and other objects in them. Pictures, bedspreads and curtains may have the same effect if not selected carefully.

Considerable attention also is being given to floor coverings. The cold, bare look is being replaced with attractive coverings. These, too, must be selected with care since parallel lines, tiny squares and some geometric designs cause some persons to feel dizzy when they look at them. Floor coverings must not only be durable but also able to withstand frequent cleaning. The floor usually is highly contaminated, and hence, solutions with germicidal properties are commonly used for routine floor cleaning.

In recent years carpeting has become more popular in hospitals. Patients and personnel in general find it aesthetically pleasing and comfortable. However, there still appears to be some difference in opinion as to whether carpeting can be cleansed sufficiently well so as to eliminate the danger of its becoming a haven for microorganisms.

Lighting. Good lighting, both natural and artificial, is another important environmental factor for the patients and the workers. While it is true that the nurse cannot alter windows or some lighting fixtures, certain modifications can be made. Light bulbs, shades or lamps can be requested if necessary and adjustments made so that what is available is put to best use.

Adequate lighting for work and reading is essential for the preservation of sight. The type of lighting used is important because of its effect on mood. Some lighting not only helps a person to feel cheerful, it also helps him look better. Other types of lighting (particularly "daylight" fluorescent bulbs) can do the reverse. Consultants in hospital architecture are emphasizing the importance of large, almost full-length windows that can be shaded as needed. In addition to providing much more natural light, they make it more pleasant for patients who enjoy looking out-of-doors.

An important point about lighting is that personnel in any health agency need far more light to see and to work effectively than do the patients. The glare from overhead lights or from windows that do not have shades partially drawn and the reflection from light objects, such as white uniforms and bed linen, can become almost intolerable to the person sitting in a chair or resting in bed. Older patients are particularly disturbed by lighting irregularities. While diffuse light in the room may be easier for personnel, it still may not be appropriate for the patient if he wishes to read. The light may be coming from such an undesirable angle that it is almost impossible for the patient to see comfortably close at hand. Ideally, a light at the patient's bed should be sufficiently adjustable so that it can serve the patient and also be used by nursing and medical personnel when needed for treatment of the patient.

A dim light is valuable as a comfort and a safety measure at night. The light should be situated so that it does not shine into the patient's eyes, no matter in what position he may wish to sleep. It should give sufficient lighting to the floor around the bed so that if the patient wishes to get up, he can do so with safety. Elderly persons are in particular need of some light at night, since this helps them to orient themselves should they awaken and be confused as to their whereabouts.

Temperature and Ventilation. Most well people are comfortable in a temperature range of 68° to 74° F. and with a humidity range of 30 to 60 per cent. However, illness may affect these comfort ranges, and the nurse will wish to make adjustments accordingly when possible. Older persons in general prefer a warmer room and usually are more sensitive to drafts than are younger people.

Many hospitals now have air conditioning, which is of great help in maintaining a comfortable environment. However, attention to the patient's covering and clothing is necessary, especially if the air circulating mechanism creates drafts.

The Furniture

Furniture now being sold for hospital use is often as attractive as any for the home. A trend which makes it more enjoyable and also safer for patients is to furnish units according to the type of care required by the patient. For example, self-care units furnished for the ambulatory patient have lower beds, desks, comfortable chairs and reading lamps, television sets and other homelike items. New units also often provide dining areas and cafeterias where patients may eat together.

Intensive care units are designed for the safety of the patient as well as for ease in caring for him. Comforts of everyday living are not as important in such units.

Home care for patients also is a part of the services of some health agencies. Nurses may be required to help arrange a functional unit in the home. This can be a challenge when it involves using the available furniture so as not to incur expenses. Both the patient's problems and the family's activities have to be considered in such planning.

The Bed. The bed frame should be made of a durable material having a finish that can withstand repeated washings and that will not chip. The height of a hospital bed, while of real concern to the patient, is determined by the requirements of those who must care for him. Early ambulation for patients, and also the current practice of encouraging patients into self-care activities as soon as possible, have led hospitals to purchase beds which can be lowered to a height more convenient for the patient getting in and out of bed by himself. If the height of the bed is not adjustable, a step stool should be provided in the unit for the patient's use. If a patient is to remain in bed for a long period of time at home, a hospital bed may be bought or rented; or the bed can be raised on solid objects, such as blocks of wood, for the convenience of those caring for him.

Most hospital beds have an adjustable headrest capable of being raised or lowered by means of a hand crank at the foot of the bed. In addition, the patient's knees may be flexed by means of another mechanism. The entire lower portion of the bed also may be raised so that both legs may be elevated at the same time. Usually, this is done by lifting the lower portion of the frame and supporting it by a metal prop.

Electrically operated beds are gaining in popularity. These beds can be placed in a variety of positions and at various heights with ease. Except for the switch that turns on the mechanism for operating the bed, the controls are mechanical on some, decreasing the danger of sparks or electrical shocks.

Hospital beds are constructed with small wheels usually with locks on them to prevent unintentional rolling. Some hospitals transport patients in their beds to other departments, eliminating the need for stretchers.

There are variations of the traditional hospital bed, which are discussed in Unit Four in connection with certain nursing care, an example being the rocking bed.

The Mattress. There is no one type of mattress recognized as being best for all situations and circumstances. A good mattress adjusts to body contours to the degree that it permits good alignment. A so-called "soft" mattress which permits the body to sag at points of heaviest weight is not conducive to rest—in fact, such a mattress may cause fatigue and backache.

As with the selection of a bed for use in the care of patients, the mattress should be able to withstand considerable use. If springs are a part of the mattress, they should be of superior structure and strength so that they will not break or lose their resilience easily. Broken springs are uncomfortable for the patient.

The covering of the mattress should be a quality material that will not tear easily or separate at the seams. It is not general practice to sterilize a mattress after each patient use. Since all mattresses have some filling, like horsehair, cotton or kapok, it is best to keep the mattress protected. Agencies having an infection control committee will have a procedure for caring for "contaminated" mattresses.

Mattresses with plasticized covering or plastic covers are also in use. Contamination of the mattress filling is reduced, and the mattress may be cleaned after use by washing. However, plastic covers have a disadvantage in that the smooth surface causes the linens to slip, especially when the head of the bed is elevated, and a contour sheet is not used.

A relatively new type of mattress on the market has a coil spring and a two-piece zippered cover. According to manufacturers' claims, the cover can be laundered or sterilized—an important factor in infection control. It is also waterproof and fire-retardant.

Foam rubber mattresses are useful in situations where pressure from a more rigid mattress may be harmful to the patient.

Pillows. Like mattresses, pillows may be filled with any one of a variety of materials and therefore vary in the comfort that they give. Usually, they are made of feathers, hair or kapok. Foam rubber pillows are in limited use, except by some persons who have allergies. A disadvantage is that they do not mold as easily as other pillows. Another disadvantage is that the rubber pillow, like the rubber mattress, is inclined to absorb and retain body heat.

In addition to the comfort that most persons derive from having a pillow under the head, pillows are extremely valuable in maintaining good posture for the bed patient. That is why variation in pillow sizes and type of filling is desirable.

Since pillows are used for all areas of the body for support and comfort, it is essential that they too be protected, for there is always the possibility of their becoming contaminated by secretions or drainage. They are always in close contact with the respiratory passages of the user; therefore, transmitting an infection from one person to another can occur unless care is taken. As a cardinal practice in good medical asepsis, pillows should be aired, vacuumed or sterilized after use. In addition, they should be protected by plastic coverings when used by a patient who has a respiratory infection.

Overbed Table. A great convenience for the patient is the overbed table, which enables him to eat, read, write or work more comfortably whether in or out of bed. The overbed table also makes it possible for him to change his position by leaning forward and resting on the table. It has conveniences for the nurse during the administration of treatments but its primary purpose is for the patient's use. A variety is available for purchase, but some tables have advantages over others. The type of overbed table which is supported by a wide foot piece that fits under the bed and has only one post has advantages when bed sides are in place or other cumbersome equipment is being used at the bedside. Most overbed tables are designed so that they can be lowered for the patient while he is in a chair and tilted to support a newspaper or a book. Some have mirrors underneath the tilt portion for the patients' use when they comb their hair, shave or apply make-up. Newer ones have space for storage of items such as make-up or shaving materials.

Small bed tables placed directly in the bed over the patient's thighs are used in some instances. They are particularly helpful in the home. In the care of children who are in cribs, such bed tables are very practical and useful.

The Bedside Stand. In the hospital, a bedside stand is provided for storing individual patient care equipment, and it is also a place for the patient to keep many of his personal items. While stands vary in size and shape, certain features are desirable for convenience and economy of time and effort for patients and nursing personnel. For example, stands which are designed without doors require less space than stands with doors. If the stand has three closed sides, the opened end of the table should be designed to be out of sight. The patient is able to manage the stand easily if it is mounted on wheels. A drawer in the table usually is used by the patient for his personal possessions; therefore, it should be placed so that it opens toward his bed. The inside of the stand usually is used for the storage of the washbasin, oral-hygiene equipment, soapdish, bedpan, urinal, bath blanket and possibly other items. Most stands have provisions for towels and a washcloth to hang on a rod.

There are additions which may be found on some stands such as a hook for the patient's urinal, a paper-bag frame and a "catch-all" which a patient may use for various purposes, such as holding occupational therapy projects, newspapers or magazines.

Bed Light or Lamps. Any number of styles of lighting fixtures are available, as a floor lamp or a bed lamp capable of being attached to the bed frame or a wall fixture above the bed. The light should be so arranged that the patient can control it himself. As mentioned previously, light intensity should vary with the work or the activity of the user. A lamp that has more than one bulb or a 3-way light bulb is ideal, since proper intensity is more likely to be obtained. Some lamps have a night light and a reading light—a desirable feature.

Chairs. Usually, a chair is included as an integral part of the patient's unit. A straight chair with good arm and back support usually is comfortable for the majority of patients. Leg heights of a chair can be managed for the very short patient by placing some suitable object underneath his feet.

Generally, chairs with arms are more comfortable for the patient, but it is also desirable to have chairs without arms available because they are more suitable when a patient must be lifted out of a bed into a chair. The arms do not get in the way of those lifting.

An upholstered chair has disadvantages for older patients and for patients who have some limitation of movement, because more effort is required to raise oneself out of it.

The Patient's Personal Care Equipment

The following are basic personal care items: basin, soapdish, mouthwash cup, emesis basin, bedpan and a urinal for the male patient.

Manufacturers provide wide selections of equipment for personal care that are both attractive and safe to use. Disposable equipment is becoming available in increasing varieties. This is an important factor in infection control. These disposable items also greatly reduce the work load of cleaning and sterilizing because they are intended for single patient use only.

If non-disposable personal care items are used, they must be of a quality to withstand frequent sterilization. This is discussed further in the next chapter.

Patient's Personal Items. Very few hospitals supply patients with such necessities as toothbrushes, combs, disposable tissues, shaving cream, razor blades and the like. Some do not supply soap or washcloths. The reasons are obvious when one considers cost, frequency of use and personal preferences. Kits containing many of the above items are being prepared commercially and sold in drugstores and hospital service shops.

Diversional Items. Items of equipment, hitherto considered as luxuries, are increasingly regarded as necessities, namely, the telephone, the radio and the television. No one wants to deny the patient these items, but they *can* become hazards. Wiring on the floor, frayed cords, loose plugs and television stands in doorways must be the concern of everyone if the environment is to be kept safe. Their proper cleansing after use, especially the telephone, is essential.

Privacy and Quiet

Privacy. An environmental essential of particular importance to most patients is provision for privacy. Anyone who is being interviewed, examined or treated, as well as anyone who is receiving care, deserves and appreciates the comfort of privacy. It is very easy for nurses and for others to begin to feel that anything routine to them is also accepted as routine by the patient. Many patients are reluctant to question any lack of privacy. Persons caring for patients, whether in a clinic, a home or a hospital, always should try to provide as much privacy as is possible.

Quiet. This is another essential concern to both worker and patient. Unnecessary noise and other disturbances have their bearing on a patient's reaction to his illness, to those caring for him and to the agency with which the patient associates them. Considerable ingenuity has gone into designing posters and signs for use in hospital corridors and waiting rooms to help reduce noise created not only by visitors but also by hospital personnel.

Buildings that are being constructed or remodeled have considerably less noise because of the use of many acoustic materials.

These are some of the noises that patients complain about most frequently: careless handling of equipment in service areas and of dishes and trays on serving carts and in the kitchen; loud talking on the telephone, in the nurses' station and during rounds; calling down the corridors; talking by visitors who are not permitted to be in with the patient but gather elsewhere near other patients or in the corridors; loud radios, television and the call system. Many if not all of these noises can be controlled to a great extent, but it takes constant awareness on the part of the nurse to see that they are.

Remember that the sick are more sensitive to noise than are well persons.

Never underestimate what patients can hear. Conversations at nurses' stations or in the corridors can be heard by patients who have little more to do than just absorb what is going on about them. Unfortunately, they may misinterpret what they hear and may become unnecessarily concerned with their welfare.

Study Situations

1. There are periodicals concerned with hospitals, their structure, furnishings and services. Browsing through them will be valuable for the nurse to see what is new, what changes other agencies are making and the effect that some of the new items or proposed changes might have on patient care.

Look through recent issues of the periodicals listed below for evidence of trends in furnishings, equipment, and so on. Note also how authors and advertisers stress safety factors in the patient environment.

Hospitals, Journal of the American Hospital Association
The Modern Hospital
Hospital Topics
Hospital Management

2. The following article is concerned with lighting in the entire hospital. How should lighting vary from one area to another? What consideration should be given to the nurse's control over light intensity for various types of patients?

- Ludwig, D. J., and Humphrey, A.: Light—the hospital's ally.
  Hosp. Topics, *42*:53-54, March, 1964.

3. A safe environment is one that is also kept free of fire hazards. Measures for fire prevention, fire drills, instruction in how to use safety features such as fire doors, emergency exits, sprinklers, etc. are usually a part of an agency's fire preventive program. Most agencies require that all personnel have such instruction. However, additional helpful ideas can be gained from the following article. What are the two chief causes of fire? What implications does this have for nursing?

- Morris, E. M.: In case of fire emergencies. Amer. J. Nurs., *68*:1496-1499, July, 1968.

CHAPTER

16

Using Principles of Infection Control

STERILIZATION AND DISINFECTION

Definitions

Asepsis is the absence of disease-producing microorganisms, called *pathogens*. *Nonpathogens,* constantly present in the environment or on the host, are microorganisms that do not cause disease. The *host* is an animal or a person upon which or within which microorganisms live.

Asepsis generally is divided into two descriptive forms: medical asepsis and surgical asepsis. Concepts of medical and surgical asepsis and related terms as used in this text are based on the following definitions.

Medical asepsis refers to practices which help to reduce the number and hinder the transfer of disease-producing microorganisms from one person or place to another. The reason for observing medical aseptic practices is that there are always microorganisms in the environment which in some individuals and under certain circumstances can cause illness. Therefore, reducing their number and hindering their transfer increase the safety of the environment. Any number of methods may be used to help to achieve this aim: dusting, vacuuming, washing, boiling, sterilizing and disinfecting are a few examples.

The efforts to help keep an environment as safe as possible come not alone from skilled health personnel, but also from all individuals in society as well as local, state and national governments and certain international agencies. Such efforts include mass immunization programs, laws concerning safe sewage disposal, regulations concerning the control of certain communicable diseases as tuberculosis, venereal diseases, and the like.

Generally speaking, medical asepsis practices are followed at all times because it is assumed that pathogens are likely to be present, the exact kind being undetermined. For example, public drinking cups are unsanitary, because pathogens may be present on the cup after use by someone harboring the organisms. On the other hand, there are times when a specific pathogen is known to be present in the environment; for instance, the German measles virus is known to be present in and on the patient having the disease, and also in his environment. In such instances, additional precautions are taken to prevent further spread of this particular organism, a procedure generally referred to as *isolation or communicable disease technic.* Isolation technic includes the use of specific measures in addition to ordinary medical aseptic practices. An example of a specific measure is the use of a gown worn by personnel caring for the patient. Isolation technic is discussed more fully later in this chapter.

Surgical asepsis refers to practices which render and keep objects and areas free from *all* microorganisms (sterile). It is concerned with the handling of objects and areas which must be kept sterile. It is used extensively in operating and delivery rooms. Surgical asepsis is employed when there is need to keep an area free from microorganisms. For example, the sterile gown and the sterile gloves that the surgeon wears during an operation protect the patient from being contaminated by the surgeon; the forceps used in handling sterile dressings protect the patient from contamination by the fingers.

Contamination refers to the process by which something is rendered unclean or unsterile. In medical asepsis, areas are considered to be contaminated if they bear, or are suspected of bearing, pathogens. In surgical asepsis, areas are considered to be contaminated if they are touched by *any* object which is not also sterile. In medical asepsis, the gown worn by the nurse or the coverall apron worn by a mother when caring for a child who has measles is to protect the nurse and the mother from contamination by the child.

A *bacteriostatic agent* prevents the growth of microorganisms. A *bactericidal agent* is one that is capable of destroying microorganisms.

Disinfection refers to the process by which pathogenic organisms (but not spores) are destroyed.

Sterilization refers to the process by which all microorganisms, including spores, are destroyed. It usually refers to methods involving the use of heat, such as boiling, steam under pressure and dry heat, but chemicals may be used also. Chemical methods of sterilization are not considered as reliable as physical methods.

Disinfectant refers to a substance used to destroy infectious or contagious agents. It is not intended to be used for destroying pathogens in or on the living person.

Antiseptic refers to a substance which inhibits the growth of microorganisms. Certain antiseptics can be used safely on the living person.

While sterilization is an integral part of surgical asepsis (sterile technic), there are innumerable instances when it is also an integral part of medical asepsis. When working against unknown pathogens, there are occasions when it is best to use measures which can be relied on to destroy all microorganisms in order to be safe. In the hospital, personal-care items which are used by patients are sterilized by boiling or steam under pressure before being offered to another patient. It is possible that the items could be made safe by washing with soap and water and rinsing well. However, since the exact nature of the contaminants is not known, it is safer to use additional precautionary measures.

One of the most important things to remember about surgical or medical asepsis is that their effectiveness is dependent on the faithfulness and the conscientiousness of those carrying them out. The failure to be exact and meticulous cannot be detected in many instances. For example, an article such as a glass, a comb, a syringe or a needle can be cleaned superficially or not even sterilized, and no one except the person responsible would really know.

Handling and Caring for Supplies and Equipment

Central Supply Units. Most hospitals in the United States maintain a central supply unit where a major portion of the equipment used in patient care is cleansed, kept in good working order and sterilized. Usually, these units are administered by nurses who are assisted by auxiliary personnel. Safety to the patient has increased as hospitals have found it economically feasible to purchase equipment for a central supply unit that could not be purchased separately for all divisions of the hospital. More nursing time is available for patient care when responsibility for cleaning and sterilizing equipment and for preparing trays for procedures has been delegated to personnel in central supply units. Also, equipment usually receives better care from persons especially taught and employed to care for it.

Disposable Equipment. In recent years, health agencies have begun using more disposable items that are sterile and ready for use. Certain items, such as scalpels, are used only for one surgical procedure and then discarded. Other items, such as bedpans, may be used repeatedly but by one patient only and then discarded upon his discharge. Almost monthly, hospital periodicals report new disposable equipment as it appears on the market. The use of such equipment has not only greatly decreased the amount of time involved in cleaning, repairing and sterilizing equipment but also has reduced problems in relation to hospital-acquired infections.

Trends toward the development of central supply units and the manufacturing of disposable items have changed many responsibilities once assumed by nurses. However, in many situations and especially in homes, nurses are responsible for the care of equipment and supplies and, therefore, need to have a good knowledge of sterilization technics.

Procedures for sterilizing and disinfecting equipment and supplies are based largely on principles of microbiology. Certain of those which affect the choice of sterilization and disinfection procedures will be reviewed briefly.

Principles Used in the Selection of Sterilization and Disinfection Methods

Nature of Organisms Present. Certain microorganisms are destroyed with considerable ease, while others are able to withstand certain commonly used sterilization and disinfection technics. Bacterial spores are particularly resistant and can withstand many germicides that readily destroy other types of organisms. *Mycobacterium tuberculosis*, the organism responsible for tuberculosis infections, is reported also to be resistant to many aqueous disinfectants including Zephiran Chloride.

Although not a great deal is known about transferring viruses by means of contaminated supplies and equipment, there are two notable exceptions: it is agreed generally that homologous serum hepatitis and infectious hepatitis viruses can be spread by the use of contaminated needles and syringes. The organisms causing the diseases can be spread with such ease that a simple prick of the skin with a contaminated needle may result in illness. Studies indicate also that the viruses causing these conditions are destroyed with certainty only by autoclaving (steam under pressure).

If the nature of the organisms on equipment and supplies is known, the selection of a safe sterilization or disinfection procedure becomes relatively easy. Unfortunately, however, in most situations where many patients with various illnesses are being cared for, the nature of organisms contaminating equipment and supplies frequently is unknown; and it would be an exceedingly difficult and impractical procedure to determine the nature of all contaminating organisms present. Therefore, when medical asepsis is being practiced, the safest method is one that can be assumed to be capable of destroying the pathogenic microorganisms. If surgical asepsis is being practiced, the only safe procedure is one that has been proved capable of destroying all organisms, regardless of their nature. It is unwise to decrease the period of time that has been considered safe for sterilizing or disinfecting equipment and supplies on the assumption that the contaminating organisms present are destroyed easily. *Time* is a key factor in sterilization or in disinfection. Anyone who fails to allow sufficient time for sterilization or disinfection is guilty of gross negligence!

In the home, where the nature of contaminating organisms occasionally may be ascertained with some certainty and where the patient may have developed immunities to certain organisms commonly found in his environment, sterilization and disinfection procedures can be modified more safely than they can in a health agency.

Number of Organisms Present. The more organisms that are present on an article, the longer it takes to destroy them. For example, an instrument that is contaminated with relatively few organisms can be rendered sterile more quickly than one contaminated with large numbers of organisms. If organisms are protected by coagulated proteins or harbor under a layer of grease or oil, it will also take longer to sterilize or disinfect the article. Articles that are cleansed thoroughly prior to sterilization or disinfection therefore will be made sterile or clean more

Table 3. Theoretical example of the order of death of a bacterial population*

Minute	Bacteria Living at Beginning of New Minute	Bacteria Killed in 1 Minute	Bacteria Surviving at End of 1 Minute
First	1,000,000	90% = 900,000	100,000
Second	100,000	= 90,000	10,000
Third	10,000	= 9,000	1,000
Fourth	1,000	= 900	100
Fifth	100	= 90	10
Sixth	10	= 9	1
Seventh	1	= 0.9	0.1
Eighth	0.1	= 0.09	0.01
Ninth	0.01	= 0.009	0.001
Tenth	0.001	= 0.0009	0.0001
Eleventh	0.0001	= 0.00009	0.00001
Twelfth	0.00001	= 0.000009	0.000001

* From Perkins, J. J.: Principles and Methods of Sterilization, p. 35. Springfield, Ill., Thomas, 1956.

easily and more quickly than an article that has not been cleansed.

Bacteriologists have found that bacteria exposed to sterilization procedures die in a uniform and consistent manner. The rate of death has been found to be governed by definite laws, so that computation of death rates of bacteria are possible. Theoretically, 90 per cent of the bacteria are killed each minute of exposure. Table 3 illustrates a theoretical example of the order of death of a bacterial population; the order of death is said to be logarithmic in nature.

Knowledge of bacterial death has important practical implications, and some bacteriologists maintain that this knowledge is applicable for heat sterilization, chemical disinfection and pasteurization.

Type of Equipment. Equipment with a small lumen, crevices or joints that are difficult to cleanse and to expose requires special care. For example, if catheters are being placed in a chemical solution, disinfection will be ineffectual if the solution does not fill the lumen of the catheters. It also must be kept in mind that certain pieces of equipment are destroyed by various sterilization and disinfection methods. For example, certain chemical solutions will dull the cutting edge of a knife blade. In using any disinfectant for such a purpose, the student should read the directions carefully. Most common sterilization and disinfection methods will ruin lens mountings in instruments such as cystoscopes. Such equipment requires special handling in order to keep it in good condition.

Intended Use of Equipment and Supplies. If equipment and supplies are being used when medical asepsis is practiced, it is sufficiently safe for them to be free of pathogenic organisms. But when surgical asepsis is required, equipment and supplies must be free of *all* organisms. Therefore, the intended use of equipment and supplies will influence the selection of a particular procedure for rendering the equipment safe.

In most hospitals today, in order to ensure safety for the patient, almost all articles used for patient care are sterilized prior to use. The nature of contamination is not always certain, as has been pointed out, and, even though in some instances it may be safe to use equipment that is clean, most hospitals follow a policy of using, whenever possible, only sterilized equipment and supplies for patient care.

Available Means for Sterilization and Disinfection. Sterilization and disinfection may be accomplished by several methods. Chemical sterilization (or disinfection) is accomplished by using solutions or gases (vapors) that destroy bacteria by chemical processes. Physical sterilization (or disinfection) usually is accomplished by the use of dry or moist heat.

Within recent years cold sterilization and disinfection through the use of ionization radiation have been investigated, but the extent to which they can be used has not yet been determined thoroughly. While considerable and encouraging advance has been made in this field, especially since World War II, much research remains to be done. Sterilizing by ionizing radiation holds great promise for the cold sterilization of heat-resistant pharmaceuticals and foods.

Ultraviolet radiation has been found to have germicidal results. It can be used as an effective agent for disinfecting indoor air and working surfaces. Ultraviolet irradiation has been especially recommended as an additive to operating-room technic. It also has been used for disinfecting working counters in laboratories, hospital rooms and elevators.

Chemical Means for Sterilization and Disinfection

Chemical sterilization employs liquid solutions or gases. Objects to be sterilized are immersed in a solution or exposed to fumes in a chamber or oven for a specified period of time. Various studies have found serious shortcomings in the use of chemicals for sterilizing purposes. In fact, some authorities state that no chemical solution can be considered completely safe for sterilization. Hence, their use ordinarily is limited to items that are heat-labile or to situations where a more reliable method is not available.

A chemical becoming more popular for sterilization is ethylene oxide gas. The gas destroys microorganisms by interfering with metabolic processes in cells and it has been found to effect lethal action on spores as well as vegetative cells. Optimal action can be attained at relatively low temperatures (130° to 150° F.) when humidity in the sterilizer is held between approximately 30 to 60 per cent. Its penetrating qualities are excellent. Although heat is a reliable and economical sterilizing agent, ethylene oxide has been found by institutions using it to be excellent for any heat-labile item, including rubber, plastic and paper.

Commonly used chemicals for disinfection purposes are discussed in other courses for nurses; hence, no attempt will be made to describe them here. The reader's attention is called to the first Study Situation at the end of this chapter, which will effect a good review for evaluating chemical disinfectants.

Physical Means for Sterilization and Disinfection

Physical sterilization and disinfection usually are accomplished by using heat, the most common methods being (1) steam under pressure, (2) boiling water, (3) free-flowing steam or (4) dry heat.

Dry heat kills organisms by an oxidation process, while moist heat coagulates protein within the cell. Sterilization and disinfection occur when heat is sufficient to destroy organisms, and, the higher the temperature, the more quickly organisms will die. Therefore, an essential factor for heat sterilization and disinfection is that equipment and supplies be exposed to the heat properly. Overloading a sterilizer or packing it in such a manner that equipment and supplies are not exposed to the heat defeats the effectiveness of the process. In the following discussion of various types of heat sterilizers, the recommended times for sterilization are based on the assumption that the packages are prepared properly and sterilizers loaded properly so that the contents are exposed to heat adequately.

Steam Under Pressure. Moist heat in the form of saturated steam under pressure is the most dependable means known for the destruction of all forms of microbial life. Steam is water vapor, and in the saturated state it can exist only at a definite pressure corresponding to a given temperature. The

Table 4. Atmospheric pressure, boiling point of water, gauge pressure at 121° C. (250° F.) and temperature when pressure is 15.12 pounds per square inch, at various altitudes*

Height Above Sea Level (feet)	Atmospheric Pressure (lbs. per sq. in.)	Boiling Point of Water ° F.	Gauge Pressure at 250° F.	Autoclave Temperature with Gauge at 15.12 Pounds	Time Factor†
0000	14.70	212.0	15.12	250.0	1.000
1,000	14.24	210.2	15.58	249.1	1.118
2,000	13.78	208.5	16.04	248.1	1.248
3,000	13.32	206.8	16.50	247.4	1.395
4,000	12.86	205.0	16.96	246.4	1.560
5,000	12.40	203.2	17.42	245.4	1.742
6,000	11.94	201.5	17.88	244.5	1.950
8,000	11.08	198.0	18.74	242.6	2.440
10,000	10.28	194.5	19.54	241.0	3.050
12,000	9.48	191.0	20.34	239.2	3.800
14,000	8.68	185.5	21.14	237.4	4.780

* Adapted from Beckett, John S., and Berman, Phoebus: Sterilization and Disinfection: With Special Emphasis on Autoclave Sterilization: A Handbook for Nurses, pp. A3-2C, North Hollywood, Calif., A.T.I. Pub. Div. 1953.

† Amount of time required for sterilization at sea level multiplied by time factor compensates for the difference, depending on altitude, in the temperature of the boiling point of water and the temperature within steam pressure sterilizers when the pressure gauge is at 15.12 pounds. For example, if at sea level it takes 10 minutes to sterilize an article, at 5,000 feet above sea level it will take 10 minutes × 1.742 or 17.42 minutes.

amount of pressure has nothing to do with the destruction of bacteria. It is the higher temperature resulting from higher pressure that destroys bacteria.

The autoclave is a pressure steam sterilizer. Most hospitals and many clinics and offices are equipped with pressure steam sterilizers today. Texts dealing with sterilization describe their operation in detail.

Many homes today have pressure cookers that operate on the same principle as pressure steam sterilizers. Foods cooked in a pressure cooker can be prepared more quickly because of the higher temperature attained by steam under pressure. Pressure cookers can be used for sterilizing equipment in the home by placing articles for sterilization on a rack or a screen above the level of water in the cooker.

The amount of time necessary to expose equipment and supplies in a pressure steam sterilizer in order to assure sterility depends on several factors: the type of equipment or supplies to be sterilized, the mannner in which they are wrapped or packaged, the way in which the sterilizer is packed, and the temperature and the pressure maintained.

It will be recalled that the temperature and not the pressure is the factor responsible for destruction of microbes. As altitude increases, a higher gauge pressure is needed in order to reach a specific temperature; and in mountainous areas persons operating pressure steam sterilizers must take this fact into consideration in order to secure sterilization.

Table 4 illustrates the effect of altitude on the boiling point of water and on steam pressure. Housewives who live in mountainous areas are aware of this difference when they find that they must cook foods longer than is necessary at sea level. Consideration for altitude becomes an important factor in sterilization procedures, as Table 4 clearly illustrates.

Dry Heat. Dry-heat or hot-air sterilization is accomplished by using equipment similar to an ordinary baking oven. Electrically heated hot-air sterilizers are preferred, since they are more reliable and more nearly accurate than other types of dry-heat ovens. Dry heat is a good method of sterilizing sharp instruments and syringes, since moist heat damages the cutting edges of sharp instruments and the ground-glass surfaces of syringes. It is also the preferred method for sterilizing needles, since the needles remain dry, and stylets, if they are used, may be left in place safely. Altitude does not affect hot-air sterilizers.

The nature of the articles, the manner in which articles are wrapped or packaged and the way in which a hot-air sterilizer is loaded will influence the time required for sterilization. Many authorities agree that, for most articles, sterilization occurs when a temperature of 160° C. (320° F.) is maintained for 1 hour or preferably 2 hours.

For equipment and supplies that will not tolerate a temperature of 160° C. (320° F.), a longer period of time at lower temperatures is required.

Boiling Water. Placing equipment in boiling water for a period of time is a common method of sterilization and disinfection. However, if spores are present on equipment, boiling water is not a practical method of sterilization, since the temperature of the water cannot rise above 100° C. (212° F.). Some spores are exceedingly resistant, and time required to kill susceptible spores is too long and too unspecific. Also, some viruses are resistant to boiling. Therefore, the nature of the organism determines the length of time required for boiling.

Clean equipment can be sterilized in boiling water in a matter of several minutes, while dirty equipment will take longer. Most authorities agree that equipment contaminated with vegetative forms of bacteria can be sterilized if submerged in boiling water for 10 to 20 minutes. These recommended periods of time are based on the assumptions that the equipment is immersed, the sterilizer is loaded properly, and the time is determined from the moment the water begins to boil.

Sometimes trisodium phosphate or sodium carbonate is added to water in which equipment is to be boiled. These chemicals help to remove grease under which organisms may harbor and also decrease the time needed for sterilization and disinfection by increasing the "wetting power" of water. When an alkali is added to water, 15 minutes usually is considered to be a sufficient period for boiling.

Equipment that will rust in water can be damaged easily by this method of sterilization and disinfection. Rusting can be minimized if the equipment is placed in the water only after it has boiled briskly for a few minutes. Boiling the water drives off dissolved oxygen; therefore, rusting, which is the result of oxidation, is minimized in boiled water.

Altitude must be taken into consideration when equipment and supplies are sterilized or disinfected by boiling. Table 4 indicates the boiling point of water at various levels. In higher altitudes, the boiling time must be increased, since the temperature necessary to boil water is lower as altitude increases.

Free-Flowing Steam. The temperature of free-flowing steam is 100° C. (212° F.) at sea level. Therefore, free-flowing steam for sterilization and disinfection should be used for the same period of time as boiling water. The free-flowing steam method has limited practical use, since it is difficult to load a free-flowing steam sterilizer in such a way that all equipment is exposed fully to the steam.

"Emergency Sterilization." There are occasions, as in an emergency, when there is insufficient time to wait the prescribed length of time for the sterilization or disinfection method. The usual procedure is to shorten the recommended period of time for sterilization or disinfection. Some persons call this an "emergency sterilization procedure." When the sterilization or disinfection time is shortened, the persons responsible for the decision must understand that a risk has been taken, that sterilization may not have been accomplished, but that the nature of the emergency warrants it.

Cleaning Supplies and Equipment

In the previous discussion, mention was made several times concerning the cleansing of equipment and supplies prior to sterilization and disinfection. Proper cleansing is important, since organisms embedded in organic material or protected under a layer of fat or grease are difficult to destroy. Furthermore, cleansing reduces the number of organisms present, and, as has been pointed out, the fewer the organisms present the easier it is to sterilize or disinfect equipment.

Persons cleaning equipment should wear water-proof gloves if the articles are contaminated with highly pathogenic materials or if there are skin abrasions on the hands. A brush with stiff bristles is an important aid for cleaning equipment, which should be done in water with soap or with a detergent.* If equipment is contaminated with organic materials, such as blood or pus, soaking in cold water with a detergent prior to washing will help to make the cleansing procedure easier. The brush, the gloves (if used) and the basin in which the equipment is cleaned should be considered as being contaminated and treated and cleansed accordingly.

Following thorough cleansing, equipment should be rinsed well and that which will rust should be dried carefully. At the same time, equipment should be examined to see that each piece is in good working order. Cleansing equipment should be done as soon after use as possible, since organic materials that are allowed to dry increase the difficulty with which equipment is cleansed and increases the likelihood of transfer of organism by air-currents.

When equipment has been cleansed thoroughly, it is ready for sterilization or disinfection.

Monel and Enamelware. Steam under pressure is the preferred method of sterilizing monel and enamelware. Dry heat also may be used. Boiling is satisfactory.

Usually, bedpans and urinals are made of monel or enamelware, and, after the contents have been removed and the equipment rinsed, they should be washed and handled in the same manner as other similar ware.

Many hospitals provide equipment designed specifically to clean bedpans and urinals. A common misconception is that all bedpan

* Except for equipment contaminated by organisms in body secretions containing proteins which are coagulated by heat, warm water is more effective than cold water as a cleaning agent because of its lower surface tension.

flushers are sterilizers. In some instances the manufacturer has labeled them as such. The mechanism flushes the contents and then releases free-flowing steam on the bedpans for a period of 1 to 2 minutes. Such equipment has been found to be satisfactory for the care of bedpans and urinals when sterilization is not necessary. However, with current concern for means by which some virus infections are transmitted, it seems that this method of caring for bedpans requires scrutiny. If the flusher is used for bedpans from many patients, cross-infection may occur, since certain viruses are not destroyed by short periods of exposure to live steam.

Glassware. Brushes especially designed to clean lumens and barrels are particularly desirable. It is important to disassemble syringes immediately after use in order to prevent the barrel and the plunger from locking. Syringes should be rinsed thoroughly and soaked so that contents will not dry in the barrel and make cleansing difficult. Steam under pressure is recommended for sterilizing glassware. Boiling is the usual method in the home, as, for example, the syringe used by a diabetic patient.

Instruments. Great care should be taken to cleanse grooves, crevices and serrated surfaces where organisms frequently harbor. Following cleansing, instruments should be dried carefully to prevent rusting.

Instruments that do not have a cutting

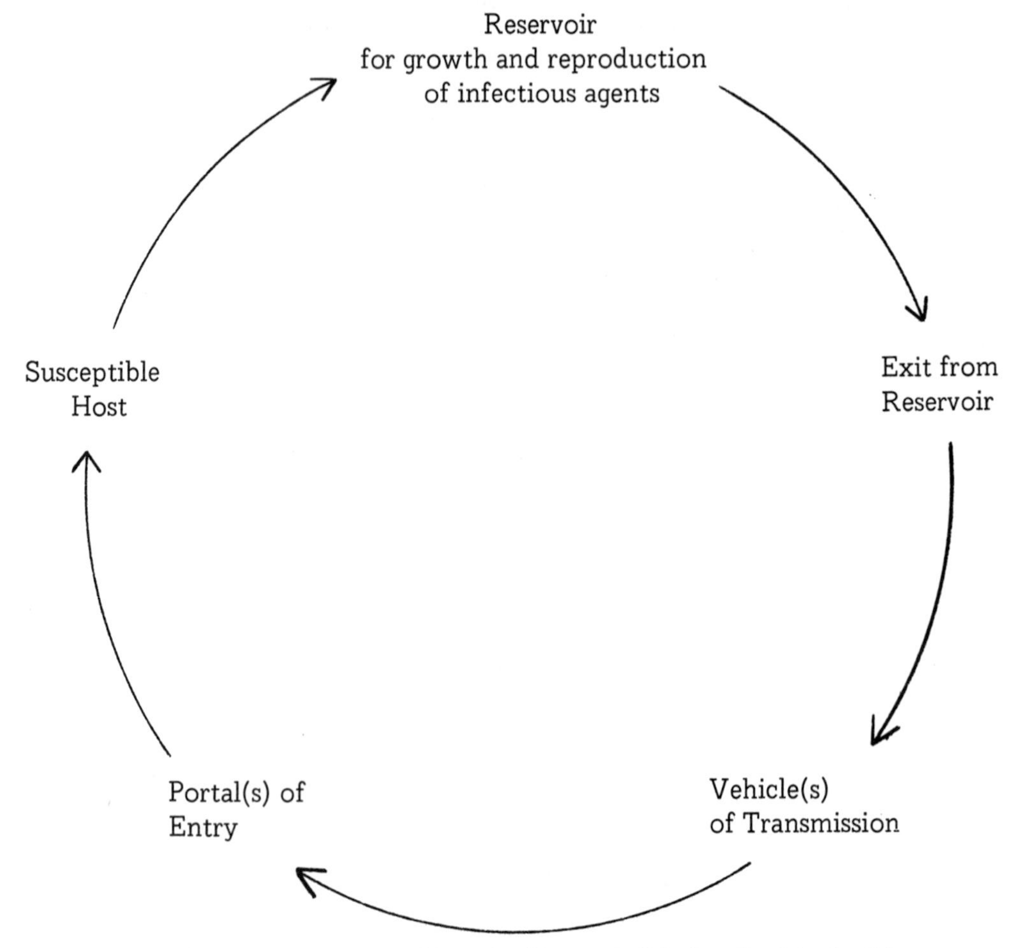

FIG. 16-1. An infection occurs as a result of interrelated factors. An infection will not develop if the sequence is interrupted. Hence, efforts to control infections are directed toward interrupting the sequence.

edge should be sterilized in a pressure steam sterilizer. Instruments with a cutting edge should be sterilized by using dry heat. For certain purposes, chemicals are used.

Needles (Other Than Suture Needles). Because of their small lumen, needles present a cleansing problem. Immediately after use, cold water should be forced through the needle with a syringe in order to rinse out contents in the lumen. Forcing alcohol or ether through the lumen will aid to remove fatty or oily substances.

Dry heat is the preferred method of sterilizing needles. Steam under pressure is also a satisfactory method. Boiling is used when the other methods are not available.

Rubber and Plastic Goods. Catheters should be rinsed thoroughly immediately following use; soaking for short periods of time also will aid in cleaning them. A soap or detergent solution should be forced through the lumen until the lumen has been cleansed thoroughly. The transparent plastic catheters make it easier to determine when the catheter is clean of gross soilage. Rubber or plastic tubing should be rinsed immediately following use.

Steam under pressure is preferred for sterilizing rubber goods. Dry heat may be used for certain types. If chemicals are used, care should be taken so that the solution fills the lumen in order that the lumen will be disinfected. Ethylene oxide gas, where available, may be used for rubber and plastic items.

MEDICAL AND SURGICAL ASEPSIS

Principles Used in Practices of Medical and Surgical Asepsis

There are two basic principles underlying practices of medical and surgical asepsis.

Certain microorganisms are capable of causing illness in man.

Microorganisms harmful to man can be transmitted by means of his direct or indirect contact with them.

Figure 16-1 illustrates the infectious process. Good practices of medical and surgical asepsis depend on observing the principles given above and include efforts to interrupt the sequence of the infectious process.

The role of sterilization and disinfection in relation to practices of asepsis has been discussed. Additional practices of medical and surgical asepsis will be covered in the remainder of this chapter. Attention also will be called to the reader to still more such practices throughout this text.

Bacterial Flora of the Hands

In 1938, Price, a noted researcher in the area of skin bacteriology, published a summary of studies conducted to determine the bacterial flora normally found on the hands. He pointed out two types—one called *transient* flora or bacteria, the other called *resident* flora or bacteria.

Transient bacteria are relatively few on clean and exposed areas of the skin. Usually, they are picked up by the hands in the normal activities of living and working; therefore, the type and the nature of the organisms will depend largely on the nature of work in which each individual is engaged. For example, a librarian may have many organisms on his hands that also can be found readily on books and papers. Similarly, one who has handled a dressing soaked with drainage may find organisms on her hands similar to those found in the drainage of the wound. Transient bacteria are attached loosely to the skin, usually in grease, fats and dirt, and are found in greater numbers under the fingernails. Transient bacteria, pathogenic as well as nonpathogenic, can be removed with relative ease by washing the hands thoroughly and frequently.

Resident bacteria are relatively stable in number and type. They are found in the creases and the crevices of the skin, and it is believed that they cling to the skin by adhesion and adsorption. Resident flora cannot be removed easily from the skin by washing with soap and water unless considerable friction also is applied with a brush, and they are less susceptible to the action of antiseptics than are transient flora. Some of them are embedded so deeply in the skin that they do not appear in washings until the skin has been scrubbed for 15 minutes or longer.

For practical purposes, it is not considered possible to cleanse the skin of all bacteria.

It was found also that transient flora may adjust to the environment of the skin if the flora are present in large numbers over a long enough period of time; they then become resident flora. For example, if one handles contaminated materials over a period of time, the organisms in the materials, although originally transient in nature, may become resident flora on the hands. If such flora contain pathogenic organisms, the hands may become carriers of the particular organisms. To prevent transient flora from becoming resident flora, it is important that the hands be cleansed promptly after each contact with contaminated materials, and especially if the materials contain pathogenic organisms. Since nurses in the course of their work often handle materials contaminated with pathogenic organisms, the importance of frequent and thorough hand washing becomes evident.

Soap and Detergents and Water as Cleansing Agents

Because soap and detergents lower the surface tension of water and act as emulsifying agents, they are good cleansing agents when used with water.

Soaps that are made with sodium salts

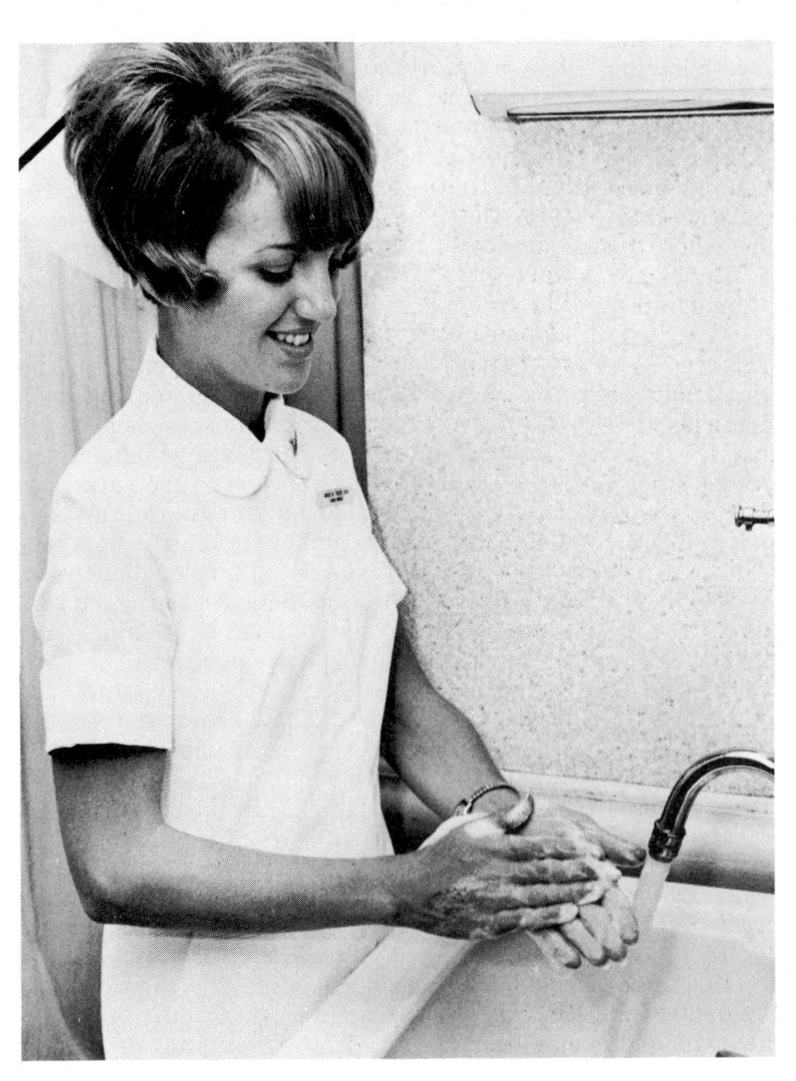

Fig. 16-2. As innumerable studies will bear out, the single most important factor in the prevention of hospital infections is good hand washing technic. It applies to all contacts of health personnel with patients. Its importance cannot be overemphasized. (Photo by Warren R. Vroom)

are hard soaps, while soft soaps are made with potassium salts. Glycerol is removed in the process of making hard soaps but is retained in soft soaps.

When soap is used in hard water, an insoluble flaky precipitate is formed when the salts of soap react with the salts found in hard water, and the reaction of the two salts makes the soap ineffectual as a cleansing agent. However, soap used with soft water is an invaluable cleansing agent.

Detergents are popular as cleansing agents. One type is the sulfonated detergents—for example, Dreft—so named because they are sulfates. The other type is the quaternary ammonium detergents which are chemically related to ammonium salts—for example, Zephiran. Detergents are effective in hard water since their salts do not react with the salts found in hard water, and they will lather readily in water of any temperature. The quaternary ammonium detergents have been found also to have some disinfectant action.

Price used various types of soap in his studies on skin cleansing. He experimented with green soap, institutional soap, castile soap and several popular toilet soaps. None of these soaps had a germicidal agent added. His studies, and other studies also, have found that all the soaps cleansed the hands equally well, and that, although certain toilet soaps may leave a pleasing odor on the skin, their cleansing effect is enhanced neither by the perfumes added nor by their price.

Since hospital-acquired infections have become a problem, it is often recommended that soaps and detergents containing a germicide be used in the hand-washing technic. The recommendation is made most frequently for operating rooms, delivery rooms and isolation units, although some persons suggest these soaps and detergents for all hospital units. Hexachlorophene (G11) and bithional (Actamer), which are phenolic compounds, have been recommended as valuable additives for soaps and detergents; pHisohex and Septisol are examples of commercial products containing these compounds. The compounds are primarily bacteriostatic and fungistatic, and with repeated use the residual effects tend to reduce skin bacteria.

A rather widely used quaternary ammonium detergent—benzalkonium chloride (Zephiran)—is reported to be a good disinfectant and detergent when the alcoholic tincture preparation is used, but it is not particularly effective in the presence of organic materials such as blood and serum or of soap, nor does it have the residual effects that the phenolic compounds do. Other germicide-detergent combinations that appear to be effective are povidone-iodine (Betadine) and undecoylium chloride-iodine (Virac).

Tap water is as effective as sterile water for skin cleansing. The few nonpathogens in tap water are not implanted on the skin during washing and therefore they rinse or wipe off with ease.

Suggested Hand Washing Technic

Studies in relation to hand washing technics have been reported in the literature since well before the end of the last century. Admonitions concerning the importance of clean hands date back even farther, to the time of the ancient Hebrews as reported in the Old Testament. In spite of much evidence to support the importance of careful and frequent hand washing, contaminated hands are considered by many authorities to be a prime factor in cross-infections to this day. Hands in health agencies are in constant use: the nurse giving an injection, the physician examining a patient, the maid folding linen, the volunteer helping a patient select reading material, the aide making a patient's bed and the engineer repairing a television control switch. Still, much hand washing appears to be more ritualistic than realistic, even though the role of hands in cross-infection is no longer debatable.

Cleansing the hands prior to performing certain procedures using surgical asepsis, such as prior to surgery or the delivery of a baby, is taught when the student learns to assist with these procedures. The suggested technic described herein is intended for use when *medical* asepsis is being practiced.

Many researchers have illustrated the value of certain antiseptics for cleansing the hands. However, if there is no reason to believe that the hands harbor pathogenic organisms in the resident flora of the skin, there would appear to be no need to use antiseptics for medical asepsis practice. Transient bacteria—the type that hands accumulate in everyday living and working—are removed easily by thorough washing with soap or a detergent and water. From a half to one minute is recommended. If the hands have been contaminated with blood, purulent materials, mucus, saliva or secretions from wounds, washing should be done for two to three minutes. *A sterile brush may be used,* if the hands are contaminated grossly, but it should be used with great care, since it is easy to brush organisms into hair follicles and skin crevices, which may lead to infection and harboring of organisms. The subungual areas should be cleansed with a sterile nail file or an orange stick, and again caution should be exercised to prevent breaking the skin. If good nail hygiene is maintained, it may not be necessary to clean the subungual areas with a stick or file with every washing, but the procedure should be followed if special circumstances warrant it.

It is preferable to wash the hands under running water at a sink with foot- or knee-controlled faucets. If the faucets are hand-controlled, a policy should be observed concerning whether they are considered to be clean or contaminated. A paper towel should be used to *open* the faucets before washing if the policy is to keep them clean; a paper towel should be used to *close* the faucets if the policy is to consider them as being contaminated. If it is necessary to use a basin, the water should be changed frequently while washing and after each person's use. The inside of a sink or a basin should be considered as being contaminated.

If bar soap is used for cleansing, the bar should be picked up at the beginning of the washing period and held in the hands during the entire washing period. Following washing, the bar should be rinsed and then dropped onto the soap dish. A soap dish that allows water to drain from the soap is preferable in order to keep the soap firm and dry between uses. It has been found that jelly-like soap can harbor pathogens that transfer from user to user. If a brush is being used, the bar of soap may be held on the back of the brush while using the brush. Simpler technics use liquid soap dispensed with a foot or knee lever or single-use bar soaps.

The hands and the forearms should be held lower than the elbows during the washing period in order that soiled water will not run up the arms. Following washing and rinsing, the hands should be dried on an individual linen or paper towel. Laundry problems when using linen, and disposal problems when using paper, have increased the use of forced hot air for hand drying in many agencies. It is suggested that a lotion or a cream be used following washing in order to keep the skin soft and pliable. Chapped and rough skin is difficult to keep clean and will break more easily with repeated washing.

If at any time during the washing period the hands accidentally brush along the inside of the sink or the basin or on the soap dish, the entire washing period should be repeated. It is suggested that a timer be placed near the sink so that the washing period can be determined with accuracy.

Keeping hands clean, regardless of the particular technic followed, is no more reliable than the individual, whose conscientiousness, concern for cleansing all areas thoroughly and respect for his own health, as well as for the health of others, will determine to a great extent the effectiveness of hand washing. For esthetic reasons as well, personnel caring for the ill should practice washing their hands immediately after caring for each patient or after handling equipment used in his care.

Examples of Common Practices of Medical Asepsis

The following examples help to illustrate the fact that medical asepsis is in constant practice:

Paper towels are used in situations where a large number of persons share common wash facilities; paper drinking cups (instead of a common drinking glass) are required by public health regulations in instances where safe drinking fountains are not available;

paper straws, such as are used at soda fountains, are wrapped individually so that they are not contaminated by constant handling; cafeterias frequently provide tongs for customers to use when taking rolls or bread; pillows and mattresses must be sterilized before they are sold, and they must have a label attached at the time of sale indicating that they have been sterilized; hairdressers and barbers are required to sterilize combs and other items after use on each customer. These are only a few examples which in every sense represent the practice of medical asepsis in daily living.

Examples from the home include the following: The homemaker washes her hands before beginning any food preparation; she roasts some meats to a higher temperature in order to ensure their safety; she washes fruits and uncooked vegetables before serving them; she teaches the children to wash their hands before eating and after going to the toilet; she provides individual items of personal care for each member of the home, such as washcloths, towels and toothbrushes.

Because certain diseases may be transmitted insidiously, there are many regulations enforced by law in most communities which aim to prevent their spread. Some of these regulations have to do with the examination of food handlers, the management of eating establishments, the disposal of garbage, the construction of sewage systems, etc. In every sense, these regulations constitute medical asepsis practices. They are defenses against the occasions when contamination may be present.

Most patients practice habits of medical asepsis which they do not recognize by such terms, but they are there. These patients have an understanding of the need for protecting themselves and the means by which it can be done. Never underestimate the patient's ability to evaluate practices of asepsis in a hospital. He is as capable of doing this as he is in judging the practices he sees in a restaurant, a food store or a motel in the light of how they may affect him. Since patients have some "know-how" in this area, it is only natural that they would expect the nurse to exemplify good health practices in all that she does. Even such activities as stripping the linen from the bed occupied by a patient, carrying linen, washing an item, visiting with a patient or holding a child provide opportunities for good health teaching.

The following examples illustrate actions which a nurse carries out, based on the fact that appropriate precautionary measures applied to daily activities and personal care aid in resisting the transmission of disease.

Wash the hands frequently but especially before handling foods, before eating, after using a handkerchief, after going to the toilet and after each patient contact. Clean underneath the fingernails frequently to keep the areas clean and free from contaminated materials.

Keep soiled items and equipment from touching the clothing. Carry soiled linens or other used articles so that they do not touch the uniform. When stooping or bending, hold the uniform so that it does not touch the floor, a grossly contaminated area.

Avoid having patients cough, sneeze or breathe directly on others by providing them with disposable wipes to hold over their mouths when close contact is necessary, as during an examination.

Clean away from yourself, especially when brushing, dusting or scrubbing articles. This helps to prevent the dust particles from settling on the hair, the face or the uniform.

Avoid raising dust. Use a specially treated cloth or a dampened cloth. Do not shake linens. Dust particles constitute a means by which bacteria may be transported from one area to another.

Clean the least soiled areas first and then the more soiled ones. This helps to prevent having the cleaner areas soiled by the dirtier ones.

Dispose of soiled or used items directly into appropriate containers or holders. Wrap items which are moist from body discharge or drainage carefully before discarding into the refuse holder so that handlers will not come in contact with them.

Pour liquids which are to be discarded, such as bath water, mouthcare rinsings, etc., directly into the drain so as to avoid splattering in the sink. Most agencies caring for the sick have sinks or hoppers which are used primarily for disposing of contaminated liquids, washings and the like.

Sterilize items which are suspected of having pathogens on them. Following sterilization, they are managed as clean items.

Practices of surgical asepsis are directed toward the elimination of all microorganisms (by sterilization) and toward preventing microorganisms from contaminating sterile areas.

Handling Sterile Transfer Forceps

Inasmuch as the hands are not sterile, it is obvious that they must not come in contact with sterile items. Sterile gloves or sterile forceps (or clamps) are used when sterility is necessary.

The practice of keeping transfer forceps in containers of disinfectant solution leaves much to be desired. Many agencies have recognized the potential danger of this practice and have discontinued its use. Only forceps taken from wrappers in which they have been sterilized can be considered safe. They are dry and not exposed to possible contamination until the wrapper is opened.

If forceps kept in a disinfectant solution are used, the container should be sterilized and fresh solution used at least daily. There is no scientific justification for only daily care; actually the more frequently this is done, the safer the forceps are likely to be. The opportunity for contamination by means of air currents, personnel and technic in handling is tremendous.

When transfer forceps are used, these principles should be observed:

A sterile object becomes contaminated when in contact with an unsterile object. If the forceps touch an unsterile item or the sides of the container not in solution, they should not be returned to the container until sterilized.

Liquids flow in the direction of gravitational pull. If the forceps are held so that disinfectant solution will touch the unsterile part of the forceps and flow back to the sterile part, the forceps are contaminated.

Examples of Common Practices of Surgical Asepsis

The examples given below illustrate common practices of surgical asepsis. Some practices exercise very extreme caution. It is far better to err on the side of safety than to take the slightest chance on possible contamination.

All items brought into contact with broken skin surfaces of the body, or used to penetrate the skin surface in order to inject substances into the body, or to enter normally sterile body cavities, should be sterile. Examples of such items are dressings used to cover wounds and incisions, needles for injection and tubes (catheters) used to drain urine from the bladder.

Never walk away from or turn your back on a sterile field. This will prevent possible contamination while the field is out of the worker's view.

Avoid talking, coughing, sneezing or reaching over a sterile field or object. This will help to prevent contamination by droplets from the nose and the mouth or by particles dropping from the worker's arm.

Hold sterile objects above the level of the waist. This will help to ensure keeping the object within sight, thus avoiding accidental contamination.

Avoid spilling any solution on a cloth or a paper sterile set-up. The moisture will penetrate through the sterile field, and capillary action could make the field unsafe. A wet sterile field is always considered to be contaminated if the surface immediately below it is not sterile.

Open sterile packages so that the edges of the wrapper are directed away from the worker, in order to avoid the possibility of a sterile surface touching the uniform.

COMMUNICABLE DISEASE CONTROL

While all phases of medicine have undergone radical changes in recent years, one of the most dramatic and encouraging is the control and the management of many communicable diseases. There are several reasons for the marked reduction in communicable diseases. The foremost probably is the discovery of immunizing agents. Helping individuals to build up a resistance to many of the common communicable diseases has become almost a routine aspect of child care in this country. The results of immunization include reducing the mortality rate in infancy and childhood, preventing serious physical limitations which frequently resulted from such illnesses and helping to improve the health of immunized individuals and to increase their life expectancy.

Of equal importance in communicable disease control is the discovery of drugs that are specifically effective against the causative organisms. While many people still become ill with some of the communicable diseases, chemotherapy not only brings the infection under control rapidly but also reduces the period of communicability—in some instances, to a matter of hours. Many of the drugs being used make it possible for patients such as those with pneumonia and streptococcic sore throat to be cared for as usual without any additional precautions.

While the incidence has been reduced and the treatment improved, there still exist some illnesses which require special consideration. Infectious hepatitis, tuberculosis and the dysenteries are examples. So also is the problem of hospital-acquired infection discussed earlier in this chapter.

General Principles for Controlling the Spread of Communicable Diseases

Isolation technics are based on this general principle: *The transfer of pathogens from person to person can be decreased when dissemination of pathogens is limited.*

Throughout this text, and in this Unit in particular, attention is directed toward preventing the spread of disease-producing organisms and examples of practices are cited. Additional nursing measures based on this principle and used when patients are ill with a communicable disease, will be discussed shortly.

Methods to limit the dissemination of known pathogens are based on the manner in which the pathogen leaves the source (patient), its portal of entry and its ability to survive outside the host.

This principle indicates that isolation technics can safely vary, depending on the specific causative organism. For example, *Mycobacterium tuberculosis* leaves the patient via the respiratory and the gastrointestinal tracts in most cases, enters the host via the respiratory or the gastrointestinal tracts and is capable of long survival inside or outside of the host. *Treponema pallidum* (causing syphilis) is transferred by direct contact, enters the host via the skin and the mucous membrane and is very fragile, living only briefly outside the host. Methods to limit the spread of these two organisms can vary markedly.

Definition of Terms

Communicable Disease or Isolation Technic—practices which limit the spread of a communicable pathogen. It involves separating infected persons from the unafflicted and rendering contaminated non-disposable items in their unit or used in their care safe for re-use.

Host—an animal or a person on which or within which a parasite lives.

Carrier—a person who has, within his body, organisms of a specific disease that may be transmitted to another person, yet who personally has no symptoms of the disease.

Infectious Disease—a disease caused by a pathogenic organism. It may or may not be contagious.

Contagious Disease—a disease that is conveyed rather easily from the sick to the well either by direct contact, through an intermediary host or by other indirect means.

It is not uncommon for the terms "contagious" and "infectious" to be used interchangeably. As the definition indicates, there is a difference.

Concurrent Disinfection—This term refers to practices that are observed routinely in the care of the patient's unit and equipment which limit or destroy the causative organism. It includes such measures as dusting, cleaning the floors, washing the equipment and the furniture in the patient's unit and caring properly for items removed from the unit, such as magazines, dishes and linens.

Here again, it seems to be worthwhile to repeat that all practices concerning the care of equipment and other items that are observed routinely as a part of medical asepsis also are considered as concurrent disinfection in that they aid to control the spread of pathogens.

Terminal Disinfection—This term refers to additional measures which may need to be taken in caring for a patient's unit and belongings after he has recovered from a communicable disease. In many instances, these measures are described in the Sanitary Code of the community. Here, again, how extensive these measures may need to be depends on the nature of the organism. For most communicable diseases, sunlight and airing and washing thoroughly with soap and water are sufficient to render the unit and other items in it safe for re-use.

Some of the practices which may be seen in both concurrent and terminal disinfection are entirely unsubstantiated and are described by some experts in microbiology as "sheer witchcraft." Any measure which is purportedly of value in rendering the unit safe for the next person should be based on scientific knowledge of the illness and the causative organism. For example, because the causative organism of tuberculosis resists disinfectants and can live for long periods in a dried state, it is wise to have the pillow, the blankets and the mattress used by the patient sterilized by steam under pressure or other effective means to make certain that it is free of contamination. On the other hand, sterilization of pillows, blankets and mattresses have been found to be not necessary for other communicable diseases transmitted via respiratory secretions; airing and exposure to direct sunlight for several hours are sufficient.

Variations in Communicable Disease Practices

Because isolation technics vary among health agencies, nurses working in one situation may be observing practices that are not followed in a similar agency in the same city or even across the street. Oddly enough,

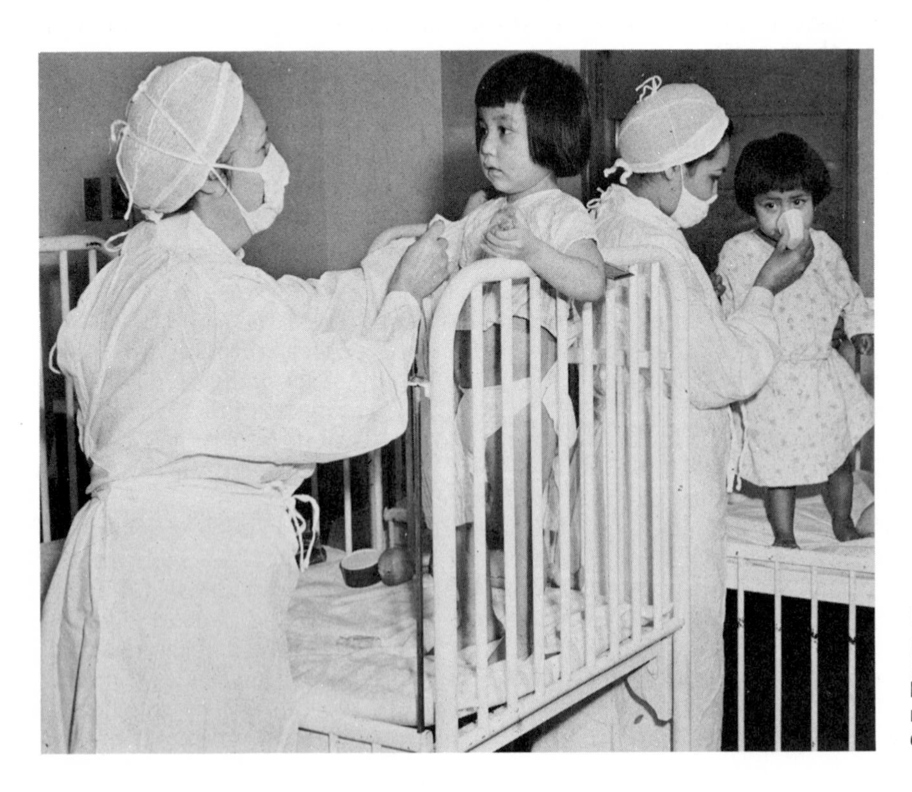

Fig. 16-3. These young patients have tuberculosis. Does the expression of the child in the foreground cause you to wonder what her thoughts are about why the nurse covers her face? (U. S. Government photograph)

the results in many instances appear to be about the same.

The combined efforts of experts in microbiology, medicine, nursing and sanitary engineering are necessary to study communicable diseases that are still posing problems and to arrive at flexible and workable technics to prevent their spread. Thus, all the facts about the illness, the causative organism, the existing facilities of the community and the problems of nursing care can be presented and evaluated. For example, some communities have sewage disposal systems which are inadequate to destroy all disease-producing organisms; therefore, action must be taken to disinfect waste materials before disposing of them in the sewage system; or if the causative agent exists only in the patient's blood, the only items that would be managed with additional care would be those that come into direct contact with the paient's blood; or, if the patient's respiratory secretions contain the causative organism, it may well be that a gown should be worn when coming in close contact with the patient and his bedding; or, if the organism is destroyed easily, the dishes may be safe if washed with hot soapy water.

An important aspect in isolation technic is gaining the cooperation of the patient. How much does the patient understand about his illness? Does he know how to protect others? Has he been helped to feel comfortable about his isolation, or is he made to feel like an outcast? If the nurse who cares for the patient is merely "carrying out a technic" mechanically and is indifferent to the patient's feelings about it, the patient is apt to sense her fear and distaste for caring for him. This can be a disastrous situation for him.

A well-informed nurse who understands how to protect both herself and her patients and a well-informed patient who is cooperating in his care are by far the best combination of communicable disease precautions.

The Isolation Unit

If a patient is to be placed in a unit by himself because his illness is considered communicable, it generally is accepted that the entire unit is contaminated. Practices that allow for so-called "clean" areas within the immediate confines of the unit are open to question. This is based on the fact that organisms present on bed linen or on the floor are easily raised into the air by activity such as walking, moving objects about, bedmaking and talking. Once present in the air of the unit, they may be carried to any object or area of the room and, under other circumstances, even to other parts of the hospital.[6] It is safer to consider the entire unit and its contents as contaminated.

One major requirement for an isolation unit is that there be facilities for hand washing in or near the patient's unit. With one type of gown technic (re-use), it is necessary to provide for hand-washing facilities within the unit.

The Use of Gowns and Masks

Gowns may be worn as a means of protecting the clothing of all who visit or attend the patient. There are two generally accepted practices in gown technics: the *throw-away* and the *re-use*.

Gowns that are used for isolation technic are made of washable cotton; most are made to be worn over the outer garments of the wearer. They are designed with the opening in the back and a tie around the waist to help to keep the gown secure and closed. Some have stockinet at the wrists; others have buttons. They may have buttons or tie strings at the neck. These minor variations do not affect the use or the value of the gown.

Throw-Away Gown Technic. Some communicable disease technics require that all who attend or visit the patient wear a gown, specifying that a clean gown must be worn whenever anyone who expects to be in close contact with the patient comes into the unit. The wearer usually picks up a gown from a supply kept outside the isolation unit and puts it on before entering the unit. There is no special way in which a clean gown must be put on. However, it should be closed well in the back so that all parts of the wearer's clothing are covered.

When the wearer is ready to leave the unit, the gown is unfastened and removed so that the wearer turns it inside out. In other words, the wearer takes off the gown and rolls it up so that the contaminated part is inside. Then the gown is discarded in a special hamper provided for it. The wearer now washes her hands thoroughly, making certain that special precautions are taken to prevent contaminating the faucets if foot- or knee-controlled faucets are not available.

While the throw-away technic produces laundering problems because of the use of so many gowns, it is a far more satisfactory technic than one in which the gowns are re-used. Disposable gowns are available and used by some agencies.

Re-use Gown Technic. Some communicable disease technics specify that a gown may be used several times and by different persons if certain precautions are observed. The re-use gown technic is based on the assumption that the inside of the gown which is in contact with the wearer's clothing can be kept clean and that the gown can be removed without contaminating the inside. When this technic is used, all who are to wear the gowns must be instructed in the exact way in which this can be accomplished. Figures 16-4 through 16-13 describe how to get into a gown which has been used, and how to get out of the gown without contaminating it so that another person may wear it safely.

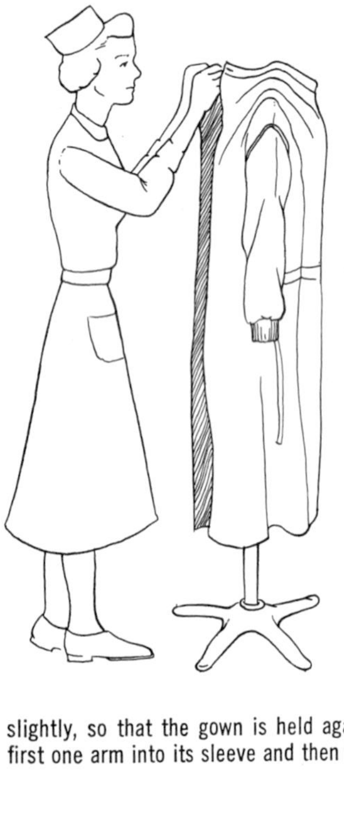

Fig. 16-4. How to put on a gown when the re-use technic is employed. The gown is on the pole, having been placed by the previous user with the insides of the gown together and the neck band folded so that it is supported upward. The neck band which is clean would of necessity be considered contaminated if it were to fall down over the gown. To put the gown on, the nurse approaches it from the back and places her hands into the inside of the gown at the neck band. She then lifts it up off the hook and holds it away from her so that the inside of the gown is toward her. To get into the gown, the nurse brings the neck band up in place and then, bending back slightly, so that the gown is held against her clothing, she slips first one arm into its sleeve and then the other.

Masks. A variety of practices is observed in the use of the mask as a barrier in caring for a patient who has a communicable disease which can be transmitted via the respiratory tract. In some instances, all personnel and visitors to the patient wear masks; in other situations personnel, visitors and also the patient wear a mask. On the other hand, it may be that only the patient wears the mask; and in certain technics, neither the patient nor the personnel wears a mask.

Purpose of Masks. Theoretically, the mask is intended to filter inspired and expired air in order to trap the organisms in its meshes.

The purpose of a mask should be understood by the wearer. For example, if masks are worn while caring for a patient with tuberculosis, the purpose is for the protection of those who care for the patient, and the mask serves to filter the air inspired by the worker. In the nursery or when opera-

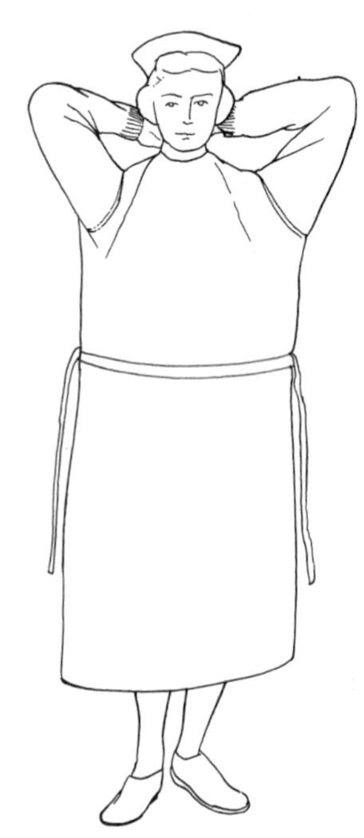

Fig. 16-5. How to put on a gown when the re-use technic is employed (Continued). Once the gown is on, the wearer's hands are still clean because they have gone only through the inside of the gown. The neck band is fastened while the hands are still clean.

tive technic is used, the purpose is to protect the infants or the patient from the air expired by the workers.

Masks generally are made of layers of gauze (preferably 6) and a weave of 42 by 42 threads per square inch. The closeness of the weave helps to make it quite effective, and the material molds well to the face and holds up satisfactorily in the laundering process.

Some masks are made of paper or plastic materials and discarded after use.

No matter how well a mask may fit the wearer's face, it is still almost impossible to prevent some air from entering around the edges where it is loose. Also, there is the possibility of the wearer's taking deep inspirations which are sufficient to suction through particles which may be in the air. If a patient who is wearing a mask coughs or sneezes, the force may be sufficient to cause the expired air to leave the mask with little filtering action taking place.

The practice of wearing a mask, removing it and then re-using it is unsound. Once the mask has been worn and it is time to remove it, it should be discarded into the laundry.

The length of time that a mask can be worn safely is a debatable question. Everyone agrees that the more frequently it is changed, the more effective it is.

Disposal of Excreta

If there is evidence that the causative organism is excreted through the urine and the feces, special precautions may be indicated. These precautions usually include treating the urine and the feces, according to the agency's policies, before disposal into the sewage system. As mentioned previously, this precaution is unnecessary in those communities where the sewage disposal technics are adequate to destroy organisms.

The problems that the disinfection of excreta brings to any nursing service usually are numerous. The psychological implications as well as the hazards of handling several pails or bedpans of excreta make it an unpopular procedure. Therefore, efforts should be made to ascertain the need for disinfecting excreta before it is done.

The disadvantages of the usual bedpan flusher have been discussed. The safest practice is to empty the bedpan, rinse it thor-

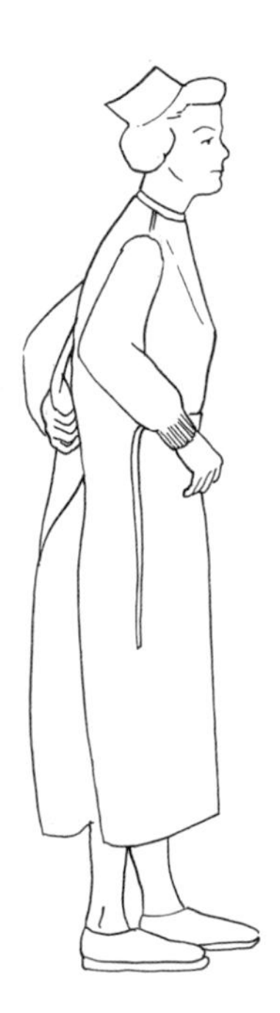

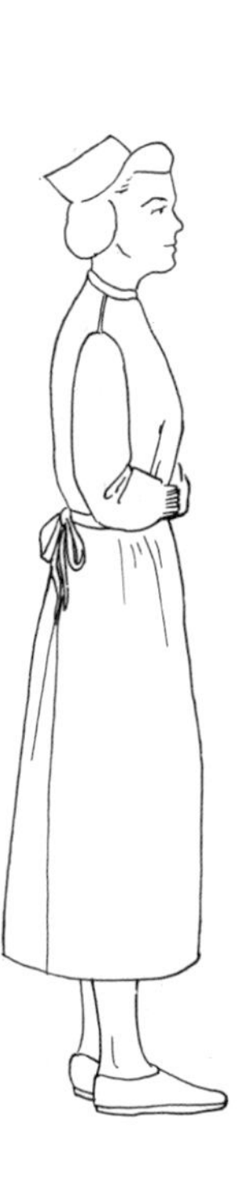

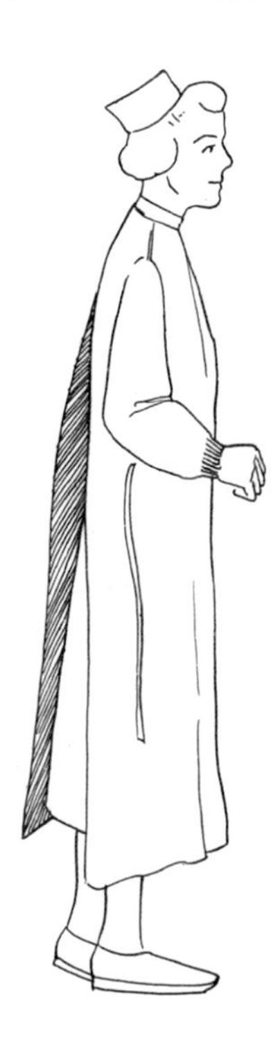

FIGS. 16-6 to 16-8. How to put on a gown when the re-use technic is employed (Continued). (Left) After the neck band is secure, the nurse takes both open ends of the gown in the back and, being careful not to have the outside and the inside of the gown come together, she rolls the ends so that the gown fits her more snugly. (Center) When the back is closed, the nurse fastens the ties at the waist so that the gown is held secure while she cares for her patient. (Right) When ready to get out of gown, the ties around the waist are loosened completely and allowed to hang freely from the places where they are attached. The sides of the gown are pulled loose from the wearer's clothing so that it will be easy to get out of the gown.

oughly with cold water, wash it with soap or detergent and water if necessary, and then sterilize it with steam under pressure before reuse.

Care of Dishes

The practices of medical asepsis as outlined earlier in this chapter indicate that proper care of dishes after use is a form of protection against illness. Most health agencies use mechanical dish washers that leave dishes free of pathogens. If this is not the case, it then becomes necessary to take special precautions when a patient has a communicable disease, especially one that is transmitted via secretions from the mouth. In some agencies, after rinsing the dishes they are boiled. Other agencies use disposable dishes so that only the silverware needs boiling. The technic of placing soiled dishes in a container of water and boiling them before being washed is a questionable practice. The heat of the water often coagulates the food particles remaining on the dishes. If the organism is contained within these solids and is particularly resistive, it may survive the washing process. Therefore, the dishes should be rinsed thoroughly first before being washed and subjected to heat. Many mechanical dish washers used in restaurants and hospitals provide for rinsing the dishes before they are washed.

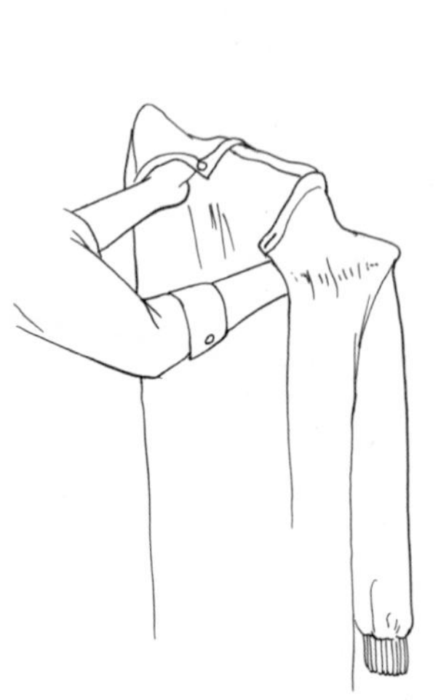

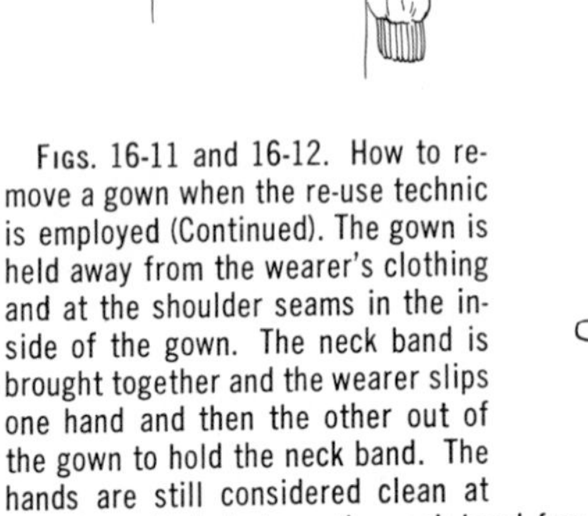

Figs. 16-11 and 16-12. How to remove a gown when the re-use technic is employed (Continued). The gown is held away from the wearer's clothing and at the shoulder seams in the inside of the gown. The neck band is brought together and the wearer slips one hand and then the other out of the gown to hold the neck band. The hands are still considered clean at this time. To help keep the neck band from falling down, it is best to hold the hands so that the neck band projects upward through the space beween the thumb and the first finger of each hand. Using the thumbs, make 2 or 3 deep folds in the gown so that the shoulder seams of the gown will be supported on the hook and the neck can be supported upward without falling down on the gown. The open ends at the back of the gown face the entrance to the unit so that the wearer walks directly to it.

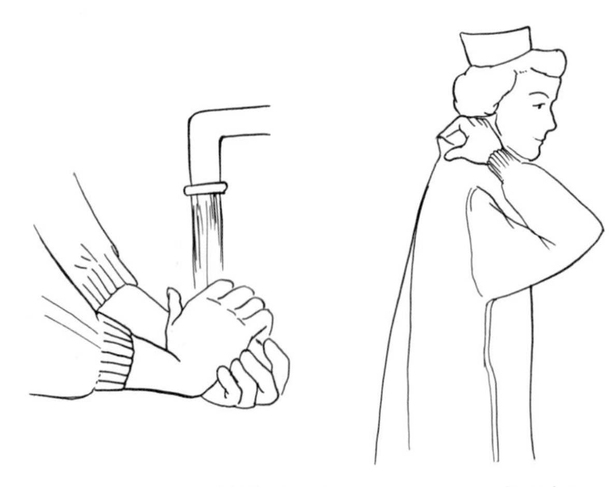

Figs. 16-9 and 16-10. How to remove a gown when the re-use technic is employed (Continued). (Left) The sleeves are then pushed up slightly on the arm to prevent wetting them when the hands are washed. (Right) After the hands are washed, the neck band is loosened. Once the neck band is loosened, the wearer slips out carefully, being careful not to touch any part of the outside of the gown with the hands.

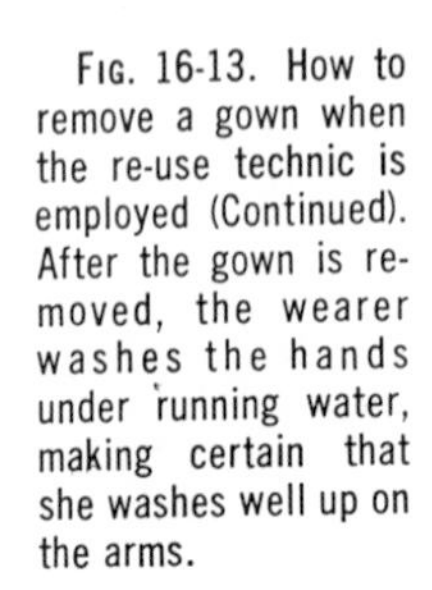

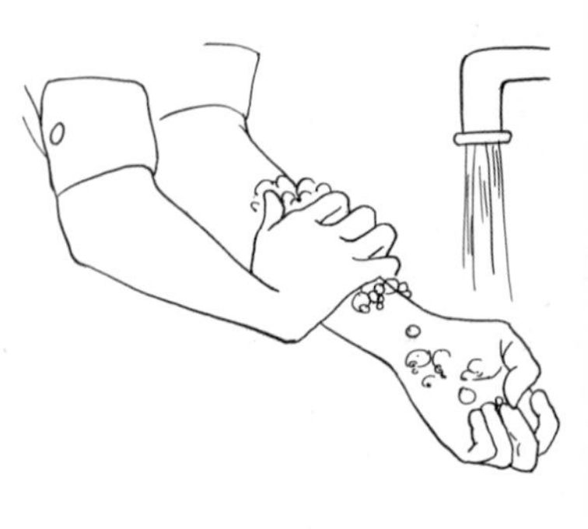

Fig. 16-13. How to remove a gown when the re-use technic is employed (Continued). After the gown is removed, the wearer washes the hands under running water, making certain that she washes well up on the arms.

Care of Laundry

Modern hospital laundering processes make it possible for almost all linens of patients with communicable diseases to be handled in the usual manner. There are some exceptions, as when linens are contaminated with organisms that are spore-forming, as the bacilli of tetanus, gas gangrene and anthrax. For such causative organisms, the linens should be sterilized by steam under pressure before they are handled by laundry workers.

For items of clothing or apparel that are not washed easily in a machine, airing in sunlight for six to eight hours is effective against organisms in vegetative forms. This would be suitable procedure for such items as blankets, decorative bed jackets and the like. Also, gas sterilizers, discussed earlier in this chapter, may be used.

Study Situations

1. The following table illustrates the scope of medical asepsis. List additional practices used commonly by individuals and by communities to limit the spread of or to destroy pathogens.

2. The following article describes various precautions to reduce cross-infections in hospitals:

- Werrin, M., and Kronick, D.: Salmonella control in hospitals.

AMER. J. NURS., *66*:528-530, March, 1966. How do the authors use the phrase, "iceberg effect," to describe cross-infection problems? What practices that may not have occurred to you when working on Study Situation 1 are discussed in this article?

3. The following article describes how

Examples of Routine Control Measures Which Destroy or Limit the Spread of Pathogens		**Additional Special Measures Against a Known Communicable Agent**
- *Practiced by the Individual* -	- *Enforced by the Community* -	
Covering mouth when coughing. Sneezing and coughing into disposable tissues. Washing hands before handling food. Washing dishes and glasses thoroughly. Using individual items of personal care, such as towels, toothbrush, comb, washcloth, etc. Wiping eyes or removing foreign particles with clean tissue or handkerchief. Expectorating into disposable wipes. Washing hands after elimination.	Disposing of garbage and sewage. Controlling pests, such as mosquitoes and rodents. Inspecting: eating establishments, pasteurization plants, plants preparing food and food-stuffs for canning or packaging, swimming pools, etc. Licensing food handlers. Regulating drinking-water plants. Regulating interstate food transportation. Establishing immunization regulation for immigrants. Recommending health programs in public schools, including immunization.	Separating infected person(s) from others: isolation. Using barriers for those caring for the ill—such as gowns and possibly masks. Using special precautions, depending on the mode of transmission of the organism; i.e., if through respiratory secretions, intestinal excretions, blood or drainage from a wound. Such precautions might include the burning of secretions, the disinfection of excreta and the sterilization of dishes. Sterilizing or disinfecting items used by the infected person. Reporting the illness to the proper community agency.

Observance of Both Routine and Special Practices in Medical Asepsis Helps to Prevent Illness in Man

Table 5. The scope of medical asepsis

problem solving was used to study cross-contamination:

- French, J. G.: Students study cross-contamination.
  AMER. J. NURS., *67*:2104-2106, October, 1967.

Identify the steps in problem solving as used in this study. What were the primary findings of the study? What was the most serious error found to be in the practice of medical asepsis?

4. The following article is suggested for reading:

- Thompson, L. R.: Evaluating disinfectants.
  AMER. J. NURS., *62*:82-83, January, 1962.

What are "in-use" tests? What reason does the author give for advocating "in-use" tests for checking the effectiveness of disinfectants? Select a disinfectant and study it in relation to the six questions posed as a guide in the article. After studying the disinfectant, indicate situations in which it most probably can be used with safety and effectiveness.

5. If in preparing a sterile field, the nurse accidentally spilled a few drops of disinfectant solution on the sterile cover, would the field be considered contaminated? Why?

If a sterile field has to be prepared at a patient's bedside unit, what precautions should be taken in relation to the following factors: drafts, movement of linens, other personnel going through the unit and bedside curtains being drawn?

6. Mention has been made of the patient's feelings about being isolated. Consider the following article:

- Bullough, B.: Where should isolation stop?
  AMER. J. NURS., *62*:86-89, October, 1962.

Note how the author describes the social isolation that Mrs. Juarez experienced and how she felt "dirty." What defense mechanisms did Mrs. Juarez use as a mode of adjusting to her isolation? What nursing help does the author suggest to keep such patients from feeling so lonely?

7. The following article describes an isolation unit:

- Kline, P. A.: Isolating patients with staphylococcal infections.
  AMER. J. NURS., *65*:102-104, January, 1965.

Note that in the unit described, rubber gloves and masks, as well as caps and gowns, were worn routinely by food service personnel when handling soiled silverware and dishes. What does the author indicate as reasons why practices of infection control are well observed in this Unit?

References

1. Benson, M. E.: Handwashing—an important part of medical asepsis.
   AMER. J. NURS., *57*:1136-1139, September, 1957.
2. Edgeworth, D.: Nursing and asepsis in the modern hospital.
   NURS. OUTLOOK, *13*:54-56, June, 1965.
3. Fitzwater, J.: Bacteriological effect of ultraviolet light on a surgical instrument table.
   AMER. J. NURS., *61*:71, March, 1961.
4. Gallivan, G. J., and Tovey, J. D.: Isolation for possible and proved staph.
   AMER. J. NURS., *67*:1048-1049, May, 1967.
5. Hicks, J. T.: Hospital-acquired infections. Part II—problems with personnel, patients and visitors.
   HOSP. MANAGE., *105*:46-50, February, 1968.
6. Hicks, J. T.: Hospital-acquired infections. Part III—the role, authority and membership of the infection committee.
   HOSP. MANAGE., *105*:55-57, March, 1968.
7. Hunter, D. T. Jr., and Baker, C. E.: Control of staphylococcal carriers in three hospitals.
   PUBLIC HEALTH REPORTS, *82*:329-333, April, 1967.
8. Jopke, W. H.: Environmental sanitation.
   HOSP., J. AMER. HOSP. ASSOC., *42*:49-58, April 1, 1968.
9. Kunin, C. M., and Henley, R. W. Jr.: Isolation procedures for the community hospital.
   J.A.M.A., *200*:295-299, April 24, 1967.
10. Lawrence, C. A., and Block, S. S.: Disinfection, Sterilization, and Preservation. 808 p.
    Philadelphia, Lea and Febiger, 1968.
11. Leonard, R. R.: Prevention of superficial cutaneous infections.
    ARCHIVES OF DERMATOLOGY, *95*:520-523, May, 1967.
12. Litsky, B. Y.: Hospital Sanitation—An Administrative Program. 167 p.
    Chicago, Clissold Publishing Co., 1966.
13. Litsky, B. Y.: The evaluation of single-use bar soaps for surgical scrub.
    HOSP. MANAGE., *103*:74-86, May, 1967.

14. Price, P. B.: The bacteriology of normal skin; a new quantitative test applied to a study of the bacterial flora and the disinfectant action of mechanical cleansing.
J. INFECT. DIS., *63*:301, November-December, 1938.
15. Skaliy, P.: Ethylene oxide as a hospital sterilizing agent.
HOSP., J. AMER. HOSP. ASSOC., *41*:100-109, November 16, 1967.
16. Streeter, S. *et al*: Hospital infection—a necessary risk?
AMER. J. NURS., *67*:526-533, March, 1967.
17. Tyler, V. R.: Gas sterilization.
AMER. J. NURS., *60*:1596-1599, November, 1960.
18. U.S. Department of Health, Education and Welfare: Public Health Service, Washington, D.C., 1966: Environmental Aspects of the Hospital. Vol. 1—Infection Control. 67 p.
19. Vesley, D., and Brask, M.: Environmental implications in the control of hospital acquired infections.
NURS. OUTLOOK, *9*:742, December, 1961.
20. Walter, C. W., and Kundsin, R. B.: The floor as a reservoir of hospital infections.
SURG. GYNEC. OBSTET., *111*:412, October, 1960.
21. Walter, C. W.: Isolation technic for containment or exclusion of bacteria for the prevention of cross-infection in hospitals.
HOSP. TOPICS, *42*:57-60, January, 1964.

Nursing Implementation: Man as an Organism

Unit 4

CHAPTER

17

Assessing the Patient's Health Status

OBSERVING THE PATIENT'S HEALTH STATUS

Introduction

In the definition of health given in Chapter 2, it was pointed out that health and illness may be considered to be on a continuum. When changes occur in any person's usual state of well-being, the human body constantly strives for psychologic and physiologic equilibrium. This is the concept of *homeostasis* or *homeokinesis*. This means that the body strives constantly to function coordinately.

Succeeding chapters in this Unit are concerned with helping the patient to maintain the best possible functioning. In other words, health team efforts are directed toward assisting the patient in the process of homeostasis. To recognize lack of coordination of body functions requires the ability to use scientific knowledge as a basis for observing the patient.

Observation as a Key Skill in Nursing

Observation has a clear-cut objective: to gain information about the status of the patient's health. It is more than just looking. Observation also entails the use of other senses: listening, touching, smelling. Skill in observation is learned, and one needs to refine the technic continuously.

The information gathered is needed to plan both the medical and nursing care for the patient. It is used for long term planning as well as for the immediate plan, and is also a means of determining if other sources of professional help may be needed, such as a medical social worker, physical therapist or clergyman.

One needs to have contact with a patient to observe him. The intercommunication system used in many agencies may be a convenience but it does little to aid in observing the person. It should also be noted that a description of a situation observed only once or infrequently may not be accurate. Additional follow-up may be needed to gain the most objective information.

The observation of a newly admitted patient usually will be more detailed than subsequent observations. However, observation continues for as long as the person is receiving care. It takes place concurrently with other activities—obtaining vital signs, explaining therapeutic measures—or for any other reason that brings the patient and the nurse in contact. The subsequent observations provide information essential to adjusting the care according to the patient's need.

Stating Observations Objectively. It must be stressed that the reporting of observations, whether verbal or written, must be objective, that is, free of personal bias and opinion. If it is not, it follows that subsequent use of the information and courses of action taken may not be helpful to the patient. It is a well-known fact that several people can observe the same situation and come away with as many different descriptions of what was observed as there were observers. Often we see only what we are looking for, or what has significance or value for us. Perhaps the reader has tried the experiment of looking at a picture that has no title and then making up a story about it. This highly subjective and biased approach can occur in nursing if skills in observation are not refined to eliminate our own opinions and value judgments.

The nurse records what she sees and does not venture a reason for it. For example, if a newly admitted patient is unshaven and unclean, this is an observation; why he appears as he does is not a matter of immediate concern. It may be, at a later time. There should be no comment that the patient has not been well taken care of or that he has been careless about his hygiene. Who knows, he might look like that when well. If it is learned that he lives in a rooming house or alone on a farm, this may become relevant when considering his care after discharge. If he will be limited in his activity, he may need someone to care for him at home.

There are descriptive terms used in connection with symptoms. *Subjective symptoms* are those described by the patient, such as a headache or a toothache. The observer cannot see the symptom, but often the patient's behavior confirms it. *Objective symptoms* are those noted by the observer, such as a rash or a swelling. It is a good practice to report objective signs associated with subjective ones.

Constitutional symptoms are produced by the effect of the disease on the whole body, as a fever. *Local symptoms* are noted in some special area or part of the body, such as a swollen jaw. *Prodromal symptoms* precede the development of disease, such as an "achy feeling" before an acute infectious disease develops.

Use proper terminology in recording observations. For example, it would not seem odd for a lay person to say he has a "bellyache." However, the nurse's report of his complaint would state exactly in what area of the abdomen he had what type of pain. Or, a patient might say he "threw up." After questioning him, the nurse would record when it occurred, what type of vomitus it was, and how much there was.

In the course of their practice, nurses learn the cause and the significance of many signs and symptoms. For example, there is a combination of signs which would indicate that a patient is in a state of shock. The nurse would record the signs and the symptoms observed but not that the patient is in shock. Diagnosing is the physician's responsibility.

Following are some suggestions for observation and frequently used terminology. Additional terms will appear throughout the text, and many more will be learned in other courses and in clinical experiences. Physicians have a routine for making a physical examination, and some nurses find it convenient to follow this same pattern. In general, it is to begin at the head and proceed to the feet. Observations of the patient's emotional and mental state can be done concurrently.

Suggestions for Observing the Patient

Mental State. Possibly the first thing that the nurse needs to know about the patient is his mental state. Normal functioning of the cerebral cortex is essential to the mental faculties of cognition, memory and association of ideas.

Explanations or questions might very well be meaningless if he is unable to comprehend them. The following terms are descriptive. Other terms, such as apprehensive, frightened, unconcerned, resentful, belligerent, preoccupied or uncooperative may very well be subjective judgments and should be avoided.

Oriented. Being aware of time, place and other environmental circumstances. *Disoriented* is the reverse.

Confused. Having a temporary interference with the clear working of the mind.

Unresponsive. Not answering by word, gesture or other indication. Generally used when a person appears to be aware but does not communicate in return with another person.

Incoherent. Speaking in a disjointed fashion, expressing thoughts that are unrelated; not completing sentences. The listener is unable to make any sense out of what is being said.

Unconscious. Showing no awareness of the presence of another. No response to sound, or voice.

All of the above terms, except *oriented* and *unconscious*, should be accompanied by a description of what the patient says or does, as, "Did not answer questions, looked toward the door as if to see what was outside;" or, "Did not appear to hear questions being asked." "Kept looking at hands, turning them over and back again." Immediate nursing action is indicated when a patient is unconscious or not oriented. This may mean the use of bed siderails or other protective measures.

Emotional State. In addition to observing the patient's mental state, it is essential to be sensitive to the emotional reactions frequently seen when illness or injury occurs, as pointed out in Chapter 9. Without this awareness it is possible that patients can be judged as resentful, belligerent, uncooperative, unconcerned or preoccupied. *Avoid such value judgments.*

Record the exact behavior observed. A patient who had been in an automobile accident was admitted on a stretcher. When she was placed in bed, she pulled the bed clothes over her head and said, "Go away. Leave me alone." The nurse approached her and said in a calm voice, "I am Mrs. Jeffrey. Is there anything I can do for you?" She was answered by a fast fist that came out from under the sheets. Who is to judge if this person is frightened, belligerent, uncooperative or what? Time was to show that her behavior, which became "worse" before it was "better," was a result of her severe emotional reaction to the experience and shock and that she had no clear awareness of it.

General Physical State. While the physician is responsible for the physical examination, the nurse assists by reporting her observations.

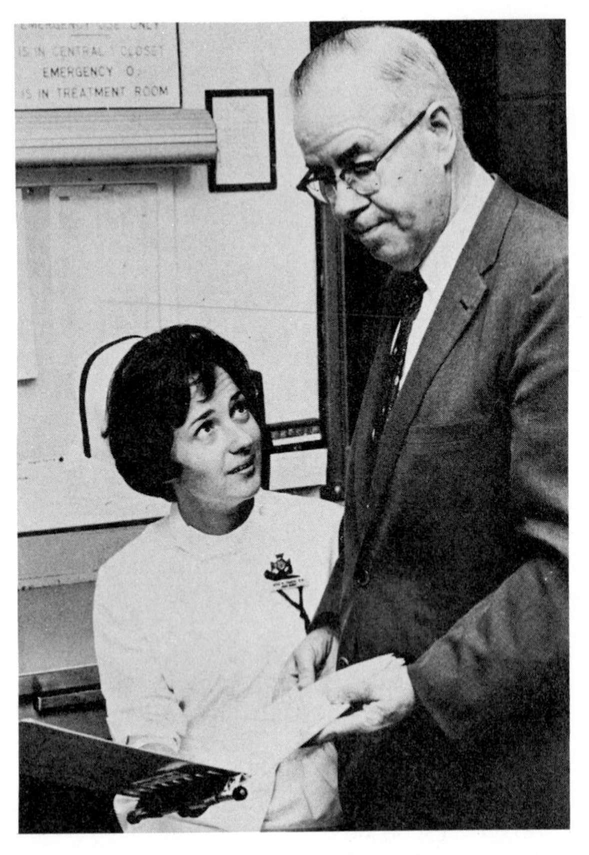

Fig. 17-1. Observation of the patient is a crucial aspect of nursing care. Then the observations must be recorded. But, there are always circumstances when the physician will need "filling in" or additional information. Before visiting his patient a physician often discusses the nurse's report of her observations with her. (Courtesy Muhlenberg Hospital, Plainfield, N.J.)

The over-all appearance of a person is a key to much information about him. It could indicate how well he cares for himself or has been cared for, possibly how long he has been ill and even the severity of the illness and his nutritional state. For example, one patient may be described as appearing to be well nourished and careful about his appearance. Another patient may be described as appearing weak and emaciated, having dull-looking eyes with dark circles under them. Some patients may show signs of neglect, especially if they have been sick for a long time. This can be noted by a disheveled appearance, uncombed and matted hair, long fingernails and toenails with dirt underneath them, soiled clothing and on a man, an unshaven face possibly with old food particles in the growth.

Look for physical limitations which may or may not have a relationship to the present health problem. These may need immediate consideration for both the patient's welfare and the nurse's ability to care for him. Hearing and sight are examples of limitations which might interfere with communications from the outset.

Record and describe on the patient's chart any device used or worn for physical limitation or support. These include such items as false teeth, hearing aids, glasses, prostheses (artificial parts, such as eye, limb or breast), canes, crutches, braces or back supports. If lost or damaged these items represent considerable expense to replace. More important, however, is the inconvenience and the possible mental and physical discomfort caused the patient.

Age. The age of the patient is required for the hospital record and is recorded on the chart by the admitting officer. Knowing the age of the patient is helpful in many situations, especially when illness or personal appearance makes the person appear to be older or younger. Whenever the patient's age becomes a factor in planning nursing care or reporting, the exact chronologic age should be used. Such terms as "young," "middle-aged" or "elderly" should be avoided, because they are subject to individual opinion.

Persons in the older age group show as much variation in their personalities and general health as do any other age groups. However, there is no question that the process of aging results in many of them having problems with memory or the ability to understand as quickly as they did when they were younger. It may take many contacts and observations before an accurate assessment of their physical and mental state can be arrived at. It is easy for a young person to judge them as uncooperative, disoriented, unable to understand or even "senile," if questions or directions are given in rapid-fire order. Frequent repetition is essential for most of these persons. It may also be necessary to vary the way in which questions or directions are given.

Weight. Not all hospitals require that a patient's height and weight be recorded on admission. However, in observing a patient the nurse may believe that the patient is underweight or overweight (obese). This may also be judgmental, and the best procedure is to state the exact weight whenever this is a factor.

Extremely thin or markedly overweight patients can present nursing care problems, especially in caring for the skin or in moving. If hospital policy does not require the recording of the weight, the nursing staff may need to obtain this information for their own use. If the patient is allowed out of bed, this does not present a problem. However, if the patient is ordered on bed rest, the physician's consent is necessary.

Nurses should also be alert to evidence of weight loss. Patients frequently lose weight as a result of anxiety about their health problem, some from fasting for many diagnostic tests and others for a variety of reasons, like different meal times, dislike for the food or its manner of being cooked.

Hearing. If impaired hearing is not recognized as soon as possible it could result in considerable apprehension on the part of the patient. He may not know quite what is going on. If a hearing aid is worn, the situation is obvious. But many persons with limited hearing do not or cannot wear a hearing aid. While the physician who performs the physical examination will note this, the observation should also be recorded on the chart by the nurse. This information also should be placed immediately on a nursing care plan.

When speaking to a person who has difficulty in hearing, make every effort to speak distinctly, face him and make certain that what has been said is really understood. Avoid shouting unless it is absolutely necessary. Many people learn to read lips if they can see them and if the other person speaks slowly and distinctly. At night, in order to avoid disturbing other patients, direct the flashlight on your face so that the patient may watch your mouth and facial expression. Another measure that is helpful with some types of hearing loss is to place the ear tips of a stethoscope in the patient's ears and speak into the bell portion.

Vision. If a patient's sight is severely limited, this should be recorded on the patient's chart and on the nursing care plan. For patients who have severe sight impairment, the concern for his safety is paramount. Place objects so that they can be seen readily and are easily accessible; offer assistance with meals, such as pouring liquids, seasoning foods or cutting food; give assistance and directions to patients who are permitted to walk about and use the bathroom facilities in order to avoid falls, tripping over objects, walking into stair wells and bumping into things. It often means telling the patient who you are until the voice is recognized.

Other Physical Limitations. While sight and hearing are especially important, all other limitations should be noted and recorded also, such as: loss of an extremity or a part of it and the use of any prostheses; loss of function in a body part such as a limb and the use of a brace, a cane or crutches. The patient should be asked if he has any areas of paresthesia (lack of sensation or tingling feeling).

Patients having had previous surgery or medical problems may wear cosmetics or supportive or protective devices or garments such as girdles, colostomy belts, brassières with breast prostheses, shoes with elastic shoelaces, easily zippered garments, elastic hose or moisture-proof underpants. Any such items are clues to the patient's problem with a limitation, and their use should also be recorded in a nursing care plan because of their significance in caring for the patient.

Some patients may speak freely about such items, even warning all to be careful of them and possibly not wanting them out of their sight. Other patients may not feel as free to talk about their problem, and with them a cautious approach is necessary. It is not a matter of ignoring the presence of such items, but rather one of asking the patient what can be done to make it easier for him and to use them while in the hospital.

Although it is not very common, some patients may have cardiac pacemakers (heart regulators). A high anterior chest scar with some protrusion is a clue. However, such patients are more likely to indicate that they have one.

It is also important to ask the patient if he has any allergies to drugs or other agents.

Skin, Including Hair and Nails. Since the skin covers almost the entire surface of the body, it is a good indicator of a person's health status. In addition to its general appearance (smooth, wrinkled, dry or well hydrated) the nurse also is concerned with evidence of injury or lack of good care. These would be evidenced by bruises, scratches, cuts, insect bites and sores. The presence of any of these is recorded. Treat all lesions on a patient with great care to avoid possible contamination of objects and transfer of infection to other persons. Because of the danger of infections in hospitals, newly admitted patients with open lesions or draining ones should be checked carefully. In many hospitals, cultures are taken; and in some, such patients are placed on special precautions until the laboratory reports are complete.

Fingernails and toenails also are an indication of the patient's general physical condition. Brittle or dry nails may well be a clue to nutrition or to the patient's illness.

Hair is also a clue to the person's state of health. It is not uncommon for the hair to lose its gloss and texture or even fall out during periods of illness.

The loss or the lack of hair creates psychological problems for many persons, especially women. Wigs, falls and other hair pieces have become popular for both those who need them and those who use them as a convenience. Many hospitals have found it necessary to record that a patient has one. The cost of replacing one is not a minor expense. Also, many are flammable and are not permitted in the operating room or other units where there is a potential fire hazard.

Some terms commonly used to describe the skin and the conditions related to it are as follows:

Flush. A deep red color, as in a blush. It is usually associated with an elevated temperature, and the face and the neck are more likely to be affected than the other parts of the body.

Cyanosis. A dusky, bluish color usually seen in the lips and the nail beds; it is caused by lack of oxygen. The appearance is similar to that which occurs when a person is chilled while in swimming or immediately upon coming out of the water.

Jaundice. Yellowness of the skin. Usually, it affects the entire body, and almost always the whites of the eyes.

Dehydration. Severe loss of body fluids which causes the skin to be loose and wrinkled. The lips and the tongue are dry and parched.

Rash. An eruption on the skin. Because the descriptive details of a rash are complex, comprising type of spots, size, elevation, coloring, presence or absence of drainage or itching, etc., they are dealt with more appropriately in a text on skin diseases. For purposes of reporting, the nurse should indicate exactly where on the patient's body a rash was noted.

Ecchymosis. A bruise. Record location, size and coloring, of which the last is an indication of how recently it occurred.

Diaphoresis. An excessive amount of perspiration, as when a person's entire skin is moist and perspiring.

Edema. Retention of fluid in the tissues with consequent swelling. (It may also occur in body cavities.) Frequently, it is noted in the feet and the lower legs, but it can occur in other body areas. The skin appears taut over these areas, and if the fingers are pressed gently into the areas, an impression remains after pressure has been released.

Wound. A break in the continuity of the skin. The wound should be described as to size, shape, depth and location. If drainage is present, it too is described as to amount and character. For example, it could be scant, moderate or profuse. Terms for describing its appearance are:

- *Serous:* light: containing the serum (clear portion) of the blood
- *Sanguineous:* containing a great deal of blood
- *Serosanguineous:* containing both serum and some blood

Purulent: containing or consisting of "pus"

Gastrointestinal Observations. Additional terms concerned with elimination are discussed in Chapters 22 and 25.

Nausea. A tendency to vomit, a feeling of being unable to keep fluid or food in the stomach. Nausea is a noun. A patient has nausea, or nausea is present; nauseous is an adjective, and to describe a patient as being nauseous is to say that he is sickening or disgusting. Record that the patient is *nauseated.*

Emesis. Vomitus, contents emitted from the stomach. If it should occur, its nature and amount are recorded, i.e., "approximately eight ounces of undigested food or approximately four ounces of green liquid." When a patient vomits uncontrollably and the contents seem to leave forcefully, it is referred to as projectile vomiting. If there is an odor, record this also, such as fecal, soured food, or alcohol odor, for example.

Distention. An enlargement or swelling-like appearance. If occurring in the stomach, there will be epigastric distention; if in the intestines, there will be abdominal distention. Tapping gently on the area usually will produce a hollow (drumlike) sound.

Respiratory Observations. If the patient has a cough, it is described as nonproductive if no matter or discharge from the respiratory tract is produced. If there is expectoration, it is called a productive cough, and the expectoration is described, i.e., mucus, thick mucus.

Mucus. A viscid watery-appearing secretion of the mucous membranes. This can be expectorated with or without cough. It is a normal process of the respiratory tract.

Sputum. Matter ejected from the mouth. It could be the result of drainage from the mouth, the nasal passages, the pharynx, the tonsils, the trachea, the bronchi or the lungs. It is seen more frequently when a cough is present. If a patient is admitted with a cough, make certain that he knows how to protect his mouth. If it is a productive cough, provide wipes and a suitable container or paper bag for disposing them safely.

Pain. Pain is a subjective phenomenon; one human being cannot accurately assess the type and intensity of pain that another human being is experiencing. The nurse will need to use both questioning of the patient and her own observations to arrive at the most objective description for purposes of recording. Pain is discussed in more detail in Chapter 25. Generally, the physician wants to know the type of pain, its exact location and the duration. Some terms used in describing pain are as follows:

Sharp: Quick, sticking and intense

Dull: Not so intense or acute as a sharp pain, possibly more annoying than painful

Diffuse: Covering a large area. Usually, the patient is unable to point to a specific area without moving his hand over a large surface, such as the entire abdomen.

Shifting: Moving from one area to another, such as from the lower abdomen to the epigastric region.

Intermittent: Coming and going. It may or may not be regular.

Additional Sources of Information as Guides to Observation

Vital Signs. Further information about the patient's health status is obtained by taking his vital signs, namely temperature, pulse, respiration and blood pressure. The methods for obtaining these are given in the following section of this chapter. Having this information frequently guides the nurse in a more structured observation or questioning of the patient, particularly in such situations as when the pulse is very rapid or blood pressure seems unusually low.

Medical History and Physical Examination. The physician's report of the patient's medical history is an additional source of information which can help guide the nurse in observing the patient and planning his care. For example, many elderly persons are subject to "blackouts." Sometimes these may last only a few seconds, and for some patients they may be the equivalent of an epileptic-like seizure. Knowing this, the nurse would try to make plans to prevent the patient from harm.

The physical examination done by the physician is also a source of information that can guide observation. The nurse's role in assisting the physician with the physical examination is presented later in this chapter.

Family Members. Whenever a patient's physical, or mental state or age makes it impossible or difficult to obtain information essential to his care, a family member and certainly the parent of a child patient may need to be questioned. For example, if the patient seems to have difficulty in breathing and sounds "wheezy," it would be necessary to know if this is a chronic illness or is associated with his present state of illness. If the patient has an elastic support on a knee, what is its purpose? When was the last time the patient passed urine? Is there a language difference? These are examples of needed information that could be supplied by a family member. It must be mentioned, however, that a family member accompanying a very ill patient to the hospital or other health agency may also be experiencing emotional stress. Therefore the nurse may need to use caution so that the person is not disturbed further. There is need to help family members as well as the patients to feel at ease.

The Therapeutic Regimen and Results of Diagnostic Measures. Understanding the physician's plan of care for the patient is essential if the patient is to be observed for positive or untoward results. For example, noting that the laboratory report on the patient's blood count shows a low hemoglobin should have meaning in relation to an observation already made or to the need for further investigation. (Hemoglobin is essential for oxygen transportation to the cells and the removal of carbon dioxide.) If the nurse noted that the patient was easily fatigued, or stated he felt tired most of the time, here is a clue. It may mean planning for the patient to take more rest periods. The patient's low white blood count should signify to the nurse that he is lacking in a vital natural defense against infection.

The succeeding chapters are also concerned with observation and assessment, and measures used for the comfort, safety and mental and physical well-being of patients, regardless of their age or clinical diagnosis.

OBTAINING THE VITAL SIGNS

Definition of Vital Signs

Alterations in body functions often are reflected in the body temperature, the pulse rate, the respiratory rate and the blood pressure. The body mechanisms governing them (a part of homeostasis) are very sensitive to changes from the normal, and that is why they frequently are referred to as *vital signs* or *cardinal symptoms*. When it is noted that the vital signs have deviated from the normal, it automatically means that the patient needs to be observed for evidence of cause and also for effects.

The introduction of monitoring devices has made it possible to keep some patients' vital signs under constant surveillance. This has been a life-saving measure for many patients, because it makes for a far more accurate means of observing the effects of the therapeutic regimen ordered by the physician.

Recording a patient's vital signs is a part of the admission procedure. These should be taken by the nurse because she is skilled in detecting deviations from normal. Before taking the vital signs, it is best to permit the patient to rest for a short period of time. The excitement of being admitted usually affects him physiologically.

Most adult patients are familiar with the procedures for obtaining body temperature, pulse and respiratory rates and blood pressure. However, an explanation of the procedures by the nurse will aid in placing the patient at ease. Explanations should always be given to children to help put them at ease.

Body Temperature

Human beings are homothermic (warm-blooded) mammals and maintain body temperature independently of the environment. The body maintains temperature through the activity of special cells in the hypothalamus. These cells act as a regulator and influence heat loss and heat production by impulses received through somatic and visceral neurons in the brain stem and the spinal cord. The control of heat is believed to be maintained through the temperature of the blood when it reaches the brain and the spinal cord.

Certain authorities also believe that the endocrine system plays a part in maintaining normal body temperature.

Body temperature is maintained by a balance between heat production and heat loss. Heat is produced by the metabolic processes of the body. It is lost by the processes of conduction, convection, radiation and vaporization. Only a minimum of heat normally is lost in excreta. When the balance between heat production and heat loss is upset, as is often the case during illness, body temperature either rises above normal or falls below normal.

Body temperature is recorded either in degrees of Centigrade or degrees of Fahrenheit, abbreviated °C. or °F., respectively. Table 6 illustrates comparable Centigrade and Fahrenheit temperatures and explains how temperatures are converted from one system to another. The thermometer is placed in the mouth to obtain an *oral* temperature, in the anal canal to obtain a *rectal* temperature or in the axilla to obtain an *axillary* temperature.

Normal Body Temperature. The average normal oral temperature for adults is considered to be 37° C. (98.6° F.) ; the average normal rectal temperature is 37.5° C. (99.5° F.) ; and the average normal axillary temperature is 36.7° C. (98° F.). Variations occur in each individual and a range of 0.3° to 0.6° C. (0.5° to 1.0° F.) from the average normal temperature is considered to be within normal limits. However, wider variations from the average temperature have been found to be normal for certain individuals.

Table 6. Equivalent centigrade and fahrenheit temperatures and directions for converting temperatures from one measure to another*

Centigrade	Fahrenheit	Centigrade	Fahrenheit
34.0	93.2	38.5	101.3
35.0	95.0	39.0	102.2
36.0	96.8	40.0	104.0
36.5	97.7	41.0	105.8
37.0	98.6	42.0	107.6
37.5	99.5	43.0	109.4
38.0	100.4	44.0	111.2

* To convert Centigrade to Fahrenheit, multiply by 9/5 and add 32. To change Fahrenheit to Centigrade, subtract 32 and multiply by 5/9.

The body temperature has been observed to be lowest during the early morning hours and highest during the late afternoon or early evening hours. An inversion of this cycle has been observed in persons who work at night and sleep during the day hours. Exercise, manner of living, amount and kind of food ingested and external cold also may influence body temperature. Newborns and young children normally have a higher body temperature than adults.

Elevated Body Temperature. An elevation in normal body temperature is known as *pyrexia*. The lay term for pyrexia is *fever*. Pyrexia is a common symptom of illness, and there is sufficient evidence to believe that an elevation in body temperature aids the body in fighting disease. For example, in an infectious disease, while the causative organisms are destroyed by a total body response, the elevated temperature apparently helps to destroy bacteria as well as to mobilize the body's defenses.

The physiologic reason for pyrexia is not understood clearly, but it is believed commonly that it is the result of a direct action on the temperature-regulating center in the hypothalamus. Heat loss is decreased or heat production is increased or both occur when body temperature rises above normal. Cells in the central nervous system may be impaired when the body temperature surpasses 41° C. (105.8° F.), and survival is rare when it reaches 43° C. (109.4° F.). When high body temperature occurs, death usually is due to failure of the respiratory center, but may be due also to inactivation of body enzymes and destruction of tissue proteins.

Pyrexia may take a variety of courses, usually depending on the pathologic process occurring in the body. Several terms are used to describe the course of an elevated body temperature. The *onset* or *invasion* is the period when pyrexia begins; it may be either sudden or gradual in nature. When the temperature alternates regularly between a period of pyrexia and a period of normal or subnormal temperature, it is called an *intermittent* temperature. A *remittent* temperature is one that fluctuates several degrees above normal but does not reach normal between fluctuations. A *continued* temperature is one that remains consistently elevated and fluctuates very little. When pyrexia subsides suddenly, the drop to normal is called a *crisis*; a gradual return to normal temperature is called *lysis*. In certain instances, when body temperature has returned to normal following pyrexia, a patient may experience a temporary *recrudescence* or *recurrence* of temperature. This may be due to increased activity or exertion, in which case there is usually little cause for alarm. However, a recurring temperature may also be a sign of relapse; therefore, the temperature warrants frequent checking.

When pyrexia occurs, body metabolism is elevated above normal, and the respiratory rate and the pulse rate will also increase, as a rule proportionately with increased body temperature. The patient usually experiences loss of appetite, headaches, general malaise, depression and occasionally periods of delirium. Observing for other signs as body temperature rises is important, such as urinary output, color of skin, condition of tongue and mouth.

Lowered Body Temperature. A body temperature below the average normal range is called *hypothermia*. Death usually occurs when the temperature falls below approximately 34° C. (93.2° F.), but exceptional cases of survival have been reported when body temperatures have fallen considerably lower. There are a few illnesses associated with hypothermia, especially those producing unconsciousness; therefore, it is important to observe a patient closely when body temperature falls below normal.

While an elevated body temperature is a protective device for the body, a lowered body temperature is also beneficial in some instances. Rates of chemical reactions in the body are slowed, thereby decreasing the metabolic demands for oxygen. Hypothermia as a form of therapy is discussed in clinical texts.

Structure of Clinical Thermometers. The glass thermometer used to measure body temperature has two parts: the bulb and the stem. Mercury is in the bulb and, being a metal, will expand when exposed to heat and rise in the stem. The stem is calibrated in degrees and tenths of a degree. The range is from about 34° C. (93° F.) to about 42.2° C. (108° F.). A wider range of temperature is not necessary, since human life rarely exists above or below these temperatures.

Fractions of a degree usually are recorded in even numbers, as .2 or .6 or .8. If the mercury apears to be a bit more or less than an even tenth, it is common practice to report the nearest tenth.

Some oral thermometers have a long slender mercury bulb, and others have a blunt bulb similar to that used on almost all rectal thermometers. The blunt bulb on the rectal thermometer is to help to prevent injury when it is inserted. The long slender bulb on the oral thermometer is thought to give a larger surface area for contact. When using a thermometer in the home or in a different agency, always check to see whether it is an oral or a rectal thermometer. Some thermometers have this printed on them; others do not.

Thermometers have not escaped the trend toward disposables. One company has produced a disposable plastic thermometer. According to the description in a leading magazine, "after use, it is placed in a portable sensing unit that reads the thermometer and records the patient's temperature on a calibrated scale."

Some agencies have adopted the procedure of using one thermometer only for each patient. The thermometer is kept in the patient's unit and is disposed of when he is discharged. Thermometers used for patients having hepatitis should always be discarded when the patient is discharged.

Selecting a Site for Obtaining Body Temperature. Most hospital policies specify the site to be used for obtaining the temperature. However, the nurse must make modifications under certain circumstances.

Oral Temperature. Oral temperatures are contraindicated for unconscious and irrational patients and for infants because of the danger of breaking the thermometer in the mouth. Oral temperatures are also contraindicated for patients who breathe through their mouths and for patients with diseases of the oral cavity or surgery of the nose or the mouth.

If the patient has had either hot or cold food or fluids, a period of approximately 30 minutes should elapse before obtaining an oral temperature to allow time for the oral tissues to return to normal temperature.[17]

Rectal Temperature. A rectal temperature is more accurate than an oral or an axillary temperature. If a patient having an oral temperature taken routinely shows a considerable change in his temperature, it is good practice to check it rectally. Some hospitals require rectal readings on patients having an

PRINCIPLES GUIDING ACTION IN OBTAINING BODY TEMPERATURE

The purpose is to measure body temperature.

Oral Method

SUGGESTED ACTION	PRINCIPLE
If the thermometer has been stored in a chemical solution, wipe it dry with a firm twisting motion, using clean soft tissue.	Chemical solutions may irritate mucous membranes and may have an objectionable odor or taste. Soft tissue will approximate the surface, and twisting helps to contact the entire surface.
Wipe once from the bulb toward the fingers with each tissue.	Wiping from an area where there are few or no organisms to an area where organisms may be present minimizes the spread of organisms to cleaner areas.
Grasp the thermometer firmly with thumb and forefinger, and with strong wrist movements shake the thermometer until the mercury line reaches the lowest marking.	A constriction in the mercury line near the bulb of the thermometer prevents the mercury from dropping below the last temperature reading unless it is shaken down forcefully.
Read the thermometer by holding it horizontally at eye level, and rotate it between the fingers until the mercury line can be seen clearly.	Holding the thermometer at eye level facilitates reading. Rotating the thermometer will aid in placing the mercury line in a position where it can be read best.
Place the mercury bulb of the thermometer under the patient's tongue and instruct him to close his lips tightly.	When the bulb rests against the superficial blood vessels under the tongue and the mouth is closed, a more reliable measurement of body temperature can be obtained.
Leave the thermometer in place for 5-7 minutes.[11]	Allowing sufficient time for the oral tissues to reach their maximum temperature results in a more accurate measurement of body temperature.
Remove the thermometer and wipe it once from the fingers down to the mercury bulb, using a firm twisting motion.	Cleansing from an area where there are few organisms to an area where there are numerous organisms minimizes the spread of organisms to cleaner areas. Friction helps to loosen matter from a surface.
Read the thermometer and shake it down as described above.	
Dispose of wipe in a receptacle used for contaminated items.	Confining contaminated articles helps to reduce the spread of pathogens.

PRINCIPLES GUIDING ACTION IN OBTAINING BODY TEMPERATURE (Continued)

Rectal Method

SUGGESTED ACTION	PRINCIPLE
Wipe, read and shake the rectal thermometer as the suggested procedure for obtaining an oral temperature indicates.	
Lubricate the mercury bulb and an area approximately 1 inch above the bulb.	Lubrication reduces friction and thereby facilitates insertion of the thermometer; this minimizes irritation of the mucous membrane of the anal canal.
With the patient on his side, fold back the bed linen and separate the buttocks so that the anal sphincter is seen clearly. Insert the thermometer for approximately 1½ inches. Permit buttocks to fall in place.	If not placed directly into the anal opening the bulb of the thermometer may injure the sphincter, or hemorrhoids if present.
Leave the thermometer in place for 2 to 3 minutes. Hold the thermometer in place if the patient is irrational or a restless child.	Allowing sufficient time for the thermometer to register results in a more accurate measurement of body temperature.
Remove the thermometer and wipe it once from the fingers to the mercury bulb, using a firm twisting motion.	Cleansing from an area where there are few organisms to an area where there are numerous organisms minimizes the spread of organisms. Friction helps to loosen matter from a surface.
Read and shake the thermometer and dispose of wipe in a receptacle used for contaminated items.	

Axillary Method

SUGGESTED ACTION	PRINCIPLE
If the thermometer has been stored in a chemical solution, wipe it dry with a firm twisting motion, using a clean tissue.	Chemical solutions may irritate the skin. The presence of solution may alter the skin temperature. Soft tissue with the aid of friction aids in removing the solution.
Read and shake the thermometer as the suggested procedure for obtaining an oral temperature indicates.	
Place the thermometer well into the axilla with the bulb directed toward the patient's head. Bring the patient's arm down close to his body and place his forearm over his chest.	When the bulb rests against the superficial blood vessels in the axilla and the skin surfaces are brought together to reduce the amount of air surrounding the bulb, a reasonably reliable measurement of body temperature can be obtained.
Leave the thermometer in place for 10 minutes or more.	Allowing sufficient time for the axillary tissue to reach its maximum temperature results in a reasonably accurate measurement of body temperature.
Remove, read and shake the thermometer and dispose of wipe.	

elevated temperature. It is usual procedure to obtain rectal temperatures for infants, for unconscious and for irrational patients. Rectal temperatures are contraindicated for patients having rectal surgery, diarrhea or diseases of the rectum.

Axillary Temperature. Obtaining an axillary temperature is rare and is used only when both oral and rectal temperatures are contraindicated or the sites are not usable or accessible. Unless the patient is capable of cooperating, the nurse will need to remain in attendance to hold the thermometer. The axillary temperature is the least accurate way of obtaining body temperature, since the axilla is easily influenced by environmental conditions and because it is often difficult to approximate skin surfaces while the bulb of the thermometer is held in place. If the axilla has just been washed, taking the temperature should be delayed, since the temperature of the water and the friction created by drying the skin will influence the temperature.

PRINCIPLES GUIDING ACTION IN DISINFECTING CLINICAL THERMOMETERS

The purpose is to disinfect a thermometer that has been used for obtaining a patient's temperature.

SUGGESTED ACTION	PRINCIPLE
Use a soft tissue for cleansing the thermometer.	Adhered organic matter interferes with disinfection.
Use a clean, soft tissue each time the thermometer must be wiped.	Soft tissue comes into close contact with all surfaces of the thermometer.
Hold the tissue at the end of the thermometer near the fingers.	Cleansing an area from where there are few organisms to an area where there are numerous organisms minimizes the spread of organisms to cleaner areas.
Wipe down toward the bulb, using a twisting motion.	Friction helps to loosen matter from a surface.
After the thermometer has been wiped, cleanse it with soap or detergent solution, again using friction.	Soap or detergent solutions loosen adhered matter.
Rinse the thermometer under cold running water.	Rinsing with water helps to remove organisms and foreign material loosened by washing. Also, certain chemical solutions are rendered ineffective in the presence of soap—for example, benzalkonium chloride (Zephiran Chloride).
Dry the thermometer after it has been rinsed.	The strength of a chemical solution is decreased when water is added to the solution.
Immerse the thermometer in the chemical solution specified.	Chemical solutions must be used in proper strength for the proper length of time in order to be effective.
Rinse the thermometer with water after disinfection.	Chemical solutions may irritate the mucous membrane of the mouth or the rectum. Also, they may have an objectionable odor and taste.
Return the thermometer to the storage receptacle.	

Cleansing Clinical Thermometers. Making a thermometer safe for use with another person presents a problem. Heat sufficient to kill pathogenic organisms will ruin thermometers by causing the mercury to expand beyond the column within the thermometer. Therefore, the method of choice is to disinfect thermometers in a chemical solution.

The suggested action and the underlying principles in the procedure on page 159 apply to either oral or rectal thermometers. However, since a lubricant is used on a rectal thermometer, cleansing to remove the lubricant thoroughly prior to disinfection is essential. If the lubricant is not removed thoroughly, organisms may harbor in a film of lubricant, and the disinfection procedure becomes ineffective. Detergents are particularly effective for emulsifying oils and fats even in cool and hard water; therefore, it is preferable to use a detergent rather than soap.

It is common practice now to have thermometers issued from the Central Supply. After being used on the patient unit (one thermometer for each patient) they are returned for cleansing and disinfection. The Central Supply unit has a machine for shaking down the mercury in many thermometers simultaneously.

Pulse

Each time the left ventricle of the heart contracts to eject blood into an already full aorta, the arterial walls in the blood system expand (distend) to compensate for the increase in pressure. This expansion of the arterial walls occurring with each ventricular contraction is called the *pulse*. The pulse can be felt with the fingertips through the patient's skin where there is a superficial artery, and by counting each expansion of the arterial wall in a given period of time, the *pulse rate* can be determined.

When the patient's pulse is being obtained, the rate, the rhythm, the volume and the condition of the arterial wall should be noted.

Normally, the rise and fall of the arterial wall or pulse wave is smooth and regular. If the ending of the pulse wave is exaggerated, the pulse wave feels double to touch, and the pulse is said to be a *dicrotic pulse*.

Pulse Rate. On awakening in the morning, the pulse rate of the average healthy adult male is approximately 60 to 65 per minute. The pulse rate for women is slightly faster —about seven to eight beats per minute more than for men. Pulse varies with age, gradually diminishing from birth to adulthood and then increasing somewhat in very old age. It has been noted also that body size and build of an individual may affect the pulse rate. Tall, slender persons often have a slower rate than short, stout ones. Very wide variations in pulse rates have been noted in normal healthy adults. The American Heart Association accepts as normal for adults a pulse rate of between 50 and 100 beats per minute.

There are numerous causes for changes in the pulse rate. The rate of the heartbeat responds readily to impulses conducted along the sympathetic and the parasympathetic nervous systems. Stimulation of the sympathetic system increases the heart rate and, therefore, the pulse rate. This system responds quickly to emotions; consequently, the pulse rate increases when a person experiences fear, anger, surprise, worry and the like. The sympathetic system also receives impulses from internal organs of the body. For example, pain in the abdomen will cause the pulse rate to quicken, usually due to sympathetic stimulation. The rate also increases with exercise as the heart compensates for the increased need for blood circulation.

Prolonged application of heat to the skin will stimulate the heartbeat and increase the pulse rate. The pulse rate increases when blood pressure decreases as the heart attempts to increase the output of blood. When blood pressure increases, the pulse rate usually will decrease. Elevated body temperature is accompanied by an increase in pulse rate—usually an increase of about seven to ten beats per minute for each 0.6° C. (1° F.) of elevation above normal.

When the pulse rate is over 100 beats per minute, the condition is referred to as *tachycardia*.

Stimulation of the parasympathetic system decreases the pulse rate. The drug, digitalis, commonly taken by patients having heart ailments, is an example of an agent that decreases the pulse rate by stimulating the vagus nerves of the parasympathetic system.

The term used to describe the pulse rate when it falls below approximately 50 beats per minute is *bradycardia.* A slow pulse rate is less common during illness than a rapid pulse rate. Therefore, when bradycardia does occur, it should be reported to the physician immediately.

Rhythm of the Pulse. Normally, the pulse rhythm is regular, and the time interval between beats is equal. The force of the normal pulse is equal with each beat. Irregular pulse rhythm is called *arrhythmia.* An *intermittent pulse* is one that has a period of normal rhythm broken by periods of irregularity or skipped beats. An intermittent rhythm may be a serious sign, as in certain heart diseases, or it may be a temporary condition due to emotional upset or fright.

Volume of the Pulse. Under normal conditions, the volume of each pulse beat is equal. The pulse can be obliterated with relative ease, by exerting pressure over the artery, but it remains perceptible with moderate pressure. When the volume of the pulse beat is difficult to obliterate, the pulse is called *bounding.* If the volume is small, the pulse is called *feeble, weak* or *thready* and is obliterated readily. A thready pulse usually is associated with a rapid pulse rate.

The Arterial Wall. When the fingertips are placed over an artery, the sense of touch will determine certain characteristics of the arterial wall. Normally, it is elastic, straight (unless the fingertips rest on a normally tortuous artery), smooth and round. With

PRINCIPLES GUIDING ACTION IN OBTAINING THE RADIAL PULSE RATE

The purpose is to count the number of times the heart beats per minute and to obtain an estimate of the quality of the heart's action.

SUGGESTED ACTION	PRINCIPLE
Have the patient rest his arm alongside his body with the wrist extended and the palm of the hand downward.	This position places the radial artery on the inner aspect of the patient's wrist. The nurse's fingers rest conveniently on the artery with the thumb in apposition on the outer aspect of the patient's wrist.
Place the 1st, the 2nd and the 3rd fingers along the radial artery and press gently against the radius; rest the thumb on the back of the patient's wrist.	The fingertips, sensitive to touch, will feel the pulsation of the patient's radial artery. If the thumb is used for palpating the patient's pulse the nurse may feel her own pulse.
Apply only enough pressure so that the patient's pulsating artery can be felt distinctly.	Moderate pressure allows the nurse to feel the superficial radial artery expand and contract with each heart beat. Too much pressure will obliterate the pulse. If too little pressure is applied, the pulse will be imperceptible.
Using a watch with a second hand, count the number of pulsations felt on the patient's artery for half a minute. Multiply this number by 2 to obtain the patient's pulse rate for 1 minute.	Sufficient time is necessary to detect irregularities or other defects.
If the pulse rate is abnormal in any way, count the pulse rate for a full minute. Repeat the counting if necessary to determine accurately the rate, the quality and the volume.	When the pulse is abnormal, full minute countings are necessary to allow for irregular timing between beats.

advancing age, the arteries become less elastic and smooth, and a normally straight artery may feel tortuous to touch.

Where the Pulse Can Be Obtained. Usually, the radial artery at the wrist is used for obtaining the pulse rate, since it is easily accessible and it can be pressed against the radius. If it is not possible to obtain the pulse at the wrist, the facial, the dorsalis pedis, the temporal or the femoral artery can be used, since they are superficial and can be pressed against a bone. It is possible to obtain the pulse rate easily and without disturbing the patient if the nurse understands how to use alternate sites. A site should be used that does not produce exertion or discomfort for the patient, since this could alter the pulse rate.

Inasmuch as external cardiac compression has become an accepted emergency measure (Chap. 21), it is very important for the nurse to know how to palpate for the carotid or femoral pulse. The carotid pulse is the one of choice because it is the easiest for the "rescuer" to use when doing either external ventilation or circulation. Use the index and middle fingers when locating the carotid pulse. Feel for the larynx, slide to the side in the area of the carotid artery, and press gently. It is easier to find with flat palpation rather than with just the fingertips.

Counting the Heartbeat at the Apex. Occasionally, a patient has a radial pulse that is difficult to count. It may be so irregular and the force of the beats so uneven that it is impossible to determine an accurate count. Even using alternate sites does not provide any more accuracy. Two nurses checking the pulse may have different counts. A more accurate estimate of the heartbeats per minute can be obtained by placing a stethoscope over the apex of the heart. The impulse of the heart against the chest wall can be heard in the space between the fifth and the sixth ribs about three inches (8 cm.) to the left of the median line and slightly below the nipple.

It is not general practice for a nurse to do this on a newly admitted patient unless this is the only way a count can be obtained, such as for a critically ill patient. Since the nurse does not know how much the patient knows about his illness, such an act might be disturbing to him. On the other hand, if the patient indicates an awareness of cardiac problems, he might expect this. The nurse will have to use judgment as to whether or not an apical count, in the interest of accuracy, might cause the patient to wonder what is wrong. In recording a pulse rate about which there is some doubt, mention should be made of the fact. A question mark alongside of the dot on the T.P.R. sheet is a practice followed in many situations. However, a description of the pulse should be recorded in the Nurses' Notes.

Apical-Radial Pulse. For many patients having cardiac impairment or receiving medications to improve heart action, the physician will request that the heartbeat be counted at the apex of the heart and the radial pulse simultaneously. This is referred to as *apical-radial pulse.* This requires two nurses. One listens over the apex of the heart with a stethoscope; the other counts at the wrist. They use one watch conveniently placed between them. After listening and feeling to be sure that they can get the best possible count, they decide on a time to start counting, for example, when the second hand is on the 15 or the 30. At this time, both start counting for a full minute. The count is recorded on the patient's chart in the place indicated by the agency's procedure.

Respiration

Respiration is the process by which oxygen and carbon dioxide are interchanged. *External respiration* refers to the delivery of oxygen to the blood and the removal of carbon dioxide from the blood via the respiratory and the circulatory systems. *Internal respiration* refers to the process by which oxygen from the blood is made available to cells in the body and carbon dioxide is removed from the tissues into the blood.

The flow of air into and from the lungs depends on pressure differences between the thoracic cavity and the atmosphere. The rate and the depth of respiration are controlled by the respiratory center in the medulla oblongata.

The chemical stimulation of an increased carbon dioxide tension in the blood is an important phenomenon of involuntary respiration. As carbon dioxide accumulates in the blood, the respiratory center is stimulated directly and also indirectly by the carotid and the aortic glomi, and the rate and the depth of respiration are increased. This involuntary chemical stimulation is responsible for the limitation of voluntary control of breathing. A new mother, not realizing this, may panic when her child has a temper tantrum and holds his breath.

When breathing is voluntary, impulses travel to the respiratory center from the motor area of the cerebral cortex. Because of this arrangement, a person can automatically control his breathing when talking and singing, and voluntarily hold his breath until the carbon dioxide tension builds up excessively in the blood.

The respiratory center responds reflexly from impulses that can be carried over any sensory nerve in the body. For example, fear, pain, unusual sights and sounds and the like will reflexly alter respiratory rates and depths. Afferent fibers of the pulmonic vagi also reflexly stimulate the respiratory center. Through this course, impulses from the lungs reflexly end each respiratory act. It is believed that certain centers in the brain also reflexly affect respirations.

When respirations are being observed, their rate, depth and character are noted, along with observation of the patient's color and the muscles used in breathing.

Respiratory Rate. Normally, healthy adults breathe approximately 16 to 20 times a minute. Wider variations have been observed in healthy persons. The respiratory rate is more rapid in infants and young children. It has been noted that the relationship between the pulse rate and the respiratory rate is fairly consistent in normal persons, the ratio being one respiration to approximately four heartbeats. Increased rate of respiration is called *polypnea*.

Respiratory Depth. At rest, the depth of each respiration is approximately the same. The volume of air normally exchanged in each respiration, the *tidal air*, varies greatly with individuals, but the average is about 500 cc. of air. The depth of respirations is described as *deep* or *shallow*, depending on whether the volume of air taken in is above or below normal. Increased depth of respirations is called *hyperpnea*.

Nature of Respiration. Ordinarily, breathing is automatic, and respirations are noiseless, regular, even and without effort. Between each respiration there is normally a short resting period.

Difficult breathing is called *dyspnea*. Dyspneic patients usually appear to be anxious, and their faces are drawn from exertion. Often, the nostrils will dilate as the patient fights for his breath. The abdominal muscles are used to aid in breathing.

Dyspneic patients frequently find relief if they sit up in bed, which places the thorax in a vertical position. This condition is called *orthopnea*. According to one authority,

> The improvement in breathing observed in this position has been interpreted as due to the following mechanism: when the thorax is in the orthopneic position (i.e., vertical) the abdominal viscera do not press against the diaphragm, and the negative pleural pressure increases; this causes pulmonary congestion to diminish. The distensibility of the lung and vital capacity increases; this causes the Hering-Breuer reflex to diminish; circulation improves, the pressure of the cerebrospinal fluid diminishes, and the blood supply to the respiratory center also improves.*

Cheyne-Stokes respirations refer to breathing consisting of a gradual increase in the depth of respirations followed by a gradual decrease in the depth of respirations and then a period of no breathing or *apnea*. Dyspnea is usually present. Cheyne-Stokes respirations are a serious symptom during illness and very often occur as death approaches.

Breathing that is unusually noisy is referred to as *stertorous*. A snoring sound is common.

There are still other terms that describe various types of respirations. Describe the specific character of the respirations rather than attempt to use a term that may be misinterpreted.

---

* Houssay, Bernardo A. *et al*: Human Physiology, ed. 2, p. 301, New York, McGraw-Hill, 1955.

Observation of the Patient. While the respiratory rate is being obtained, the color of the patient and his act of breathing should be noted. *Anoxia* is present when the patient is not receiving an adequate supply of oxygen. As a result, the skin and the mucous membranes will appear dusky and bluish. This skin coloring is described as *cyanosis*, from a Greek word meaning blue. Both abdominal breathing, involving the diaphragm and the abdominal wall muscles, and costal breathing, involving the intercostal muscles, are present. In certain disease conditions, either one or the other may be exaggerated.

Cyanosis is more marked on the body where numerous small blood vessels lie close to the skin surface, such as the nailbeds, the lips, the lobes of the ears and the cheeks. When cyanosis is not marked, these may be the only areas appearing cyanotic. In marked cyanosis all areas of the skin may appear bluish. If pallor is present, cyanosis may be masked. If the skin is flushed for any reason, cyanosis may be intensified. In persons with dark skin, cyanosis usually can be detected by examining the color of the mucous membrane of the mouth and under the tongue to see if there is a dusky appearance.

Factors Affecting Respiration. From the brief discussion earlier concerning the control of respirations, it can be seen that a variety of factors will normally influence respirations. During illness, there are still other influences. When body temperature is elevated, the respiratory rate increases as the body attempts to rid itself of excess heat. Any condition involving an accumulation of carbon dioxide and a decrease of oxygen in the blood also will tend to increase the rate and the depth of respirations.

There are conditions that characteristically predispose to slow breathing. For example, an increase in intracranial pressure will depress the respiratory center, resulting in irregular and/or shallow, slow breathing. Certain drugs will also depress respirations.

Frequency of Obtaining Temperature, Pulse and Respiration. Most hospitals have policies determined by medical and nursing personnel, governing when and how frequently temperature, pulse and respiration observations are made on patients. In addition to

PRINCIPLES GUIDING ACTION IN OBTAINING THE RESPIRATORY RATE

The purpose is to obtain the respiratory rate per minute and an estimate of the patient's respiratory status.

SUGGESTED ACTION	PRINCIPLE
While the fingertips are still in place after counting the pulse rate, observe the patient's respiration.	Counting the respirations while presumably still counting the pulse keeps the patient from becoming conscious of his breathing and possibly altering his usual rate.
Note the rise and fall of the patient's chest with each inspiration and expiration. This observation can be made without disturbing the patient's bedclothes.	A complete cycle of inspiration and expiration constitutes one act of respiration.
Using a watch with a second hand, count the number of respirations for half a minute. Multiply this number by 2 to obtain the patient's respiratory rate per minute.	Sufficient time is necessary to observe rate, depth and other characteristics.
If respirations are abnormal in any way, count the respiratory rate for a full minute. Repeat if necessary to determine accurately the rate and the characteristics of the breathing.	Full minute countings allow for unequal timing between respirations.

the admission observation, some require that all patients have at least two observations per day. Patients having elevated temperatures or those who are in the immediate postoperative period may have observations made every four hours. In some self-care, chronic illness or psychiatric units, these observations are not made unless the physician requests it. When a patient's condition is not associated with an elevated temperature, there seems to be little justification for observing these signs several times a day.

Although auxiliary personnel may make temperature, pulse and respiration observations, the point remains that the nurse responsible for the patient is ultimately responsible for these observations as well. Should a patient show untoward symptoms, the nurse should count the pulse and the respirations and, if necessary, take the temperature. They are cardinal signs and a good clue to what is happening in the body.

Nurses as well as physicians have questioned the frequency with which routine temperature and pulse and respiratory rates should be obtained on hospitalized patients. It does not seem logical to disturb patients unnecessarily to obtain temperature and pulse and respiratory rates when they have been consistently within a normal range and when the patient's condition is such that an abnormal temperature or pulse or respiratory rate would be unusual.

Blood Pressure

Although the physician measures the patient's blood pressure at the time of the physical examination, frequently it is the responsibility of the nurse to record it upon admission and to follow up with subsequent checks. This is particularly true with patients who have unusually low or high blood pressure. It is also necessary during the immediate postoperative period when the patient is reacting from anesthesia or following injury or shock. As with the other vital signs, measuring the blood pressure is a satisfactory way of determining certain physiologic changes that may be occurring.

From the study of human physiology it will be recalled that maximum pressure is exerted on the wall of the arteries when the left ventricle of the heart pushes blood into the aorta. The maximum pressure is called *systolic pressure,* and the minimum pressure (or pressure which is constantly present on the arterial walls) is called the *diastolic pressure.* The difference between the two is called the *pulse pressure.* Determining systolic and diastolic pressure is an excellent way of determining the work of the heart and the resistance offered by the peripheral vessels. Blood pressure is recorded in millimeters of mercury, abbreviated mm. Hg, and recorded as follows: 120/80, 120 being the systolic pressure and 80 being the diastolic pressure.

Factors Maintaining Normal Arterial Pressure. The cardiovascular system is a closed system, and measuring blood pressure determines the pressure in that system. There are five primary factors that normally maintain pressure:

1. The pump action of the heart. A weak pump action results in a lower blood pressure than a strong pump action.
2. Peripheral resistance. If the caliber of the peripheral vessels is abnormally small, blood pressure is increased, while peripheral vessels with a large caliber will mean a decreased blood pressure.
3. The quantity of blood. When blood quantity is low, for example following a hemorrhage, blood pressure is low; increasing the quantity of blood will increase the pressure.
4. The viscosity of the blood. Viscosity is the quality of adhering, i.e., having a sticky, glutinous consistency. The more viscous the blood, the higher the blood pressure will be.
5. The elasticity of the vessel walls. Vessels that have little elasticity offer more resistance than vessels with great elasticity. As resistance increases, so also does the pressure.

Disease conditions that affect one or more of these five factors will influence blood pressure.

Normal Blood Pressure. Studies of healthy persons indicate that blood pressure can fall within a rather wide range and still be normal. Since individual differences are considerable, it is of importance to know what is the *normal* blood pressure for any given person. However, if there is a rise or fall of 20 to 30 mm. Hg in an individual's pressure, it is of real significance, even if it is well within the generally accepted range of normal.

The normal newborn infant has a systolic pressure of approximately 20-60 mm. Hg. Blood pressure increases gradually until puberty when a more sudden rise occurs. A steady but not great rise continues from adolescence to old age in healthy individuals. Average range of pulse pressure is about 30 to 50 mm. Hg. The pulse pressure assumes an important factor in certain illnesses inasmuch as it varies directly with the amount of blood being pumped out during systole.

It has been found that nearly all persons will show normal fluctuations within the course of a day. The blood pressure is usually lowest early in the morning before breakfast and before activity commences. The blood pressure has been noted to rise as much as 5 to 10 mm. Hg by late afternoon, and it will gradually fall again during the sleeping hours.

There are several factors that will influence blood pressure in the normal healthy person. The age factor has already been demonstrated. Sex influences blood pressure, females usually having a lower blood pressure than males at the same age. Blood pressure has been observed to rise after the ingestion of food. It will also rise during a period of exercise or strenuous activity. Emotions will generally cause a rise in blood pressure. A person who is lying down will have a lower blood pressure as a rule than when he is in a sitting or a standing position.

Persons whose blood pressure is above normal are in a state of *hypertension*; a blood pressure below average is called *hypotension.*

Measuring Blood Pressure. A sphygmomanometer and a stethoscope are necessary to measure blood pressure by the *indirect method.** The stethoscope is used to listen to the sounds; the sphygmomanometer measures the pressure.

One type of sphygmomanometer consists of a rectangular inflatable rubber bag covered with a long piece of cloth so that it can be secured to the patient's arm. The bag communicates with a mercury manometer via a rubber tube. A pressure bulb is used to inflate the bag, which acts like a tourniquet on the arm. A needle valve on the bulb allows air to escape from the bag so that the pressure can be released. It is by means of this valve that the pressure in the bag can be regulated so that the blood pressure can be measured. Another type of manometer is the aneroid type. It too has a cuff, but it is attached to an instrument which gives the pressure reading on a dial indicator.

* The *direct method* of obtaining blood pressure is done by placing a needle in an artery and connecting it with a manometer. This method is used only when precise measurement is needed.

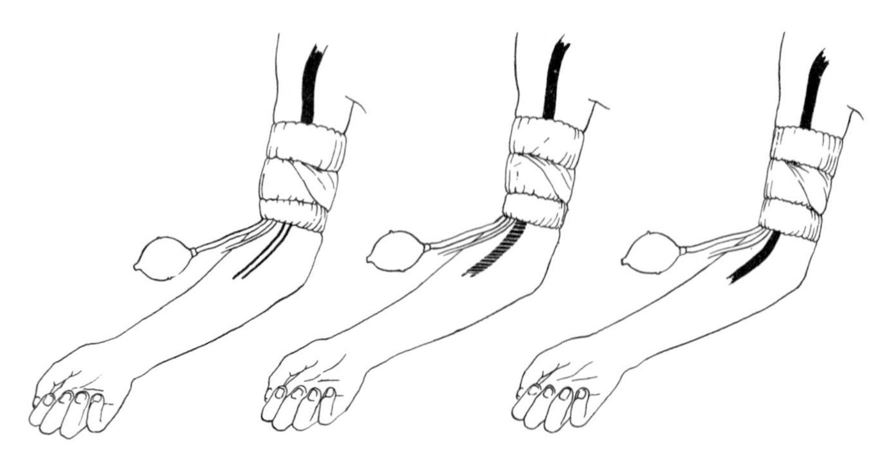

Fig. 17-2. When the cuff has been inflated sufficiently, it will occlude the flow of blood into the forearm (left). No sound will be heard through the stethoscope at this time. When pressure in the cuff is reduced sufficiently for blood to begin flowing through the brachial artery (center), the first sound is recorded as the systolic pressure. As the pressure in the cuff continues to be released, the last distinct sound heard through the stethoscope is the diastolic pressure. At this time, blood flows through the brachial artery freely (right).

PRINCIPLES GUIDING ACTION IN OBTAINING THE BLOOD PRESSURE WITH A MERCURY MANOMETER

The purpose is to measure the patient's systolic and diastolic blood pressure by an indirect method.

SUGGESTED ACTION	PRINCIPLE
Have the patient in a comfortable position with the forearm supported and the palm upward.	This position places the brachial artery so that a stethoscope can rest on it conveniently in the antecubital area.
Place yourself so that the meniscus of mercury can be read at eye level, and no more than 3 feet away.	If the eye level is above or below the meniscus, parallax* will give an inaccurate reading. A distance of more than 3 feet will result in an inaccurate reading.
Place the cuff so that the inflatable bag is centered over the brachial artery (it lies midway between the anterior and the medial aspects of the arm) so that the lower edge of cuff is 2 cm. above antecubital fossa.	Pressure applied directly to the artery will yield most accurate readings.
Wrap the cuff smoothly around the arm and tack end of cuff securely under preceding wrapping.	A twisted cuff and wrapping could produce unequal pressure and thus an inaccurate reading.
Use the fingertips to feel for a strong pulsation in the antecubital space.	Accurate blood pressure readings are possible when the stethoscope is directly over the artery.
Place the stethoscope on the brachial artery in the antecubital space where the pulse was noted.	Sound transmission can be distorted when source and reception are misaligned.
Pump the bulb of the manometer until the mercury rises to approximately 20 to 30 mm. above the point where it is anticipated that systolic pressure should be.	Pressure in the cuff prevents blood from flowing through the brachial artery. (Lack of blood causes a numb sensation in patient's lower arm.)
Using the valve on the bulb, release air 2 to 3 mm. per heart beat and note on the manometer the point at which the first sound is heard; record this figure as the systolic pressure.	Systolic pressure is that point at which the blood in the brachial artery is first able to force its way through, against the pressure exerted on the vessel by the cuff of the manometer.
Continue to release the air in the cuff evenly and gradually. Sounds may become a bit "muffled".†	The artery is open, but still partly occluded.
Note the reading on the manometer when the last distinct loud sound is heard. Record this figure as the diastolic pressure.	Diastolic pressure is that point at which blood flows freely in the brachial artery and is equivalent to the amount of pressure normally exerted on the walls of the arteries when the heart is at rest.
Allow the remaining air to escape quickly, remove the cuff and cleanse the equipment according to hospital procedure.	

* Parallax is the apparent change of position of an object when seen from two different points. For instance, if the mercury level were higher than eye level, the reading would be higher than it actually is.

† Increase drop to 5 to 6 mm. for patients who have a known wide pulse pressure until near the expected diastolic.

The width of the cuff, that is, the distance the cuff extends up and down the limb (the arm being used most frequently), is a factor in obtaining an accurate blood pressure reading. If the cuff is too small, such as an average cuff used on an obese person, the reading could very well be higher than the actual pressure in the artery. Pressure is not evenly transmitted. If a cuff is too large, as an adult cuff used on the thin arm of a child, the reading may be less than the pressure in the artery. In this instance, pressure is being directed toward a smaller surface area and therefore is more concentrated. It is recommended that the cuff width be 1.2 times the diameter of the limb. Inasmuch as a large selection of cuffs is not available, the one coming closest to this measurement should be used. (See illustrations in the American Journal of Nursing.[1])

The stethoscope is needed in order to listen to the sound directly over the artery as the pressure in the cuff is released and the blood is permitted to flow through. The bell or conelike construction in the tip of the stethoscope magnifies the sounds in the artery, and these sound waves are transmitted by means of the tubing to the listener. By listening to the sounds and watching the mercury column or dial, the blood pressure reading is obtained. Make certain that the eartips of the stethoscope are directed into the external canals of the ears and not against the ear itself. Individual differences in persons using a stethoscope will determine if the ear tips should be directed one way or the other into the ears. Every nurse should experiment to determine which method is best for her.

If the patient has been active, a short period of rest is indicated before taking the reading. Where extreme accuracy in measurement is required, the physician may ask that repeated readings be taken in the same arm, at the same time of day and with the patient in the same position, i.e., lying down or sitting. Changes in these circumstances can affect the readings. This is especially important if the patient has hyper- or hypotension.

This procedure requires accurate hearing and sight on the part of the person taking the reading. Not everyone is qualified to perform it with consistently reliable results.

Frequency of Measuring Blood Pressure. The patient's blood pressure usually is obtained on admission to a health agency and not again unless there is reason for additional readings. If the patient has an illness involving the circulatory system, daily or even more frequent readings may be ordered by the physician. Postoperative readings may also be ordered.

As with temperature, pulse and respiration, the nurse will have to exercise judgment. If a patient shows a change in condition, a blood pressure reading would be helpful to the physician when reporting to him.

Patients who are in need of almost constant recording of vital signs are usually placed in the intensive care facilities where this can be done by means of the monitoring systems.

Try to take the blood pressure reading as quickly as possible in order to prevent venous congestion. Remember the cuff acts as a tourniquet. Venous congestion in the arm below the cuff will also affect the reading.

When necessary to repeat the procedure in order to be certain an accurate one was obtained, allow the venous circulation in the lower arm to return to normal 20 to 30 seconds or more if necessary.

If a patient is to have frequent blood pressure readings taken and the cuff is left in place, always check to see that it has not rotated out of position before taking the next reading. Make certain cuff cannot be inflated in between readings.

ASSISTING WITH THE PHYSICAL EXAMINATION

Introduction

The necessity of at least an annual physical examination is accepted by the public as being an important part of health care. Its role in detecting and preventing disease is readily recognized. Unfortunately, too few people bother to practice what they know is good health care. Therefore, few persons have a regular physical examination unless their employer requires it.

Many health organizations are encouraging people to assume a more positive attitude toward health by making certain diagnostic facilities available to them, such as chest x-rays, "screening" procedures for detecting diabetes, films on self examination of the breast, and so on. Magazines and newspapers abound in information about health and illness; so do radio and television. The lay person can be quite knowledgeable about medical information and therapy and many may be tempted to do some self-diagnosing and treating. This can sometimes be disastrous. Periodic health check ups are a good preventive measure.

A physical examination is a routine part of the admission of a patient to the hospital. The nurse may be needed to assist the physician during the entire procedure if the patient's condition makes this necessary. Or, the nurse may assist with certain phases of it. Understanding the procedure and the values of it should aid nurses in teaching patients and their families.

Measuring the Patient's Height and Weight

After a patient is admitted, it is common practice in most health agencies for his height and weight to be measured. Even though the patient may have been weighed recently at home, it is preferable to weigh him on admission so that subsequent weights can be taken on the same scale, thus making comparisons more nearly accurate. The patient's height is measured at the same time; he should be asked to remove his shoes for this procedure. It is good medical aseptic technic to place a paper towel on the scale before the patient stands on it with his bare feet and to use a clean towel for each patient.

Weighing the patient and measuring his height may be delayed if he is too ill, unless the physician needs to know the weight for purposes of therapy. To make weighing easier for very ill patients, some hospitals have portable scales or scales mounted on wheels. The scale can then be rolled to the patient's bedside and he need only step out of bed onto the scale.

Many factors enter into a consideration of what is normal weight, such as age, body build, height and sex. Therefore, it is dif-

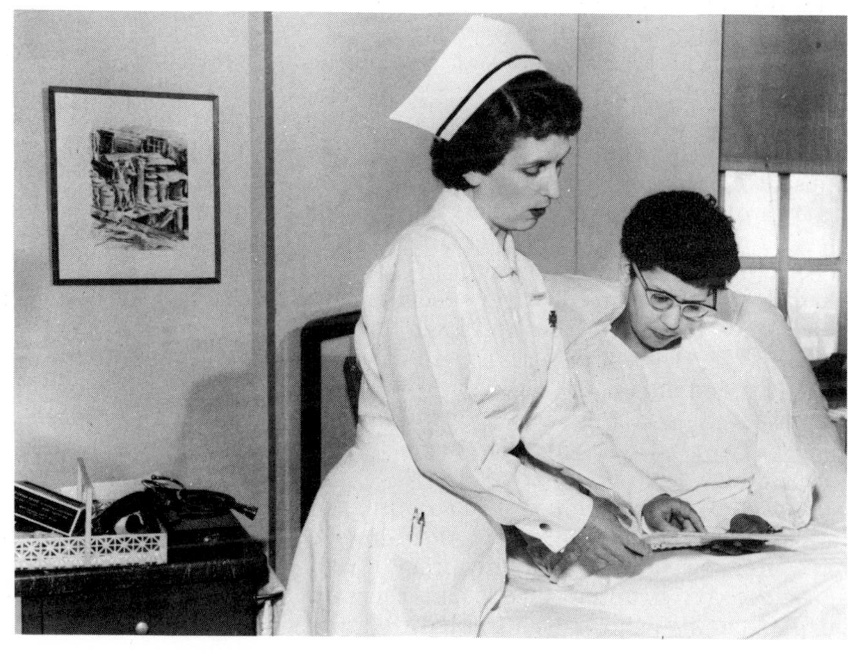

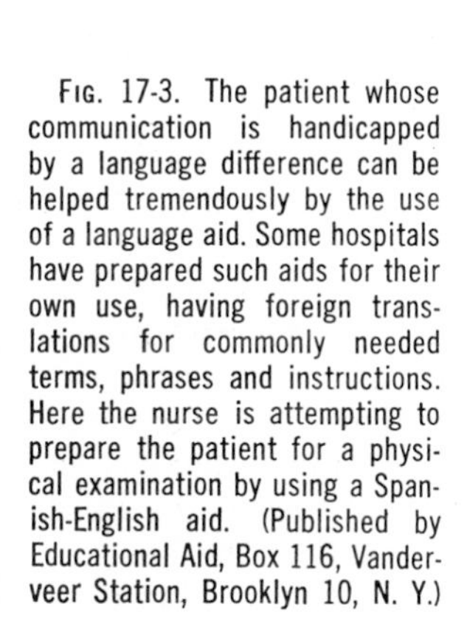

Fig. 17-3. The patient whose communication is handicapped by a language difference can be helped tremendously by the use of a language aid. Some hospitals have prepared such aids for their own use, having foreign translations for commonly needed terms, phrases and instructions. Here the nurse is attempting to prepare the patient for a physical examination by using a Spanish-English aid. (Published by Educational Aid, Box 116, Vanderveer Station, Brooklyn 10, N. Y.)

ficult to determine where abnormality begins. Many physicians believe that a 10 to 15 per cent variation from the average described in weight tables falls within normal limits.

The patient's height and weight are recorded in the appropriate places on the patient's chart.

Preparation for the Physical Examination

A physician is responsible for performing the physical examination. The nurse's role is to assist the physician, help the patient to assume the positions essential for examination, drape the patient and remove the equipment that the physician used. The physical examination may be done in the patient's room or in an examining or a treatment room.

Most hospitals and clinics have a tray or basket for holding the necessary equipment. The following items are usually kept in readiness: ophthalmoscope (for examining the eyes), otoscope (for examining the ears), ear speculum, nose speculum, head mirror, flashlight, stethoscope, sphygmomanometer, tape measure, tongue depressors, tuning fork, skin pencil, percussion hammer, tissue wipes and waste container, safety pins, cotton, and test tubes for hot and cold water. For rectal and vaginal examinations, the following items are necessary: bivalve vaginal speculum, sterilized or disposable gloves, powder and lubricant.

As part of a physical examination, several laboratory examinations commonly are requested by the physician. Each agency has its own procedure or laboratory manual concerning the type of container in which to collect the specimen, the amount of specimen needed, preparation of the specimen, the laboratory to which the specimen is sent, and the like. The nurse's responsibilities will vary, depending on the agency's procedure. Necessary items for laboratory examinations should be readily available, such as test tubes, slides and cotton applicators.

In preparing for the physical examination, it may also be necessary for the nurse to have items available for draping. Some agencies have draping sheets, but the same purpose can be achieved with a bath blanket, a draw sheet or the top bedcovers if the patient is examined in bed. The purpose is to avoid exposing the patient except for the part being examined. In some instances, it is also essential to prevent the patient from drafts or being chilled. This is particularly true with the very ill patient and the elderly patient.

When the patient is very ill or has difficulty moving, the nurse will need to help to place the patient in the position that the physician requests. While the examination is being conducted, the nurse keeps the patient draped properly, exposing areas of the body as indicated.

Positioning the Patient

Erect Position. This is the normal standing position. The patient wears slippers, or the floor is protected. The draping may be a gown, a small sheet or a bath blanket, so arranged that the physician may inspect body contours, posture, muscles and extremities with ease. The nurse assists the patient to hold draping in place as necessary.

Dorsal (Horizontal Recumbent) Position. In this position, the patient lies flat on his back with his legs together, in bed or on the examining table. His head may be supported with a pillow and his legs extended or slightly flexed at the knees to relax the abdominal wall. He should be covered with a bath blanket or a draw sheet. Parts of the drape are folded back to expose the area being examined. The dorsal position is assumed most commonly for examination of the abdomen, the chest anteriorly, the breasts, the reflexes, the extremities, the head, the neck, the eyes, the ears, the nose, the throat, etc.

Dorsal Recumbent Position. This position is used primarily for digital examination of the rectum or the vagina of a female patient. For the physician's convenience the patient should be brought close to the edge of the bed. This should make it easier for him to examine the patient and to avoid leaning on her leg. The patient lies on her back with the legs separated and the knees flexed; the soles of the feet rest flat on the bed or table. One pillow may be placed under the head. A bath blanket or a large sheet is placed diagonally over the patient with opposite corners protecting the legs and wrapped around the feet so that the drape will stay in place. The third corner of the drape covers the patient's chest, and the fourth corner is placed between her legs. A disposable pad placed under the patient's buttocks avoids soiling linen. When the physician is ready, the corner of the drape between the patient's legs is raised and folded back on the abdomen to expose the part being examined. (See Fig. 17-4.)

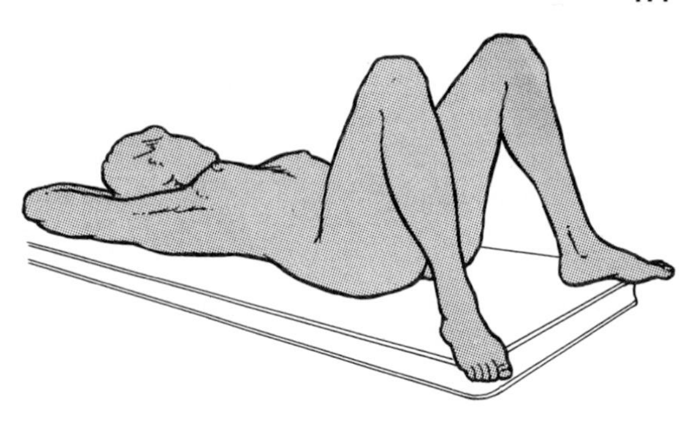

Fig. 17-4. Dorsal recumbent position.

Lithotomy Position. This position, also used primarily for female patients, is the same as the dorsal recumbent position except that the patient is usually on a table equipped with foot stirrups. The patient's buttocks are brought to the edge of the table. The knees are flexed, and the feet are supported in the stirrups. A disposable pad is placed under the patient's buttocks, and draping is the same as for the dorsal recumbent position. The position is also assumed usually for digital examination of the rectum or instrument examination of the vagina. (See Fig. 17-5.)

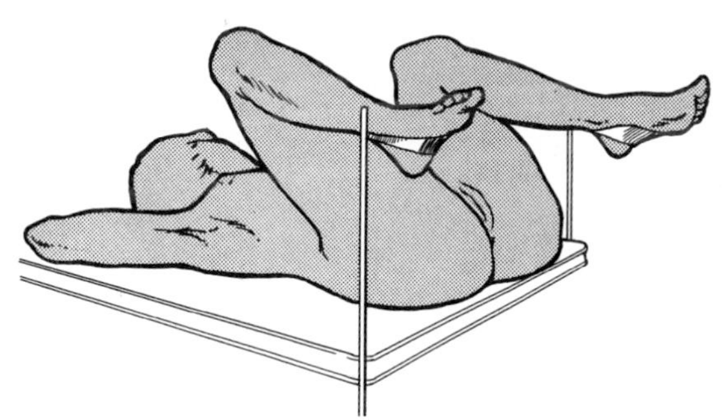

Fig. 17-5. Lithotomy position.

Sims (Lateral) Position. In the Sims position, the patient lies on either side, but, in most instances, the physician prefers that he lie on the left side. In the left Sims position, the patient lies on his left side and rests his left arm behind his body. The right arm is forward with the elbow flexed and the arm resting on a pillow placed under the patient's head. The patient's body inclines slightly forward. The knees are flexed, the right one sharply on the abdomen and the left one less sharply. This position usually is assumed for a digital examination of the rectum or the vagina. The drape may be a bath blanket or a draw sheet placed over the patient. A disposable pad is used under the buttocks. When the physician is ready, one corner of the drape is folded back on the patient's hip to expose the area being examined. (See Fig. 17-6.)

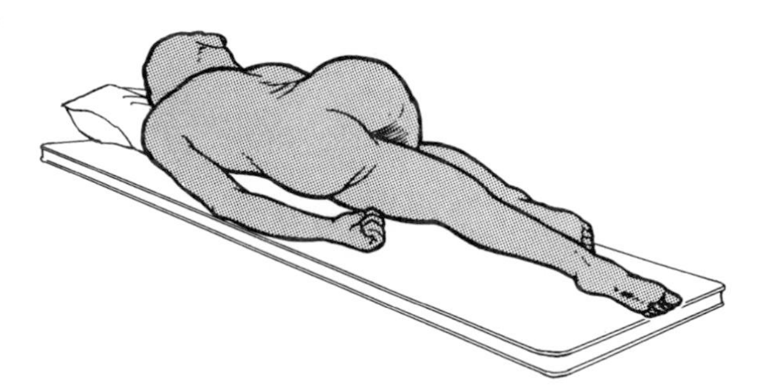

Fig. 17-6. Sims's position.

Knee-Chest (Genupectoral) Position. The patient rests on his knees and chest in this position. The head, turned to one side, rests on a small pillow. A small pillow also may be placed under the chest. The arms are above the head or they may be flexed at the

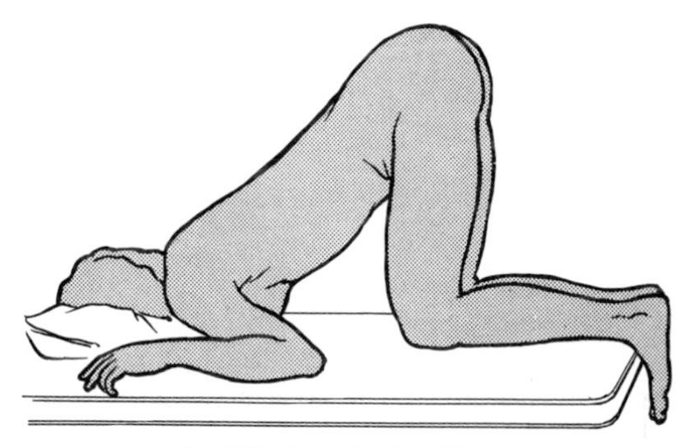

Fig. 17-7. Knee-chest position.

elbows and rest alongside the patient's head. The lower legs are placed perpendicular to the thighs. The knee-chest position frequently is assumed for an instrument examination of the rectum. The drape is placed so that the patient's back, buttocks and thighs are covered. Only the area to be examined is exposed. This is a very difficult position for most patients to assume, especially for the elderly patient. Therefore, the nurse assisting with the examination should have all equipment ready and should not assist the patient into position until the physician is ready. (See Fig. 17-7.)

The dorsal recumbent, lithotomy, Sims and knee-chest positions are used to examine areas of the body which cause embarrassment to most patients. The examinations can be made easier for the patient if the nurse takes every precaution to prevent exposure and to give explanations and directions slowly and carefully. Even when a patient is properly draped for an examination, there may be concern on his part that someone can see into the unit or come into the room. The nurse should make every effort to see that either or both do not happen.

Some women patients are greatly distressed if told that a pelvic examination is necessary. To be told that millions of other women have had this examination is of no consolation to the patient. If there ever is a time when the understanding of how the other person feels about his situation can guide action, this is one of them. A patient feels this way as a result of socio-cultural influences she has had or perhaps for other reasons. It requires a non-committal attitude in order to find a way of proceeding which will not be psychologically traumatic to the patient.

Assisting the Physician with the Physical Examination

For male patients, the physician usually does not ask the nurse to assist. However, it is the policy of many agencies to require a nurse to be present at the time a female patient is examined. Most require a nurse's presence when a pelvic examination is done. This is primarily for the comfort of the patient but also as protection for the physician and the agency.

Each physician will conduct a physical examination in a manner most convenient for him. The following brief description acts as a guide for the nurse to anticipate the manner in which the physician usually will proceed and what he will include in the examination.

Methods of Examining. There are four general methods that the physician uses to obtain information during a physical examination.

Inspection utilizes the eye of the examiner; inspecting the patient is looking at the patient and observing him.

Percussion involves striking a particular area of the body, either with the fingertips or with a percussion hammer, in order that the examiner may listen for sounds or determine resistance of the tissue. Percussion is used when the physician taps the patient's chest wall in order to determine the sound created. If fluid is present, the sound will be dull; when the physician passes the level of fluid, a hollow sound will be heard.

Palpation uses the sense of touch as the examiner feels or presses on the body. For example, the physician uses palpation when he examines the abdomen to feel the various abdominal organs.

Auscultation uses the sense of hearing for interpreting sounds in the body and usually is performed with the aid of the stethoscope. The physician uses auscultation when he listens to the patient's heart sounds with the stethoscope.

Sequence of the Examination. *Case History.* The physician obtains a history from the patient soon after admission or immediately prior to the physical examination. He will ask for a description of the patient's chief complaints and note the date of onset of illness, the probable causes, the factors that appeared to precipitate the illness and the progress of the illness. He will also inquire about all his past illnesses. The patient's personal history includes type of occupation, marital status and personal habits. The physician will also ask about his family's medical history.

It is common practice for the physician to take the case history without the presence of a nurse. In some instances, this is desirable because the patient may be reluctant to answer some questions in the presence of a third person. However, no nurse should avoid the experience if time and circumstances permit. It is an excellent way to get to know the patient better.

General Observations. The general observations that the physician will make during the physical examination include the patient's constitution and stature; symmetry of the body; state of nutrition; posture and gait; positions assumed while standing, sitting and lying; nature of speech; mental reactions and emotional state; texture, pigmentation and color or skin; and texture and distribution of hair.

Examining the Head and the Neck. The contour of the skull is examined, and occasionally the physician may wish to measure the size of the cranium with a tape measure. The physical characteristics and the facial expressions and the condition of the hair and the scalp are noted. The head and the neck are palpated for nodules. The thyroid gland in the neck, the larynx and the trachea are palpated.

Examining the Eyes. Eyelids and eyeballs are inspected, and movements of the eyes are noted. A flashlight may be used to determine the reaction of the pupils to light. The interior of the eyeball is inspected from the corneal surface to the eyegrounds with the aid of an ophthalmoscope. Sight and field of vision are examined with the aid of a reading test chart and a perimeter chart. Unless there is reason for a detailed examination of sight and field of vision, test charts and perimeter are not used for the routine physical examination.

Examining the Ears. The general contour is noted. The external auditory canal and the eardrum are observed with the aid of an otoscope or an ear speculum and head mirror. The mastoid area is palpated and inspected. Tuning forks are sometimes used to test acuity of hearing. The most accurate way to test hearing is with an audiometer, but unless there is indication for careful study of hearing, an audiometer is not used for the routine physical examination.

Examining the Nose. The nose is inspected and palpated. A flashlight or a head mirror and a nasal speculum are used to inspect the nostrils and the septum. Sense of smell is determined by having the patient smell commonly recognized substances. The physician will indicate whether he wishes to have substances on hand to test the sense of smelling.

Examining the Lips, the Mouth and the Throat. Examining the lips is usually by inspection. A tongue depressor and a light are used for inspecting the mouth, teeth, gums, tongue, hard and soft palate, tonsils, pharynx and larynx.

Examining the Breasts. The breasts are examined for symmetry, position and size. Palpation is used to determine the presence of tumors. The nipples are examined by inspection and palpation.

Examining the Chest. Contour, size and shape are inspected, and respiratory movements are noted. Palpation is used to make observations concerning the transmission of vibrations within the respiratory tract to the fingers of the examiner. Percussion is used to set up vibrations in underlying tissue; the type of sound produced is significant to the physician, since certain sounds over air-containing and airless tissue are characteristic of health and others are characteristic of disease. Auscultation with a stethoscope is used to hear and evaluate breath sounds. During auscultation of the chest, the patient may be asked to cough, and he should be provided with tissue wipes to cover his mouth when so doing.

Most physicians agree that a physical examination is incomplete without x-ray pictures of the chest to aid in observing the lungs. Some health agencies have a policy that patients have a chest x-ray made on admission. Routine chest x-ray is helpful in early cancer detection and has aided immeasurably in diagnosing tuberculosis long before the patient might have become aware of having the disease. X-rays also aid in inspecting the contour and the size of other organs in the chest, and of the ribs.

Examining the Cardiovascular System. By

using inspection, palpation, percussion, auscultation and roentgenography, the physician investigates the size and the shape of the heart, abnormal pulsations, heart sounds, murmurs and the like. A more extensive study of heartbeat can be done with the use of an electrocardiograph, an instrument operated by a trained technician, that records the particulars of the pulse beat. Pulse rate is noted by palpating a peripheral artery. Elasticity and thickness of artery walls and the course of an artery are determined by palpation.

Occasionally, the physician will ask the nurse to count the pulse rate at the radial artery as he counts simultaneously at the apex of the heart (apical-radial count). Differences in count often indicate the presence of pathologic changes of the heart.

Although the nurse very often measures the patient's blood pressure on admission, the physician will also wish to take the blood pressure.

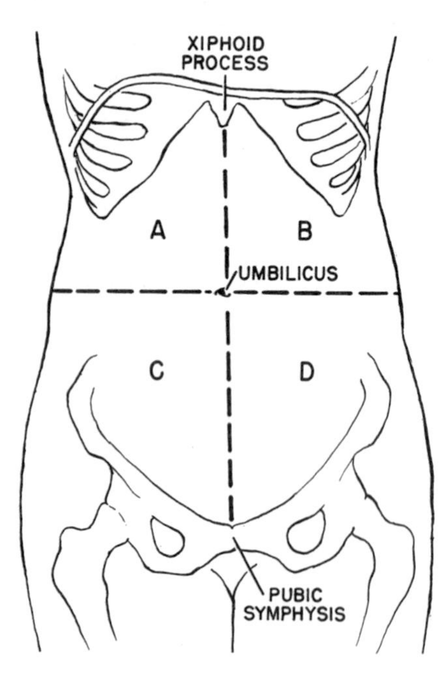

FIG. 17-8. Quadrants of the abdomen: (A) the right upper quadrant—RUQ; (B) the left upper quadrant—LUQ; (C) the right lower quadrant—RLQ; (D) the left lower quadrant—LLQ.

Examining the Abdomen and the Back. Inspection will determine the general contour of the abdomen, the condition of the skin and the distribution of pubic hair. By palpation, normal organs or abnormal masses may be noted. Percussion is used to outline organs. Auscultation of the abdomen has little practical value except for examining the pregnant woman to determine the fetal heart rate.

In order to describe the location of signs and symptoms of the abdomen, systematic areas of the abdomen have been defined. The most common method of subdividing the abdomen is by describing four quadrants. A line drawn from the tip of the sternum to the pubic bone through the umbilicus and a horizontal line crossing the other at the umbilicus divides the abdominal area into four quadrants. These quadrants are called the right and the left upper quadrants and the right and the left lower quadrants. They are frequently abbreviated RUQ, LUQ, RLQ, and LLQ, respectively. Figure 17-8 illustrates these four divisions.

The back is inspected and palpated to determine its contour and the position of the spine.

Thorough examinations of the abdomen, the pelvis and the back usually include x-ray examinations, but x-rays are used infrequently unless a pathologic condition appears to exist. Contrast media, such as dyes and barium, are used for x-ray examinations of abdominal and pelvic organs. X-ray of the spine is scheduled when detailed examination of the spine is indicated.

Examining the Genitalia, the Perineum, the Anus and the Rectum. These areas are examined by inspection and palpation. Rectal and vaginal examinations rarely are done on children and young adults unless specific complaints are referred to these areas. A bivalve vaginal speculum is used to examine the vagina and the cervix. The physician will use gloves for this part of the examination. Powder sprinkled on his hands aids him in putting them on.

Unless symptoms are referred to the rectum, instruments rarely are used, digital examination being used most commonly. The physician will use gloves and a lubricant.

The physician examines the genitals and the rectum of the male patient alone or with a male nurse in attendance. Physicians usually recommend that men over 40 years of age have a rectal examination by proctoscopy or sigmoidoscopy annually and preferably semiannually to aid in the early detection of cancer. This requires special preparation for cleansing the colon, so it is done as a separate examination.

Examining the Musculoskeletal System. Inspection and palpation are used to examine the musculoskeletal system. General contour is noted, and joints are inspected. Occasionally, the physician may wish to measure extremities with a tape measure. X-rays frequently are used as an aid in examining the skeletal system.

The Neurologic Examination. During the neurologic examination, the physician examines the reflexes and the various senses. Usually, the percussion hammer is used to test reflexes. A skin pencil is employed frequently to mark certain neurologic as well as musculoskeletal findings on the patient's body. The senses of touch and pain are examined with cotton and with a pin. Placing test tubes containing hot and cold water on the skin is used to test heat and cold receptors.

Following the physical examination, the nurse assists the patient as necessary. For reasons of both safety and courtesy, a very ill, uncomfortable or older patient should be assisted off an examining table. If the patient has been examined in his room, the nurse arranges the bed linen and helps to make the patient comfortable.

The nurse should follow the agency's procedure for the care of equipment used during the physical examination. See that all items used on the patient are properly cared for in terms of medical asepsis, i.e., tongue blades and applicators disposed of and instruments cleansed, or sterilized if possible.

Study Situations

1. For those interested in historical items, read about the thermometer, an item we take for granted.

- Keezer, W. S.: The clinical thermometer. AMER. J. NURS., *66*:326-327, February, 1966.

2. How accurate an account of the patient's T.P.R. can be expected when obtaining these signs are a matter of routine and various persons are taking them? Read the two following articles reporting on studies done many years ago. The problem and the question still exists today.

- Kory, R. C.: Routine measurement of respiratory rate. J.A.M.A., *165*:448, October 5, 1957.
- Schmidt, M. A.: Are all T.P.R.'s necessary? AMER. J. NURS., *58*:559, April, 1958.

3. If you react to scholastic examinations as most persons do, you are aware of being in a different physiologic state. Take your pulse and respiratory rates when you feel you are at ease. Compare them with your findings just before an examination or after any episode that created fear or anxiety. What is happening physiologically? How can you use a knowledge of the reaction and its explanations when caring for patients?

4. This comment is made in the article below: "Patient assessment is the responsibility of the professional nurse. She initiates the assessment as soon as possible after the patient is admitted and continues to assess and evaluate, modifying the plan of care as the patient's behavior or functional abilities change."

Note the guide on page 83. It should increase your understanding of the extent to which observation skills must be developed in order for nursing to be therapeutic and for care to be individualized.

- McCain, R. F.: Nursing by assessment—not intuition. AMER. J. NURS., *65*:82-84, April, 1965.

5. It was pointed out in Chapter 5 that reporting and recording are basic to the practice of nursing. It was mentioned also

that recording by nurses leaves much to be desired. The following article is directed toward improving recording by nurses. Even if automated devices are used in the recording aspects of patient care, the nurse still must know how to obtain and assess observations made.

- Walker, V. H. *et al*: A care plan for ailing nurses' notes.
  AMER. J. NURS., *65*:74-76, August, 1965.

6. The need for exact descriptions of a patient's state of consciousness is essential for accurate diagnosis and treatment. Read the article below for further understanding of patients who have disturbances of consciousness. A suggested outline for assessing is given and an example of how it is used is also given. How could such an outline be used in conjunction with a patient's nursing care plan if the patient had a disturbance of consciousness?

- Gardner, M. A.: Responsiveness as a measure of consciousness.
  AMER. J. NURS., *68*:1034-1038, May, 1968.

7. Special reference was made to the elderly patient and the need for closer observation to establish his mental state. How does the article listed below describe confusion? What can be some of the causes of confusion? How can a family member help in such a situation, and why is it necessary for the family member to sit close to the patient and touch the patient frequently?

- Patrick, M. L.: Care of the confused elderly patient.
  AMER. J. NURS., *67*:2536-2539, December, 1967.

8. Read this article for further discussion on how the nurse needs to use many sources of information in order to arrive at a nursing diagnosis; how the making of a nursing diagnosis is an independent, important function in nursing.

- Rothberg, J. S.: Why nursing diagnosis?
  AMER. J. NURS., *67*:1040-1042, May, 1967.

9. In the April, 1964, issue of the American Journal of Nursing there is a group of articles under the title heading of "Cancer in Situ of the Cervix." All of them are concerned with early detection and treatment, a goal of all health personnel. Of particular interest, and to reinforce the concept of man as a person, read:

- Alpenfels, E. J.: Cultural clues to reactions in society. pp. 83-86.

Note that the author (an anthropologist) suggests the "marriage between the field of medicine and that of anthropology." How does she justify this?

Also read: Gilmer, R., and Hassels, A.: Nurses' practices and attitudes toward cancer.

References

1. Correcting common errors in blood pressure measurement. (Programmed Instruction). AMER. J. NURS., *65*:133-164, October, 1965.
2. Eisenberg, S. W., Napoli, R. P., and Radding, B.: Proctosigmoidoscopy. AMER. J. NURS., *65*:113-115, January, 1965.
3. George, J. H.: Machines in perspective. Electronic monitoring of vital signs. AMER. J. NURS., *65*:68-71, February, 1965.
4. Hammond, K. R. *et al*: Clinical inference in nursing: Revising judgments. NURS. RES., *16*:38-45, Winter, 1967.
5. Komorita, N. I.: Nursing diagnosis. AMER. J. NURS., *63*:83-86, December, 1963.
6. Levine, M. E.: Adaptation and assessment. A rationale for nursing intervention. AMER. J. NURS., *66*:2450-2453, November, 1966.
7. Manthey, M. E.: A guide for interviewing. AMER. J. NURS., *67*:2088-2090, October, 1967.
8. Mumford, E., and Poslusny, E.: A brief program: The nurse as observer. NURS. OUTLOOK, *15*:56-60, October, 1967.
9. Newman, M. A.: Identifying and meeting patient's needs in short-span nurse-patient relationships. NURS. FORUM, *5*:76-88, No. 1, 1966.
10. Nichols, G. A., and Verhonick, P. J.: Time and temperature. AMER. J. NURS., *67*:2304-2306, November, 1967.
11. Nichols, G. A., and Verhonick, P. J.: Placement times for oral thermometers: A nursing study replication. NURS. RES., *17*:159-161, March-April, 1968.
12. Nichols, G. A. *et al*: Oral, axillary, and rectal temperature determinations. NURS. RES., *15*:307-310, Fall, 1966.
13. Nichols, G. A., and Glor, B. A. K.: A replica-

tion of rectal thermometer placement studies. NURS. RES., *17*:360-361, No. 4, July-August, 1968.

14. Peterson, L. W.: Operant approach to observation and recording. NURS. OUTLOOK, *15*:28-32, March, 1967.
15. Purintun, L. R., and Bishop, B. E.: How accurate are clinical thermometers? AMER. J. NURS., *69*:99-100, January, 1969.
16. Taylor, J. W. *et al*: For effective thermometer disinfection. NURS. OUTLOOK, *14*:56-57, February, 1966.
17. Thomas, B. J.: Clues to patients' behavior. AMER. J. NURS., *63*:100-102, July, 1963.
18. Verhonick, P. J., and Werley, H. H.: Experimentation in nursing practice in the army. NURS. OUTLOOK, *11*:204-206, March, 1963.
19. Walker, V. H., and Selmanoff, E. D.: A note on the accuracy of the temperature, pulse and respiration procedure. NURS. RES., *14*:72-76, Winter, 1965.

CHAPTER 18

Maintaining Nutrition

Because of her close contact with patients, the nurse is a key person in helping to maintain or to improve their nutrition. This is a responsibility that frequently requires her to coordinate and to augment the plans of several persons contributing to the patient's care. Though the physician prescribes the diet, a dietitian prepares the menus, the dietary personnel serve the meals, and the nursing personnel may assist patients to eat, a nurse is still responsible for knowing what the patients eat and how they react to their diets.

General Principles of Nutrition

All body cells require adequate nutrition. Food is basic to life, and there are food substances essential to health. In other words, probably we could eat only what we like and remain alive, but if these foods did not contain the variety of nutrients needed by the cells of the body, physiologic functioning would be impaired.

The nutrients essential to health are carbohydrates, proteins, fats, vitamins and minerals. Water is essential to maintain fluid balance in the body. All of these are required to build and repair tissue, to furnish energy and to make essential substances, such as enzymes and hormones. They are made available to the body by the process of digestion. The digestive process breaks them down mechanically (chewing and intestinal movements) and chemically (oral and gastrointestinal secretions) so that they can be absorbed into the blood and the lymph.

Food requirements vary among individuals. From birth to old age nutritional requirements continually vary. They are dependent on the demands of the body for growth and tissue repair and also are affected by such factors as activity, climate, emotional status, pregnancy, illness, and so forth. Requirements differ, too, among individuals who would seem to have the same nutritional needs. There are differences in the way their foods are digested, assimilated and used by the body.

Appetite is nature's first defense against hunger. Hunger is a sensation which tells us that our body needs nourishment. Appetite is a very individualistic thing and is influenced by myriad factors, some of which will be discussed later in this chapter.

The nurse's responsibility in relation to the patient's nourishment is essentially threefold: to assist as necessary with seeing that patients receive and eat their prescribed diets; to take such steps as are possible to stimulate and/or maintain the patient's appetite; and to teach patients as indicated concerning dietary needs.

The Ordering and the Serving of Food in a Health Agency

Health agencies have procedures for transmitting the physician's order for a patient's diet to the dietary department. The nurse will need to acquaint herself with the details of the nursing department's responsibility, such as forms to use to order diets, time limits for ordering, changing diets or canceling diets.

Patients on regular or relatively minor restrictive diets often are given menus from which they may select the foods they prefer for the next day's meals. While the type of tray, tray cover, dishes and silver used are not within the nurse's realm of control, the general appearance of the tray should be the best possible when it is served. Some agencies increase the attractiveness of the tray by using name cards and holiday favors. In the home care of patients, the nurse can do much to please the patient, such as adding a flower, using different colored cloths and napkins, serving one course at a time and adding surprises like cookies or candy if the patient is permitted to have them.

As mentioned in Chapter 13, some hospitals having self-care units permit the patients to be served in a cafeteria or dining room. A dietitian is present to help patients on special diets to make a selection from the foods available. Even if dining rooms are not available, provisions for groups of patients to eat together, as in a solarium, is a thoughtful gesture. This is true especially for Sundays, holidays and special occasions. It is the rare person who prefers eating alone.

Modifying the Usual Pattern for Serving Food. Whenever it seems that some modification in the usual dietary routine or the diet itself would make the patient feel better, the nurse should consider how this might be accomplished. For example, if it is noted that an elderly patient leaves the meat untouched, investigation might show that he has loose-fitting dentures and cannot chew meat. A request might be made to serve him ground meats. Or when cultural patterns affect food preferences to the extent that the pa-

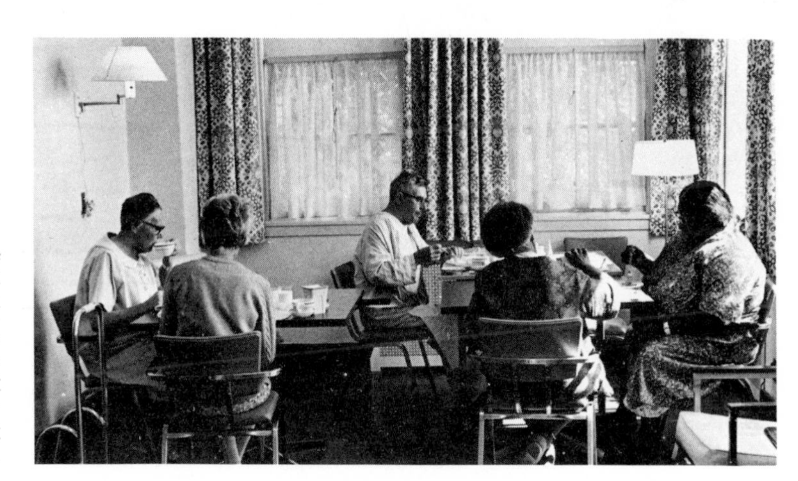

FIG. 18-1. One of the many advantages of a continuing care unit is that patients may eat their meals at tables and with other persons, if they so choose. The food is placed on attractive place mats even though it is brought from the kitchen on trays. It is not uncommon for three or four persons at the same table to have entirely different meals, if each one has different diet orders.

tient is not getting an adequate diet, it may be necessary to consult with the dietitian so that substitutes can be made.

Some patients find the time span between meals unsatisfactory. Three meals served within an eight- to nine-hour period and then a 15-hour wait for the next meal is not usual routine at home. They may want a snack at bedtime. Some agencies provide this, but many do not. Having the patient save some item, as a piece of cake or fruit, from one of his trays may be an answer. Hunger is distressing, and anything to avoid this should be considered.

Occasionally, patients wish to substitute something served on the trays, and this can be managed through the kitchen on the unit. For example, the patient may have a jar of powdered coffee and he needs only the hot water. Or, he may have a favorite canned item, and all that is required is that it be opened and served.

Size of the food portions may also be a source of discomfort to some patients. For those who eat little and leave a part of the food served, there is no problem. But patients who are accustomed to eating larger portions will feel dissatisfied with the meal. Extra portions usually can be arranged with the dietary department.

Sometimes, patients' wishes cannot be granted because of hospital policies or because it would mean doing for one what cannot be done for all. For example, there are patients who would like meals brought from home. Some of the implications can be readily imagined: family members coming in at times other than visiting hours to leave the food; requests being made to heat foods; dishes being left in rooms until family members take them home; food stored in bedside stands and conflicts with the patient's regular diet. However, an occasional item of food which can be eaten immediately or shortly afterward, such as a sandwich, a piece of homemade pie or cake or a jar of cooked fruit might please the patient very much. If hospital policy does not permit the admission of any food, then the nurse is obliged to comply.

Not all likes and dislikes can be acted upon, but when a patient shows obvious distress, some effort should be made in his behalf.

Helping To Maintain or Improve the Patient's Appetite

For most people eating is a pleasure. When we recall how much a part of our life and leisure time is associated with food, we can readily see why this is so. Family celebrations, holiday meals, parties, picnics, coffee breaks, informal visits and watching sports events, movies and television usually include food in one form or another. We even tend to associate certain foods with particular events, such as hot-dogs at baseball games, champagne at weddings, and the like.

As mentioned earlier, appetite is affected by many factors. Disturbances of appetite can interfere with gastrointestinal secretions and hence, digestion. Persons who have been upset while eating or directly afterward have been known to vomit completely undigested food hours later. Not only may his physical condition affect his appetite, but what the patient can see, hear, smell or taste may influence it as well.

Below are some suggestions nurses will want to consider in relation to maintaining and/or stimulating the patient's appetite.

See that the patient is in a comfortable position for eating.

Be sure that the patient is clean and free from damp or soiled garments.

Alleviate pain or discomfort, as far as possible.

Correct such annoyances as a loose or a tight dressing.

Give the patient an opportunity to void if he desires.

Avoid treatments, such as enemas, dressings and injections, immediately before or directly after mealtimes if possible.

See that the room is comfortable from the standpoint of temperature and ventilation.

See that the patient is dressed adequately and comfortably.

Remove or keep out of sight objects which would be unpleasant to look at while eating, such as urinals, bedpans, dressing trays or carts, drainage containers, suction machines, and the like.

Screen patients who may be very ill, in pain or receiving therapy (such as a transfusion or gastric suction) and will not be served a meal. Many patients receiving infusions or transfusions are served meals and should not be screened.

Make certain that the immediate environment itself is in order, such as removing soiled linen, treatment trays that have been used, dead flowers, etc., and that the furniture is orderly. Many persons who must remain in bed prefer not to have their baths before breakfast if it means having the bed disarranged and bathing items left about the unit.

Make certain that the person serving the meal is pleasant and courteous and that care has been taken to avoid spilling liquids or disarranging dishes.

Cooperate with dietary personnel so that the meals can be served as quickly as possible. This helps to keep hot foods hot, and cold foods do not melt or become wilted.

If the patient is nauseated, the above measures are especially helpful. There is more discussion on nausea and vomiting in Chapter 25.

Assisting Patients to Eat

Some patients will need assistance with eating and drinking. Physical limitations and the need to conserve strength are some of the reasons. For some patients, such as those in casts or in traction or those with some loss of hand or arm strength, it may be a matter of preparing foods and placing them conveniently. It would include such things as opening the shell of a cooked egg, buttering bread, cutting meat and preparing other foods so they can be eaten easily.

If it is difficult for a patient to drink from a cup or a glass, a drinking tube should be used. Disposable drinking tubes are preferred to glass or plastic because considerable care is needed to keep the nondisposable tubes clean. Accumulated food particles in a drinking tube at room temperature make a good growth medium for microorganisms.

Some patients are unable or not permitted to feed themselves and must be fed by someone else. When feeding a patient, a nurse or an assistant should be relaxed and in a comfortable position, so that the patient does not feel rushed. The person feeding should inquire if the patient is accustomed to say-

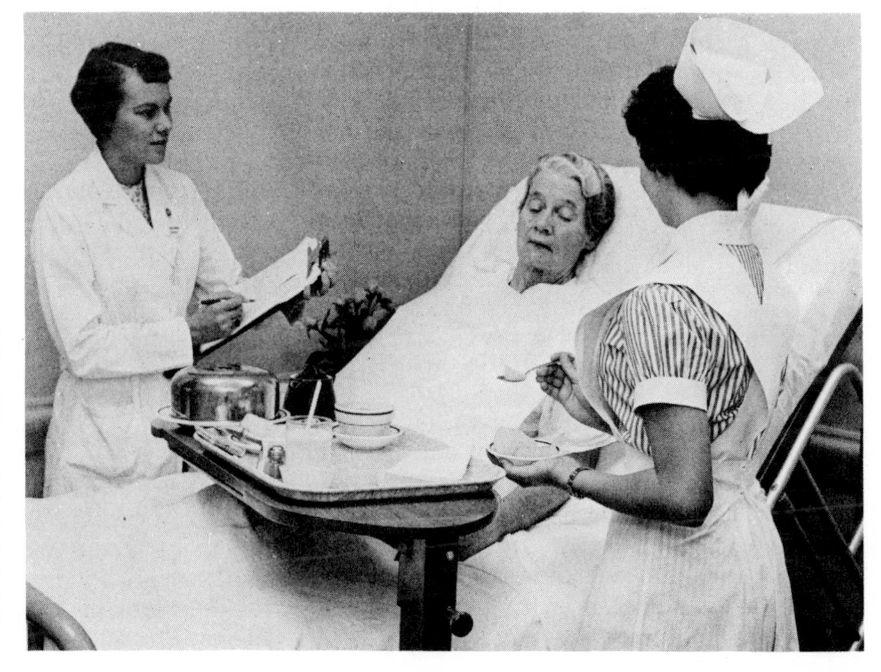

Fig. 18-2. As mentioned in the text, helping to maintain the nutritional intake of a patient is a multidiscipline effort. The physician prescribes the diet, the dietitian prepares the menu, and the nursing staff assists in helping the patients to eat well. This patient must be fed. She has a disposable bib over her gown which is more practical and esthetically acceptable than a face or bath towel. The student nurse has removed the completed main course from the tray and now has the dessert and the beverage before the patient. Keeping the tray and the food appealing to the sight helps the appetite. The dietitian who has stopped by is interested in learning the patient's reaction to the food served.

ing grace. If so, permit him to do so and join by remaining respectfully silent. A comment on his nursing care plan which indicates that the patient says grace would help to individualize his care.

Ask the patient which foods he would like to eat first and other preferences he might have. For example, he might like his coffee with his meal or after it, a piece of bread after each piece of meat or some potato and meat together. Serve the food at the rate the patient wishes it.

If the patient is permitted some slight activity and has some hand and arm functioning, permit him to hold a piece of toast or a roll or to hold the drinking tube in the beverage while he sips it. If there is a beverage that he would like at the end of a meal and it can be placed so that he need only hold the drinking tube, consider doing this. It will prolong the pleasure of the meal and give him some feeling of independence. Avoid having to leave a patient after starting to feed him. If you must, use diplomacy so that he does not feel abandoned.

If a patient being fed is blind or if his eyes are bandaged, it is best to use some method of signaling when the next mouthful of food is ready or when it is wanted. Touching the patient's arm when the food is ready or having the patient move his hand when he wants more can make the situation much easier for both.

Teaching in Relation to Nutrition

Several general principles in relation to nutrition were stated earlier in this chapter. No effort is made in this text to review content which the student studies in courses in nutrition and diet therapy. However, because the nurse is often the pivotal person in relation to teaching patients needing help with nutritional problems, it behooves her to keep abreast of knowledge in the nutritional sciences. In problem areas, the dietitian will gladly assist the nurse and she should be consulted freely.

Below are a few examples of problems nurses may encounter with suggestions in relation to helping patients.

Food fads are common, and frequently the nurse is faced with helping a person separate fad from fact. People read about or are told about diets to lose weight, increase fertility, prevent cancer, high blood pressure and heart disease and all sorts of things. Even if they do not like the diet they will stick with it if they are convinced that it will bring results. Such persons will need considerable teaching and supportive evidence in order to give up erroneous concepts.

Very often, patients who are on modified diets claim to have lost their appetites; what they are permitted to eat does not give them any pleasure. It is difficult to be denied foods and seasonings we like, and more difficult still for a person to deny himself these pleasures when he no longer feels ill. To have an appetite for foods and to keep reminding yourself that you cannot have them takes considerable self-control. That is why many patients do not adhere to their diets after discharge from the hospital. The nurse has a responsibility to try to help make the special diet as appealing to the patient as possible. If a patient is to be on a special diet after being discharged from the hospital, arrangements should be made to teach and to plan with him long before the day arrives. Having the dietitian meet with the patient and offering him suggestions and illustrative materials can often do much to help. Moreover, the patient is much more likely to follow the diet when he knows the reason for it. There are helpful materials such as food composition charts, calorie charts, exchange lists of foods, sample menus, recipes using seasoning substitutes and lists of stores where special foods can be purchased.

Having to eat foods for which you have no appetite can lead to some desperate action. Patients on low sodium or calculated carbohydrate and fat diets have had salt, sugar or candy brought to them by family or friends. Patients on restricted calorie diets have been known to hide candy and sneak bites as an alcoholic might take "nips." Or, there is the example of the diabetic patient who wandered about the ward eating the desserts of patients who did not want theirs. The teaching implications are evident.

It is important to support such patients by at least indicating an awareness and an understanding of their feelings. Reprimanding is not nursing. The patient needs help and support from all—his family, the physician, the dietitian and the nursing personnel. Nursing care plans for such patients would provide a consistent approach which could help them.

The person who lives alone may have a problem with adequate nutrition. This is particularly true with the older age group. Often, they do not wish to cook for one person since they find it no fun to eat alone and maintain that they have no appetite anyway. When a person is known to live alone, inquire about provisions for meals before the patient is discharged. Explore all possible means for the provision of regular and adequate meals and stimulating the patient's desire for food. The so-called TV dinners and the many canned foods are one answer if they are available and if the patient can afford them. Recently, in some areas food service to the home has been instituted for the ill, the handicapped or the incapacitated. Meals with friends and relatives are possible suggestions also.

Two elderly women who lived alone and within walking distance of each other's homes had an interesting arrangement. They ate lunch together several times a week on a "dutch treat" basis. Each would bring her own lunch, and the other supplied the hot water and the milk for their tea. Although often their lunches were their main meal for the day and consisted of sandwiches made from leftover meat and a fruit as well as a beverage, just knowing that they would be eating with someone else made the preparation of the meal a pleasure.

In our country most people have sufficient money to provide their families with adequate nutriton. Nevertheless, opinion holds that many persons do not eat balanced, nutritious meals. Many people are simply unaware of the body's nutritional needs; therefore, a teaching program may be indicated.

There are some persons who cannot discipline themselves concerning food consumption and eat compulsively. Health problems associated with obesity can be numerous. The problem of obesity is multi-faceted, and reprimanding holds no place in its solution. Although teaching is important, the nurse, as well as other health personnel, will want to give as much emotional support as possible in helping the patient to overcome the tendency to overeat.

The "affluent society" notwithstanding, an abundant food supply is not available to all in this country. It is disheartening to know that many children and adults are chronically hungry and suffering from severe malnutrition. Sometimes teaching better food selection and using nutritious but inexpensive foods is helpful. In other situations, social agencies may need to assist.

Study Situations

1. In the following article, list the suggested remedies the authors give as solutions to eating problems when hospital routines interfere:

- Newton, M. E., and Folta, J.: Hospital food can help or hinder care.
  AMER. J. NURS., *67*:112-113, January, 1967.

2. The following article describes food and feeding interestingly:

- Rubin, R.: Food and feeding—a matrix of relationships.
  NURS. FORUM, *6*:195-205, #2, Spring, 1967.

How does the author relate appetite and self-appraisal? What implications do you see for nurses when the author writes, on page 201, "It is the context in which the food is offered that is significantly meaningful."?

3. Read the following article:

- Manning, M. L.: The psychodynamics of dietetics.
  NURS. OUTLOOK, *13*:57-59, April, 1965.

How does the author define the word, psychodietetics? Note particularly the last two paragraphs in the article. How does the author believe nurses can aid most in overcoming obstacles patients have in relation to eating habits and dietary selections?

4. The following article illustrates how problem solving was used to aid in meeting one patient's eating problem:

- Nickels, E., and Clement, W. R.: Search

or research? An experimental analysis of nursing behavior.
NURS. OUTLOOK, *13*:70, February, 1965.
How does the author deal with the statement sometimes made of health personnel who "need to keep people sick."?

References

1. Braley, I.: Hospital prepared meals for homebound aged persons.
HOSPITALS, *37*:82, August 16, 1963.
2. Golub, S.: Can mamma's food be bad?
AMER. J. NURS., *65*:87, August, 1965.
3. Kornblueh, M.: The cafeteria food game.
NURS. OUTLOOK, *15*:41, February, 1967.
4. ———: How does your diet rate?
NURS. OUTLOOK, *13*:61-62, July, 1965.
5. Mitchell, H. S. *et al*: Cooper's Nutrition in Health and Disease. ed. 15. 650 p.
Philadelphia, Lippincott, 1968.
6. Moore, M. L.: When families must eat more for less.
NURS. OUTLOOK, *14*:66-69, April, 1966.
7. Newton, M. E., and Folta, J.: Hospital food can help or hinder care.
AMER. J. NURS., *67*:112-113, January, 1967.
8. Phillips, M., and Dunn, M.: Toward better understanding of other lands, other people—their folkways and foods.
NURS. OUTLOOK, *9*:498, August, 1961.
9. Stare, F. J.: Good nutrition from food not pills.
AMER. J. NURS., *65*:86-89, February, 1965.
10. Wilson, S. J.: I like eggs.
AMER. J. NURS., *66*:1343, June, 1966.

CHAPTER 19

Providing for Personal Cleanliness

Patients differ in practices of personal cleanliness according to social, environmental and cultural influences and personal idiosyncracies. Variations in the performance of personal hygiene care certainly are permissible. The time of day for brushing the teeth and for bathing or the frequency of shampooing the hair and changing bed linens and sleeping garments are relatively unimportant. The important thing is that personal care be carried out conveniently and often enough to be effective.

During illness, the nurse helps the patient to continue sound hygienic practices. For example, the patient may feel that it is too much bother to brush his teeth while he is feeling ill, and he may neglect to do so without help or an explanation of its importance. If the nurse notes that the patient is unaware of certain hygienic practices or that he uses an unsound practice, she has an opportunity for teaching. In certain instances, daily hygienic practices may need to be modified because of the patient's condition. For example, the patient who has an elevated temperature may need special mouth care in order that his lips and his tongue and the mucous membrane of his mouth may not become dry and crack. Or the patient who has dry skin may need lotion rubbed into the areas of the elbows and the heels to prevent irritation.

Nurses often are asked about hygienic fads and superstitions, which offers the nurse opportunity for health teaching. Such discussions often help the nurse to understand her patient better and may very well reveal attitudes that affect the patient's health or his recovery.

General Principles for Care of the Skin and Mucous Membrane

Practices concerned with the care of the skin and the mucous membrane are guided by this basic principle: *Unbroken and healthy skin and mucous membrane serve as first lines of defense against harmful agents.* The general functions of the skin include protection, secretion, excretion, heat regulation and sensation. Mucous membrane lining the body orifices has the same general functions except that it is less important in aiding excretion. When the skin and the mucous membrane are healthy and intact, they function at their optimum.

This chapter is concerned with practices that aid to keep the skin and the mucous membrane healthy and intact and to minimize irritation. For example, in the selection of soaps, detergents, make-up, deodorants and depilatories, products should be used that minimize chemical irritation on the skin and the mucous membrane in order to prevent injury. Mechanical irritation is minimized when friction is used judiciously, as when rubbing the patient's skin or smoothing the linen on which the patient lies. Patients with sensitive or tender skin, as infants and older patients, are handled very carefully to prevent skin breaks and irritation. Physical irritation is minimized when the nurse applies emollients and avoids drying agents such as alcohol when the skin is already dry. It is also minimized when the nurse keeps the skin dry and cool and the mucous membrane moist. Chemical and mechanical irritation is reduced when body secretions and dirt are removed by bathing. Microbial invasion is reduced by keeping the skin and the mucous membranes intact through prevention of mechanical, physical and chemical irritation.

Resistance to injury of the skin and the mucous membrane varies among individuals. Individual resistance is influenced by factors such as age, general health of the patient and the amount of subcutaneous tissue. The very young person and the older person have particularly sensitive skin and mucous membrane. When body cells are poorly nourished or hydrated, as in the emaciated or the dehydrated patient, the skin and the mucous membrane are more susceptible to injury. Very thin and very obese people tend to be more subject to skin irritation and injury.

Body cells adequately nourished and hydrated are more resistant to injury. In Chapter 18, the importance of nutrition to good body functioning was discussed. Cells in the skin and the mucous membrane need adequate nourishment and hydration. The better nourished the cell, the better its ability to resist injury and disease.

A corollary to adequate nourishment and hydration of cells is that *adequate circulation is necessary in order to maintain cell life.* When circulation is impaired for any reason, the cells involved are nourished inadequately; hence, they are more subject to injury. The importance of this principle will be illustrated more clearly in relation to the prevention of bedsores, discussed later in this chapter.

Care of the Skin

The skin consists of two rather distinct layers. The superficial portion is called the *epidermis* and is made up of layers of stratified squamous epithelium. The deeper layer is called the *dermis* and consists of smooth muscular tissue, blood vessels, nerves, fat, hair follicles, certain glands, and fibrous and elastic tissue. The skin covers the entire body and is continuous with mucous membrane at normal body orifices.

The skin serves to protect underlying body tissue and organs from injury; it prevents microorganisms from invading the body; water, including nitrogenous wastes, is excreted through the skin; and the skin houses sense organs of touch, pain, heat, cold and pressure. The skin also plays an important part in the regulation of body temperature.

Heat is lost from the body through vasodilatation and evaporation of perspiration, and heat is retained through vasoconstriction and the phenomenon known as "goose pimples," which are formed by the contraction of muscular tissue in the dermis, thus making the hair stand on end.

The cutaneous glands include the sebaceous, the sweat, the ceruminous and the mammary glands. The sebaceous glands secrete an oily substance called sebum which lubricates the skin and the hair and keeps the skin and the scalp pliant. The sweat glands secrete perspiration. The wax in the ears, consisting of a heavy oil and pigment, is secreted by the ceruminous glands. Milk is secreted during the postpartum period, by the mammary glands.

Age is a factor in caring for the skin. Because an infant's skin is injured easily and subject to infection, he should be handled and bathed gently to prevent injury. Young children's skin becomes more resistant to injury and infection but requires frequent cleansing because of toilet and play habits.

During adolescence, the skin should be kept immaculately clean and free from irritation to aid in the control of acne, a common condition during these years. During adolescence and up to approximately 50 years of age, secretions from skin glands are at their maximum. Hence, frequent bathing is necessary to prevent body odors and the accumulation of secretions and dirt.

As age advances, the skin becomes less elastic and thinner. Subcutaneous fat decreases. Wrinkles appear, most of which are deep in the dermis. Since less oil is secreted from sebaceous glands, the skin becomes dry, often scaly and rough in appearance.

The primary purpose of cleansing the skin is to remove dirt, oils, perspiration and transient bacteria. Although the skin may be cleansed in various ways, the best way is to bathe with soap or a detergent and water. Soap or detergents should be sufficiently mild to prevent irritation. Youngsters and oldsters require special attention concerning the selection of an appropriate soap or detergent, since their skin is more subject to injury and to irritation. If the skin at any age is very dry, lubricating creams should be used; in extreme cases creams may be needed as cleansing agents. Bath oils aid dry skin. Alcohol or any other defatting agent should be avoided on dry skin.

Illness very often alters the condition of the skin and makes special care necessary. Severe fluid loss through fever, vomiting or diarrhea reduces the intracellular and the extracellular fluids of the body. This produces a physical state referred to as *dehydration.* Dehydration makes the skin appear loose and very often flabby. The skin can be lifted easily, and it may not spring back as it does when the patient is well. Also, excessive perspiration may present a problem during illness. Some illnesses are accompanied by pigmentation of the skin. The most commonly seen change in the skin color is that of jaundice. This symptom of several pathologic conditions is a yellow to deep green-yellow pigmentation of the skin. Other diseases may produce tiny hemorrhagic spots on the skin or mottled areas, and the skin appears as though the underlying blood vessels were barely covered.

Soaps, Detergents and Creams. A great variety of soaps is available on the market today. However, there is very little difference in their quality, despite advertising claims. The expensive soaps, with their color, perfume and endorsements, have not been found to be superior to the less expensive soaps as cleansing agents. Detergents are satisfactory cleansing agents for the skin, especially when the water is hard, cold or salty. Persons who are sensitive to soap often find that they can use detergents without difficulty. Detergent bars are now available, but there is no contraindication for using the mild granulated or liquid detergents on the skin. The laundry-type detergents may cause burning and irritation of the skin.

For those who are sensitive to both soap and detergents, cleansing creams may be used. An emulsion type of cream consisting of mineral oil and water is usually very satisfactory, and the wide variety available makes selection for individual preferences an easy process. If sensitivity is not a problem but the skin is dry, the skin should be washed with a mild soap and warm water *before* applying a cream or a lotion except in extreme cases. Dry skin may become even drier during cold weather. At best, creams cannot cleanse the skin thoroughly of oils and dirt and therefore can function only as a less effective substitute for soap and water cleansing.

Deodorants. Keeping the body clean is the prime requisite for preventing body odors. Deodorants may be used *after* the skin is clean. Boric acid or zinc stearate usually are used in deodorants that destroy odor only. The deodorants that check perspiration as well as destroy odor usually contain aluminum chloride, tannic acid or zinc sulfate. These deodorants should be used with care in order to prevent irritation of the skin. There are toilet soaps that, according to manufacturers' claims, kill skin bacteria and therefore eliminate body odors. However, deodorants, medicated soaps, toilet waters and powder cannot replace the need for bathing.

Cosmetics and Creams. Cosmetics frequently enhance the appearance of a clean and healthy skin (although certain cultural and religious groups would not agree with this opinion). For older people, make-up used judiciously helps to disguise blemishes, improves skin coloring and makes wrinkles appear less obvious. Creams and lotions made by reputable concerns are safe to use, but it has not been demonstrated that their cost is commensurate with their quality. The choice is chiefly a matter of personal preference. Vanishing cream is similar to soap and therefore often acts as a good powder foundation for persons with an oily skin.

The skin has absorbent ability, but to a limited degree. Advertising claims for creams that "nourish" the skin and the underlying tissue are misleading. Nourishment is transported to the skin through the blood; absorption by skin tissue cells is negligible.

From time to time, powders containing harmful ingredients have appeared on the market. However, those occasions are rare and usually are discovered promptly. For persons sensitive to one type of powder, the variety is large enough so that often another brand with a different type of base, dye or perfume can be found. Powder puffs should be kept clean.

Superfluous Hair. Custom dictates what hair on the body is superfluous. In American culture, axillary hair is considered superfluous for women but it is not so considered, for example, in some European and Oriental groups. Hence, superfluous hair has more important psychological implications than physical.

Superfluous hair can be removed in a variety of ways. Tweezers for plucking are commonly used for the eyebrows. Scissors and clippers are used on hair on the head.

The safest and the most economical way to remove unwanted hair is to use a razor. It has not been proved that repeated shaving causes excessive growth and coarseness of hair. Depilatories which either destroy hair shafts or mechanically remove hair often irritate the skin and cause infection, although many persons find them safe to use.

The only way to remove hair permanently is by electrolysis, a process by which the hair follicle is destroyed with a mild electric current. This is an expensive and tedious process and requires a careful and experienced operator.

Older people tend to have softer and finer hair. Superfluous hair on the face is common and the nurse can give advice concerning its removal if the patient finds that it is a problem.

A three per cent solution of hydrogen peroxide may be used as a bleach for superfluous hair, especially on the face. The bleached hair is hardly noticeable and often solves the problem easily and inexpensively.

The Prevention of a Decubitus Ulcer

A decubitus ulcer is a circumscribed area in which cutaneous tissue has been destroyed, and there is a progressive destruction of the underlying tissue. The terms decubitus ulcer (or simply decubitus), pressure sore and bedsore are used interchangeably. The plural of decubitus is decubiti. Reddened, irritated and tender skin is the forerunner of broken skin and the formation of decubiti. Any reddened or irritated skin should be reported promptly and given special attention to prevent further irritation.

Decubiti result from interference with circulation and nutrition in the area. There are several factors that can result in poor circulation and nutrition. Usually, not one factor but a combination of factors is responsible for the development of a decubitus ulcer.

Any patient who is debilitated by illness and in a poor nutritional state is less likely to have the same protection from the skin that he has when in good health. Older patients whose skin is wrinkled because of loss of its subcutaneous fat are more prone to develop decubiti than the young. The skin forms folds and becomes irritated quickly. Some patients who have lost considerable weight also may have loose, flabby skin with very little turgor.

The patient's specific illness may have a great effect on the rapidity with which a decubitus might occur. If circulation is impaired, if fever is present, or if the function of the cells is altered, destruction of tissues may be relatively easy.

Skin that is dry and without its usual amount of resistance is irritated easily by feces, urine and drainage from wounds. Keeping the patient clean and free from irritation is of extreme importance in the prevention of decubiti. Dressings may need to be changed more frequently and arranged to keep drainage from irritated areas. Patients who are incontinent (unable to control urinary or bowel excretions) require special consideration. As a precautionary measure, it is now common practice for the physician to request that an indwelling catheter be inserted into the patient's urinary bladder if the patient is in constant danger of urinating.

The skin always has microorganisms on it. While the skin manages well with its own flora, the presence of organisms from infected wounds or from feces is potentially dangerous if the skin is irritated. If the skin is moist and warm, and the area dark, conditions become ideal for the growth of transient bacteria. Infection of the skin may occur, and, once the area is broken, the problem of healing it complicates the patient's plan of care and his illness. Patients who are in danger of developing decubiti should be washed locally following each bowel evacuation.

Patients who must lie for long periods of time on sheets over rubber or protective materials perspire, and evaporation of the moisture is prevented. The constant presence of the moisture along with continuous pressure predisposes to decubitus formation. Good results have been reported from placing patients especially prone to bedsores on a piece of "sheepskin." The "wool" is cropped close. The air spaces in the wool help keep the patient's skin dry. The wool also eases pressure on the area. Although actual sheepskins can be purchased, they are expensive and individual agencies have substantial evidence gained through testing that they cannot be rendered sterile by machine washing. This would make them unsafe for use by more than one patient. Synthetic "sheepskins" are more commonly used and then discarded after use or when soiled.

In addition to keeping the skin surfaces clean and dry, light rubbing of the areas which receive a great deal of pressure is helpful. These areas are the heels, the elbows, the coccyx, the scapulae and the back of the head. The iliac crests are also danger areas if the patient is very thin and must be on the abdomen much of the time. These areas should be examined frequently and rubbed with alcohol if the skin is not too dry. If the skin is dry, a lotion or an ointment offers additional protection to the skin. Lanolin frequently is recommended for dry skin areas.

One of the best protective measures is to prevent pressure against any one area of the body. Pressure constricts vessels and hence impedes blood supply. This can be done by frequently alternating the patient's position. The position in bed that is most likely to cause the greatest amount of pressure to the largest number of areas is the back-lying positon. Congestion of blood reduces the activity of the cells, since oxygen and other nutrients are not brought in and waste products are not removed adequately. If this local state is maintained for hours at a time, death of tissue cells occurs, and a decubitus has been produced. To keep patients from having pressure exerted against any one area for long periods of time, nurses frequently provide for the patient to turn or be turned at frequent intervals. The details for such a plan should then be indicated in the patient's plan of care.

Decubiti are apt to develop on the ankles and heels of some patients. Good results have been reported from the use of polystyrene foam blocks to protect these areas from pressure.[1] The blocks, one for each ankle, are cut in half, hollowed to fit the ankle, padded (preferably with sheepskin), and gripped together around the patient's ankles. The device keeps the foot above the mattress level, thus preventing pressure and irritation. Hyperextension of the knees can be eliminated by placing a pillow under them.

Still another device, reportedly successful in relieving pressure on the body, is the "water bed." A hollow foam rubber mattress is filled with a plastic bag of water on which to "float" the patient. To avoid chilliness, extra bed covering may be necessary. Pressures on the body are markedly less, allowing decubiti to heal, or preventing their development in patients who are susceptible to them.

There are sources of irritation to the skin which could predispose to the formation of a decubitus for which the nurse must be alert. They include wrinkled bedclothes which cause pressure, crumbs and other objects in the bed, top linen so applied that it restricts freedom of movement, and pressure and irritation from casts, adhesive, tubing, arm boards and the like.

A decubitus, while often called a bedsore, is not confined necessarily to those persons who are in bed constantly. Some patients who are able to be out of bed but remain in a chair for a good portion of the day are also likely to develop decubiti if not cared for properly. Old as well as young patients are vulnerable.

When a decubitus ulcer develops, the plan of treatment is the physician's. The great variety of methods that have been used to treat decubiti indicates that not one has been found to be entirely effective. Unquestionably, the best treatment is to prevent their formation.

Bathing the Patient

The primary purpose of the bath is to clean the skin. Some persons may require daily or even more frequent bathing while others may bathe less frequently and still be clean. The condition of the skin, the type of work, the place of work, the type of activities and the weather conditions are all guiding factors in establishing bathing habits.

Values of a Bath. For most patients, a bath can be very refreshing when they are feeling restless and uncomfortable. Depending on the situation and the temperature of the water used for the bath, the patient may feel stimulated and ambitious following it, or he may relax to the point that sleep follows soon after. To those who enjoy a bath, the feeling of cleanliness and relaxation that accompanies it is satisfying. Hence, warm water usually is used for bathing, since the warmth tends to relax muscles. The cooling effects of the bath, even when warm water is used, result from evaporation of water from the body surface.

The cleansing bath can also affect physiologic activities. Friction applied to the skin will affect the peripheral nerve endings and the peripheral circulation. If firm movements are used in stroking the various areas, muscles will be stimulated, and circulation will be aided. This action on the circulation often results in increased kidney function. It is not uncommon for a patient who has been given a bath in bed to need to void immediately following it.

The activity involved in bathing also can be of great value to the musculoskeletal system as a form of exercise. If the bath is taken or given with this advantage in mind, it is possible to exercise all of the major muscle groups and place almost all joints through *full range of joint motion.* Here, again, the accompanying physiologic effects are of advantage to the patient. As the muscle groups contract, blood within the veins is assisted to return to the heart. The activity of the muscle groups helps to maintain muscle tone.

If, during the bathing process, there is a definite attempt to include some planned exercise, respirations also will be involved. Increasing the rate and the depth of respirations has physiologic advantages, such as increasing the oxygen intake and preventing congestion within the lung tissue.

Whether given by the nurse or taken by the patient, a bath can be so managed that it functions as a cleansing procedure as well as a conditioning activity for the body. Middle-aged and elderly patients often will say that they are too stiff to reach down and wash their legs while in bed, to get into a bathtub, to brush their hair, to button or tie a bed gown in the back. They may very well be correct, but investigation often will show that there is no pathologic basis for this limitation. Their knees are stiff, and they cannot reach in back because they have not attempted to do so for a long time. Many of these patients can be helped to increased activity by nurses who can explain the values of good body mechanics.

Bathing offers the nurse one of her greatest opportunities for observing and getting to know the patient and for health teaching. While it is possible to have numerous contacts with the patient during the course of the day, few are as prolonged as the time spent in preparation for and assistance with the bath. The nurse is able to evaluate both the physical and the mental status of the patient.

Bathing Routines. Hospitals usually have routines for bathing patients. Nurses should bear in mind that these routines, which usually are for the convenience of hospital personnel, sometimes may not be liked by some patients. However, most patients will understand the reasons for such routines and, upon explanation, will adjust to them.

Some people prefer a shower to a tub bath, and vice versa. Some bathe in the morning on arising and others in the evening before retiring. Some bathe daily, others every other day, and still others once a week, or even less frequently. It is impossible to satisfy all these habits in hospital situations, but, when practical, it is appreciated by the patient if his ordinary routines can be observed. This is more likely to be possible for the ambulatory patient when shower and tub facilities are available. Some ambulatory patients are permitted to take their baths or showers in the evening or the afternoon if they desire. This information should appear on the patient's nursing care plan, and a nurse caring for him for the first time would not need to disrupt a routine already sanctioned.

No matter where or when the patient is to be bathed, the nurse still has the responsibility for assisting the patient as needed, seeing that he has his necessary articles and checking to see that safety and privacy measures have been considered. Protecting the patient from possible sources of injury or harm include avoiding drafts, making certain that the water is a safe, comfortable temperature and providing means for preventing slipping in the tub or the shower. The patient should never be left out of easy calling distance of the nurse, and the doors of bathrooms should not be locked. These precautions apply to patients of all ages.

The Shower Bath. Even if the patient can manage by himself, the nurse should make certain that all is in order before permitting him to use the shower. If the patient is weak, he should be watched closely and every precaution taken to avoid an accident. A shower stall having guide rails on the wall both inside and outside the stall offers safety. It is best if there are two levels of rails in the stall; one placed low enough so that, if a patient prefers to sit on a stool while in the shower, he can assist himself to stand. Sitting in the shower is much safer for the older patient or the patient who is still weak. Also, sitting on a chair or a stool makes it easier for the patient to wash his legs with less likelihood of slipping.

The Tub Bath. For the physically limited person, the advantages of the tub bath are often defeated by the disadvantages of the tub itself. It is not a particularly easy device to get in and out of. In some instances, the addition of an attachment to the tub or a rail on the wall will make it easier to enter and leave. Another arrangement that has helped many patients is the use of a chair alongside the tub. The patient sits on the chair and eases to the edge of the tub. After putting both feet into the tub, it is then easier for him to reach the opposite side of the tub and ease down into the tub. Occasionally, it is easier if the patient has a towel or a mat in the tub and then, instead of easing down directly, to kneel first and then to sit down. In some instances, it is best for the bath water to be run after the patient is seated and then drained before the patient attempts to get out of the tub. A hydraulic lift which can be installed in home bath tubs can be used to assist. The person sits on a seat, swings over the tub and then lowers himself into the tub. The reverse is done for getting out of the tub.

In addition to its cleansing and refreshing value, the tub bath has the added advantage of assisting patients who have musculoskeletal limitations to move and exercise the affected areas easily.

The Bath Taken in Bed. Some patients must remain in bed as a part of their regimen, even if they are permitted to care for themselves, feed themselves, play games, read and possibly do some prescribed exercises. If they have not had a bed bath given to them previously, they may need some suggestions on how to proceed to bathe themselves.

In addition to providing the patient with all of the necessary articles for oral hygiene and for washing, the nurse prepares the unit so that it is more convenient for the patient. This includes removing the top bed linen and replacing it with a bath blanket so that the patient does not get the bedding wet. The necessary articles should be placed conveniently, usually on the bedside or overbed table. Clean clothing should be placed within easy reach. Make-up items for the woman patient should be left where she can obtain them after she has finished her bath. Male patients may wish to shave either before or after they have bathed. This requires providing clean hot water.

Patients in bed will have varying degrees of physical ability to bathe themselves. Some patients will be able to wash only the upper parts of their bodies. The rest of the bath is then completed by the nurse or someone on the nursing staff. Other patients will be able to wash all but their backs. Some patients are able and are encouraged, as a part of their bed exercises, to wash their backs as well. Washing every area of the body while in bed requires considerable manipulation and exercise. This activity in itself is a good conditioner for someone who is not up and about. With good teaching the nurse can help the patient to understand its values.

The Bath Given in Bed. For patients who are restricted in their activity and for those who are unable to move, the bath is refresh-

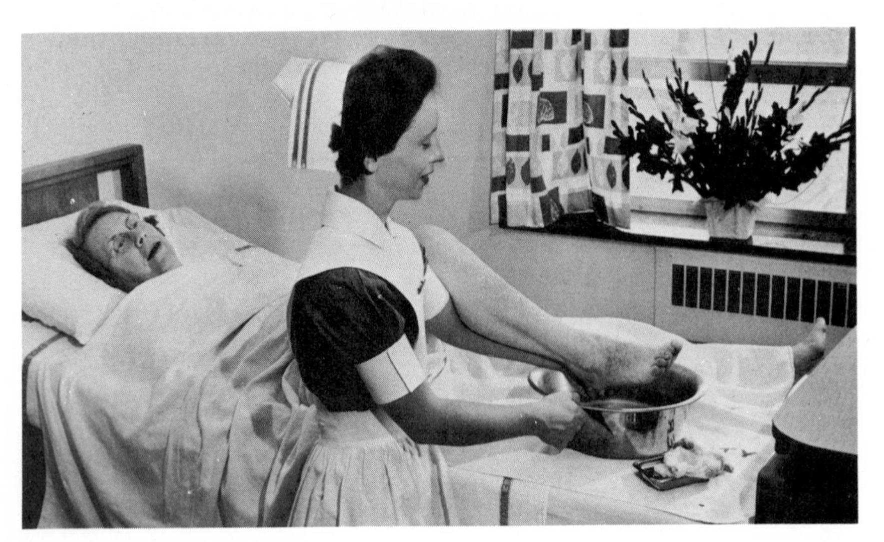

Fig. 19-1. The bed bath for the helpless patient is often refreshing and relaxing. Here, the student nurse skillfully is holding and supporting the patient's leg in preparation for placing it in the basin of water. Note that the patient is well draped, the bed protected with the towel and the equipment placed conveniently and ready for use.

ing and physiologically stimulating. For the very ill and inactive patient, bathing with modifications of water temperature and types of strokes used can bring considerable relief from discomfort.

Before starting the bath, it is best to offer the patient the bedpan.

The following description of a bath assumes that the patient is able to be raised or lowered in bed and that, while there is limitation of movement, it is possible for the nurse to manage the patient alone. It also assumes that only routine hygienic care is needed. Bathing procedures vary. The following suggested actions with reasons are given as guides.

Male nursing personnel usually are responsible for finishing the bath for male patients unable to do so for themselves. The nurse is responsible for this care for the female patient. Finishing the patient's bath must be done with tact and understanding, but to neglect this part of personal care represents poor quality nursing.

Back Rub. Following the bath, most hospital procedures suggest giving the patient a back rub, either with alcohol or with an emollient preparation. The values are similar to those discussed in relation to a bath. A back rub relaxes the patient, stimulates muscles and peripheral circulation and acts as a general body conditioner. Agencies differ concerning back rub practices. One of the Study Situations at the end of this chapter describes one in which the reader will be interested.

Making an Occupied Bed. It is usual procedure to plan to change linens at the time that the bed bath is given, since the top bedding will be already off. The occupied bed is made by rolling the patient over to the far side of the bed and tucking the soiled bottom linens and the rubber or plastic draw sheet toward the center of the bed and well under the patient. The clean linens are then placed so that one half of the bottom of the bed can be made. The patient can then be rolled over onto the freshly made part of the bed. The soiled linens are removed, and the clean linens are pulled through tightly. A smoother bed will be possible if the pull on

SUGGESTED PROCEDURE FOR BATHING A PATIENT IN BED

Obtain all articles needed for hygiene and bed making. For the patient's psychological comfort, provide for privacy.

Arrange the articles in order of use for convenience in working.

Remove the top bedding and fold linen to be replaced on the bed so it is ready when needed without being rearranged. Place bath blanket over patient to avoid exposure and to provide warmth.

Assist the patient to the side of the bed for convenience and ease in working.

Elevate the head of the bed slightly while oral hygiene is being done, to avoid having the patient aspirate liquids.

Lower the head of the bed and remove either all pillows or all but one. Assist the patient to raise the head and the shoulders in order to remove the pillows.

Arrange washcloth in a fashion to prevent corners from dragging over the patient's skin. Use firm but gentle strokes.

Wash the patient's face, ears and neck. When washing the eyes, wipe from the inner canthus outward and use a separate portion of the washcloth for each eye.

Wash and dry the patient's arms. Wash and dry the patient's chest. Then wash and dry the abdomen, including the area of the thighs near the groin.

Drape the bath blanket around the upper thigh to prevent exposure of the patient while washing the leg.

Lift the patient's leg at the bony prominence at the ankle and the heel and then support the leg on your arm until you can place it carefully into the basin of water. Wash each leg separately.

Change the water.

Roll the patient to the side-lying position and bring him close to the edge of the bed.

Place the towel along the back and turn the bath blanket back to expose the patient's back. Wash the back of the neck, the shoulders, the back, the buttocks and the posterior upper thighs. Use firm, long strokes.

Rub the patient's back with alcohol and then powder or rub with lotion if he prefers or if his skin is dry.

Roll the patient back to the back-lying position.

Wash the genital area. If the patient is able to do this, provide water, soap and towel within easy reach and leave the unit. Remove equipment which can be cleaned while the patient is busy.

Comb the patient's hair after the bed is made. The old pillow case or towel can be used to protect the bed from combings.

the clean linen is done directly behind the patient's back. The weight of the patient will then hold the linen in place. The bottom of the bed is then completed. The patient is usually turned back toward the center of the bed, and the top of the bed is made. The use of contour bottom sheets has greatly reduced the amount of time needed to tighten sheets.

There are variations in the procedure for making the occupied bed. However, these small differences have no real effect on the patient's comfort. In some instances, it is necessary for nurses to devise unique ways to change the linens on a patient's bed because of the nature of the patient's condition, orthopedic appliances on the bed or treatments that may be in progress.

Care of the Hair

General Considerations. The hair is one of the accessory structures of the skin. Each hair consists of the shaft which projects beyond the surface of the skin and the hair follicle which lies under the surface of the skin. Hair grows in the follicle and, as is true of other parts of the body, receives its nourishment from the blood which circulates through each follicle.

Good general health is essential for attractive hair, and, like the skin, cleanliness aids in keeping it attractive. Illness affects the hair (excessive hair loss, brittleness and decreased rate of growth) especially when endocrine abnormalities, increased body temperature, poor nutrition or anxiety and worry are present.

The hair is exposed to the same dirt and oil as the skin. It should be washed as often as necessary to keep it clean. For most persons, a weekly shampoo is sufficient, but more often or less frequent shampooing may be indicated for others. Daily brushing of the hair aids in keeping it clean and in dis-

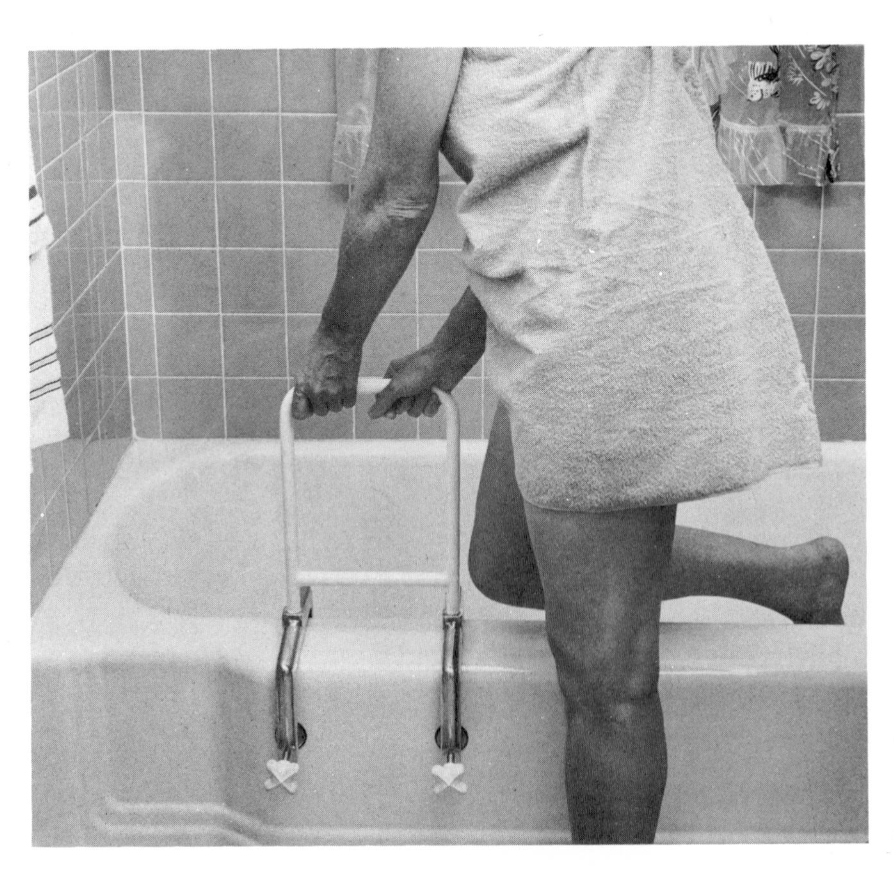

Fig. 19-2. An aid which helps the patient to get into and out of the bathtub offers considerable security to the aged or the physically limited patient. (Bollen Products Co., East Cleveland, Ohio)

tributing hair oil along the shaft of each hair. Brushing also stimulates the circulation of blood in the scalp.

A comb used for arranging the hair does not replace brushing. Personal preference dictates the selection of a comb, but sharp and irregular teeth which may scratch the scalp should be avoided. The comb and the brush should be washed each time the hair is washed and as frequently as necessary between shampoos.

If the hair is dry, oils may be used. Pure castor oil, olive oil or mineral oil are satisfactory, but perfumed preparations may be used with safety if sensitivity of the skin is no problem. If the hair is oily, more frequent washing is indicated.

Baldness. There is no known cure for baldness or *alopecia*, despite the promises of many advertisements. Baldness is believed to be hereditary, and no amount of external treatment is likely to help. Alopecia is rare in women and common in men. Wigs or toupees, frequently worn by persons who are bald, require the same care as normal hair, but less frequent washing is required since they are not lubricated with oil from the sebaceous glands.

Dandruff. This may be due to excessive scaling of the skin on the scalp or to an infection on the scalp. If dandruff is heavy and persistent and irritates the scalp, a physician should be consulted. Proprietary preparations have not been found to be effective for "curing" dandruff. Daily brushing and washing as necessary, in most cases, will aid in keeping the scalp free of dandruff.

Shampoo Preparations. Certain shampoos on the market, recommended for dry hair, are designed to remove all substances except the natural oils. However, if the hair is dry and unmanageable after washing, a few drops of oil rubbed into the hair produces satisfactory results. Detergents are more effective than soap when used with hard water. Liquid and cream shampoos rinse from the hair with greater ease than does bar soap.

Permanent Waves. Home permanent waves have become very popular with women who have learned how to use them, and they often mean additional comfort for patients confined for long periods of time. In some situations, as in a chronic illness unit, the nurse may be asked to assist a patient with a home permanent wave. If there is consent on the part of the patient's physician, and the nurse feels that she has the necessary competence, the procedure could result in considerable satisfaction for the patient.

Pediculosis. Infestation with lice is called pediculosis. There are three common types of lice: *Pediculus humanus*, var. *capitis*,

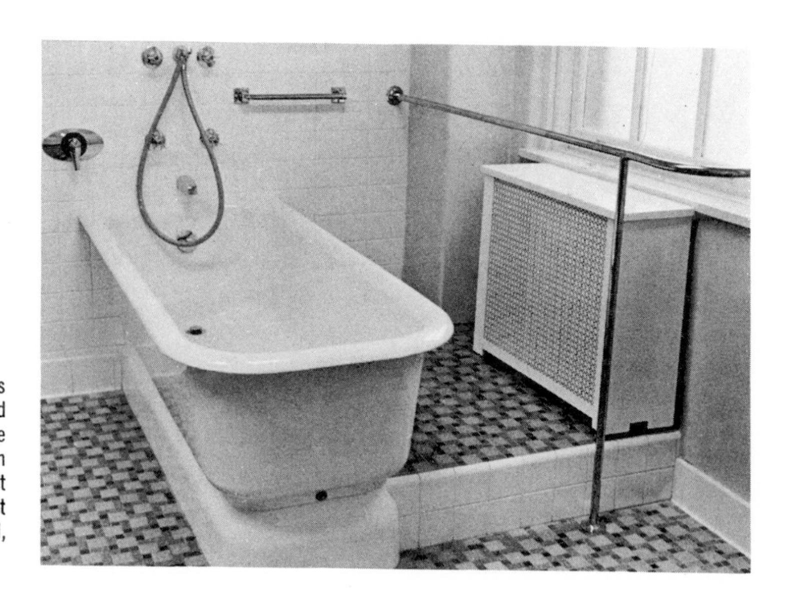

FIG. 19-3. An example of a bathtub that is used in continuing care units. It is situated so that the patient may step up on one side and get into it easily, yet it is on floor level on the other side so that the nurse can stand at a level convenient to her if she must assist the patient. (Courtesy Muhlenberg Hospital, Plainfield, N. J.)

which infests hair and scalp; *Pediculus humanus*, var. *corporis*, which infests the body; and *Phthirus pubis*, which infests the shorter hairs on the body, usually the pubic and the axillary hair. Lice lay eggs, called *nits*, on the hair shafts. Nits are white or light gray and look like dandruff, but they cannot be brushed or shaken off the hair. Frequent scratching and scratch marks on the body and the scalp suggest the presence of pediculosis. Although anyone may become infested with lice, the continued presence of pediculosis is usually a result of uncleanliness.

Pediculosis can be spread directly by contact with infested areas or indirectly through clothing, bed linen, brushes and combs. The linen and the personal care items of patients with pediculosis require separate and careful handling to prevent spreading from person to person.

There are any number of preparations, called *pediculicides*, for the treatment of pediculosis, some of which will destroy the nits as well as the lice. Several treatments are usually necessary before all the nits are destroyed. The procedures and the medications used for the treatment of pediculosis vary from hospital to hospital and with the personal preference of the physician. Shaving off the infested hair is frequently done, especially when pubic and axillary hair are infested. Although shaving is a relatively simple way of handling pediculosis, shaving the scalp is rarely done.

Care of the Patient's Hair. The care of the hair may present no special problems with a

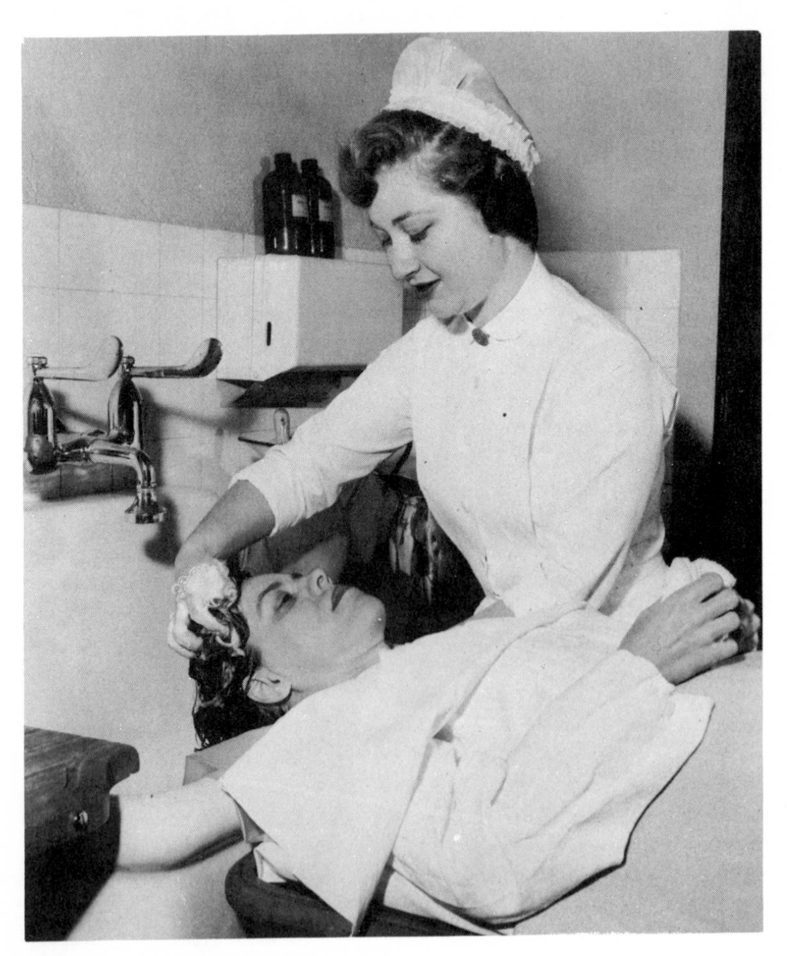

Fig. 19-4. A convenient way for the patient to have her hair shampooed is to place her on the stretcher and move her to a sink or a hopper. The patient's neck is resting on the edge of the hopper, which has a bath towel covered with a small plastic sheet on it. This makes it more comfortable for the patient and also provides for the shampoo and the water to run off easily. A much more thorough washing and rinsing can be done this way, and the entire procedure is easier for both the patient and the nurse.

male patient. However, with the female patient, it does mean time and attention to an important part of grooming. During the acute phase of illness, the female patient may beg to have her hair left undisturbed. To do so, especially if the hair is long, may prove to be disastrous. Hair which becomes entangled is difficult to undo. Hours of careful combing of tiny sections of hair may be necessary if a patient's hair is not combed for even one day. The best way to protect long hair from matting and tangling is to ask the patient for permission to braid it (some patients may not wish to have their hair arranged in braids). Patients usually will consent to such a procedure if it provides them with more comfort during a time when they are unable to manage the arranging of their own hair. Parting the hair in the middle on the back of the head and making two braids, one on either side, prevents the discomfort of lying on one heavy braid on the back of the head.

Occasionally, a patient's hair is almost hopelessly matted, and cutting the hair may be necessary. Before a patient's hair is cut, it is usual procedure to have the patient sign a written consent. It is also considered good policy for the nurse to discuss the necessity for cutting the hair with an immediate member of the patient's family.

Nurses should be aware of the fact that most women have a hair style that is most satisfying to them. If it is necessary to comb and arrange a patient's hair, the nurse should ask the patient how she wishes it to be arranged. Doing so in the fashion the patient considers best is often a big boost to her morale.

Many health agencies have beauticians and barbers to assist with the care of the patient's hair, including shampooing it. However, this convenience does not relieve the nurse of her responsibility to see to it that the patient's hair is cared for properly.

If a beautician is not available, shampooing a patient's hair becomes a nursing responsibility. This procedure usually requires the physician's consent. If the patient is ambulatory, there is no real problem. If the patient is confined to bed but is able to be moved onto a stretcher, she can be transported to a convenient sink for a shampoo. The hair is washed and rinsed over the sink while the patient remains lying on the stretcher.

For patients who must remain in bed for a shampoo, the patient's head and shoulders are moved to the edge of the bed. A protective device is placed under the head. This may be a Kelly pad or an improvised trough made from a large rubber sheet which has been built up on both sides by rolling a towel into each side. To prevent the bed from getting wet and to ensure a thorough cleansing and rinsing of the hair, it is necessary that the patient and the trough or pad be so placed that the water constantly drains. Newer devices for shampooing hair in bed are now available. They have a rigid frame which reduces the likelihood of the water flowing into the bed. Procedures for shampooing a patient's hair in bed depend on the equipment and the facilities available in the agency. Following a shampoo, the patient's hair is dried as quickly as possible to avoid chilliness.

Oral Hygiene

General Considerations. The mouth is the first part of the alimentary canal and an adjunct of the respiratory system. The ducts of the salivary glands open into the vestibule of the mouth. The teeth and the tongue are accessory organs in the mouth and play an important role in beginning digestion by breaking up food particles and mixing them with saliva. The mucous membrane which lines the mouth is not so sturdy as skin; therefore, care is needed while cleaning the mouth to prevent injury.

General good health is as essential as cleanliness for maintaining a healthy mouth and teeth. The relationship, for example, between good teeth and a diet sufficient in calcium and phosphorus along with vitamin D, which is necessary for the body to utilize these minerals, is well established. Equally well proved is the fact that frequent cleansing of the mouth and the teeth aids in reducing dental caries, or decay and in preventing gum inflammation and deterioration.

The old saying, "an ounce of prevention is worth a pound of cure," can be applied very aptly to the care of the teeth. Most dentists recommend a dental examination every six months and preferably every three months, but frequent dental examinations are not a substitute for good oral hygiene.

Toothbrushing. It has been shown that bacteria in the mouth react with food particles to form an acid which predisposes to dental caries. Therefore, frequent cleansing of the teeth and the mouth becomes one of the first prerequisites for maintaining a healthy mouth and teeth. Cleansing can be done by using a toothbrush and by rinsing the mouth thoroughly with clear water. Most people prefer brushing the teeth on arising and before bedtime. After eating, rinsing the mouth with water is satisfactory, but using a brush is desirable. Most children eat frequently between meals, and it is particularly important for them to be taught to

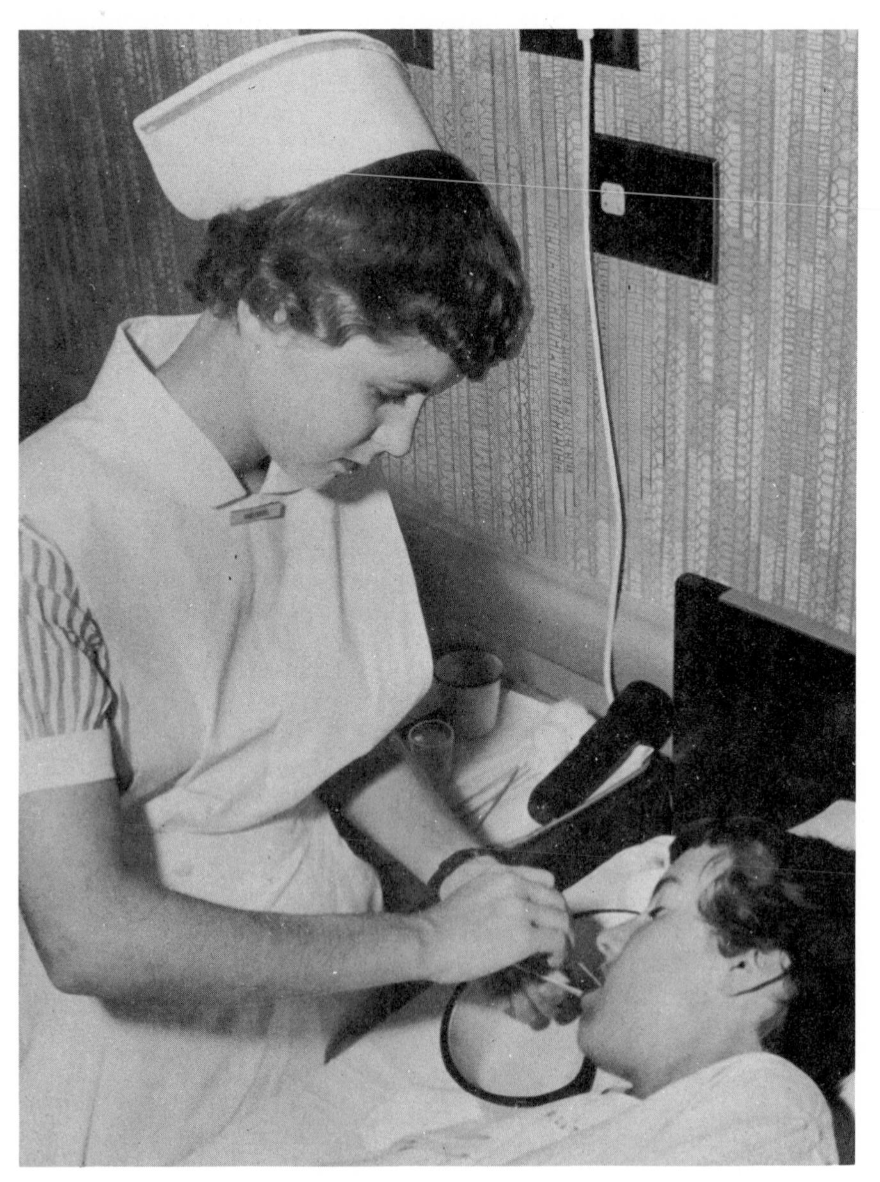

FIG. 19-5. In giving mouth care to the unresponsive patient, every precaution should be observed to prevent having fluid accumulate in the mouth because of the danger of aspiration. A safe way is to position the patient's head so that any fluid placed in the mouth will run toward the lips. Here, a pillow is used to support the patient on her side, thus keeping the head to the side and facing slightly downward.

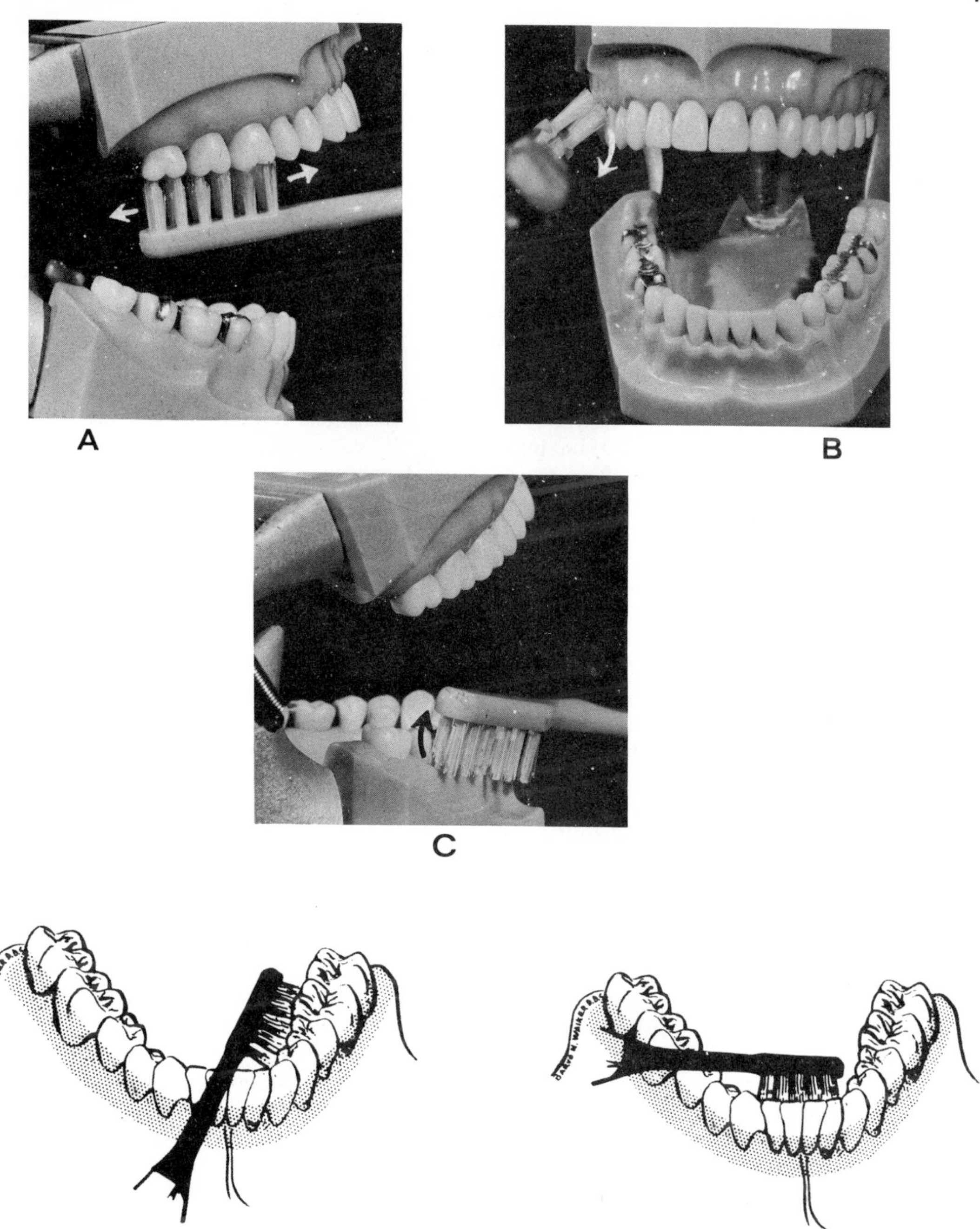

Fig. 19-6. Correct technic of brushing teeth. A, B, and C, outer aspect. (Kesel, R. G., and Sreebny, L. M.: Toothbrushing, Am. J. Nurs. 57:186-188). D and E, inner aspect. D, for molars, brush is held against teeth and moved in an upward motion. The brushing stroke is a slow and careful back and forth motion on the gingival margin. E, for incisors, brush can be held in a vertical position also so that the teeth and gingival margins are brushed from two directions. (Prichard, J. F.: Advanced Periodontal Disease: Surgical and Prosthetic Management. Philadelphia, W. B. Saunders, 1966.)

rinse their mouth with water very often. Many persons are unaware of the need for such frequent cleansing, and the nurse often finds herself in an excellent position to teach patients of its importance.

The toothbrush should be small enough to reach all teeth, and it should have firm short bristles. Preferably, the tufts should be widespread to allow easy access to all surfaces of the teeth and easy cleansing and drying of the brush. There is difference of opinion concerning how the teeth should be brushed. However, it is agreed that care should be exercised so that the tufts do not injure gum tissues. If food is tightly wedged between the teeth, dental floss may be used, provided that care is exercised not to injure the gums. The tongue also should be cleansed with the brush. Automatic toothbrushes (electric or battery operated) have been found to be simple to use and as good as hand brushes in removing debris and plaque.

Water spray units (Water Piks) are available to assist with oral hygiene. Although the unit does not take the place of a properly used brush, it has its uses and is unlikely to do harm to the gums and teeth. The unit, attached to a faucet, sprays water under pressure upon areas to which it is directed. It is especially helpful as an additional aid to the brush for flushing material from around braces and dental bridges.

Toothpastes and powders aid the brushing process, usually have a pleasant taste and often encourage brushing, especially among children. Most dentrifices are safe to use, but those containing harsh abrasives may scratch the enamel of the teeth and therefore are not recommended. Salt, sodium bicarbonate or precipitated chalk are just as effective for cleansing the mouth and the teeth and are far less expensive than proprietary products on the market. Dentrifices containing stannous fluoride have proven to be effective in aiding to decrease dental caries, and, hence, are recommended by many dentists.

"Bad breath" or halitosis is often systemic in nature. For example, the odor of onions and garlic on the breath comes from the lungs where the oils are being removed from the blood stream and eliminated with respiration. When halitosis results from a systemic cause, oral treatment can only mask the odor temporarily at best. Mouthwashes may be pleasant to use, and some persons prefer a mildly flavored mouthwash to a salt or a sodium bicarbonate solution, but they cannot remove halitosis when odors are being eliminated by respiration.

If the cause of halitosis is due to poor oral hygiene, cleansing will reduce the odor. Certain mouthwashes claim antiseptic value which supposedly decreases the bacteria in the mouth. However, such claims are not well founded; mouthwashes have little more, if any, value than plain water. If they are used in a concentrated form, they may injure oral tissue, and infection and additional odor may result.

Oral hygiene is equally important for persons with dentures. The removable type are removed and cleansed with a brush. There are brushes designed for dentures which are helpful for cleaning in small areas. There also are preparations in which to soak dentures to aid in removing hardened particles. Some dentists recommend that removable dentures remain in place except while they are being cleaned. If the patient has been instructed to remove his dentures while sleeping, a disposable denture cup is convenient and easy to use. From an esthetic standpoint, dentures should not be placed in cups, glasses or other dishes that are used for eating purposes. Keeping the dentures out for long periods of time permits the gum lines to change, thus affecting the fit of the dentures.

Water Fluoridation. The addition of fluoride compounds to drinking water that is fluoride-deficient, for the prevention of dental caries, has been under study for approximately 25 years. In general, studies have indicated that fluoridation has aided in reducing dental caries and that it is a safe public health measure. However, in certain areas, public opposition has been sufficient to prevent water fluoridation, so that it has not yet become a common practice.

Giving Oral Hygiene. While the care of the mouth described earlier is still applicable during illness, there are numerous occasions when it must be modified to meet changes in the mouth. These changes usually are an alteration in the amount of secretion in the mouth and the formation of a coating on the tongue. If the patient is able to assist with his own mouth care, it may very well be a matter of providing him with the materials necessary to cleanse his mouth more frequently. If the patient is helpless, the nurse will help make certain that special attention is given to the patient's mouth as often as necessary to keep it clean and moist. It is not unusual to provide special mouth care as often as every hour, especially for patients who are unable to take fluids or are not permitted fluids by mouth. For those patients who are permitted foods, the mouth should be cleansed before meals so that the patient may enjoy them.

Medicated mouthwashes may be used for special mouth care, especially if the patient likes the taste of an aromatic solution. However, it will be recalled that plain or salted water will help equally well to loosen mucous particles and to cleanse the mouth mechanically. If the mucous is very tenacious, a solution of half water and half hydrogen peroxide is effective for cleansing.

It may be necessary for the nurse to use some means for opening the patient's mouth for cleansing if the patient is unconscious. A tongue blade usually works satisfactorily. Several methods are possible for cleansing the mucous membrane of the mouth after it is opened, but each has certain limitations. If gauze is wrapped about a tongue blade and secured with adhesive so that it does not come off, the resulting applicator is usually too large to clean all surfaces of the mouth well. If small gauze squares are held with a clamp, it is easier to reach all surfaces, but there is danger of damaging the membrane with the clamp. Large cotton applicators, prepared so that the cotton will not come off the stick, seem to be effective. The cotton is less irritating than gauze, and the size can be varied easily, depending on the situation. The patient's toothbrush may be used, but care must be exercised not to injure the mucous membrane. If the brush is stiff and hard, running hot water over it softens the bristles and there is less tendency to injure gum tissues.

Whenever placing an object such as a toothbrush or an applicator into a patient's mouth, a mouth gag should be used to hold it open if the patient tends to close his mouth. One should not use the fingers to hold a patient's mouth open. The mouth constantly harbors organisms, and a human bite is a potentially dangerous wound.

When introducing fluid into the mouth of an unresponsive patient, keep the head in such a position that even a small amount will not be aspirated by the patient. When dipping the applicator into the solution to be used for cleaning the mouth, make certain that it is moist but not so wet that solution will pool in the mouth.

After cleaning the surfaces of the mouth, clean the teeth, using the patient's toothbrush, and then clean the tongue, using gauze held on a clamp or wrapped over a tongue blade or the patient's toothbrush. The tongue is not as subject to injury as the mucous membrane of the mouth. After the entire mouth has been cleansed, moisten the mucous membrane with water. Cold cream or lanolin may be applied to the lips to help prevent cracking. The skin on the lips is very thin, and evaporation of moisture from them takes place rapidly, especially when the patient has a fever.

If the patient is able to take fluids by mouth, an excellent aid to oral hygiene and comfort is frequent moistening of lips and mouth with water.

If the patient has removable dentures, they should be cleansed more often than usual. If they are kept clean, the patient is more likely to keep them in the mouth. However, if permitted to get coated with mucus, they will annoy the patient, and he will wish to have them removed. Extreme care should be taken when managing a patient's artificial dentures. They represent a considerable financial investment, and damage or loss is not only expensive but embarrassing for the patient.

When artificial dentures are cleansed, they should be held over a basin of water so that should they slip from the person's grasp, they may not drop onto a hard surface. The patient's emesis basin with water in it can be used. This also facilitates rinsing them during the cleansing process.

When the patient's teeth are not in the mouth, they should be stored in a suitable container and in a safe place. As mentioned previously, from an esthetic standpoint, dentures should not be placed in drinking cups, glasses or other dishes used for eating purposes.

Care of the Nails

Like the hair, the nails are an accessory structure of the skin. They are composed of epithelial tissue. The body of the nail is the exposed portion; the root lies in the skin in the nail groove where the nail grows and is nourished.

The fingernails may be trimmed by filing or cutting in an oval fashion. Trimming the nails too far down on the sides is contraindicated because of possible injury to the cuticle and the skin around the nail. Great care must be exercised if a nail scissors is used to prevent injuring tissue surrounding the nail. Hangnails are broken pieces of cuticle; they should be removed by cutting. Hangnails can be prevented by pushing the cuticle back gently with a blunt instrument or with a towel after washing the hands when the cuticle is soft and pliable. Cleansing under the nails is accomplished best by using a blunt instrument, being careful to prevent injuring the area where the nail is attached to the underlying tissue.

The toenails are trimmed straight to prevent them from becoming ingrown. Otherwise, care is similar to the care of the fingernails. The reader will be interested in a Study Situation at the end of this chapter that discusses common foot care problems.

Some authorities believe that nail polish and polish remover have drying effects and predispose to splitting of the nails. Creams and oils may be used to aid in preventing excessive dryness.

Care of the Eyes

The eyes very frequently reflect the state of health. The nurse will observe that, during illness, the eyes may water more freely and appear glasslike. As health returns, the eyes regain their normal appearance. Secretions from the eyes may adhere to the lashes, dry and become crusty, or there may be slight discharge from the mucous membrane. If discharge is present, it may accumulate in the corners of the eyes, especially during sleep. Water or physiologic saline should be used to wipe the eyes clean, unless the physician prescribes another solution. Wipe from the inner canthus (corner near nose) to the outer canthus. This is to minimize the possibility of forcing the discharge into the area drained by the nasolacrimal duct. Use a clean portion of the patient's washcloth each time the eye is wiped. Soft, disposable tissues may also be used, especially if there is any question about the cleanliness of the washcloth.

Artificial Eyes. Most patients who wear an artificial eye will prefer to take care of it themselves, and they should be encouraged to do so when possible. However, the nurse should provide the necessary equipment, which usually includes a small basin and solution for rinsing the prosthesis. Normal saline or tap water can be used. Most persons have their own method for cleansing the eye and the area around it. The nurse should ask the patient how he does this and make it possible for him to continue with his usual practice.

If the patient needs assistance, an artificial eye may be removed by putting pressure below the eye until the suction is broken, and then the eye will slip out easily. Another method is to place suction on the artificial eye itself and remove it. A simple method is to use the rubber bulb of an eye dropper. The bulb is compressed to expel the air and placed near the center of the eye. When pressure on the bulb is released, the bulb will cling to the eye and it then can be removed by gentle lifting. The artificial eye is cleansed with normal saline. Care should be taken to avoid scratching an artificial eye. The eye is replaced by pulling down on the lower lid and slipping it in position.

Care of the Ears and Nose

Cleaning the Ears. Other than cleaning the outer ears, little more is needed for routine hygiene of the ear. After the ears are washed, they should be dried carefully with a soft towel so that water and wax are removed by capillary action. Forcing the towel into the ear for drying may aid in the formation of wax plugs.

If a wax plug is present in the auditory canal, it is removed by gentle syringing of the ear. The physician's approval is necessary for this procedure. Using items such as bobby pins or a hairpin to remove wax is extremely dangerous since the eardrum may be punctured.

Cleansing the Nose. The best way to cleanse the nose is to blow it gently. Irrigations are contraindicated unles ordered by a physician because of the possible danger of forcing material into the sinuses. Objects should be kept away from the nose to prevent aspiration if the object is small and to prevent injuring the mucous membrane of the nose.

If the external nares are crusted, applying mineral oil aids in softening and removing the crusts. Disposable paper tissues are recommended for nasal secretions.

Study Situations

1. In the following article, the author likens a back rub to a conductor of messages:

- Temple, K. D.: The back rub.
  AMER. J. NURS., *67*:2102-2103, October, 1967.

How does the author describe a back rub as helpful in aiding to develop good interpersonal relationships with patients? Describe briefly the four back rub technics illustrated in the article.

2. Two devices for bathing the bedridden patient are described in the following articles:

- Linsay, M. E.: Shower cart and area. (Trading Post).
  AMER. J. NURS., *63*:101, September, 1963.
- Sciaraffa, J. A., and Chevillon, C. F.: New bed-bath system.
  AMER. J. NURS., *65*:102, April, 1965.

What advantages do these devices offer over the bath given in bed?

3. A podiatrist discusses care of the feet in the following article:

- Simko, M. V.: Foot welfare.
  AMER. J. NURS., *67*:1895-1897, September, 1967.

According to the author, what nursing measures may be observed for the following foot problems: corns or calluses, profuse perspiration, and blisters? Note particularly the precautions that should be taken when caring for toenails of persons with vascular disorders.

4. Principles of good dental care for all persons are discussed in this article:

- Schreiber, F. C.: Dental care for long-term patients.
  AMER. J. NURS., *64*:84-86, February, 1964.

The suggestions for the care of dentures are helpful since their care often confronts the nurse.

References

1. Butterworth, R. F., and Golding, C.: A device for treating pressure sores around the ankles. GERIATRICS, *20*:413-414, May, 1965.
2. Carney, R. G.: The aging skin. AMER. J. NURS., *63*:110, June, 1963.
3. Hass, R. L.: The case for fluoridation. AMER. J. NURS., *66*:328-331, February, 1966.
4. Hoover, D. R., and Robinson, H. B. G.: Effect of automatic and hand toothbrushing on gingivitis. J. AMER. DENT. ASS., *65*:361, September, 1962.
5. Lefkowitz, W.: Effectiveness of automatic and hand brushes in removing dental plaque and debris. J. AMER. DENT. ASS., *65*:351, September, 1962.
6. Levenson, M. F.: Bite if you can't brush. AMER. J. NURS., *66*:2012-2013, September, 1966.
7. Newton, M.: Feminine hygiene. AMER. J. NURS., *64*:100-102, December, 1964.
8. Weinstein, J. D., and Davidson, B. A.: Fluid support in the prevention and treatment of decubitus ulcers. AMER. J. PHYS. MED., *45*:283-290, December, 1966.

CHAPTER

20

Providing for Posture and Exercise Needs

PRINCIPLES OF BODY MECHANICS

Introduction

No one would question the relationship of rest to health, or of good nutrition to health. So, also, is there a direct relationship of body mechanics to the effective functioning of the body. Body mechanics has been described as the efficient use of the body as a machine and as a means for locomotion. Good health depends not only on how expertly we choose our foods, but also on how carefully and efficiently we utilize our body parts in relation to internal and external forces. For example, a truck driver may eat adequately nutritious meals; but if he does not understand how to use his body properly to lift a heavy object onto his truck, he may injure himself. Or the homemaker may be well aware of the essentials of proper menu planning, and she may have many modern conveniences to assist her. But improper use of her body in activities performed throughout a good part of her day, such as reaching, bending, stooping or standing, may tire her.

The importance of understanding body mechanics is universal, not only for an ill person but also for everyone at all times. The basic principles of body mechanics should be in evidence in every activity and even during periods of rest. Because correct use of the body is another phase of prevention of illness and the promotion of health, the nurse has a major teaching responsibility, both directly and indirectly, by example.

To remember to use the correct muscle groups for the correct activity is indeed a chore when one already has developed a life pattern of using muscle groups in another way. However, as with all habits, it takes time to learn a new pattern, especially when the process involves breaking down an established one. In the final analysis, good body mechanics will pay dividends in good health and appearance and body function, which in turn produces happiness and comfort on the part of the person using them. Good body mechanics is not accomplished by following a set procedure; it is achieved through knowledge which guides actions in every activity performed and is a fundamental concept of nursing.

To be able to evaluate the patient's musculoskeletal needs and to teach by example, the nurse must understand and utilize the principles of body mechanics. Every activity in which she engages will require understanding and use of these principles, from as simple a thing as moving a chair closer to the patient's bedside to lifting a patient out of bed.

Terms and Concepts of Body Mechanics

All that is involved in body mechanics is sometimes referred to as basic *orthopedic principles in nursing care.* Orthopedics means the correction or the prevention of deformities. Since body mechanics is concerned with prevention of injury to or limitation of the musculoskeletal system, these terms could understandably be interchangeable.

Nurses have long recognized that body mechanics principles are applicable to all areas of nursing and not just to the patient who has a bone fracture or some other skeletal pathologic change. For example, the patient who is on complete bed rest is in danger of losing muscle tonus. Should the bed rest be prolonged there is the danger also of developing contractures if he does not have exercise and joint motion and if provision is not made for maintaining good posture.

Tonus, a normal quality of healthy muscle, is a steady state of contraction present except during sleep. Muscles usually contract by shortening their fibers, but in some types of muscle contraction the length of the muscle fibers remains the same while the tension within the muscle increases.

A *contracture* results from a prolonged state of muscle contraction, usually observed in flexor muscles rather than in extensors because generally flexors are stronger. Flexor muscles when they contract decrease the angle of a joint formed by two adjacent bones. Extensors increase the angle. Knee and elbow contractures are common complications when bedridden patients have not had proper preventive exercises.

While the plight of the patient in bed might be easy to comprehend, everyone who is up and about faces problems as well. A person who is hyperactive may very well exhaust himself and become fatigued. Or, on occasions when patients are depressed or for one reason or another become quite inactive, they may have diminished muscle tonus because of inactivity. This is due to the fact that the use of muscles is essential for maintaining muscle tone. Inactivity leads to *hypotonia* or *atony*, decrease or absence of tone, respectively. Continued inactivity also leads to *atrophy*, a decrease in size (and a loss of normal function) in a muscle.

The woman who is going to have a baby, if taught how to adapt to her weight changes, is able to continue her routine activities more easily. If she understands how to use her muscles effectively during pregnancy, she also helps prepare herself for an easier labor and delivery.

The nurse who understands how to help maintain musculoskeletal functioning is able to care for patients in such a way that their recovery may be speeded, their limitation from inactivity reduced to a minimum and their convalescence shortened.

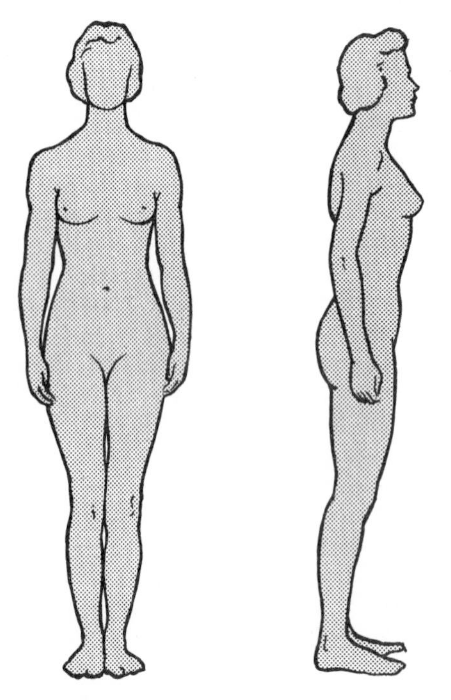

Fig. 20-1. (Left) Anterior view of the body in good alignment. (Right) Lateral view of the body in good alignment.

A first step in understanding body mechanics is to consider posture.

Posture or good body alignment is that alignment of body parts which permits good musculoskeletal balance and operation and promotes good physiologic functioning. Good posture is essential in all positions: standing, sitting or lying down. M. C. Winters describes the body as being in good functional alignment when

> . . . the feet are at a right angle to the lower legs and face forward in the same direction as the patellae; the weight-bearing line passes through the center of the knee and in front of the ankle joints; the knees are extended but are not tense or hyperextended; the thighs are extended on the pelvis; the spine is elongated, and the physiologic curves are within normal limits; the chest is upward and forward and the head is erect[18] (Fig. 20-1).

Posture in itself is a key point in body mechanics and should not be considered as merely the simple procedure of holding oneself erect. Good standing posture involves maintaining balance, which constitutes an effort even though we are not consciously aware of it. To balance the body and maintain good alignment in the standing position, and to engage in various activities such as lifting, stooping, pushing and pulling, require more effort on the part of the body than sitting or lying. This everyone knows from experience, but probably few persons stop to analyze the reasons. There are forces which are present constantly and must be overcome. There are laws of physics which, if utilized properly, will help to reduce the amount of effort expended in maintaining good posture and balance, and in lifting and moving.

Concepts most helpful to the understanding of body mechanics are those concerned with the effect of gravity on balance—balance of all objects, not alone that of humans. Figure 20-2 illustrates these.

The center of gravity of an object is defined as the point at which its mass is centered. In humans, when standing, the center of gravity is located in the center of the pelvis approximately midway between the umbilicus and the symphysis pubis.

The line of gravity is a vertical line which passes through the center of gravity.

To understand further what is involved in the struggle to maintain balance and good posture, it is also necessary to know that there is an accelerating tendency of all bodies toward the center of the earth, referred to as gravity (equal to the earth's attraction minus the centrifugal force arising from the rotation of the earth on its axis; equal to about 32.16 feet per second). This constant pull toward the earth's center is a phenomenon which nurses should understand, since it is a factor in innumerable nursing activities, such as gravity suction, the flow of fluids, drainage of body areas and the stability of objects.

From the diagrams in Figure 20-2, several basic points can be made—namely, that an object is more stable if its center of gravity is close to its base of support; if the line of gravity goes through the base of support; if it has a wide base of support.

While these three points are important facts to be considered with every inanimate object, they are equally important to humans. To prove that these three points have a direct relationship to stability, try standing with the feet close together and then begin to lean forward. As soon as the line of gravity is out of the base of support, you will place one foot forward in order to avoid falling. When standing, a person provides a base of support wide enough so that the line of gravity goes through the base, and he thereby stabilizes himself.

But the act of standing is not merely one of providing a base of support. Synergistic muscle groups contract sufficiently to steady the joints, such as those formed by the head of the femur in the acetabulum of the hip and the knee joint formed by the lower end of the femur and the upper end of the tibia. Usually, muscles work in groups, and synergistic action is smooth coordinated action.

An additional point developed from the three basic ones mentioned is that the stability of an object is also dependent on the height of the center of gravity and the size of the base of support. The wider the base of support and the lower the center of gravity, the greater is the stability of the object. For example, a can of evaporated milk requires little manipulation in order to stabilize it on a table; however, a candle, perhaps, could be made to balance itself, but in order to ensure its remaining erect it is necessary to provide a base of support for it.

In humans, as was mentioned, muscular effort is necessary to maintain the erect po-

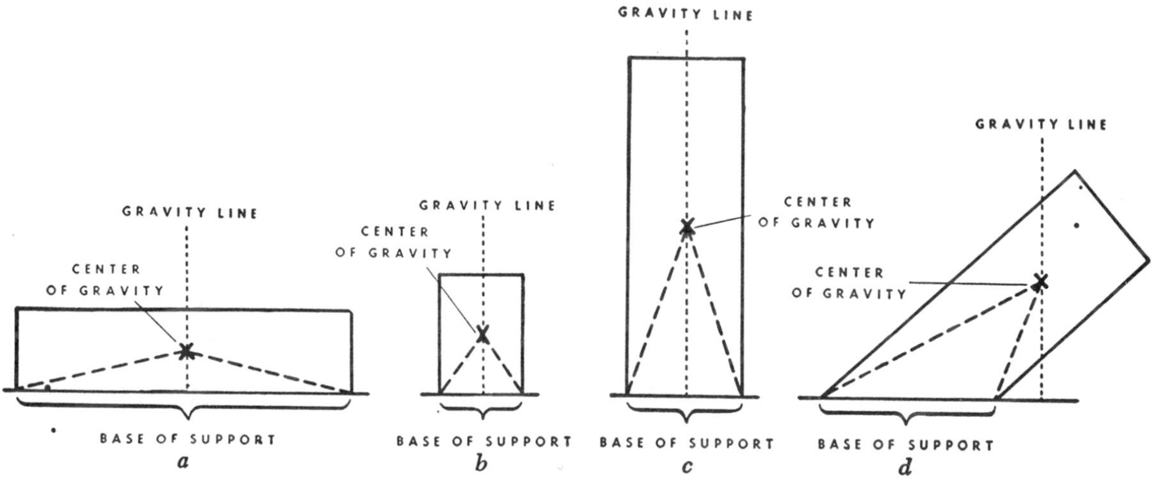

FIG. 20-2. The effect of the base of support and gravity on balance. (Winters, M. C.: Protective Body Mechanics in Daily Life and in Nursing, p. 20, Philadelphia, W. B. Saunders)

sition. Therefore, the amount of effort required by the muscles is related directly to the height of the center of gravity and the size of the base of support. Again, as an example, the ballet dancer while on her toes is utilizing more effort to maintain herself erect than when she has her feet directly on the floor.

The Need for Body Activity

The values of exercise and good posture have long been recognized. From past experience, we know that sitting in a chair in a class for a period of an hour or more with the shoulders and the head brought forward may cause fatigue and altered breathing. If, in addition, the muscles of the legs have not contracted during that period of time, there may be a certain amount of swelling of the feet. This is because skeletal muscles serve many functions in addition to movement, heat production and maintenance of posture. When the muscles contract they squeeze veins. This squeezing action helps to move the blood back to the heart. Together with breathing which changes the pressure within the closed chest cavity and the tiny valves located along the inner surface of the veins, venous circulation is maintained even against the pull of gravity. If inactivity eliminates most of this squeezing action and if poor posture prevents normal breathing, then venous circulation is slowed down. Fatigue will develop as a result of too much waste material accumulating and too little nourishment going to the muscles. Muscle fatigue usually is attributed to the accumulation of too much lactic acid in the muscles.

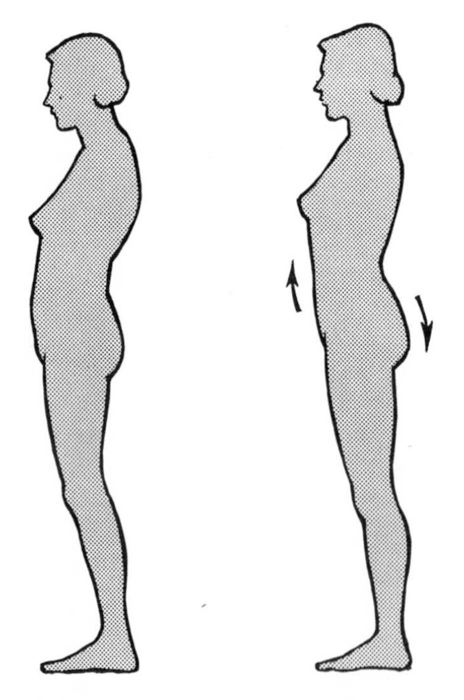

Fig. 20-3. (Left) Slouch position, showing abdominal muscles relaxed and body out of good alignment. (Right) Internal girdle "on." Abdominal muscles contracted giving feeling of upward pull and gluteal muscles contracted, giving a downward pull.

Posture while both standing and lying, as well as exercise and maintenance of balance, are only initial phases of body mechanics. While there is concern if the body is not kept in good alignment and active, there is equal concern when the body is put to use. When motion of the body is extended to include activities such as moving and lifting, there are additional aids which should be considered, since efficient use of the muscles will conserve energy and reduce the possibility of strain.

How to Use Muscles Effectively

One of the primary factors in efficient musculoskeletal activity is that the longest and the strongest appropriate muscles should be used to provide the energy needed. When muscles which cannot provide the best strength and support are forced into exertion, strain, injury and fatigue frequently result.

Origin is the name given to the less movable attachment of a skeletal muscle to a bone. *Insertion* is the name given to the more movable attachment of the muscle to the bone, in other words, the attachment to the bone that is being moved.

In addition to using the longest and the strongest muscles of the arms and legs properly, the muscles in the pelvic area also must be prepared for any vigorous activity. This preparation of the muscles to stabilize the pelvis, to support the abdomen and to protect the body from strain comprises two activities—namely, putting on the internal girdle and making a long midriff.

The internal girdle is made by contracting the gluteal muscles (buttocks) downward and the abdominal muscles upward. The internal girdle is helped further by making a long midriff. This is done by stretching the muscles in the waist. One has the feeling of standing up tall, and of trying to increase the length of the waistline. It is especially important that the muscles involved in the internal girdle and the long midriff assist the long strong muscles of the arms and the legs in activities such as lifting, moving and carrying heavy objects. (Fig. 20-4)

Another factor in musculoskeletal physiology is that persistent exertion without adequate rest is harmful. Muscles must have alternate periods of rest and work. Therefore, activities should be conducted accordingly, especially if the task is a strenuous one.

Using the combination of the longest and the strongest muscles of the arms and the legs, the internal girdle and the long midriff in lifting or moving heavy objects is as much a protective measure as it is an efficient use of muscles. Both the back and the abdominal wall are susceptible to injury. It will be recalled that the spinal column is composed of a series of irregularly shaped bones called the vertebrae. These are separated from each other by cushions of cartilage (disks) and held together by strong bands of connective tissue called ligaments. Viewed from the side, the vertebral column looks somewhat like a double S. It has a concave curve at the neck (cervical) and a convex one at the chest (thoracic), another concave curve (lumbar) and then a convex one at the end of the spinal column (sacral). Muscles are attached to the vertebrae and permit flexion and extension as well as a certain amount of lateral movement in certain areas.

When severe strain is placed on the muscles attached to the vertebrae and the force is transmitted to any one of the curves in the spinal column, injury can result. Many low-back (lumbar) injuries are caused by such strain, i.e., lifting heavy objects incorrectly. The so-called whiplash injury occurring in the cervical area is a frequent result of an automobile accident in which the car is hit from the rear and the person's head is thrown backward suddenly and forcefully. Even in the course of everyday activities, strain and fatigue can be felt in the thoracic or the cervical regions if we sit with the head flexed forward for periods of time when reading or writing. If our backs were absolutely straight many of these injuries would not occur, but then neither could we enjoy the degree of mobility that we have.

While the back is susceptible to injury because of its general structure and muscle groups, the abdominal wall also can be injured by improper use of muscle groups. Weakened musculature of the abdominal wall

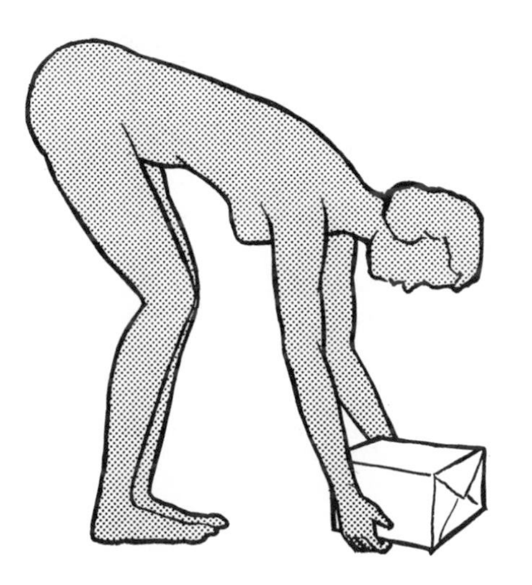

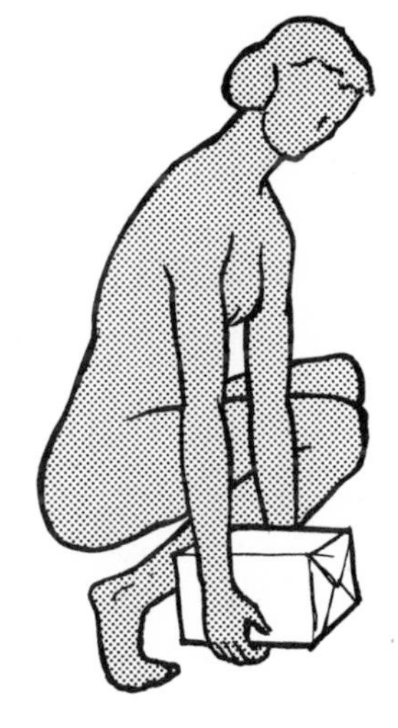

Fig. 20-4. (Left) Poor position for lifting (pull exerted on back). (Right) Good position for lifting (use of long and strong muscles of arms and legs).

from decreased tone or from cutting muscle fibers as in surgery can contribute to making the back more susceptible to injury. Because the organs in the abdomen are not protected by any anterior or lateral bony cage, they rely on strong and supportive abdominal muscles. If they are not protected, the organs can cause a protrusion of the abdominal wall which in turn can result in an exaggeration of the lumbar curve (sometimes called swayback). Exaggerated back curves are sufficiently serious that they can cause some individuals to be excluded from occupations where lifting is required. They may also be prevented from engaging in some sports or other activities.

The abdominal wall has its own points of inherent weakness. These are areas subject to hernias (ruptures, in lay terminology). A hernia is the protrusion of an abdominal structure through an area of weakness in the musculature. (Technically, the term "herniation" can be used to describe such occurrences elsewhere in the body, but for purposes of this discussion it is concerned with the abdominal wall.) These areas of weakness are at the umbilicus, the inguinal canals which transmit the spermatic cords in the male and the round ligaments in the female and at the femoral rings which transmit the femoral vessels to the legs. A hernia can occur in any of these areas if a strain imposed on the abdominal muscles exceeds the capability of the muscles at these points. Some persons having had abdominal surgery have suffered incisional hernias because of weak musculature and improper use of the muscles when lifting or moving heavy objects. Those who have hernias often describe the discomfort they experience when sneezing or coughing and their need to protect the area on such occasions by pressing their hands against it.

When practiced consistently, using the longest and the strongest muscles of the extremities and putting on the internal girdle and the long midriff can become almost an automatic act. Many nurses have saved themselves from injury by just such action. It is not an infrequent occurrence in nursing to have a patient or a visitor feel faint and start to slide to the floor or to have a patient almost fall out of bed while reaching for something. The nurse must act instantly and put herself in the best protective position in order to avoid injury to herself as well. It could be disastrous for the nurse to attempt to hold some one up or for that matter to ease him down when in a position that is putting strain on her back or the abdomen.

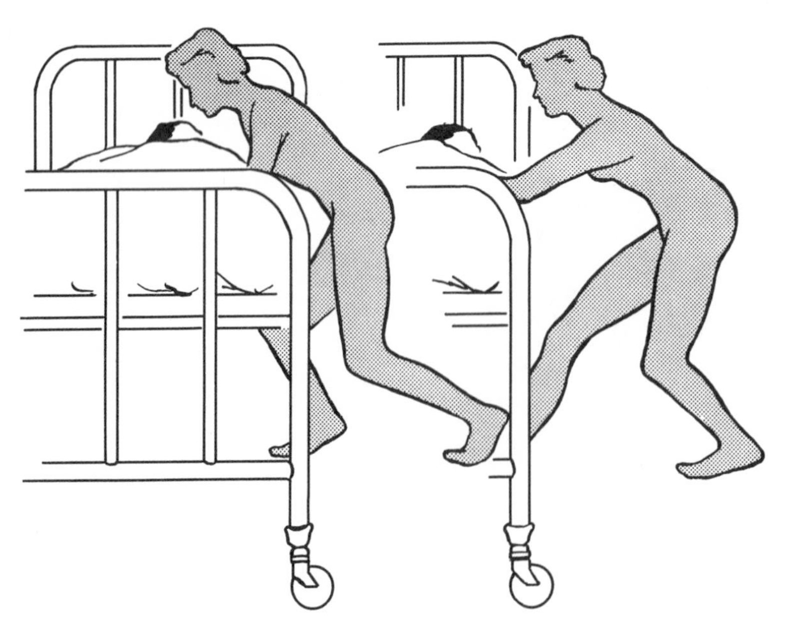

Fig. 20-5. (Left) Shows good position prior to sliding patient to edge of bed; wide base of support with one knee under edge of bed and both knees flexed; arms under patient as far as possible; person close to patient and leaning over him. (Right) Rocking backward to use own body weight to assist in the "pull," person will be in position shown at right.

The nurse will need to teach many patients how activities can be done with greater ease and less fatigue. There is an efficient and safe way or a wrong way of performing such taken-for-granted acts as picking up a baby from a play pen, shoveling snow, raking leaves, skiing, dancing, lifting a turkey out of the oven or unloading heavy objects from the trunk of a car.

Principles of Physics Guiding Body Mechanics

Essential to the performance of acts of moving, lifting and carrying which reflects good body mechanics is the correct application of some of the basic laws of physics. If applied effectively, they will conserve energy, reduce the amount of effort exerted and prevent injury. A few guides based on laws of physics are as follows:

Push, pull, slide or roll an object on a surface rather than lift it. Lifting involves overcoming the pull of gravity.

Work as close as possible to an object which is to be lifted or moved. This brings the center of gravity of the body close to the center of gravity of the object being moved, thereby permitting most of the burden to be borne by the large muscles.

Use the weight of the body as a force for pulling or pushing by rocking on the feet or leaning forward or backward. This reduces the amount of strain placed on the arms and the back.

Summary of Actions Guided by Body Mechanics Principles. The following actions are guides to the efficient use of the musculoskeletal system during periods of activity and inactivity:

Maintain good posture in all activities—walking, sitting or lying—and thereby promote physiologic functioning, and good general appearance.

Use the longest and the strongest muscles of the arms and the legs to help provide the power needed in strenuous activities.

Use the internal girdle and a long midriff to stabilize the pelvis and to protect the abdominal viscera when stooping, reaching, lifting or pulling.

Work close to an object to prevent unnecessary reaching and strain on the muscles.

Slide, roll, push or pull an object rather than lift it in order to reduce the energy needed to lift the weight against the pull of gravity.

Use the weight of the body both to push an object by falling or rocking forward and to pull an object by falling or rocking backward.

Place the feet apart in order to provide a wide base of support when increased stability of the body is necessary.

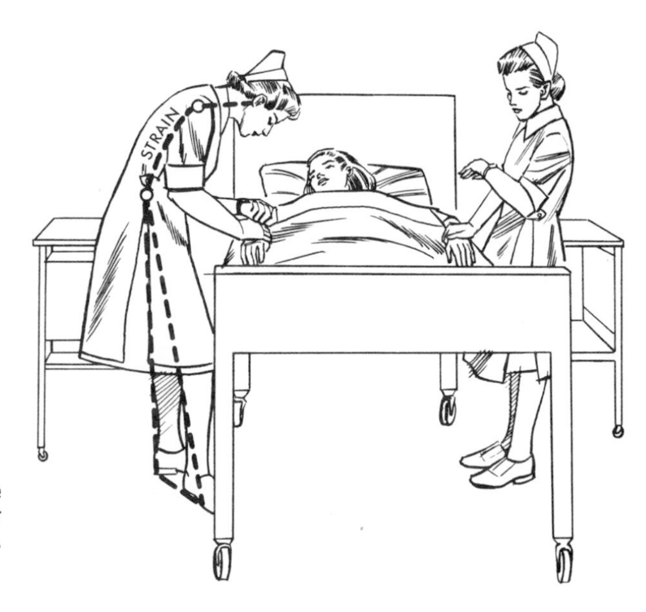

Fig. 20-6. Incorrect and correct body mechanics on the part of the nurse obtaining the patient's pulse rate. (After Body Mechanics in Nursing Arts by Bernice Fash, p. 44. McGraw-Hill Book Company, Inc.)

Flex the knees, put on the internal girdle and come down close to an object which is to be lifted.

Nursing care which prevents impairment of musculoskeletal functioning is highly therapeutic. How the nurse helps in this area is discussed in the succeeding parts of this chapter. They relate to the various activity needs of patients.

HELPING THE PATIENT TO MAINTAIN OR ATTAIN AN AMBULATORY STATUS

Maintaining an Ambulatory Status

For many patients, fortunately, prolonged periods of bed rest are no longer considered necessary. The benefits of keeping a patient "up and about" as much as possible are evident. Activity, even as mild as a stroll around the room or down the hall, is a protective measure for all body systems. It improves circulation and respiration, helps maintain muscle tonus, and aids in elimination from the urinary bladder and intestines. One needs only a mild session with an upper respiratory infection and rest in bed for a day or two to emerge with "sea legs."

Most persons do not wish to be kept in bed and so present no problem. Keeping some persons *in* bed does present a problem many times. Occasionally some persons, especially elderly ones, will decrease their ambulatory activities. Many factors contribute to this, such as arthritis, aches and stiffness. Some of their problems are in a sense self-induced by lack of exercise of certain joints and muscles over a long period of time. These persons should be encouraged to move about, take walks, climb stairs, do toe-heel exercises and perform any other activity that helps keep them in condition to be on the move.

Patients who have surgery may need some encouragement to take that first walk the day of or following their surgery. Incisional discomfort, a running intravenous infusion, or fear of harming themselves act as deterrents. However, most patients understand that it is to their benefit to do so. Assistance in moving them and supporting them in their first efforts will make the process easier.

Physical Conditioning in Preparation for Ambulation

Patients who are not confined to bed and have a good night of sleep and possibly short periods of rest during the day may not require special considerations for physical activity. However, there are other patients who will have to be prepared for the day when ambulation is resumed. Even if they are active in bed, preparation for walking will have to be a consideration. Certain protective exercises can be done in bed which strengthen the over-all efficiency of the musculoskeletal system.

Quadriceps Drills (Sets). One of the most important muscle groups used in walking is the quadriceps femoris. This muscle group helps to extend the leg on the thigh and flexes the thigh. In addition to walking, it helps lift the legs as in stair climbing. The "sea legs" following even short periods of bed rest result from disuse of these muscles. To help to reduce weakness and make first attempts at walking easier, bed patients should be encouraged to contract this muscle group frequently. It is done by asking the patient to contract the muscles which pull the kneecap up toward the hips, during which the patient has the feeling that he is pushing the knee downward into the mattress and pulling the foot upward. This should be held to the count of four: 1-and-2-and-3-and-4. The exercise should not be done so that fatigue of the muscle group results. It is a very simple exercise that can be done two or three times hourly.

Push-Ups or Sit-Ups. In preparation for getting out of bed, the muscle strength of the arms and the shoulders also should be improved. It provides the strength needed to hold on to or get into a chair and to move about better. It is a part of the preparatory exercises for all patients who must learn to walk on crutches.

A trapeze attached to the bed of a patient who has limited use of the lower part of his body helps him to move about in bed. However, this does not strengthen the triceps, which is the muscle group necessary for crutch walking or moving from bed to chair. More suitable exercises are sit-ups or push-ups, frequently considered by some physical therapists to be two different types of exercises.

The exercise may be done by having the patient sit up in bed without support and then lift the hips up off the bed by pushing the hands down into the mattress. If the mattress is soft, it may be necessary to use blocks or books under the hands. The other form of the exercise is to have the patient lie face downward on the bed. The arms are brought up so that the patient pushes his head and chest up off the bed by completely extending his elbows. This is repeated several times each time the exercise is done, and the exercise is repeated several times a day. Some patients would find the latter method more difficult to do.

Daily Activities for Purposeful Exercise. In addition to teaching the patient specific exercises, many other activities can be carried out with benefit to the patient. These include such things as placing the bedside stand so that the patient may use shoulder and arm muscles to reach what he needs instead of placing it so as to require little effort to take things from it; placing the signal cord so that the patient must engage in either arm or shoulder action in order to reach it; encouraging the patient to sit up and reach for the overbed table, to pull it close to him, and then to push it back in place, encouraging a patient to try to wash his back, and having him put on his socks while still in bed. There are innumerable ways in which patients can be helped to exercise, and when they understand the purpose, they very often adopt other exercises for themselves.

Preparing for the Patient to Get Out of Bed

In addition to the attention given to the patient's physical state, the nurse is concerned with the necessary items needed, such as a chair or a wheel chair if the patient is going to stand but not walk about, a walker or crutches. If the patient is going to walk, it is best for him to wear his shoes or supportive slippers. Having to walk with loose slippers or with shoes that have little support adds to the difficulty of the procedure if there is any physical limitation. This applies to all patients, whether young or old, and whether sick for a long or a short time. Patients who are asked to walk immediately following surgery or after long illness are not able to walk as steadily as they would be if their feet were covered properly.

While it is not possible to set the exact manner in which any one patient should be dressed when out of bed, several points should be mentioned. The amount and the type of clothing worn by the patient will depend on the temperature and the air movement in the environment. It is the nurse's responsibility to protect the patient from

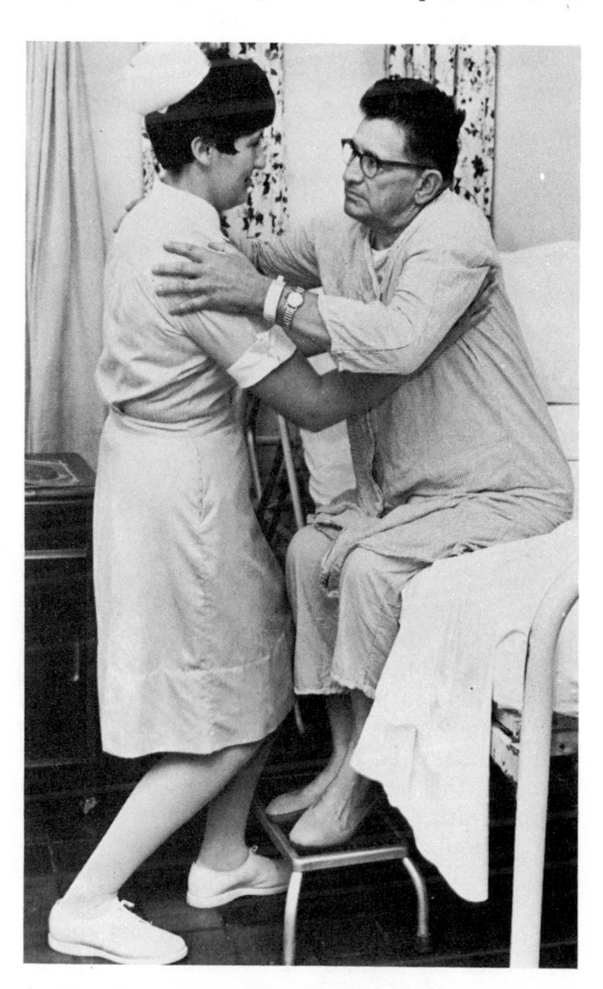

Fig. 20-7. Assisting the patient out of bed. The nurse's hands are in a position to support the patient in the event that he becomes weak and also to assist him to the standing position. (Photo, Warren R. Vroom)

discomfort due to overdressing and against the danger of having him becoming chilled because he is insufficiently clothed. Changes in the physical state as a result of illness usually make patients more susceptible to environmental factors such as drafts. Patients who may be permitted to sit out in the open on porches or patios may need to be given some sort of head covering. For most patients, it is usually better for their morale if they can be dressed in their usual attire. Agencies for the chronically ill make every effort to reduce the association with illness by having their patients dress in clothes either from home or provided by the agency.

Assisting the Patient Out of Bed

If a patient has sufficient strength to stand and to support his own weight, getting him out of bed is a relatively simple matter. However, during the time that the patient is being assisted out of bed, he should be observed for signs of faintness and difficulty in breathing. It is not uncommon for patients to become faint due to an alteration in blood pressure. It is best to assist the patient to the sitting position slowly and to provide a short period of rest between each move. Taking the pulse is a good way to determine the patient's reaction to the activity. If the pulse rate is more rapid than usual, proceed with caution.

If the patient is too weak to walk, the preparation of the chair should precede the preparation of the patient. If a wheel chair is used, the wheels should be locked. If this is not possible, place it against the wall or have it held in place by another person.

The patient is brought to the side of the bed and assisted to the sitting position. The head of the bed should be elevated to help support him in this position. As soon as the patient feels comfortable in this position, the nurse supports his shoulders and legs and pivots him around so that his legs are off to the side of the bed. The feet should be placed on a chair or footstool so that he can support his body and so that pressure against the posterior thigh is reduced. If the feet are not supported, the patient does not feel comfortable, and there is always danger of his sliding off the bed. This position frequently is used preparatory to ambulation and is referred to as *dangling*.

While the patient is sitting on the edge of the bed, it is easy to dress him in his robe and to put on his shoes. A footstool should be so placed that it will be in place for the patient to step down on it.

Helping a Patient Out of Bed: Body Mechanics of the Nurse. With the footstool in place, the nurse stands directly in front of the patient. The patient places his hands on the nurse's shoulders. The nurse places her hands in the patient's axillary region with thumbs pointing upward. In this position, she is able to support the patient's shoulders should he begin to fall. If the nurse's hands are held against the chest instead of up in the axillary region as described, she would need to press the patient's chest tightly if he were to fall. This would be extremely uncomfortable for the patient.

Permit the patient to stand on the footstool for a few seconds to make certain that he is not feeling faint, and then assist him to step down to the floor. If the nurse is tall and the patient is short, it may be necessary for the nurse to put one foot behind, flex her knees and come down with the patient.

Continue to face the patient and turn him around so that his back is toward the chair. Lower the patient to the edge of the chair first. While doing this, the nurse should have one foot forward and the knees flexed and again come down with the patient. Assist the patient to sit well back in the chair and adjust the footrests if it is a wheel chair.

If a high-low bed is used, the nurse should prepare the patient and permit him to dangle his legs while the bed is in the high position. This creates less strain on her arms, and she is in a better position to support the patient. When the patient is ready to stand, the low position would eliminate the need of a footstool. However, if the patient is very weak, the nurse is in a better position to support him and to use her long and strong arm and leg muscles, if she does not lower the bed and follows the procedure described above.

Assisting the Patient to Walk

Many patients who have been confined to bed for a long period of time find that they must almost learn to walk all over again. An activity which needed no special teaching or encouragement in childhood now becomes a real challenge. Often, it is the nurse who plays a major role in the patient's recovery and mental outlook, his hope and faith, especially when he must stick to a rigid and often difficult schedule of re-educating muscle groups. Physicians have said that a patient able to raise his leg only one inch from the bed is considered to possess sufficient power to permit walking.

Where a major problem of muscle re-education presents itself, the patient will need the assistance of experts in physical medicine. However, nurses are often asked to assist patients out of bed and to help them to walk when the presence of a physical therapist is not possible. There are several aspects to this problem of ambulation with which the nurse should be familiar.

Walking. The normal pattern of walking is to move alternate arms and legs. For example, the right arm and the left leg move forward, and then the left arm and the right leg move forward. If a patient is able to be supported from the rear at the waist while he practices these movements and has no real limitations to the muscle groups of the hips, the legs and the feet, he will soon be walking well again.

If the patient is quite weak and is reluctant to try to stand with support only at the waist, it may be necessary to support him under the arm until he feels that he is able to try the other method. A patient who seems to be very weak can be assisted to regain a sense of balance and stability by supporting himself on a walker or the backs of two chairs. Then when the patient walks, if he needs some additional support for a while, the nurse should walk alongside him, keeping her arm which is near the patient under his arm. It is an arm-in-arm position. The advantage of this position is that, if the patient begins to feel faint, the nurse's arm is in a position to slide up into the patient's axilla. The nurse throws one foot out to the side to make a wide base of support and rests the patient on her hip.

To assist patients in the retraining process of walking, there are a number of supportive measures available. Patients may be given canes, walkers or crutches, or assisted to the supportive bars now being installed on hospital patient unit corridors.

Crutch Walking

Sometimes, it is necessary for patients to use crutches for a period of time in order to avoid using one leg or to help strengthen one or both legs. This procedure is taught best by a physical therapist; however, there are numerous instances when the nurse is called on to measure patients for crutches and to teach them to use them. Even if a patient is being taught to crutch-walk by a physical

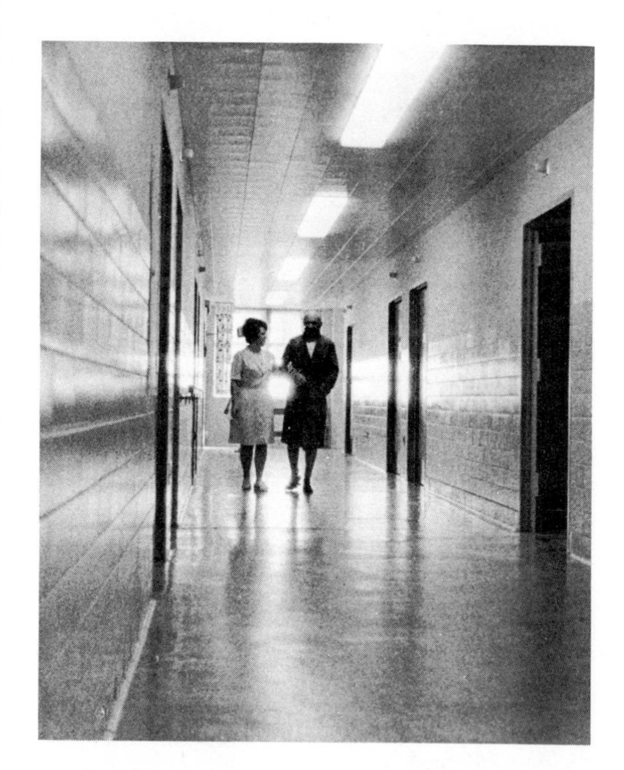

Fig. 20-8. For the patient who has just gotten that invitation, "Let's try a walk down the hall this morning," it may seem more like walking the last mile. All the more reason why bed exercises and quadricep sets are so important. (Courtesy of Muhlenberg Hospital, Plainfield, N.J.)

therapist, it is necessary for the nurse to understand the patient's progress and the gait he is being taught. There are many hours when the therapist is not around, and the nurse should be able to be of some assistance to the patient.

There are several ways in which crutches can be measured, but the two methods described here are considered satisfactory. These are done when the patient is in bed. One way is to measure from the anterior fold of the axilla straight down to the heel and then add two inches. The other way is to measure from the anterior fold of the axilla diagonally out to a point six inches away from the heel. The measurement for the crutches includes the shoulder pads and the suction tips at the bottom. Then the crutches will need to be adjusted for the hand grip of the patient. This may be done when the patient is in the upright position. The hand grip should be placed so that the elbows are slightly flexed while the patient is using them. The elbows should not be extended.

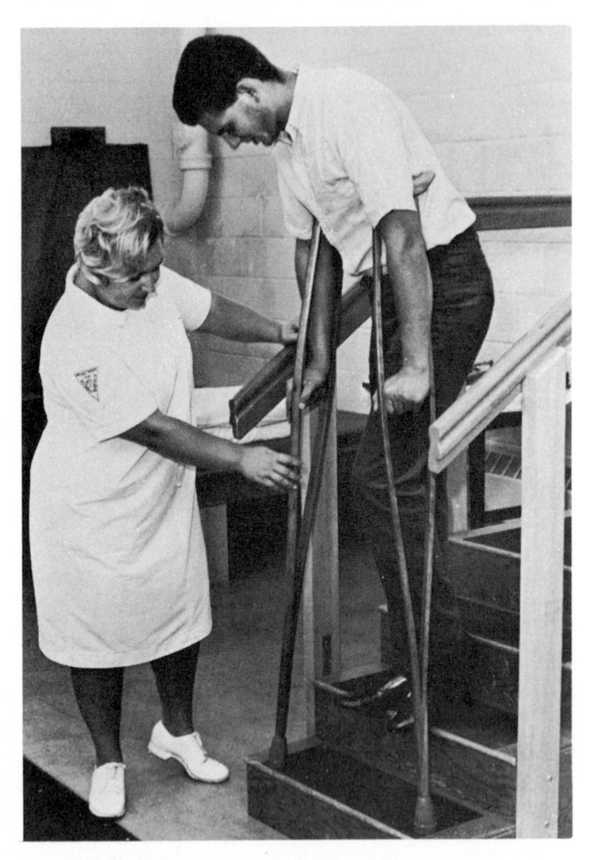

Fig. 20-9. It is important for the nurse to understand which crutch gait the patient is learning from the physical therapist. (Photo, Warren R. Vroom)

Essentially, there are three gaits: 4-point, 3-point and 2-point. There is also a swing-through gait which is used by some patients when they become more accustomed to the crutches and wish to get about quickly and by patients who have had a leg amputated.

Four-Point Gait. Weight-bearing is permitted on both feet, and the pattern is as follows: right crutch, left foot, left crutch, right foot. It is the normal reciprocal walking pattern.

Two-Point Gait. Weight-bearing is permitted on both feet and the pattern is a speed-up of the 4-point gait: right crutch and left foot forward at the same time, left crutch and right foot forward at the same time.

Three-Point Gait. Weight-bearing is permitted on only one foot. The other leg cannot support, but it acts as a balance in the process. It is used also when partial weight-bearing is allowed on the affected extremity. The pattern is as follows: both crutches and the non-supportive leg go forward, and then the good leg comes through. The crutches are brought forward immediately, and the pattern is repeated.

Exercises Preparatory to Crutch-Walking. Before the patient is asked to use the crutches, several exercise drills will help him to be more confident and skillful. The patient must begin by strengthening the arm and the shoulder muscles. The sit-up exercise described earlier is most helpful. The muscles of the hand must also be strengthened. Squeezing a rubber ball 50 times a day by flexing and extending the fingers helps to do this.

The patient should be assisted into a chair which is close to the wall. Then he should be helped to stand against the wall and the crutches placed in his hands. Next, standing slightly away from the wall, he should sway on the crutches from side to side. This accustoms the hands and the arms to weight-bearing.

After this, he should be asked to lean against the wall and pick one crutch up about six inches from the floor and then place it down. This should be repeated with the other crutch and the whole exercise done six to eight times. Then, still leaning against the wall, he should be asked to pick up both crutches from the floor and place them down. This too should be repeated several times.

After these exercises, it will be possible to judge the patient's ability to hold and manage the crutches without the added concern for movement. If the patient is judged capable of proceeding into the practice of a gait, if possible begin with the 4-point gait.

Patients using crutches with the axillary support should be cautioned about exerting pressure against the axillae. When patients first begin to use crutches, they should be taught that the support should come primarily from the arms and the hands. The crutches should not be forced into the axillae each time the body is moved forward.

There are crutches available which have no axillary support. A supportive frame extends beyond the hand grip for the lower arm to help guide the crutch. Such crutches are more likely to be used by patients who have permanent limitations and will always need crutch assistance for ambulation.

PROVIDING PROTECTIVE MEASURES FOR THE PATIENT CONFINED TO BED

Introduction

One of the greatest challenges in nursing is the care of the patient confined to bed. This is particularly so if the person's illness renders him immobile. He is truly dependent upon others to do for him what he cannot do for himself and to help keep him in the best possible physiologic and psychologic state. A review of the first part of this chapter would be helpful, because it is essential that the nursing personnel caring for helpless patients be aware of and use principles of body mechanics to protect themselves as well. One person can manage a helpless patient safely and easily if knowledge of body mechanics principles is applied.

General Principles Guiding the Nursing Care of the Bedfast Patient

The body requires alternate periods of rest and activity. Going to bed for the purpose of resting, as for sleep, is truly therapeutic. However, prolonged periods of confinement to bed, whether prescribed or induced by a state of illness, can bring about undesirable results. Close observation of the patient, careful planning for activity within the patient's scope of endurance, and the use of protective measures become an essential part of the patient's nursing care.

The body strives constantly to function coordinately. Optimal functioning of the body, psychologically and physiologically, depends upon all systems being "go." When certain systems are not functioning well, others will be affected. Therefore, when locomotion and movement of the body cease, or are reduced to a minimum, there is urgent need to prevent disruption of other functions.

The Danger of Bed Rest. As was mentioned in the previous part of this chapter, keeping the patient as active as his physical condition allows is now a goal in the treatment of any patient. Obviously, being able to walk about is of great psychological value. Therefore, when a person must be confined to bed it can be expected that this will strongly affect his behavior.

The physiologic damage that can result from prolonged bed rest is not confined to damage of the musculoskeletal systems, such as muscular weakness, difficulty in walking, foot drop or contractures that limit joint movement. The effects can be far more damaging than the illness the patient had at the onset. For example, circulatory stasis can cause the formation of thrombi (blood clots), or there can be a dilation of blood vessels in the abdomen; respiration can be affected and inadequate exchange of gases will result; lymphatic disturbances can cause edema (swelling due to the accumulation of fluid in the tissues); impaired digestion; constipation; breakdown of tissues, such as bed sores; even chemical imbalance resulting in brittleness of bones. These are but a few of the complications that must be prevented in the bedfast, inactive patient.

However, many patients who have not been in bed long have come to the hour of their discharge only to find that nursing personnel or a family member had to dress them. They could not button a shirt, tie a shoelace, or reach back and hook a brassiere. These limitations in activities of daily living cause distress to the patient. It is true that many of these limitations are temporary and that the patient will regain his previous abilities. However, in most instances, patients need not reach the point where such activities cause discomfort and concern for even a short period of time.

If the frequent opportunities for observation are used well, the nurse can be a key person in helping to recognize beginning limitations, which can be acted on immediately or prevented from developing further. To help determine to what extent the patient will be self-sufficient, nurses need to encourage the patient to engage in routine activities of daily living, referred to as A.D.L. The extent to which any individual can perform day-to-day actions is an indication of his capacities. These include walking and nonwalking activities, such as being able to sit up alone in bed, roll over from side to side while in bed, or climb a flight of stairs. Also included are such routines as being able to brush the teeth, comb the hair, cut meat into small pieces, lift a cupful of liquid, button a collar button and tie shoelaces. Experts in physical medicine are able to measure scientifically a patient's capacities to meet at least 150 physical demands.

Physicians' orders for bed rest can have many different interpretations. In some agencies there are descriptions of what is meant by different types of bed rest: e.g., absolute rest, including being fed; bed rest, but may feed and bathe self; bed rest, with bathroom privileges only. An exact understanding of the patient's activity regimen is needed to plan his nursing care.

Devices for the Safety and the Comfort of the Patient Confined to Bed

Resting in bed usually is very comfortable if the body is held or supported in a restful position. Merely being in a horizontal position does not ensure rest. It is as important to be in good alignment and posture when lying down as it is when standing or sitting. To sit with the knees crossed may be comfortable for a short while, but it soon becomes uncomfortable and fatiguing. Having the knees crossed while sitting is not too

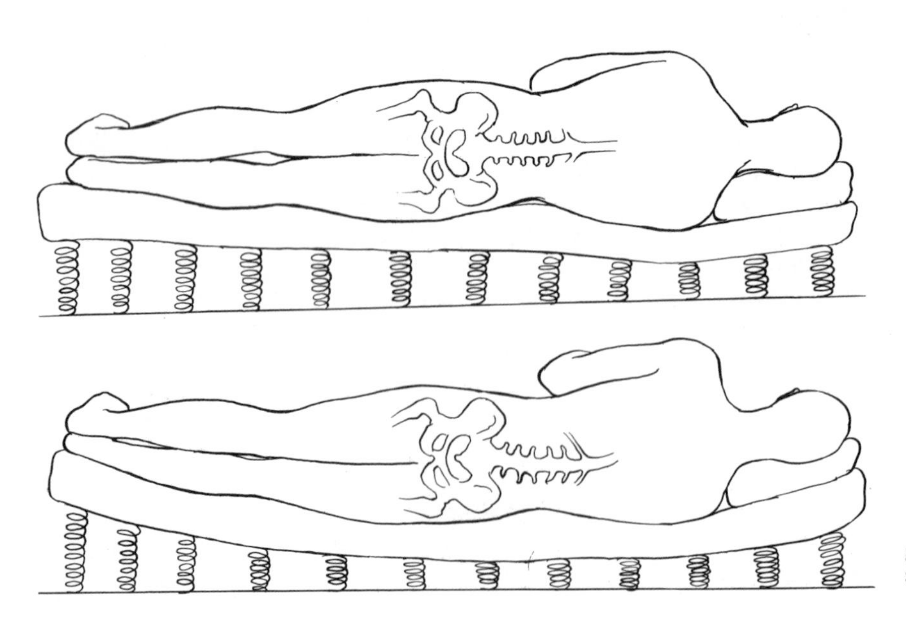

Fig. 20-10. The effects of a good and a poor mattress and spring on body alignment.

different from having one leg adducted and rotated inwardly while lying on the side. It is only when the body is supported properly and the position changed frequently enough to rest certain muscle groups and utilize others that rest in bed can serve its best purpose.

There are many devices which help to maintain good body alignment and muscle tonus in bed and to alleviate discomfort or pressure on various parts of the body.

Pillows are used primarily to help keep a patient comfortable. They are used also to keep the patient in position, to provide support and to elevate the head or the extremities. Variety in sizes of pillows increases their usefulness. Home and hospital pillows are usually the full- or large-size pillow. Small pillows are ideal for some areas of support or elevation.

Mattress. For a mattress to be comfortable and supportive, it must be firm but have sufficient "give" to permit good body alignment. Figure 20-10 shows the effect of a supportive and a nonsupportive mattress on body alignment. If a patient were to remain in a bed such as is depicted at the bottom of the illustration, he might very well complain of backache and other discomforts.

A well-made and well-supported foam-rubber mattress retains a uniform firmness and therefore helps to protect the patient. These mattresses are made of natural or synthetic rubber, or both in combination. A large volume of air is incorporated. The foam-rubber mattress conforms to the contours of the body and supplies support at all points. Its greatest advantage is that it does not form slopes and valleys as the inner-spring mattresses are likely to do. Nor does the foam rubber mattress create as much pressure against bony prominences, such as the ankles, the elbows, the scapulae and the coccyx.

Bed Board. If the mattress does not provide sufficient support, a bed board may help to keep the patient in better alignment. Bed boards usually are made of plywood. The size varies with the needs of the situation. If sections of the bed can be raised, such as the head and the foot of a hospital bed, it may be necessary to have the board divided and held together with hinges. For home use, a full bed board may not be obtainable. If a smaller board is used temporarily, it should be cut so that it extends the entire width of the mattress. However, every effort should be made to obtain a full-length board.

Alternating Pressure Mattress Pad. While mattresses should be firm to help maintain good alignment of the body, their firmness also may be cause for concern. Constant pressure on any one body area is the forerunner of a decubitus. A number of devices, such as the alternating pressure mattress pad, have been designed to help to reduce this constant pressure. The principle on which they operate is that sections of the pad distend with air or fluid while other sections remain flat. Then those that remained flat distend, and the other sections deflate. In this way, no one area of the body is receiving constant pressure. These pads are placed over the regular bed mattress. Caution is necessary with such a pad because puncture by sharp instruments and pins can cause a leak of the fluid or the air.

The alternating pressure pad is not disturbing to the patient. The fact that it does produce occasional tickling sensations which cause muscular contractions is considered to be beneficial. For the most part, however, patients become adjusted to them and do not seem to realize that they are on the pad.

High-Low Tilt Bed. Another useful device is the bed adjustable as to height and angle. The value of having an adjustable-height bed has been discussed earlier. These beds also permit the angle to be changed so that the head is higher than the feet, or vice versa. Such beds are extremely helpful for patients forced to lie flat. They have several advantages, one of which is the fact that when the head is up the patient is able to see about him without extreme flexion of the neck. Also, the patient is assisted to a more nearly vertical position without the effort of standing. The shift in the position of the abdominal organs and the alteration in the circulation in the extremities and other body areas are preparation for the day when weight-bearing and standing will begin.

Rocking Bed. The rocking bed, while used in the care of patients with vascular or respiratory diseases, is also of great value in the care of other immobile patients. This bed is mounted on a frame rather than the usual bedstead. By means of a motor, the bed can be made to rock rhythmically up and down in seesaw fashion. There is a footrest on the bed to help keep the patient from sliding and also to help to keep the feet in good alignment. If the patient is in a moderate sitting position there is little danger of the patient's sliding. The bed is adjusted to rock at the same frequency of the patient's respirations. The rocking aids respiration by shifting the abdominal viscera, which in turn helps to move the diaphragm upward and downward, helping air to be drawn into and forced out of the lungs.

Also, the constant alteration of position aids the flow of blood. The same principle (pull of gravity) is in operation when the tilt bed is used. In some vascular diseases, it is helpful if venous circulation is assisted during the time the patient must be confined to bed.

Other patients, because of their inactive state, also need some measure to assist or improve circulation. It will be recalled that venous blood is assisted in its return to the heart by the contraction of muscle groups in the legs. Pressure against the veins helps to move the blood along its course. If activity is at a minimum, elevation of the extremities is helpful in that the position aids the blood in its return flow.

Chair Bed. Another type of bed used in the care of patients requiring bed rest is one that can be made into a chair position. These beds were designed primarily for the patient who has a heart ailment. In some instances, they are referred to as the cardiac bed.

The popularity of the chair bed is not assured. It is cumbersome, and nowadays it is not uncommon for patients with impaired heart function to have bathroom or commode privileges.

Rubber Air Rings, Cushion Rings and Doughnuts. Inflated rubber rings, cushion rings and handmade doughnuts for relieving pressure on bony prominences by lifting them from the mattress surface, have been quite popular. Their disadvantage lies in the fact that, in protecting one area, they create pressure in immediately surrounding areas. This pressure, in turn, impairs circulation to the area of most concern and thus reduces the supply of oxygen and nutrients.

There are more effective means of relieving pressure on bony prominences and protecting the patient from developing pressure sores. A piece of sponge rubber large enough to be supportive placed adjacent to the pressure point so that it fills the space and thus reduces some of the pressure is effective. Small pillows, if available, are also helpful in elevating an area such as the heels, so that the pressure is reduced. Pieces of synthetic sheepskin are useful and protective.

Rubber air rings have some value for patients who are having sitz baths following rectal and perineal surgery. In such instances, they provide comfort for the brief period when the patient must sit in the tub. They are not recommended as a device for the prevention of a bedsore on a patient's coccygeal area.

Foot Boards. A board placed at the foot of the mattress and perpendicular to it is often used to help to keep the top bed covers from pressing on the feet. Foot boards are usually made so that they can be wedged between the mattress and the bedframe or so that an extension slides under the mattress. The board should be of sufficient height to hold the bedclothes above the toes when the feet are held in the walking position (dorsal flexion). If the board is too high, it may prevent the top linen from resting on the patient's thighs and legs, thus causing a feeling of chilliness. A foot board may be used to help to keep the feet in dorsal flexion if a firm support is used to build up the area from the board to the patient's feet. However, a more suitable method for supporting the feet is to use a foot block.

Foot Blocks. A foot block is a firm object placed on the mattress at the foot of the bed so that the patient's feet can rest against it in the correct position, dorsal flexion. A foot block can be made from a box or a carton. The block is covered with a pillow case or some other suitable piece of linen before being placed against the feet.

Like other devices, foot blocks cannot meet the needs of all patients equally well. They must be adjusted to the patient. If the patient is short, a foot block may need to be of considerable size in order to reach the patient's feet. If the patient is tall, a small foot block is necessary. If a foot block is not readily available or if it is not suitable for the patient, an improvised foot support can be made from a pillow and a large sheet. The pillow is rolled in the sheet, and the ends of the sheet are twisted before being tucked under the mattress. The ends should be tucked under the mattress at an angle toward the head of the bed to help to keep the pillow in place. A pillow foot support does not provide the firmness of a carton, a box or the foot block, nor does it assist in stimulating proprioceptor senses, muscle contractions and circulation; but it will suffice for a few hours until a better support can be obtained.

If the patient is in a sitting position while in bed, the foot block must be placed at an angle. This is to prevent hyperextension of the knees which would result if the feet were kept in dorsiflexion while the trunk was flexed forward.

Cradle. If pressure of the top bedding is a problem, or if the top bedding must be kept off the patient's lower extremities, a device called a cradle is used. There are any number of sizes and shapes of cradles. If used, the cradle should be fastened securely to the bed so that it does not slide or fall on the patient.

Sandbags. Some patients must have an area of the body held in position by a firm supportive device. For example, the patient may have a tendency to rotate his leg outward. In order to prevent his lying in this position for extended periods of time, the leg can be held in good alignment by placing sandbags alongside the outer surface of the leg from the hip to the knee. Sandbags have numerous uses and their value is enhanced if they are available in various sizes. When properly filled, they are not hard or firmly packed. They should be pliable enough to be shaped to body contours and to give support. They should not create pressure on a bony prominence.

Trochanter Rolls. If sandbags are not available to help prevent a patient's legs from rotating outward, it is possible to improvise a support that will serve the same purpose. Fold a sheet lengthwise and place the narrow dimension under the patient so that it extends from the patient's waist to his knees. A large, bulky piece of linen should not be used because of the discomfort it will cause to the patient's back. Under each end of the sheet, which extends on either side of the patient, place a rolled bath blanket or two bath towels. Roll the sheet around the blanket so that the roll is under. In this way, it cannot unroll itself, and the weight of the patient helps to hold it secure. When the trochanter roll is in place properly, the patient will be lying on a piece of linen which has a large roll on either side of it. Fix these rolls close to the patient and tight against the hip and the thigh so that the femur does not rotate outwardly. If the roll is not sufficiently long, very little support can be expected.

Hand Rolls. If patients are paralyzed or unconscious, it may be necessary to provide a means for keeping the thumb in the correct position; namely, slightly adducted and in apposition to the fingers. To do this for short periods of time, any number of improvisations can be made. For example, a rubber ball of the appropriate size or sponge rubber may be used. However, if the hands are going to need protective support for many days or weeks, consideration should be given to the preparation of a plastic or aluminum splint which can be made by the department of occupational or physical therapy. In this way, the thumb is held in place no matter what position the hand is in. Patients who are not moving their fingers should be encouraged to do finger exercises with special attention to having the thumb touch the tips of each finger.

Bed Siderails. One of the greatest safety concerns of nursing personnel is to prevent patients from falling out of bed. Hospital accident reports show a high proportion of such events; hence, in many agencies, it is routine to use extra protection on the beds of unconscious and disoriented patients and, on the beds of elderly patients. The terms "bedrails" and "siderails" are used synonymously with the term "bed siderails."

There is no question that the presence of siderails often has an unfortunate psychological effect on rational and oriented patients and on their families. Therefore, the use of them requires explanation beyond passing it off as "routine." The patient should be helped to understand how the siderails offer protection if he is weak, or receiving certain drugs and cannot prevent himself from falling, should he roll to the edge of the bed.

Bed siderails, even if they are the full length of the mattress, may not deter some patients from getting out of bed. Many a patient has gone to the foot of the bed and gotten out that way.

A study done in one hospital showed that out of 614 accidents reported in one year, 283 were falls out of bed. Of these falls, 106 occurred even when siderails were in place. Injuries from falls when siderails are in place usually are far more serious, since the patient drops from a point two or three feet higher than the mattress.

The adjustable-height bed seems to be one answer for certain types of patients, such as, the ambulatory elderly patient. These patients usually go to the bathroom frequently, and if, when they bring their feet over the side of the bed, they are able to place them directly on the floor, they are safer and more stable. If, on the other hand, they must dangle from the height of the usual hospital bed, they may slide off the edge, lose their balance and fall to the floor. Many nurses note that the incidence of falls when the bed is lowered to the usual height of the home bed is practically nil.

While bed siderails are used primarily for the patient's safety, they do have a secondary value for many helpless patients. For example, siderails make it possible for the patient to roll himself from one side to the other or even to sit up without calling for assistance. This in itself is a very good activity measure to help to retain or regain muscle efficiency.

Protective Positions for the Patient Confined to Bed

Unless medical orders specify restriction of activity, bed patients can be prevented from developing physical limitations by changes in position. The protective side-lying, back-lying and face-lying positions are intended to help to maintain good body alignment. To place the patient in any of these positions, it is essential to understand the position of body parts when in good *posture*. Briefly, these can be recalled: for a person in the standing position the feet perpendicular to the legs (dorsal flexion); the knees in a slight degree of flexion (5° to 10°); the patellae facing forward; the hips straight; the arms alongside the body, the forearms slightly adducted toward the body; the hands pronated; the thumbs adducted into the hands; the fingers in the grasp position; the head held erect on the shoulders so that vision is horizontal with the floor.

The Protective Back-Lying (Supine) Position. In the back-lying position, two areas of the body are in need of particular attention. These are the feet and the neck. Of course, if the patient is unable to move at all, then all areas of the body require attention.

The greatest danger to the feet occurs when they are not held in the dorsal flexion position. The toes drop downward, and the feet are in plantar flexion. This position of the feet occurs naturally when the body is at rest. If maintained for extended periods of time, plantar flexion can cause an alteration in the muscles, and the patient may develop a complication referred to as *dropfoot*. In this position, the foot is unable to maintain itself in the perpendicular position, heel-toe gait is impossible, and the patient will experience extreme difficulty in walking. If it is severe enough, the patient will not be able to walk at all. Intensive physical therapy over a long period of time may be required, and, in some instances, surgery has been necessary to help to lengthen the shortened muscle group. The use of a foot support aids in avoiding this complication.

During the time that a patient is in bed, pillows almost always are used to support the head. It will be noted that the patient frequently uses the pillows to tilt the head forward in order to improve his field of vision. This produces flexion of the cervical spine. Often one may see patients who are out of bed continue to walk about with this same flexion of the cervical spine. Since the back-lying position is the one in which the patient often spends the greatest length of time, the thorax, the neck and the head should be supported properly.

If the patient is active in bed and able to move his arms, use his hands and roll from side to side, these activities are protective in themselves and reduce the need for some supporting devices. However, if the patient is unable to move, supportive measures are necessary. A means for keeping the patient in good alignment while on his back follows. The decision as to whether one, more or all measures are necessary is dependent on the condition of the patient, his illness limitations, his activity status and his body build.

The Protective Side-Lying Position. Lying on the side is a welcome relief from prolonged periods of lying on the back. Patients who have difficulty turning themselves from side to side appreciate a frequent change of position, which is also essential for alternate rest and activity of muscle groups. The side-lying position removes pressure from the prominent areas of the back.

While on the side, the feet are usually in a lesser degree of plantar flexion because the toes are not being pulled downward by gravity. The neck is also held in a more erect position. The primary concern for the patient in this position is the degree of inward rotation of the upper thigh and the upper arm. The pull created by both of these extremities can become very fatiguing. If, in addition, the upper arm pulls the shoulder girdle forward and compresses the thorax, respiration is impaired.

THE PROTECTIVE BACK-LYING POSITION

COMPLICATIONS TO BE PREVENTED	SUGGESTED PREVENTIVE MEASURE
Exaggerated curvatures of the spine and flexion of the hips	Provide a firm supportive mattress. Use a bed board if necessary.
Flexion contractures of the neck	Place pillow (s) under the upper shoulder, the neck and the head so that the head and the neck are held in the correct position.
Internal rotation of the shoulders and extension of the elbows (hunch-shoulders)	Place pillows or arm supports under the forearms so that the upper arms are alongside the body and the forearms are pronated slightly.
Extension of the fingers and abduction of the thumbs (clawhand deformities)	Make hand rolls or use small towels for the hands to grasp. If the patient is paralyzed, use thumb guides to hold the thumbs in the adducted position.
External rotation of the femurs	Place sandbags or a trochanter roll alongside the hips and the upper half of the thighs.
Hyperextension of the knees	Place a small soft roll or sponge rubber under the knees, sufficient to fill the popliteal space but not to create pressure and not to exceed 5° of flexion.
Plantar flexion	Use a foot block or make an improvised firm foot support to hold the feet in dorsal flexion.

A suggested means for keeping the patient in good alignment while in the side-lying position follows. Again, the decision as to whether one, several or all measures are necessary depends on the condition of the patient, his illness limitations, his activity status and his body build. (See Figs. 20-11, 20-12, and 20-13.)

A large pillow may have to be placed against the patient's back to help to prevent him from rolling backward.

The Protective Face-Lying (Prone) Position. Lying on the abdomen, face down, can be a valuable and relaxing position. Unfortunately, many patients are unwilling or unable to be placed in this position.

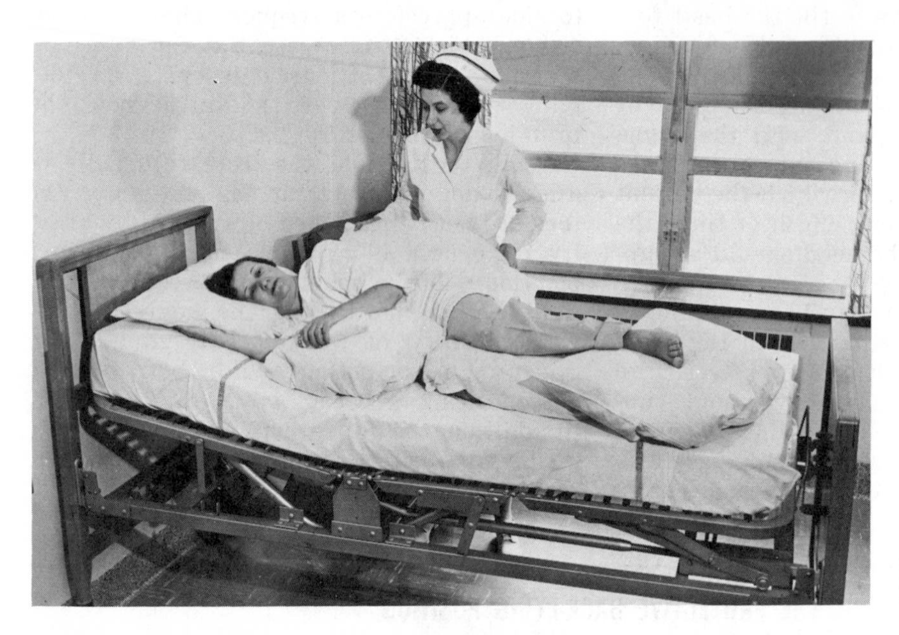

Fig. 20-11. Nurse placing a pillow to keep patient from rolling back.

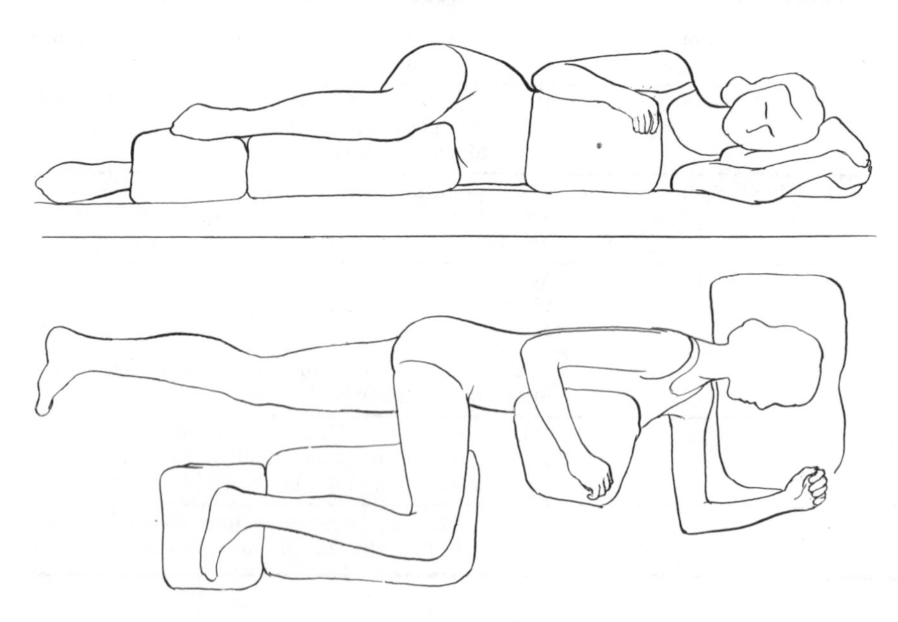

Fig. 20-12. (Top). Diagram illustrating anterior view of patient in protective side-lying position.

Fig. 20-13. (Bottom). Diagram illustrating side view of patient in protective side-lying position.

THE PROTECTIVE SIDE-LYING POSITION

COMPLICATIONS TO BE PREVENTED	SUGGESTED PREVENTIVE MEASURE
Lateral flexion of the neck.	Place a pillow under the head and the neck.
Inward rotation of the arm and interference with respiration	Place a pillow under the upper arm.
Extension of the fingers and abduction of the thumbs	Provide a hand roll for the fingers and the thumbs.
Internal rotation and adduction of the femur	Use 1 or 2 pillows as needed to support the leg from the groin to the foot.

From the standpoint of alignment, the prone position offers the fewest sources of concern. If the patient is comfortable in the position and enjoys it, the feet are the only area of real concern. Unless supported or allowed to go over the end of the mattress, they are forced into plantar flexion, and the legs rotate inward or outward. Because the position is helpful, nurses should encourage patients to assume it on their own if they have complete freedom of activity. If the patient needs assistance, the time of the bath is often a good one for placing the patient in the prone position as when washing the

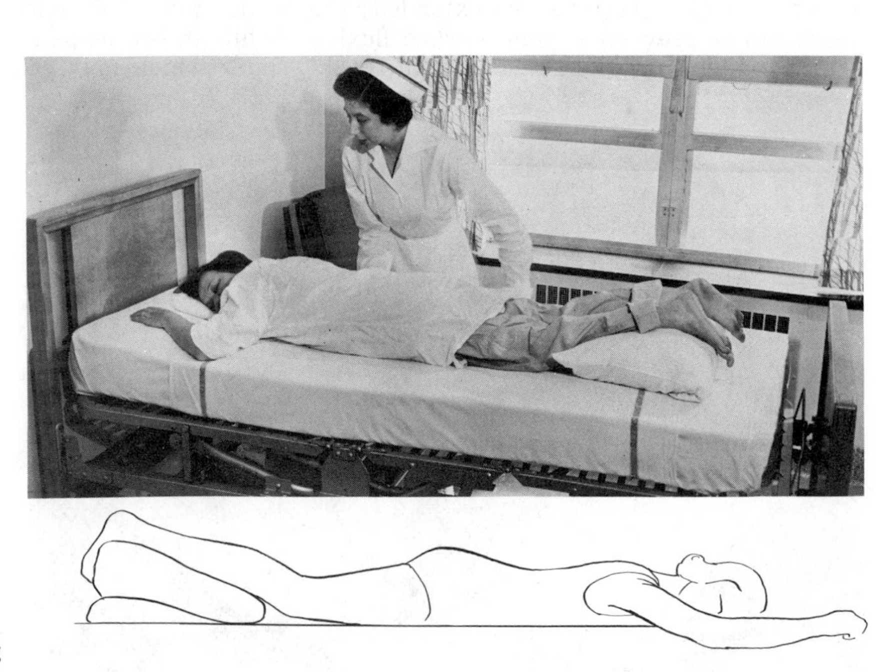

Fig. 20-14. (Top) Nurse placing patient in protective prone position.
Fig. 20-15. (Center). Diagram illustrating correct protective prone position.
Fig. 20-16. (Bottom). Diagram illustrating incorrect prone position.

THE PROTECTIVE FACE-LYING POSITION

COMPLICATIONS TO BE PREVENTED	SUGGESTED PREVENTIVE MEASURE
Plantar flexion	Move the patient down in bed so that his feet are over the mattress; or support his lower legs on a pillow just high enough to keep the toes from touching the bed.
Flexion of the cervical spine	Place a small pillow under the head.
Hyperextension of the spine. Impaired respiration	Place some suitable support under the patient between the end of the rib cage and the upper abdomen if this facilitates breathing and there is space there.

back. In some instances, patients are ordered to be placed prone for specified periods of time each day.

The advantages of the face-lying position are as follows: the shoulders, the head and the neck are placed in the erect position; the arms are held in good alignment with the shoulder girdle; the hips are extended; the knees can be prevented from marked flexion or hyperextension; and the arms can be abducted and flexed. In a sense, it can be said that the body can be "straightened out" when placed in the face-lying position. (See Figs. 20-14, 20-15, and 20-16.)

Protective Exercises and Activities for the Patient Confined to Bed

Keeping the patient in good alignment while in bed helps to prevent unequal muscle pulls which may cause limitations of move-

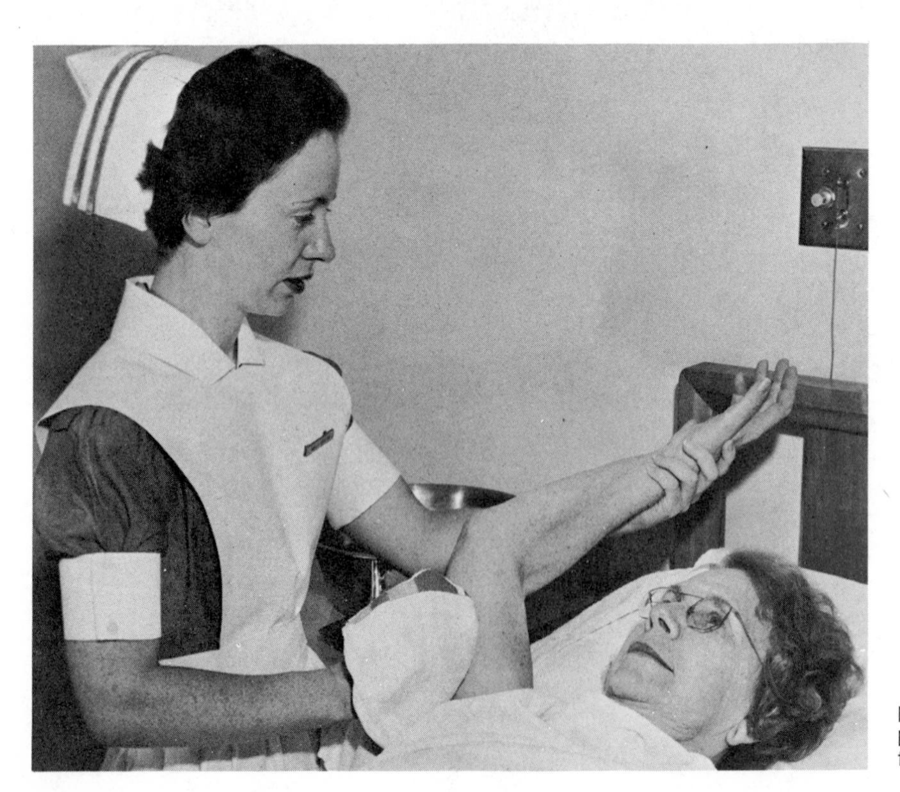

Fig. 20-17. Nurse extending patient's arm during bath as a part of placing shoulder through full range of joint motion.

ment. It is often the only activity possible for some patients, such as those who are paralyzed or unconscious. However, when a patient is permitted some exercise, additional measures should be considered to help keep him in good condition.

As little as several days in bed is sufficient time to produce muscular weakness and difficulty in walking. Therefore, efforts to assist patients to maintain good muscle tone must often begin with the first day of confinement to bed. When this is not possible, carefully planned exercises eventually must be started and increased gradually in frequency and endurance on a day-to-day basis. For some patients, it will require the services of a physical therapist.

The goal of the activities discussed here is to keep the patient in the best possible physical state while bed rest is enforced. This, in turn, should help to prevent physical limitations and to reduce the length of the convalescing period. Where the following exercises are not considered as routine nursing measures, the patient's physician must be consulted first.

Full Range of Joint Motion. The framework of the body is the skeleton. The bones of the skeleton are of various sizes and shapes and are held together by ligaments. These points of approximation are the joints. It is by means of the muscles and the joints that body motion is possible. The type of movement possible at the various joints of the body depends on the shape of the terminal portion of the bones and the number of bones forming the joint. It will be recalled that there are six classifications of movable joints: gliding, saddle, hinge, pivot, ball and socket, and condyloid. Knowing the classification and the structure of a joint is essential to understanding the type of movement it is capable of performing.

As mentioned previously, if muscle groups are altered, as in the formation of a contracture, movement of the joint is altered, and physical limitation occurs. It is essential that the nurse understand the range of motion of the various joints so that preventive measures can be instituted, especially for the patient who is unable to assist in his own care to any great extent. Engaging in routine tasks, such as bathing, eating, dressing and writing, helps to utilize muscle groups which keep many joints in effective range of motion. When all or some of these activities are impossible for various reasons, attention should be given to the joints not being used, either at all or to their fullest extent.

If a patient is incapable of moving himself, it may be necessary for his joints to be placed through full range of motion several times a day. This can be done during the bath or while changing his position. However, the mere procedure of the bath does not ensure that all joints will have been put through range of motion. It is possible to wash the extremities without fully abducting, extending and flexing the joints. Therefore, purposeful planning for full range of joint motion is necessary. (See Fig. 20-18.) For the helpless patient, this activity is necessary several times a day. In the regimen for some patients who have suffered strokes, a physician's order may be written for full range of motion for specific joints, as the shoulders, the hips and the thumbs four times a day. The extent to which such exercise is necessary depends on the patient's illness, physical state, and potential for recovery.

Occasionally, it is necessary to teach a patient to observe a daily routine of range of motion. In such instances, emphasis may be placed on moving the joints in directions least likely to be used by the patient. The following could be included:

While sitting up in bed without support:
- moving the head backward so that the cervical spine is hyperextended
- flexing the trunk laterally from side to side
- rotating the trunk
- flexing the arms up over the head
- extending the arms to the side of the body and then swinging them in circular fashion

While lying face downward on the bed:
- hyperextending the spine by lifting the head and the chest off the bed without the aid of the arms
- hyperextending the arms by lifting them off the bed toward the ceiling

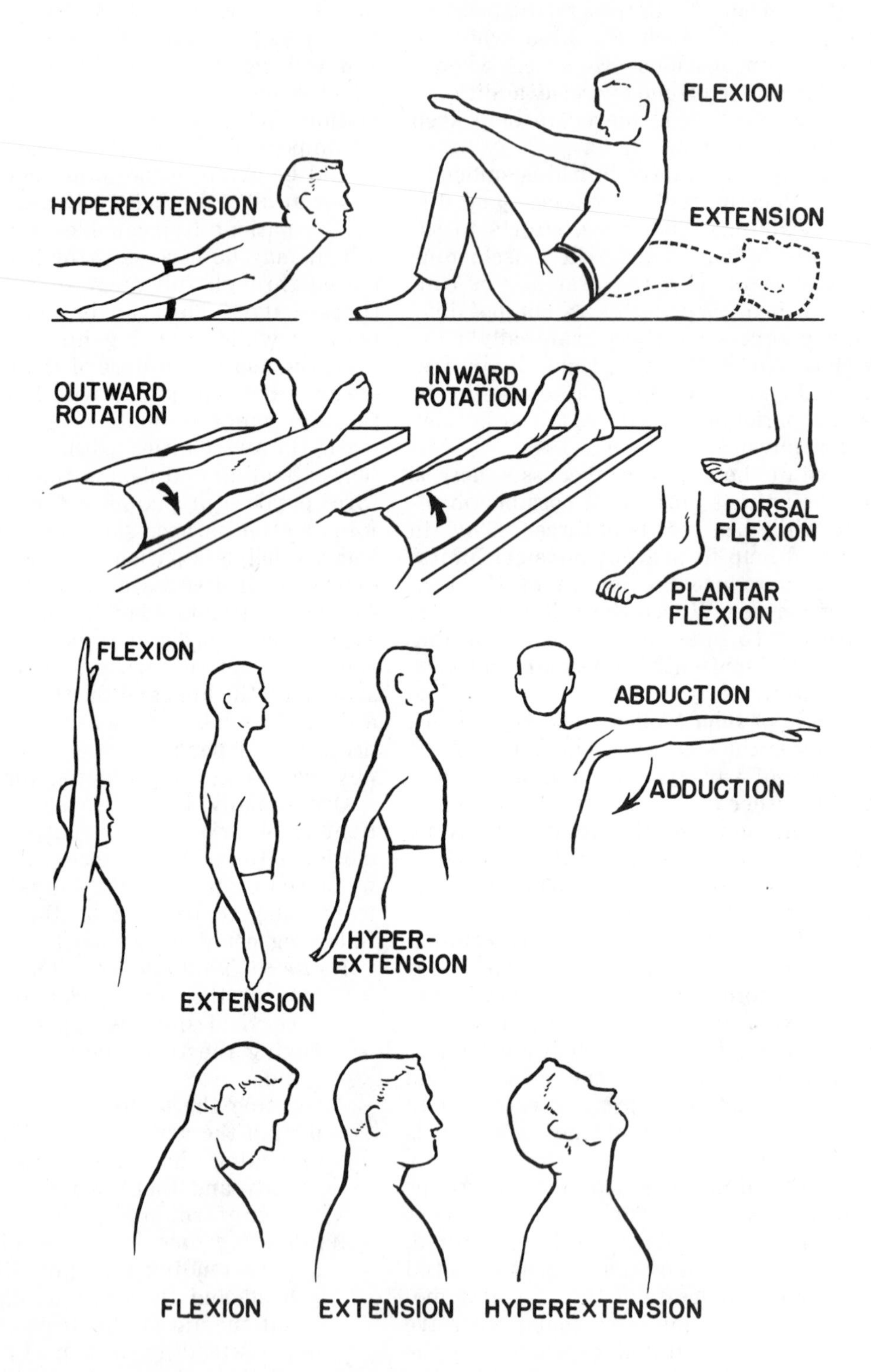

FIG. 20-18. Examples of exercises to help maintain range of motion.

hyperextending the legs by lifting them up off the bed toward the ceiling

While lying on the back:

flexing the knees by drawing the legs up against the thighs

rotating the ankles inward and outward

flexing and extending the toes.

Attention to the thumb is of special importance. If the thumb is abducted permanently so that it cannot be brought into contact with each one of the fingers, the patient will be limited seriously. Without the full use of the thumb, it is difficult to put buttons through a buttonhole, turn a doorknob and hold various everyday devices securely.

The question might be raised as to the danger involved if the nurse were to place patients who had orders for limited activity through range of motion. In defense of this modest but valuable activity, it must be recalled that the effort of using muscle groups to move a joint is much less than the effort expended to raise oneself while in the horizontal position to get on and off a bedpan.

Whenever any of the protective positions, exercises or devices are used to help to prevent physical limitations or to restore functions, a comment should be entered on the nursing care plan. It should explain what, how and when so that all who care for the patient observe the same routine.

Means by which to Move, Lift or Carry a Helpless Patient

Frequently, it is necessary to move a helpless patient either in the bed or from the bed to a stretcher or a chair, or vice versa. In addition to keeping him in good alignment while being moved, it is necessary that he be protected from injury. Such protection involves understanding how to support muscles and joints which the patient cannot control voluntarily.

When moving a patient, care should be taken to avoid grabbing and holding an extremity by a muscle group. The caution, "avoid grabbing the muscle bellies," is quoted frequently. An extremity should be held at the location of the insertion of the muscle tendons.

When a patient is to be moved or lifted, his comfort and safety and that of the persons involved should be considered as being equally important. First of all, those who lift patients must be realistic about the effort involved. Two small-statured, 100-pound women must realize immediately that they are physically incapable of lifting a 250-pound patient. He may be pushed, pulled or slid in bed, but lifting him from one area to another is another matter. Labor laws in some states specify that the maximum a woman can be expected to lift is 35 to 40 pounds. This may act as a guide in some situations, but it is not a specific guide; in certain situations and under some circumstances a woman can safely lift considerably more weight.

By using good body mechanics and the principles of mechanical laws, moving and lifting helpless patients can be made relatively easy. It is essential that the nurse understand such procedures so that she is not entirely dependent on assistance from others. Waiting for assistance which may not be necessary often means that patients cannot be moved as often as or when they would like to be. This is also true of helpless patients in home situations. If the family is taught how to move the patient easily, home care is accepted more readily.

Using Two Persons To Move a Helpless Patient Up in Bed. Children and light-weight adults are relatively easy to slide toward the head of the bed without the assistance of a second person. Average-weight adults of about 140 to 150 pounds begin to pose a problem. Many nurses have devised ways of moving heavy patients up in bed without assistance, but these methods are usually at great risk to the nurse. When moving a heavy, helpless patient up in bed, two persons should be available.

If the patient is able to push with his feet, the procedure is simple and easy. The wheels of the bed are locked first. One nurse stands on one side of the bed and the other nurse on the other side, near the patient's chest and head. Both nurses face the head of the bed. The patient is asked to flex his knees. Each nurse places the arm nearest the patient under the patient's axilla. One nurse assumes responsibility for supporting the patient's head. The other nurse places the pillow up against the head of the bed so that the patient does not hit the bed frame. Both nurses flex their knees, place one foot forward, come down close to the patient and upon a signal given by one of the nurses, the patient pushes with his feet, and the nurses rock forward, thus moving the patient up in bed.

If a patient is unable to assist by pushing with his feet, the nurses will need to hold him so that the heaviest part of his body is moved by them and not by the patient. The wheels of the bed are locked. Then, the patient's knees are flexed and held in position if necessary. The pillow is placed against the head of the bed. The nurses standing at either side of the bed face each other at a point between the patient's waist and hips. Both nurses give themselves a wide base of support, flex their knees and lean close to the patient. They join hands under the widest part of the patient's hips and under his shoulders. At a given signal, both rock toward the head of the bed and slide the patient on the bed. The procedure may need to be repeated if he is heavy and is far down in bed. Care should be taken to avoid injury to the patient's neck and head.

Using a Draw Sheet Pull To Move a Helpless Patient Up in Bed. While the method described previously may be necessary or convenient, the amount of effort expended by the nurses can be reduced. A draw sheet or a large sheet may be placed under the patient so that it extends from his head to below the buttocks. The sides of the sheet are rolled close to the patient so that they may be grasped easily. The wheels of the bed are locked. The patient's knees are flexed. The nurses stand at opposite sides of the bed at a point near the patient's shoulder and chest and face the foot of the bed. They have a wide base of support with the leg nearest the bed behind them and the other leg in front. Holding the sheet securely at a point near the patient's neck and the lumbar region, they first

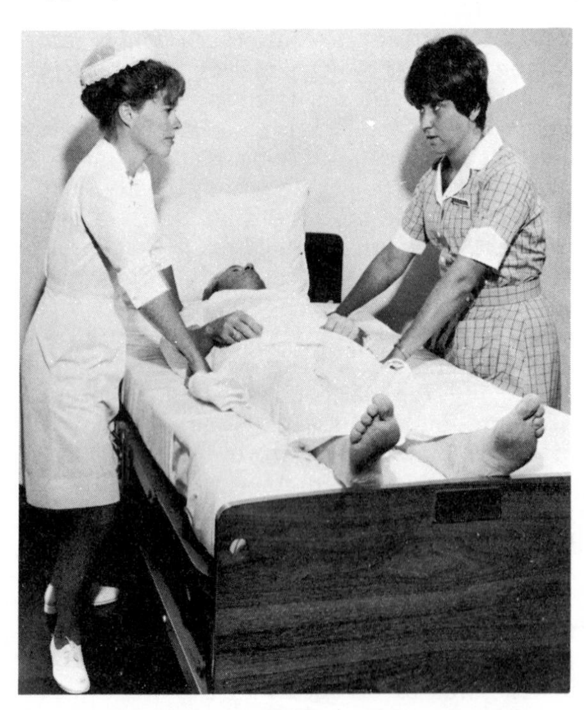

Fig. 20-19. Nurses in position to rock back and slide patient up in bed. Each one has a hand grasping the rolled draw sheet under the patient near his neck in order to support it. When they have a grasp of the sheet close to the patient's body in the hip area, one will give the signal and they will rock back.

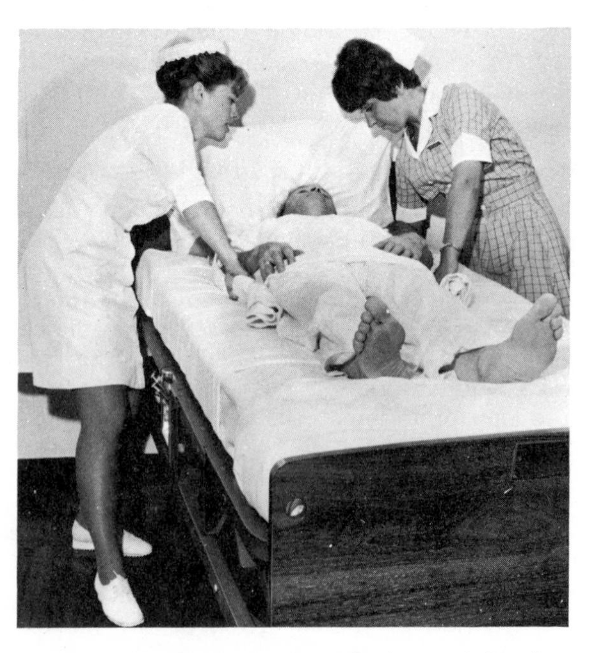

Fig. 20-20. Nurses in position following completion of the draw sheet pull.

lean forward and then rock backward. As they rock backward, the weight of their bodies helps to slide the draw sheet and the patient. At the completion of the rocking motion, each nurse usually has the elbow nearest the patient on the mattress.

The procedure can be done with the nurses facing the head of the bed. It seems easier when the backward rock is used. In the forward rock there seems to be a certain amount of upward pull necessary. Figures 20-19 and 20-20 illustrate the draw sheet pull.

Moving a Patient From the Bed to a Stretcher. Considerable care must be taken, when moving a patient from the bed to a stretcher, or vice versa, to prevent injury to the patient. If he is unconscious or helpless, the extremities and the head must be supported. The most convenient way to move the patient is to use a sheet underneath him and then carefully pull on the sheet to slide the patient from one surface to the other. However, there are instances when patients must be lifted and carried. This can be done by *(Text continued on page 234.)*

THE THREE-MAN LIFT

The purpose is to move a patient from one place to another while maintaining his horizontal position. (From bed to stretcher is used for this procedure.)

SUGGESTED ACTION	RELATED BODY MECHANICS FOR THE NURSE
Place the stretcher at a right angle to the foot of the bed so that it will be in position for the carriers after they pivot away from the bed. Lock the wheels of the bed.	
Arrange the persons lifting the patient according to height, with the tallest person at the patient's head.	The tallest person usually has the longest arm grasp, making it easier for him to support the patient's head and shoulders.
Stand facing the patient and prepare to slide the arms under him. The person in the middle places the arms directly under the patient's buttocks; the person at the head has one arm under the patient's head, neck and shoulder area and the other arm directly against the middle person's arm; the person at the patient's feet has one arm also against the middle person's arm and the other arm under the patient's ankles.	The greatest weight is in the area of the buttocks. Having the middle person's armspread smaller than that of the other two persons helps to prevent strain on this person. Having the arms of the first and the third persons touch the arms of the middle person provides additional support in the heaviest area.
Slide the arms under the patient as far as possible and get in a position to slide the patient to the edge of the bed.	Place one leg forward, the thigh resting against the bed and the knees flexed, and put on the internal girdle.
Lean over the patient and on signal simultaneously rock back and slide the patient to the edge of the bed.	Movement is accomplished by rocking backward and attempting to "sit down"; the weight of the nurses and the power of their arms, hips and knees move the patient.
Place the arms farther underneath the patient. Prepare to "logroll" the patient onto the chests of all three at the same time the patient is being lifted from the bed.	Place one leg forward, flex the knees and put on the internal girdle. "Logrolling" the patient onto the carriers brings the centers of gravity of all objects closer, thereby increasing the stability of the group and reducing strain on the carriers.
Pivot around to the stretcher and, on signal, lower the patient onto the stretcher.	Flex the knees, have one foot forward, and bring your own body down with the patient, thus letting the large leg and arm muscles do the work of lowering the patient.

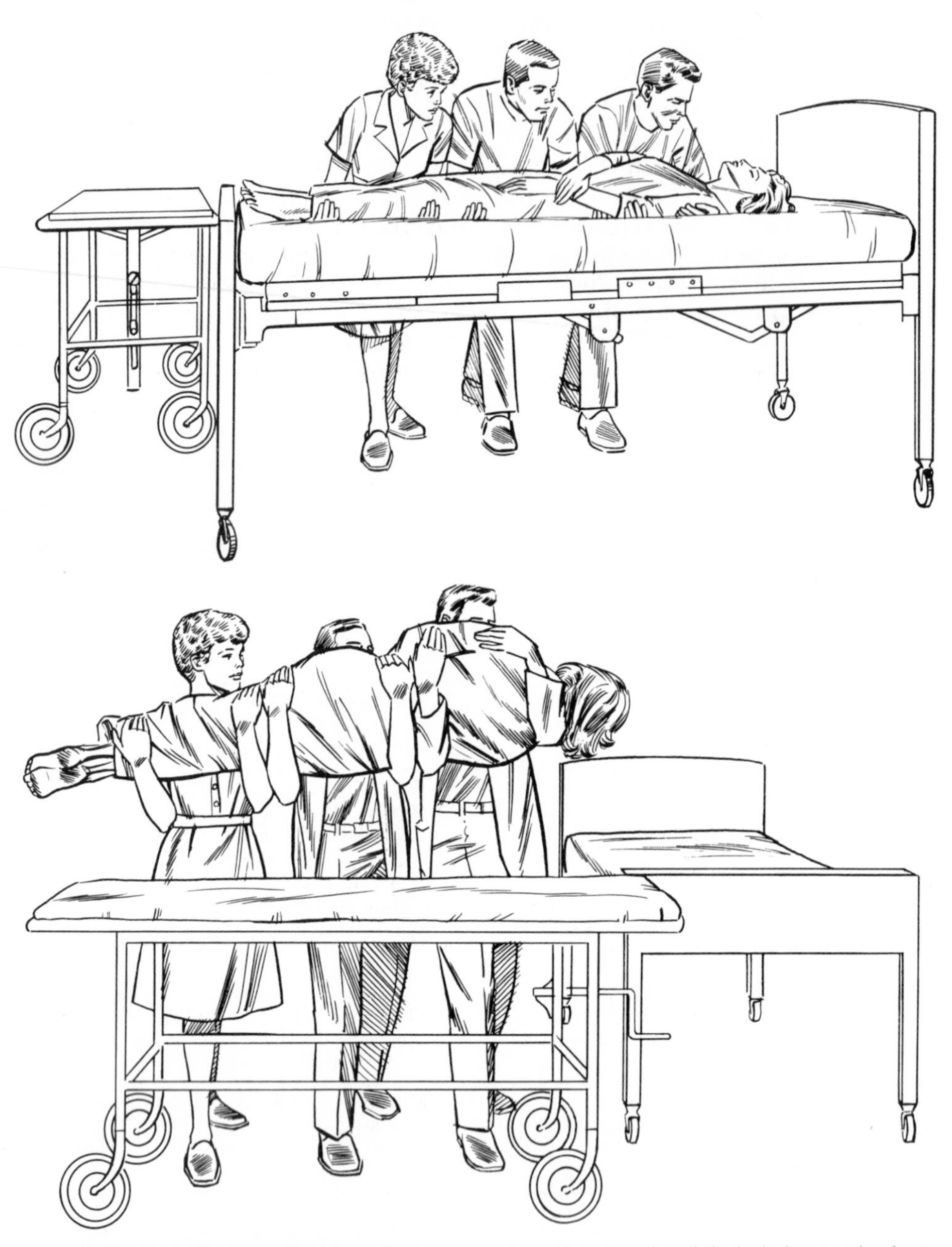

FIG. 20-21. (Top). The 3-man lift. The patient has been brought to the edge of the bed, the stretcher is at a right angle to the foot of the bed and the 3 persons preparing to lift the patient have their arms well under the patient with the greatest support being given to the heaviest part of the patient. Each has a wide base of support and each is leaning over close to the patient in preparation for the lift.

FIG. 20-22. (Bottom). The 3-man lift (Continued). On a given signal, the 3 persons rock back and simultaneously lift the patient and logroll her onto their chests. They then pivot and place the patient on the stretcher. As the patient is being lowered onto the stretcher, all 3 carriers maintain a wide base of support and flex their knees.

SINGLE PERSON MOVING A HELPLESS PATIENT FROM BED TO CHAIR

The purpose is to move a helpless patient out of bed when his weight makes it impossible for the only available person to lift him.

SUGGESTED ACTION	RELATED BODY MECHANICS FOR THE NURSE
Place the chair facing and against the bed at a point near the patient's buttocks to receive the patient and to use as a brace.	
Slide the upper portion of the patient's body to the edge of the bed. (This makes the patient lie diagonally on the bed.)	Place the arms under the patient's head and shoulders. Place one foot forward and rock backward.
Place the arms well under the patient's axillae from the rear. (The patient's head and shoulders will be resting on the nurse.)	Support the upper portion of the patient's body on yourself to reduce the weight of the patient to be moved.
Move around to the back of the chair, pulling the patient into the chair while so doing.	Lean against the back of the chair to keep it from moving and to brace yourself. Rock back and pull the patient into the chair.
Pull the chair away from the bed until the patient's feet are on the edge of the bed, being careful not to pull the chair out from under the patient.	Flex the knees, grasp the chair near the seat and rock back.
Support the patient's legs while lowering the feet to the floor.	Flex the knees while lowering the patient's feet to the floor.

Make certain that the wheels of the bed are locked and that the chair is protected from slipping.

SINGLE PERSON MOVING A HELPLESS PATIENT FROM CHAIR TO HOSPITAL BED

The purpose is to move a helpless patient from a chair into a hospital bed when his weight makes it impossible for the only available person to lift him.

SUGGESTED ACTION	RELATED BODY MECHANICS FOR THE NURSE
Bring the chair to the side of the bed so that the patient is facing the center of the bed, if the bed is higher than the chair.	Slide the chair to the bed. It requires less energy than lifting it one side at a time.
Stand to one side of the chair and behind the patient. Place the arms well under the patient's axillae and bring the patient close to yourself.	This position makes it possible for the nurse to use the long, strong muscles of the arms and the shoulders.
Place the foot that is near the chair back and the other foot forward. Come close to the patient and, using a strong upward rocking motion, quickly lift the patient's trunk out of the chair and onto the bed. (The entire trunk and buttocks must be on the bed.)	This is the crucial step, and its success depends on the nurse's using her strong leg and arm muscles during the upward rocking movement. The higher the bed, the more difficult it is to get the patient on the bed.
Support the patient against the bed, if necessary, while sliding the chair away with the foot.	Rest against the patient's thighs to help to hold him on the bed.
Lift the patient's legs up onto the bed and place the patient in position.	Roll and slide the patient, while placing him in position, to conserve energy.

means of a three-man lift. If it is done properly, the patient will feel secure, and those lifting will not suffer strain.

When returning the patient to the bed from the stretcher, the same principles are observed. However, the carriers should lower the patient close to the edge of the bed first. Then, one member of the team supports the patient on the edge of the bed to prevent his falling off while the other two members of the team go around to the opposite side of the bed and place their arms underneath the patient in preparation for sliding him to the center of the bed. Once the two persons on the opposite side of the bed have a good grip on the patient, the third person is able to join them and assist in sliding the patient to the center of the bed. Sliding the patient requires much less effort than attempting to place him directly in the center of the bed. If this is attempted, the group usually is unable to hold the patient, and he is dropped onto the bed.

The three-man lift is used in various other situations, such as lifting a patient who has fallen to the floor and is unable to get up by himself, or lifting a patient out of a chair into the bed. Once the principles of such a lift are mastered, it becomes relatively easy to analyze situations in which it may be used.

For patients who present special problems because of their excessive weight or a cast,

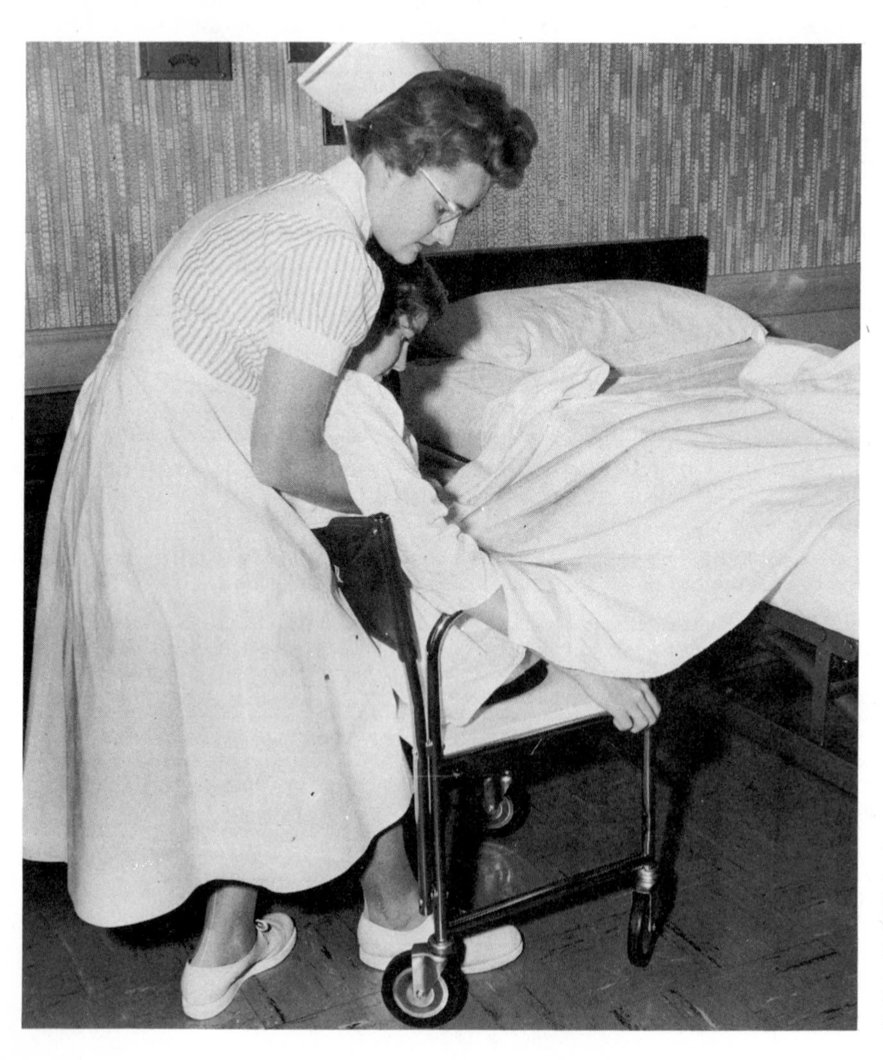

FIG. 20-23. Sliding a patient who cannot stand onto the chair commode is relatively easy if proper body mechanics are used by the nurse. (See suggested procedure.) For the patient it is a real treat to be able to be out of bed, physiologically and psychologically.

MOVING A HELPLESS PATIENT FROM CHAIR TO BED AT HOME (Bed and Chair Level About Equal)

The purpose is to move a helpless patient from a chair into a bed at home when his weight makes it impossible for the only available person to lift him.

SUGGESTED ACTION	RELATED BODY MECHANICS FOR THE NURSE
Bring the chair directly alongside the bed with the patient facing the foot of the bed. Place a pillow on the arm of the chair.	Slide the chair rather than lifting one side at a time. If the floor has a polished surface, slide the chair on a small rug or rags.
Lift the patient's legs onto the edge of the bed.	Flex the knees and lower the body and support both the patient's legs when coming to an erect position.
Go behind the chair, grasp the patient under the axillae from the rear and roll him onto the bed.	Face the back of the chair and the bed at an angle. Have a wide base of support and rock to move the patient onto the bed.
Move the chair and help the patient into the desired position.	Slide the chair with the foot and brace yourself against the bed to prevent the patient from falling off.

the three-man lift may not be sufficient. It may be necessary to have an additional person who is used to help support the heaviest or most cumbersome part of the patient. The persons distribute their arms while carrying so that the heaviest part is well supported.

Moving a Helpless Patient From Bed to Chair. There are occasions when a patient is permitted to be out of bed but loss of various body functions makes it impossible for him to assist in the process. If the patient is able to help by using his arms for support, the problem is reduced considerably. However, some patients cannot use their arms, and nurses must be prepared to face this problem. In the hospital several persons usually are available to lift the patient from the bed to the chair. To a great extent the procedure is dependent on the size and the weight of the patient and the style of chair that the patient is to use. Chairs complicate the procedure because the backrest and the arms get in the way of the persons lowering the patient.

It is possible for only one person to get a helpless patient into a chair, though two peo-

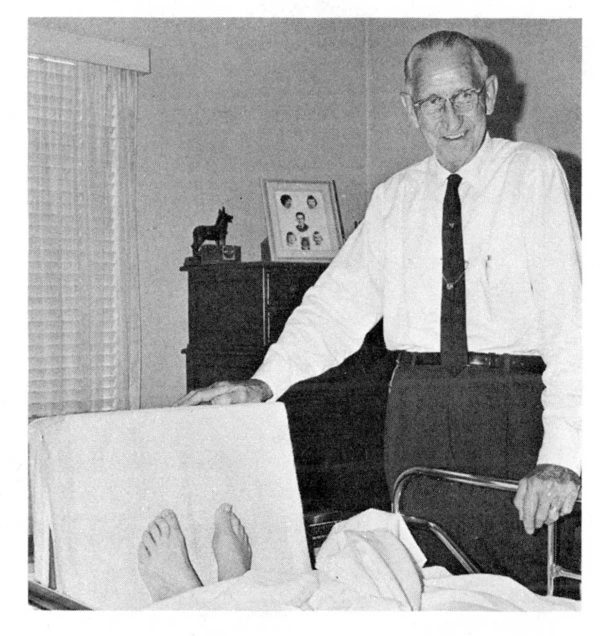

Fig. 20-24. This man prepared a foot board for his wife and is obviously very pleased with the results, since they met with the approval of the visiting nurse. (Courtesy Good Samaritan Hospital, Phoenix, Arizona)

ple simplify matters. The single-person technic is a valuable procedure for nurses to know for the home care of invalids. Often, only one family member is available to assist the patient out of bed and to return him to it. It is easier if the level of the bed is fairly close to the chair seat. It may be helpful in the hospital to remove the casters from the bed, or to elevate the bed at home. (See Fig. 20-23.)

Self-help Devices for Patients Having Activity Limitations

While it is recognized that abilities totally lost cannot be re-created those abilities which remain should be developed to their fullest capacities. Patients who have lost the full use of a muscle group can be helped to learn new ways in which to continue their activities of daily living when they are no longer confined to bed. Of considerable help to such patients are the numerous self-help devices which are being designed and manufactured. Some of these items are so helpful that they are made available through mail order houses and department stores. Persons who never had to participate in a planned rehabilitation program but have had gradual loss of muscle power through advancing age or repeated minor illnesses find such items of real value.

Examples of self-help items used in personal care include elastic shoe laces which eliminate the need for tying laces, long-handled shoehorns which eliminate the need for bending down to put on shoes, handbrushes and toothbrushes which need not be grasped, and a nail clipper which can be worked by a foot pedal.

For the handicapped homemaker there are numerous items which facilitate activities associated with cooking and cleaning, such as a one-handed eggbeater, a safety cutting board which holds food in place while it is

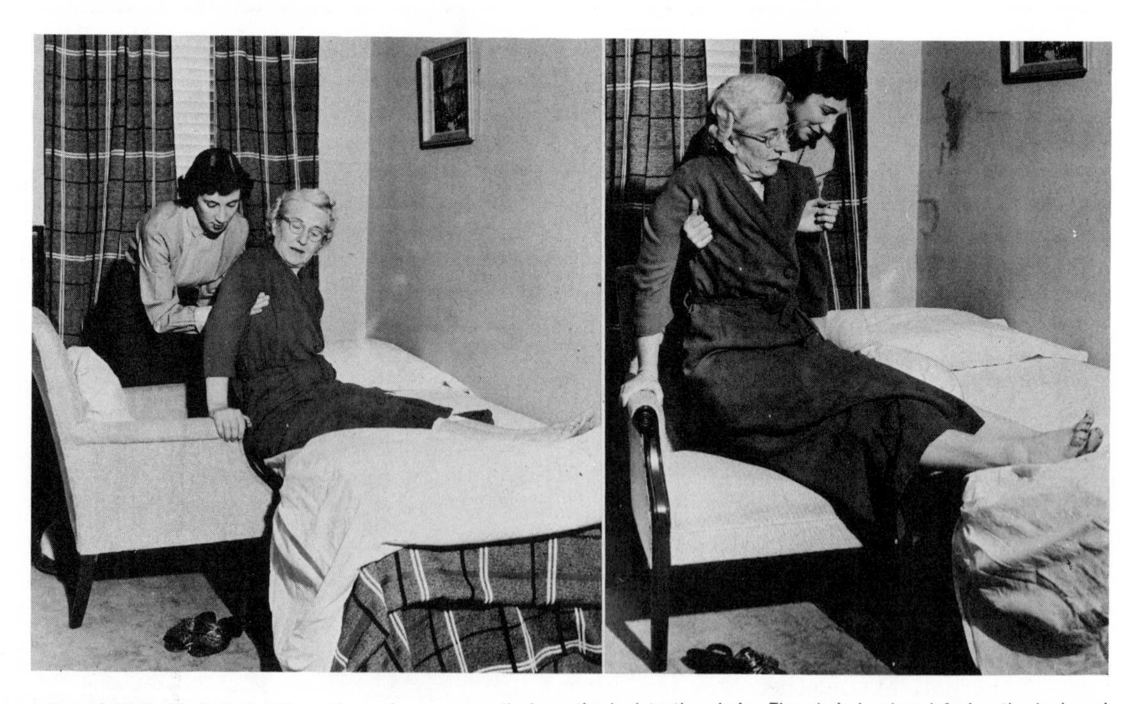

Fig. 20-25. (Left). Assisting the patient who cannot walk, from the bed to the chair. The chair is placed facing the bed, and the patient is assisted to the edge of the bed so that she is able to support herself on the arms of the chair. With assistance from a family member, she is guided and supported as she slides into the chair.

Fig. 20-26. (Right). Assisting the patient who cannot walk, from the chair to the bed. The chair is placed next to the bed. A pillow is wedged alongside the arm of the chair nearest the bed, and the patient's feet are bought up on the bed. The family member then assists the patient to lift up in the chair and guides and supports her onto the arm of the chair and the pillow before completing the move into bed.

being pared or cut, a long-handled dustpan, a one-handed food chopper, an automatic pressure saucepan, mixing bowls with a suction base, and an interchangeable grater, slicer and shredder held securely on a frame. Many of these items are of value to anyone. They reduce the amount of energy expended and therefore lessen fatigue.

Study Situations

1. What are some of the activities of daily living that would be seriously affected if you did not have full use of your thumb? As starters, try opening a door knob, writing, or buttoning a blouse.

2. The following article discusses a form developed to evaluate a patient's condition and progress in several areas: mental attitude, mobility, physical independence and skin condition. For each area of observation note the gradations possible. Consider how such a form would show almost at a glance a patient's progress, or lack of it and thus an indication of care given or needed.

- Simon, J. R.: Systemic ratings of patient welfare.
  NURS. OUTLOOK, *9*:432-436, July, 1961. See also Ballantyne.[1]

3. When turning a patient on the side is not possible, tilting also affords physiologic benefit. In the following article a device for tilting the bed to a 12° angle on either side is described and illustrated:

- Larson, E. R.: Turning the bed patient.
  AMER. J. NURS., *63*:100, February, 1963.

4. Some families have a member who is physically incapacitated and requires hours of care a day. Often such families are will-

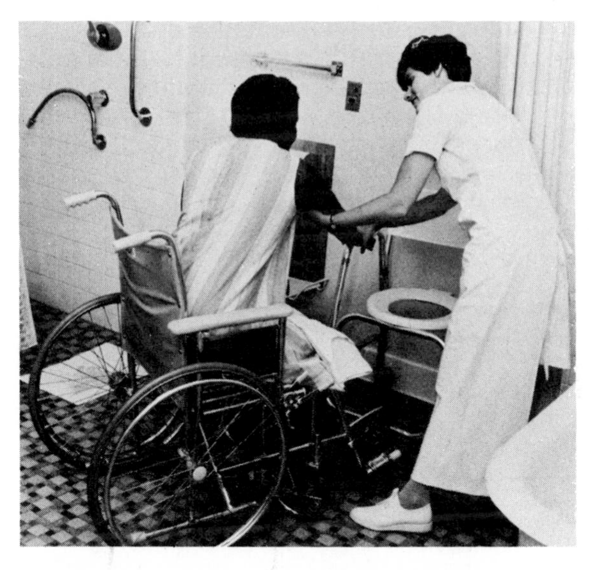

FIG. 20-27. Many hospitals now have continuing care (or interim care) units. Here patients who are not acutely ill but not able to be self-sufficient at home can learn to take care of themselves. In this training unit this patient is receiving some assistance from the nurse. She will be helped onto the shower chair which is secured against the wall. After she is undressed she can be wheeled into the shower which has a low water spigot so that her head does not become wet. There is a disposable mat at the doorway to the shower, and the nurse wears a long plastic apron to protect her uniform and legs. (Photo Warren R. Vroom)

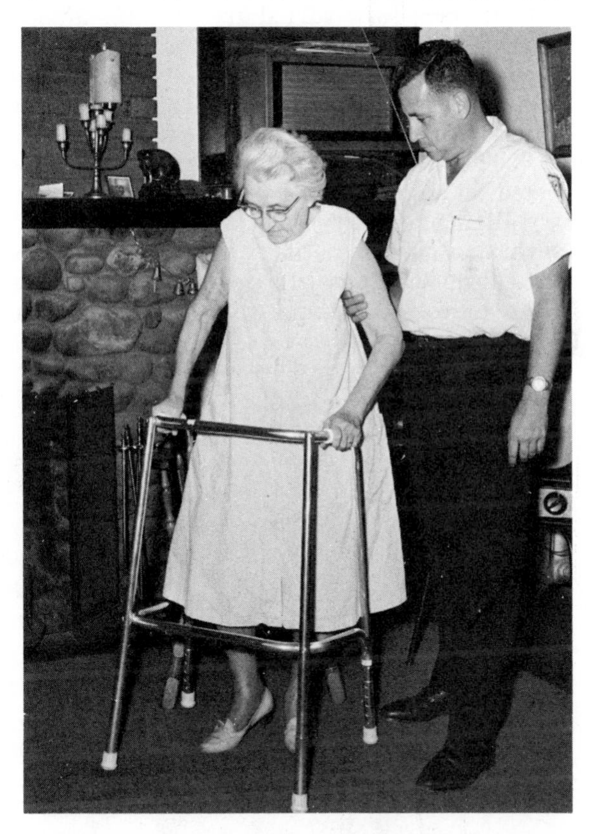

FIG. 20-28. After discharge from the hospital many patients require supervision of other health workers in addition to a visiting nurse. In this instance, the physical therapist is helping the patient in her struggle for more mobility. The nurse will be aware of this as she visits the home, and she too can supervise the patient in her efforts. (Courtesy Good Samaritan Hospital, Phoenix, Arizona)

ing to manage and capable of doing so with the supervision and aid of a visiting nurse. For other families, and under some circumstances, this is not possible. Another person, a substitute for a family member, is often the answer. Who is this person? How is the role of this person defined by the American Nurses' Association?

- Goeppinger, J.: Why a home health aide? Amer. J. Nurs., *68*:1513-1516, July, 1968.

5. As you sit in different types of chairs, analyze their effect on you from the standpoint of areas of stress or fatigue, such as on the leg muscles, in the lower back or in the chest area. Since people are not identical in body structure it is unfortunate (and inevitable) that library and classroom chairs are all alike. How varied are postures among your fellow students! No wonder many of them are uncomfortable. Note also the position of left-handed persons who must write in right-handed desk chairs.

6. Take each one of the physics principles listed on page 211 and test it. For example, try lifting a chair and then sliding it; lift several books from the table with the arms extended, and then lift them with the arms close to your side and your body near the table; open a self-service elevator door by standing alongside it (not facing it); place your hand in the door, and rock back to open it. Then try opening it with your arm strength alone while facing the door.

7. When persons have impaired function of both arms and legs, they are susceptible to falls and other types of accidents. See the case reports in the following article for suggestions other nurses have made to patients to help to prevent accidents in the home. Any one of these situations can exist in a hospital as well.

- Westaby, J. R. *et al*: Integrating accident prevention in total patient care. Nurs. Outlook, *11*:600-603, August, 1963.

8. What happens to persons who have limitations in ambulation? How does it affect their lives, such as their ability to use public transportation or where they can live? Read what the author of the following article found out from patients when she recognized a problem and sought to "collect data."

- Schwartz, D.: Problems of self-care and travel among elderly ambulatory patients. Amer. J. Nurs., *66*:2678-2681, October, 1966.

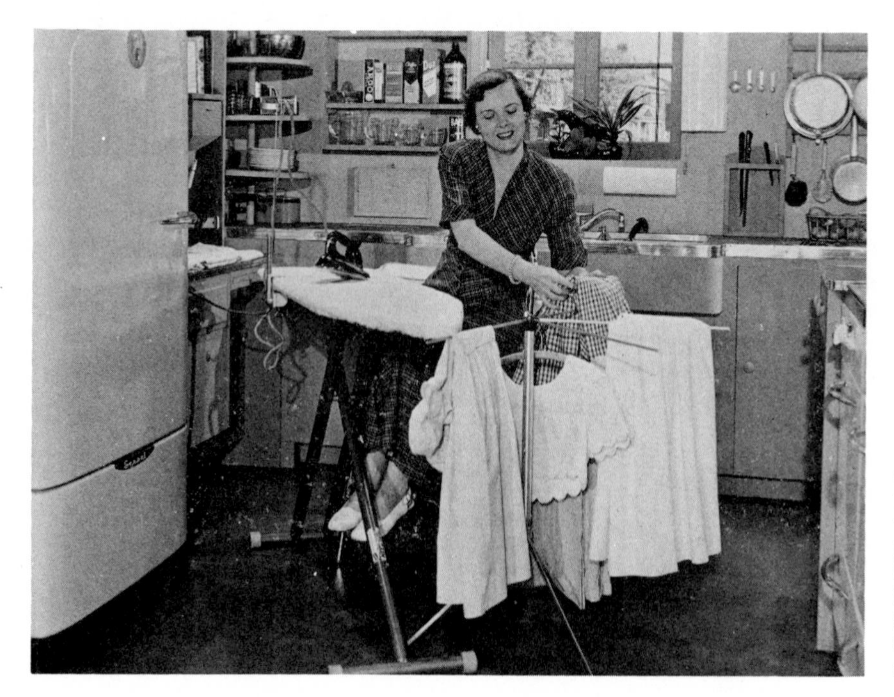

Fig. 20-29. Knowing how to conserve energy is often the key to a homemaker's ability to maintain health. The nurse should be prepared to teach her patients how they can reduce fatigue and thereby conserve their health. (From the publication Heart of the Home, American Heart Association, Inc., New York)

References

1. Ballantyne, D.: Evaluating ADL at the bedside.
AMER. J. NURS., *66*:2440-2441, November, 1966.
2. Day, Sr., M. A. C.: Postural reflex patterns: An exploratory study.
NURS. RESEARCH, *13*:139-147, Spring, 1964.
3. Fash, B.: Body Mechanics in Nursing Arts. pp. 3-24, 48-59.
New York, McGraw-Hill, 1946.
4. Huddleston, O. L.: Therapeutic Exercises—Kinesiology. 205 p.
Philadelphia, F. A. Davis, 1961.
5. Jensen, J. T.: Introduction to Medical Physics, Body Mechanics. pp. 34-43.
Philadelphia, Lippincott, 1960.
6. Kelly, M. M.: Exercises for bedfast patients.
AMER. J. NURS., *66*:2209-2213, October, 1966.
7. Kendall, H. O., and Kendall, F. P.: Developing and maintaining good posture.
PHYS. THER., *48*:318-336, April, 1968.
8. Kerr, A.: Orthopedic Nursing Procedures. pp. 7-16 and 17-32.
New York, Springer Publishing Co., (revised 1960).
9. Kottke, F. J., and Blanchard, R. S.: Bedrest begets bedrest.
NURS. FORUM, *3*:57-72, #3, 1964.
10. Larson, C. B., and Gould, M.: Calderwood's Orthopedic Nursing. pp. 1-59, ed. 6.
St. Louis, C. V. Mosby, 1965.
11. Nordmark, M., and Rohweder, A.: Scientific Foundations of Nursing, 388 pp.
Philadelphia, Lippincott, 1967.
12. Rehabilitative Aspects of Nursing. A Programmed Instruction Series. New York, National League for Nursing, 1966.
13. Seven basic rules for proper lifting procedure.
HOSP. MANAGE., *100*:54-55, November, 1965.
14. Smith, E. G.: Albianna fashions: Wardrobe with a purpose.
AMER. J. NURS., *66*:1320-1321, June, 1966.
15. Smith, R.: Let's dress the disabled for living.
NURS. OUTLOOK, *13*:59, December, 1965.
16. Stilwell, E. J.: Pressure sores—one method of care.
AMER. J. NURS., *61*:109, November, 1961.
17. Wiebe, A. M.: Orthopedics in Nursing, Chapter 4: Posture and Body Mechanics and Their Relation to Health. Chapter 7: The Nurse's Role in Health Promotion, Prevention of Disability, and Rehabilitation.
Philadelphia, W. B. Saunders, 1961.
18. Winters, M. C.: Protective Body Mechanics in Daily Life and in Nursing: A Manual for Nurses and Their Co-workers. 150 pp.
Philadelphia, Saunders, 1952.

CHAPTER 21

Maintaining Respiratory Integrity

Introduction

The mechanism of external respiration involves the exchange of gases; oxygen from the air delivered to the blood and carbon dioxide removed. Preservation of the integrity of the respiratory system—that is, the state of being in sound functional capacity—is vital to physical well-being. Yet most persons do not consider respiratory maintenance in the total picture of personal hygiene. Unless pathology is present, breathing is quiet and automatic. It does not command the attention that other bodily activities do: i.e., watching weight, concern about bowel functioning, applying creams or lotion to the skin, or taking tranquilizers to reduce tension.

From time to time we are made aware of respiratory functioning, such as when we "catch" our breath after being forced into a fast walk or run, or when we climb up the stairs; or if hiccoughs (singultuses) occur and we hold our breath or blow into a paper bag.

The need for attention to respiratory functioning is now considered as much a part of basic nursing care as any other measure.

Some of the physiologic factors of respiration were discussed in Chapter 17 and will not be repeated here. The problems of respiratory care when pathology is present are more appropriately found in clinical texts containing descriptions of the disease and its treatment. However, respiratory arrest constitutes a crisis; therefore, cardiopulmonary resuscitation is also included in this chapter.

General Principles in Relation to Respiratory Care

Respiration is the exchange of gases between the living organism and its environment. Oxygen is inhaled and carbon dioxide discharged, while internal respiration takes place at the cellular level.

All living body cells require oxygen. It follows then that the means by which the body receives this necessity of life should be kept in the best possible state.

Incomplete expansion of the lungs can result in atelectasis (collapse or partial collapse of lung tissue). The areas of the lungs affected by atelectasis cannot fulfill the function of respiration.

Adequate hydration is essential to respiratory functioning. Fluid is essential to the production of the watery mucus, which is normally present in the respiratory tract and is being constantly propelled towards the upper respiratory tract by ciliary action. This is an important mechanism because it helps remove foreign particles and "debris" from the lungs. This covering of mucus also protects the underlying tissues from irritation and infection.

Anatomically, the respiratory system consists of the nose, pharynx, larynx, trachea, the bronchial tree (bronchi with its ciliated cells, bronchioles) and the lungs. Gas exchange takes place in lung tissue. Because all parts are interdependent, it is toward the maintenance of the entire system that nursing measures involving breathing, coughing and adequate hydration are directed. Other measures, such as exercise, frequent turning and changing of position are related and are discussed in other parts of the text.

Not all lung tissue is active to the same degree with each respiration; that is, ventilation depends upon the extent of perfusion in the area. Blood flow in the lungs is influenced by gravity. Therefore, the amount of blood present in any given area of lung tissue depends partially upon whether the person is sitting up or lying down, prone, supine or on either side. The use of lung tissue is also dependent upon activity. Greater activity results in increased cardiac output

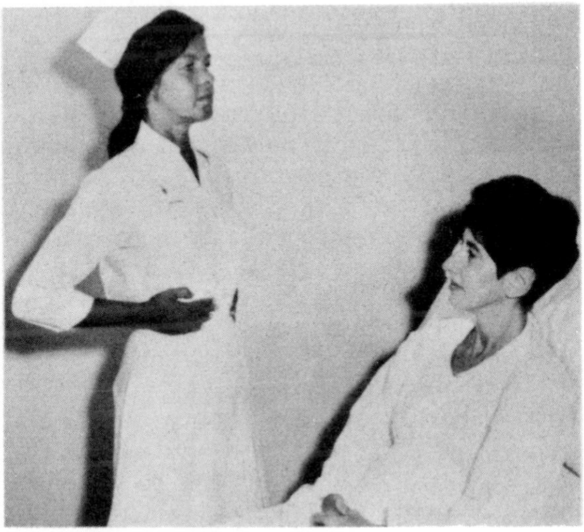

Fig. 21-1. The nurse demonstrates to the patient deep breathing exercises. She is showing her how to take a deep inspiration so that she can feel the pull between the ribs.

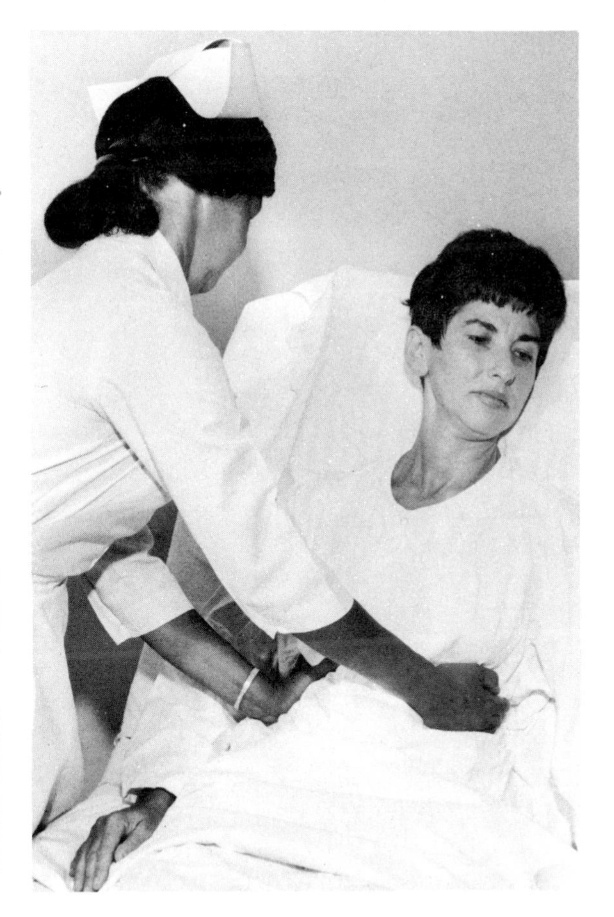

Fig. 21-2. The nurse is showing the patient how she can support the lower chest when doing deep breathing or coughing exercises.

and, consequently, increased blood supply to the lungs. The implications for the nursing needs of patients who are bedfast, or sitting in chairs most of the day, should be obvious.

Respiratory maintenance is now considered basic to preventive nursing care. It is not limited to the inactive patient or to the preoperative patient. Other factors also affect respiration, such as drugs, pain, fear, and even sights and odors that seem disagreeable; therefore, the presence of any of these may indicate a need for preventive nursing measures. In recent years, progress in respiratory care has given rise to another paramedical group, the thoracic physiotherapists or inhalation therapists. These practitioners instruct patients in breathing and coughing exercises[5]; in addition they administer treatment to patients who have pulmonary pathology. For example, patients who have need to dislodge accumulated secretions in the lungs may require technics such as tapping, cupping, vibration and postural drainage. Where such therapists are not available, nurses help to fill the gap. However, *preventive* respiratory care is always a part of good nursing.

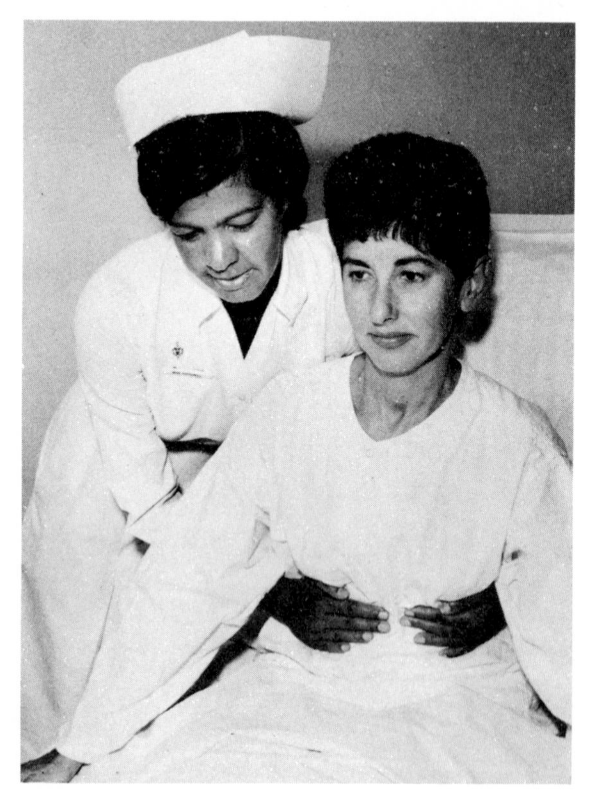

FIG. 21-3. The nurse is assuring the patient that if she has discomfort that there are means for helping her to do deep breathing and coughing exercises. As for example, the nurse will go behind the patient and support her while she does deep breathing and coughing exercises.

Although the actual teaching of preventive respiratory exercises such as deep breathing and coughing (see Figs. 21-1 through 21-3) is not difficult, experience has shown that having the patient follow through and do them is. Frequent reminders throughout the day are necessary for most patients.

Deep Breathing and Coughing Exercises

Breathing. Habits of breathing that are not in the best interests of bodily functioning may develop. Some persons, for one reason or another, develop a pattern of shallow breathing or walk with a "caved-in" chest. The result may be decrease of lung distensibility. A means of combating this is taking deep breaths (hyperinflation). Daily periodic hyperinflation is essential in such instances.

One study[11] reports on the findings of three technics: the single deep breath, the deep breath and hold, and multiple deep breaths. The deep breath and hold was found to be most effective for increasing arterial oxygen concentration.

Although there are some variations in what is considered to be *the* best method for therapeutic deep breathing, physiologic principles guide the actions that are essential. For one, the person should be instructed to inhale slowly and evenly to the greatest chest expansion possible for him. Next, he should hold his breath for at least three seconds. Studies indicate that a longer period does not produce any more benefit than the three second hold. Then the person permits normal recoil of the chest. As to the frequency with which this should be done, the patient's condition is the best possible guide. For some persons two to three times every two to three hours is satisfactory. For patients in danger of pulmonary complications it may need to be as often as every hour.

Involuntary deep breathing often occurs during sleep. Persons who snore, although a problem to those who have to listen, may benefit by their condition in that they frequently take deeper breaths. Also when they try to "saw through a knot in the wood," they alter the respiratory rate and depth.

Coughing. The cough mechanism consists of an initial irritation, a deep inspiration, a quick tight closure of the glottis together with a forceful contraction of the expiratory intercostal muscles, and the upward push of the diaphragm. This causes an explosive movement of air from the lower to the upper respiratory tract. To be effective, a cough should have enough muscle contraction to force air to be expelled and to propel a liquid or a solid on its way out of the respiratory tract. When a cough does not occur as a result of reflex stimulation of the cough-sensitive areas, it can be induced voluntarily.

Providing for Adequate Hydration

In addition to hyperinflation and ridding the lungs of accumulating secretions through deep breathing and coughing, attention must be given to adequate fluid intake. The patient's fluid intake should be within the limits of his regimen. In those circumstances in which the air is dry (low humidity), artificial means for humidification will be necessary. The inspiration of dry air removes the normal moisture in the respiratory passages which is essential to protection from irritation and infection.

Cardiopulmonary Resuscitation

Cessation of breathing may be due to respiratory or cardiac failure. Emergency treatment must be instituted *immediately*. It is the opinion of many medical authorities that as many persons as are capable of learning how to safely administer resuscitation technics be taught to do so. In most health agencies there is an on-going program for teaching such technics to all health personnel. Such teaching programs are extending into the community, over and beyond such groups as police, firemen and rescue workers.

Recognizing When Resuscitation is Indicated. Cessation of breathing can be of cardiac or pulmonary origin. If of cardiac origin, breathing usually stops within 30 to 45 seconds. If of respiratory origin, cardiac action may continue, but become more and more feeble. Resuscitation *must* begin immediately. No time must be wasted in asking "what happened?", or calling "give him air," or taking blood pressure, and so on. Brain damage may occur quickly from a lack of oxygen. Irreversible damage may occur in about four minutes, but for some persons, such as those with vascular disease, damage may occur sooner.

Feel for a carotid or femoral pulse. These areas are considered best. In *cardiac arrest, pulsation in these areas is absent*. Also, the patient lapses into unconsciousness within a matter of seconds (10 to 15). Dilation of the pupils follows. In pulmonary arrest, chest and abdominal wall movements are absent. Dilated pupils occur as a delayed symptom. A distinguishing difference between a person who has "fainted" and a person in cardiac arrest is that the person who has fainted has a pulse—weak, but palpable.

The person recognizing the need for emergency resuscitation should institute action immediately and have someone else get medical aid. In hospital situations there is a plan which calls a team of doctors, nurses and other therapists into action at any time of the day or night. The person or persons resuscitating the victim continue their efforts until this team arrives. In the community the same holds true. The rescuers continue their efforts until the emergency squad arrives.

Resuscitation Technics

Artificial Ventilation. This is the procedure of forcing exhaled air into the lungs of the victim. It can be done by means of an S tube, mouth-to-mouth, or mouth-to-nose.

The S tube, so named because of its shape, can be inserted into the patient's mouth over the tongue. It has a flange on it so that the patient's mouth can be sealed. Be sure the mouth is clear of any obstructive material. The rescuer then takes a position facing the top of the victim's head, and tilts the head back as far as possible in order to try to open the airway. In some instances this act alone may result in spontaneous breathing as evidenced by movement of the chest and the presence of breath sounds.

Insert the long end of the tube for an adult, and the short end for a child. Use both hands, one on either side of the tube. With thumbs, pinch patient's nose closed and with other fingers hold chin up to hold head back and flange tight over mouth. Take a *deep* breath and blow into the mouthpiece. When the victim's chest rises, take mouth off of tube and allow him to exhale. Take another deep breath and repeat. Do not blow forcefully for a child.

An S tube is usually standard emergency equipment on all units of a health agency. Some agencies have gone so far as to have one in each patient unit. It is a good idea to have one in the home emergency first aid supplies as well. There has been no specific part of this text marked for "home emergencies" or "home first aid," but a point can be made here. No matter where one lives, temporary first aid items should be a part of the environment. This goes beyond emergency treatment of burns and insect bites, and other minor accidents. Instructions for artificial ventilation should also be readily available.

Mouth-to-Mouth resuscitation. As with the S tube, clear the mouth if necessary, and tilt the patient's head back as far as possible. Again, the rescuer takes a deep breath, pinches the victim's nose closed, and then places his mouth over the victim's mouth, making a tight seal and then exhaling. The volume of air should be sufficient to cause the patient's chest wall to rise. Remove mouth and allow the chest to return to "normal." Repeat once every five seconds or at least 12 times a minute.

Mouth-to-nose resuscitation. If the rescuer cannot get a good coverage of the mouth so that there is a tight seal, close the patient's mouth and force exhaled air into his nose. The mouth should be open for exhalation because the palate may obstruct, preventing air from leaving through the nose.

Air can be forced into the stomach; therefore, look for signs of bulging of the stomach. If it occurs, press gently but firmly over the epigastric area. It is wise to turn the patient slightly on his side in the event stomach contents are emitted. This facilitates clearing the mouth and prevents aspiration of emitted material.

After two deep inflations, check the pulse. The carotid is considered best. Continue to keep the head back while feeling for the pulse. Resume ventilating.

Artificial circulation. If no pulse is detected, the person is judged as being in a state of cardiopulmonary arrest. Circulation must be maintained by externally applied compression of the heart. An initial emergency measure is to give the person a sharp, quick blow over the sternum. This may be sufficient to stimulate cardiac action. However, do not waste time doing this repeatedly.

When external cardiac compression is performed it must be accompanied by artificial ventilation.

For external cardiac compression to be effective, the patient should be on a *firm* surface. Place him on the floor if necessary. The rescuer should be at either side of the patient. The point of concentration is the sternum. Place the heel of one hand (part closest to wrist) on the lower part of the sternum, but *not* over the xiphoid process (tip of the sternum) in order to prevent internal injury to the patient. The entire palm of the hand is not used because it covers too large an area and could cause damage to the rib cage. Place the other hand over the first one. For each compression movement the sternum should be depressed one and one-half to two inches, then relax pressure completely. Do not lose contact with the point of compression over the sternum. The rate of compression should be at least 60 times per minute in adults and 100 times per minute for children.

Palpate for the femoral or carotid pulse at frequent intervals to determine if the compression is being effective. If artificial circulation is being done effectively it can sustain a reasonable cardiac output in most patients.

Artificial ventilation and circulation must be done alternately during the period of emergency. One person can do both. That is, give two to three rapid mouth-to-mouth or mouth-to-nose breaths (this will usually supply the lungs with enough oxygen for about 15 seconds) then do cardiac compression for 15 seconds, doing about one compression per second. If a second person is available, one can concentrate on the artificial ventilation and the other on the artificial circulation. In this case the ratio is one breath to five compressions.

Emergency care continues until the arrival of medical personnel. The physician is then responsible for definitive therapy which includes the use of drugs, such as for stimulating heart action and stabilizing blood pressure or preventing acidosis; the use of oxygen; defibrillating equipment, and so forth. These measures are covered in detail in clinical texts and periodical literature. The implications for nursing care are considerable, not the least of which are: understanding what this episode means to the person, giving emotional support to him and his family, observing for evidence of resulting physiologic disturbances, and maintaining a protective environment.

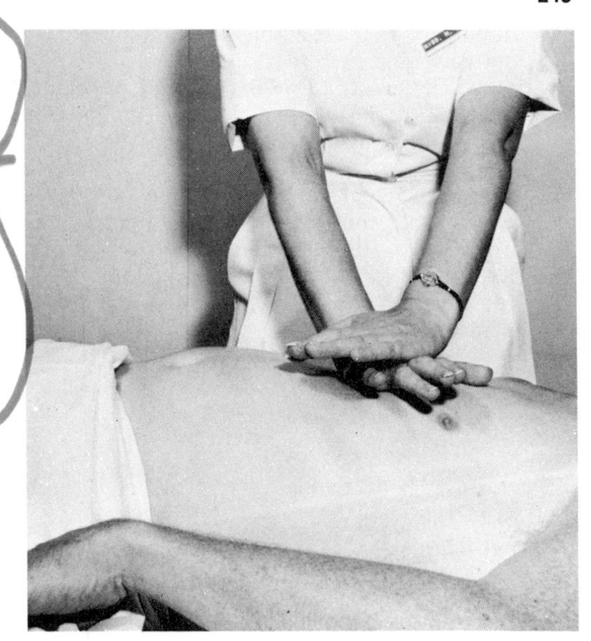

Fig. 21-4. Hands in position for cardiac massage, above the tip of the sternum.

Study Situations

1. When the word "rehabilitation" is used it most frequently is associated with the regaining of musculoskeletal functioning. When respiratory functioning is impaired, rehabilitation is also essential. C.O.L.D. in the following article stands for chronic obstructive lung disease. Although it is clinically oriented, it does have many illustrations of exercises for the maintenance of respiratory integrity.

- Kinney, M.: Rehabilitation of patients with C.O.L.D.
  Amer. J. Nurs., *67*:2528-2535, December, 1967.

2. In the February, 1966, issue of the American Journal of Nursing, Sister Regina Elizabeth's article "Sensory Stimulation Techniques," pp. 281-286, describes how to induce or inhibit coughing. See how some students sought to investigate her findings. How does their study relate to problem solving?

- Hedges, J. E., and Bridges, C. J.: Stimulation of the cough reflex.
  Amer. J. Nurs., *68*:347-348, February, 1968.

References

1. American Thoracic Society—Medical Sect of N.T.A.: Principles of respiratory car Amer. Rev. Resp. Dis., *95* (No. 2) :32 February, 1967.
2. Bendixen, H. H. *et al*: Respirator 252 pp. St. Louis, C. V. Mosby Co., 1965.
3. Betson, C.: Blood gases. Amer. J. Nurs., *68*:1010-1012, Ma
4. Cardiopulmonary Resuscitation—A Ma for Instructors. pp. 11-16, 26-28, 29-30. American Heart Associaton, 1967.

5. Hanamey, R.: Teaching patients breathing and coughing technics.
NURS. OUTLOOK, *13*:58-59, August, 1965.
6. Healy, K. M.: Does preoperative instruction make a difference?
AMER. J. NURS., *68*:62-67, January, 1968.
7. Hanson, J. S. *et al*: Comparative exercise—cardiorespiratory performance of normal men in the third, fourth and fifth decades of life.
CIRCULATION, *37*:345-360, March, 1968.
8. Kurihara, M.: Assessment and maintenance of adequate respiration.
NURS. CLINICS N. AMER., *3* (No. 1):65-76, March, 1968.
9. Olson, E. with Thompson, L. F.: The hazards of immobility—effects on respiratory function.
AMER. J. NURS., *67*:781-782, April, 1967.
10. Paisner, L.: The therapeutic alphabet.
AMER. J. NURS., *66*:531, March, 1966.
11. Ward, R. J. *et al*: An evaluation of postoperative respiratory maneuvers.
SURG., GYNEC. OBSTET., *123*:51-54, July, 1966.

CHAPTER

22

Maintaining Bowel and Bladder Integrity

Introduction

A recurrent theme in this Unit is the concept of homeostasis: the coordination of the body's mechanisms for optimal functioning. Observation of and questioning of patients in relation to bowel and bladder elimination often tends to be careless or neglected in nursing care. These functions usually are taken for granted unless something goes radically wrong. However, as in maintaining respiratory integrity, preventive measures are equally important in promoting normal patterns of elimination.

A brief review of anatomy and physiology of elimination from the intestines and urinary bladder follows. Some basic nursing measures are included. The measures needed to combat problems of elimination are discussed further in Chapter 25.

General Principles in Relation to Bowel and Urinary Elimination

Efficient physiologic functioning requires that waste substances be eliminated from the body. Elimination is essential to life itself. Mechanisms of elimination include not only bowel and bladder, but other organs, namely the lungs and the sweat glands.

Patterns of elimination from the large intestine and the urinary bladder vary among individuals. Despite individual differences, as long as the intestines and the urinary bladder are eliminating wastes efficiently, there is no great need for concern.

Stress-producing situations and illness may interfere with normal habits of elimination. Persons under stress often encounter problems in elimination. For example, a patient confined to bed may find it so difficult to use a bedpan or a urinal that he may be unable to have a bowel movement or to urinate normally.

In addition to the stress associated with hospitalization, normal elimination (especially from the large intestine) often is affected by change in diet, certain medications, therapeutic and diagnostic measures and reduction in the patient's normal activities.

Patterns of elimination from the urinary bladder do not vary among individuals so markedly as bowel habits. Most people urinate just before bedtime, upon arising and several times during the day, depending on their diet, fluid intake, activity, and the like.

Elimination from the Intestines and Measures to Maintain Normal Functioning

Food is ingested and digested by the alimentary canal. The end-products of digestion which the tissue cells of the body assimilate are absorbed through the mucous membrane of the alimentary canal. The residue that the body does not select for utilization becomes waste products and is excreted by the skin, the lungs, the intestines and the urinary tract. The process of excretion of wastes is essential for life and must continue during illness as in health.

Large Intestine. The large intestine is the lower or distal part of the alimentary canal. It extends from the ileocecal valve to the anus. Waste products of digestion are received by the large intestine from the small intestine.

The length of the large intestine in adults is approximately 50 to 60 inches, but variations have been observed in normal persons. The width of the colon varies in different parts. At the narrowest point, the colon is approximately one inch wide; at the widest

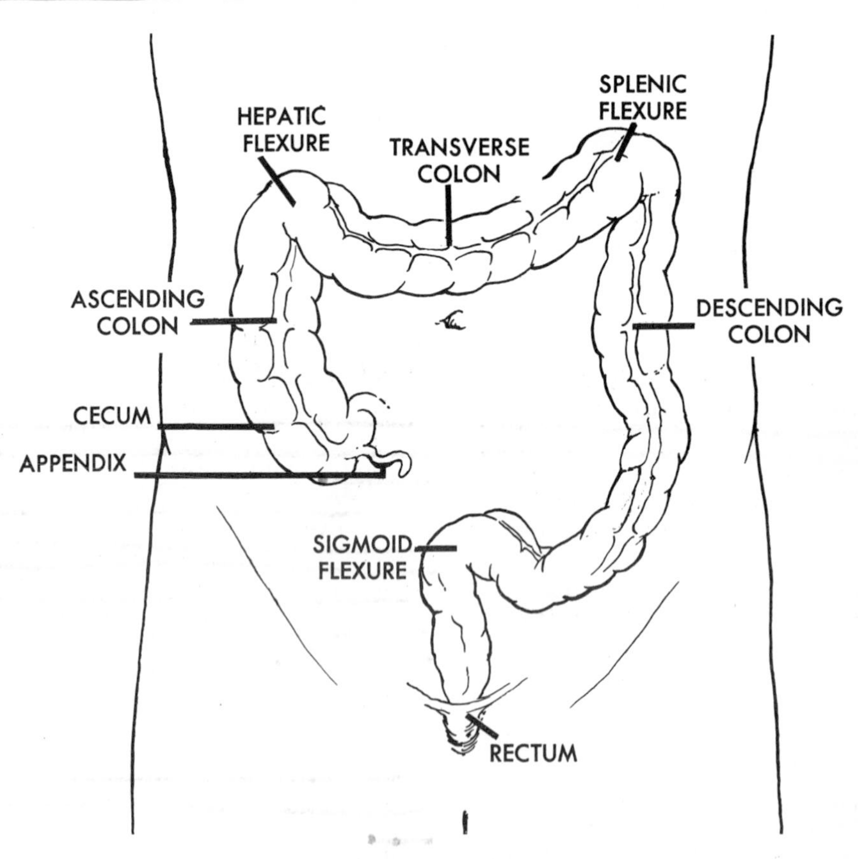

FIG. 22-1. Diagram of the large intestine.

point, about three inches. Its diameter decreases from the cecum to the anus.

The barrier between the large intestine and the ileum of the small intestine is the *ileocecal* or *ileocolic* valve. This valve normally prevents contents from entering the large intestine prematurely and prevents fecal matter from returning to the small intestine.

The waste contents pass through the ileocecal valve and enter the cecum, which is the first part of the large intestine. It is situated on the right side of the body, and to it is attached the *vermiform process* or *appendix*. When waste products enter the large intestine, the contents are liquid or watery in nature. While they pass through the large intestine, water is absorbed. This absorption of water accounts for the formed, semisolid consistency of the normal stool. When absorption does not occur properly, as when the fecal matter passes through the large intestine at a very rapid rate, the stool is soft and watery.

From the cecum, the contents enter the colon, which is divided into several parts. The *ascending colon* extends from the cecum up toward the liver, where it turns to cross the abdomen. This turn is referred to as the *hepatic flexure*. The *transverse colon* crosses the abdomen from right to left. The turn from the transverse colon to form the descending colon is referred to as the *splenic flexure*. The *descending colon* passes down the left side of the body from the splenic flexure to the *sigmoid* or *pelvic colon*. When the waste products reach the distal end of the colon they are referred to as *feces*, and, when excreted, the feces are usually called the *stool*.

The sigmoid colon contains feces ready for excretion and empties into the *rectum*, which is the last part of the large intestine. The rectum is approximately four to six inches long. Normally, transverse folds of tissue, usually three, are present in the rectum.

The three transverse folds may help to hold the fecal material in the rectum temporarily. In addition, there are vertical folds. Each vertical fold contains an artery and a vein. Distended veins are called *hemorrhoids*. If hemorrhoids are present, caution must be exercised when a thermometer is inserted. Objects introduced into the anus or rectum should always be lubricated to reduce friction. If force is applied, injury to the mucous membrane may occur. The rectum is usually empty except during and immediately prior to defecation. Waste products are excreted from the rectum through the anal canal and the anus, which is about one to one and one-half inches long.

The muscular layer of the large intestine plays an important part in excretion. The internal circular muscles are thicker than they are in other parts of the gastrointestinal tract. The outer longitudinal fibers are also thicker and are arranged in three muscle bands called *taeniae coli*. When muscles of the large intestine contract, they are capable of producing strong peristaltic action to propel fecal matter forward. Peristalsis is a kind of wormlike contraction of the musculature.

The contents of the large intestine act as the chief stimulant for the contraction of intestinal musculature. The pressure of the contents against the walls of the colon causes muscle stretch. This in turn causes stimulation of the nerve receptors, which in turn is followed by contraction of the walls of the colon, peristalsis and haustral churning.

Stimulation occurs by both mechanical and chemical means. The bulk of the contents acts as a mechanical stimulant; as bulk increases, the pressure in the intestine increases, causing the muscles of the large intestine to contract. Bacterial action in the intestinal tract is responsible for chemical stimulation. Certain bacteria act on carbohydrates, causing fermentation, while other bacteria are responsible for the putrefaction of proteins. The end products of fermentation and putrefaction are organic acids, amines and ammonia, which stimulate muscular contraction chemically. Various gases formed by bacterial action also stimulate muscle contraction by increasing pressure within the colon. Emotional disturbances also have been observed to produce muscle contraction in the large intestine. Such contraction occurs by reflex action.

Waste products in the large intestine are

propelled by mass peristaltic sweeps one to four times each 24-hour period in most individuals. The fecal mass is moved during these sweeps. This movement is unlike the frequent peristaltic rushes that occur in the small intestine. Mass peristalsis often occurs after food has been ingested. This accounts for the urge to defecate that frequently is observed following meals.

Anal Canal and Anus. The internal sphincter in the anal canal and the external sphincter at the anus control the discharge of feces and gas.

The internal sphincter consists of smooth muscle tissue and is involuntary. The innervation of the internal sphincter occurs through the autonomic nervous system. Motor impulses are carried by the sympathetic system (thoracolumbar) and inhibitory impulses by the parasympathetic system (craniosacral). It will be recalled that these two divisions of the autonomic nervous system function antagonistically to each other in a dynamic equilibrium.

The external sphincter at the anus has striated muscle tissue and is therefore under voluntary control. The levator ani reinforces the action of the external sphincter and also is controlled voluntarily. Interference with the normal functioning of elimination from the intestines can occur as easily in health as it can during illness. It can be affected by amount and quality of fluid or food intake, degree of activity and emotional states.

The Act of Defecation. Defecation is an evacuation of the bowels and is usually referred to as a bowel movement. There are two centers governing the reflex to defecate. One is situated in the medulla, and a subsidiary one is in the spinal cord. When parasympathetic stimulation occurs, the internal anal sphincter relaxes, and the colon contracts. The defecation reflex is stimulated chiefly by the fecal mass in the rectum. When the rectum is distended, the intrarectal pressure rises, the defecation reflex is stimulated by the muscle stretch, and the desire to evacuate results. The external anal sphincter, controlled voluntarily, is constricted or relaxed according to will. If the desire to defecate is ignored, defecation can often be delayed voluntarily.

During the act of defecation, several additional muscles aid the process. Voluntary contraction of the muscles of the abdominal wall, fixing of the diaphragm and closing of the glottis aid in increasing intra-abdominal pressure up to four or five times normal pressure that aids in expelling the feces. Simultaneously, the muscles on the pelvic floor contract and aid in drawing the anus over the fecal mass.

Normal Defecation. Normally, the act of defecation is painless. *Normality is associated with the regularity and type of stool.* If the bowels move at regular intervals and the stools are normal, functional problems of frequency of elimination occur infrequently. However, nurses find that most patients show concern if they do not have a daily bowel movement. The normal frequency of bowel movements cannot be stated arbitrarily. Although most adults pass one stool each day, healthy persons have been observed to have more frequent or less frequent bowel movements. Some persons have a bowel movement two or three times a week, others as often as two or three times a day.

Normally, the stool consists principally of food residues as cellulose which is not digested and other foodstuffs which the body has not utilized completely; microorganisms of various kinds; secretions from intestinal glands; biliary pigments; water and body cells. Unless the diet is high in roughage content, little of the total amount of feces is food residue. The normal stool is a semisolid mass. The amount of stool varies and depends to a large extent on the amount and the kind of food ingested. The color of the normal stool is brown, due chiefly to urobilin, which is a result of the reduction of bile pigments in the small intestine. A change in color is significant, since it frequently indicates impaired physiologic functioning. The stool has a characteristic odor due chiefly to skatole and indole produced by bacterial action on tryptophan. The diet may influence odor, as will certain drugs.

Normally, the stool assumes the shape of the rectum. Change in the shape of the stool is significant if such change persists. For example, pencil-like stools frequently indicate a change in the lumen of the colon and may be due to a growth.

Nursing Responsibilities. Nursing personnel are responsible for observing the patient's stool. Color, odor, consistency, shape and amount are noted, and anything unusual such as the presence of blood, pus, parasites, mucus, etc., should be reported promptly.

It is important for the nurse to know the patient's normal patterns of elimination in order to recognize any abnormality.

The frequency with which stools are passed should be noted. It will be recalled that frequency normally varies with individuals, and this should be taken into account when making judgments concerning the frequency of bowel movements.

Passing little or no gas or unusual amounts of gas are often important symptoms. Difficulty with passing a stool or pain during defecation also should be reported to the physician.

The nurse should understand that the establishment of bowel habits begins in childhood. Bowel habits have many psychological implications, depending on accepted practices in various cultural groups. These practices are concerned with consideration for privacy, cleanliness, frequency and other factors. Having a bowel movement is usually easier when the person is relaxed both physically and mentally. Individual patterns of living will guide the selection of a convenient time. The urge to defecate often occurs following a meal. After breakfast is a common time for persons who are awake during the usual daylight hours.

Encourage the patient to eat an adequately nutritious diet and plenty of fluids. At the first sign of bowel disturbance, either constipation or frequent stools, investigate the patient's food and fluid intake. Exercise is also helpful in maintaining normal bowel functioning. To the extent that the patient's regimen permits, encourage activity to prevent decreased bowel functioning. Disturbances of bowel elimination are discussed in Chapter 25.

Elimination from the Urinary Tract and Measures to Maintain Normal Functioning

As with the gastrointestinal system, the efficiency of the urinary system is vital for the maintenance of good physiologic functioning. During illness, considerable emphasis is placed on the patient's ability to excrete urine normally. Close observation is essential if deviations are to be detected early.

The urinary tract is one of the routes by which wastes are excreted. Certain inorganic salts, nitrogenous waste products, and water are removed from the blood stream, accumulated, and excreted through the proper functioning of the urinary tract.

Kidneys and Ureters. The kidneys are located on either side of the vertebral column behind the peritoneum and in the posterior portion of the abdominal cavity. They are responsible for maintaining the composition and the volume of body fluids. The kidneys function in a selective manner; that is, they single out constituents of the blood for excretion for which the body has no need. Despite varying kinds and amounts of foods and fluids ingested, body fluids remain relatively stable if there is proper kidney function. The waste solution containing organic and inorganic wastes which the kidneys produce is called *urine.*

The nephron is the unit of kidney structure. Urine from the nephrons empties into the pelvis of each kidney. From each kidney, urine is transported by rhythmic peristalsis through the ureter to the urinary bladder. The ureters enter the bladder obliquely, and a fold of membrane in the bladder closes the entrance to the ureters so that urine is not forced up the ureters to the kidneys when pressure exists in the bladder.

Urinary Bladder. This is a smooth muscle sac which serves as a reservoir for varying amounts of urine. There are three layers of muscular tissue in the bladder—the inner longitudinal, the middle circular and the outer longitudinal. The three layers are called the detrusor muscle. At the base of the bladder, the middle circular layer of muscle tissue forms the vesical or internal sphincter. This sphincter guards the opening between the urinary bladder and the urethra. The urethra conveys urine from the bladder to the exterior of the body.

Urinary bladder muscle is innervated by the autonomic nervous system. The sympathetic system carries inhibitory impulses to the bladder and motor impulses to the vesical sphincter. These impulses result in relaxation of the detrusor muscle and constriction of the vesical sphincter, causing urine to be retained in the bladder. The parasympathetic system carries motor impulses to the bladder and inhibitory impulses to the vesical sphincter. These impulses result in contraction of the detrusor muscle and relaxation of the sphincter, causing urine to escape from the bladder.

The bladder normally contains urine under very little pressure, and, as volume of urine increases, the pressure increases only slightly. This adaptability of the bladder wall to pressure is believed to be due to the characteristics of muscle tissue in the bladder and makes it possible for urine to continue to enter the bladder from the ureters against low pressure. When the pressure becomes sufficient to stimulate stretch receptors located in the bladder wall, the desire to empty the bladder becomes apparent.

Urethra. The urethra differs in men and women. In men, the urethra is common to both the excretory system and the reproductive system. It is approximately five and one-half to six and one-half inches in length and consists of three parts—the prostatic, the membranous and the cavernous portions. The external urethral sphincter consists of striated muscle and is located at the distal end of the cavernous portion of the urethra. The external sphincter is under voluntary control.

The female urethra is one and one-half to two and one-half inches in length. Its function is to convey urine from the bladder to the exterior. Striated muscle at the meatus or exit of the female urethra is under voluntary control. There is a difference of opinion concerning whether the muscle at the meatus can be called a true sphincter, since the muscle tissue is not well developed as it is in the external sphincter of the male. However, most literature refers to muscle at the meatus in the female as the external sphincter.

The Act of Micturition. The process of emptying the urinary bladder is known as *micturition*; the terms *voiding* or *urination* are used also. Nerve centers for micturition are situated in the brain and the spinal cord. Voiding is largely a reflex act (involuntary).

Following stimulation of the stretch receptors in the bladder, the detrusor muscle contracts, the vesical sphincter relaxes, and the desire to void becomes apparent. When restraint of voiding is removed, the muscles of the perineum and the external sphincter relax, and micturition occurs. The act consists of relaxation of the vesical sphincter, contraction of the detrusor muscle, slight contraction of the muscle of the abdominal wall and a lowering of the diaphragm. The act of micturition is normally painless. During micturition, the pressure within the bladder is many times greater than it is during the time the bladder is filling. The voluntary control of voiding is limited to initiating, restraining and interrupting the act.

Restraint of voiding is believed to be subconscious when the volume of urine in the bladder is small. But when voiding is delayed, the bladder continues to fill. Discomfort may then be felt when undue distention occurs and the urgency to void becomes paramount.

Increased abdominal pressure, as occurs for example with coughing and sneezing, sometimes forces the escape of urine involuntarily, especially in the female since the urethra is shorter. Strong psychic factors, such as marked fear, may also result in involuntary urination. Under certain conditions, it may be difficult to remove the restraint to void, such as when a urine specimen is requested from a shy or embarrassed person.

When the higher nerve centers develop after infancy, the voluntary control of micturition develops also. Until that time, voiding is purely reflex in nature. Persons whose bladders are isolated from control of the brain because of either injury or disease also void by reflex only.

Normal Urine. Healthy adults excrete approximately 1,000 to 1,800 cc. of urine in each 24-hour period. However, this amount may vary, depending on several factors. If large amounts of fluids are being excreted by the skin, the lungs or the intestine, the amount excreted by the kidneys will decrease. The amount of urine will depend on the amount of fluid ingested: the greater the fluid intake, the larger will be the amount of urine produced, and vice versa. Diet influences the amount of urine. Persons on high protein diets will produce more urine than those on a regular diet. Children and infants excrete more urine in proportion to their weight than adults do.

The word *diuresis* is used most often to mean an increase in the production and the elimination of urine. Certain fluids act as diuretics and will cause an increase in the production of urine. Examples are coffee, tea and cocoa. Certain drugs also produce diuresis.

The color of normal urine is golden yellow or amber. If the urine is scant in amount and concentrated, the color will be darker; if it is dilute, the color will be lighter. Urine has a characteristic odor. Some foods and drugs will alter the odor.

Normal urine is clear. On standing and cooling, there may occur cloudiness and a sediment which are due to the presence of urates and phosphates that precipitate as the reaction of urine changes from acidity to alkalinity. Normal urine will clear again rapidly if acid is added and the urine is heated to body temperature.

Laboratory examination reveals that the specific gravity of normal urine varies on the average between approximately 1.015 and 1.025, but it has been observed to vary between 1.002 and 1.040 in healthy persons. The inorganic constituents of normal urine include ammonia, sodium chloride and traces of iron; and phosphorus, sulfur, sodium, potassium, calcium and magnesium in combination with oxygen. Organic constituents include urea, uric acid, creatinine, hippuric acid, indican, urine pigments and undetermined nitrogen. Traces of urobilin, sugar, fatty acids, carbonates, mucin and cystine may be present.

The urine of persons on a normal diet is slightly acid. Vegetarians excrete a slightly alkaline urine. Normally, the urinary tract is sterile; therefore, urine is free of bacteria. Bacteria are found at the end of the urethra, and if they are washed into a urine specimen, usually they will be identified by laboratory examination.

Frequency of Urination. The frequency of voiding depends on the amount of urine being produced. The more urine that is being produced, the more often voiding is necessary, and vice versa. Normally, from two-thirds to three-fourths of the urine output is voided by ambulatory persons during the daytime hours. Unless the fluid intake is very large, most healthy persons do not void during their normal sleeping hours. The first voided urine of the day is usually more concentrated than urine excreted during the remainder of the day.

Some persons normally void small amounts at frequent intervals because they habitually respond to the first early urge to void. This habit is insignificant and is not necessarily an indication of disease.

Nursing Responsibilities. Nursing personnel are responsible for observing the patient's urine when this is essential to his health problem. The color, odor, amount, appearance and the frequency with which voiding occurs are noted. Anything unusual is reported to the physician. Difficulty or pain associated with the act of micturition also is reported promptly.

Adequate fluid intake is a prime factor in maintaining urinary elimination. The patient should be encouraged to drink plenty of fluids if his intake is not restricted. Question the patient about his fluid intake if there are signs of concentrated urine.

Some patients find it difficult to void while in bed. Even the sitting bed position is not helpful. They may need to have their legs over the side of the bed while sitting on the bedpan. Some male patients on bed rest may need permission from the physician to be able to stand to use the urinal.

Providing for Use of the Bedpan and the Urinal

Men patients confined to bed use the urinal for voiding and the bedpan for defecation; women use the bedpan for both. When a woman patient is unable to sit up in bed—for example, when she is in a body cast—a female urinal may be used. Having to use the bedpan and the urinal is considered embarrassing by most patients. In addition, the bedpan is often difficult to use. It "fits" no one. Privacy is important to almost all patients when they use either a bedpan or urinal.

Most bedpans are made of metal. This is important to remember when the room is cold. The bedpan may be warmed by running warm water inside it and then rotating the water around the sides of the pan.

Bedpans of nylon resin are now coming into use. They feel warm to touch and can be sterilized by conventional methods. Also, these bedpans eliminate the problem of noise associated with handling of metal bedpans.

Unless contraindicated, the head of the bed should be raised slightly before placing the patient on the bedpan. This makes it easier for the patient to lift himself onto the pan. If he is flat in bed, it is necessary for him to hyperextend his back in order to lift himself up onto the bedpan.

After providing privacy, fold a corner of the top bed linen over onto the patient so that it is easy to slip the bedpan under him. It is not necessary to expose a patient for this procedure. When the patient is on correctly, leave the toilet tissue within easy reach, check to see that the signal bell is convenient, and leave the patient alone if physical condition warrants. The patient should be instructed to signal when finished.

If the patient is very weak, it may be necessary for the nurse to place one hand under his buttocks and assist him to raise himself. If the patient cannot help to lift himself, raise the head of the bed slightly, turn the patient over on one side, place the bedpan against his buttocks, and hold it in place while the patient is rolled back onto the bedpan.

Before emptying the bedpan, the contents should be noted carefully. The excretory products are a vital clue to the patient's physiologic state. Any abnormalities in the nature of the stool or the urine or in the act of elimination should be reported promptly and recorded on the patient's chart.

After a patient has used the bedpan, offer a wash cloth which has been moistened with water and soap, and a towel.

Commodes can be used for patients allowed out of bed but unable to use the bathroom toilet. Commodes are chairs (straight back or wheel chairs) with open seats and a shelf or a holder under the seat on which a bedpan is placed.

If the patient is allowed to use the bathroom toilet, the nurse still is responsible for noting any abnormalities of elimination when stools are a factor in the patient's health problem—i.e., diarrhea and gallstones. Other patients may need to be taught to report abnormalities to the nurse and instructed not to flush the toilet until the nurse has seen the stool and the urine.

A weak patient should be assisted to the bathroom. Remain in attendance if there is any danger of the patient's falling. Bathrooms should not be locked, and a signal bell should be within easy reach of the patient so that help can be summoned easily if the patient feels weak and in need of assistance.

Many a dangerous situation has been created in the absence of a signal bell or bedpan. Patients confined to bed have gotten out to go to the bathroom to void. Some had to climb over or around bedside rails, and others removed oxygen masks or canopies. For example, an elderly woman was admitted to the hospital in a comatose state. The physician ordered her on *absolute* rest and oxygen as well as other medications. Several hours later when a nurse went in for one of the frequent checks on the patient, the latter was nowhere in sight. She was found in the bathroom. Asked how she got out of bed she said she had crawled around the bottom of the bedside rails. As to why she did it, she said simply: "I had to go." It was recognized that this patient was beginning to have lucid moments; henceforth, she was offered a bedpan frequently.

Offering a bedpan or urinal frequently can save many a patient from a fractured hip or a dislodged infusion. If a patient appears very ill or is sedated, he may not think to ask in time. Remember: the nurse is responsible for the patient's safety at all times.

Measuring Fluid Intake and Output

In many instances, the physician will request that the patient's fluid intake and urinary output be measured. A study of daily fluid intake and output and their relation to each other is important in assisting the physician to determine the patient's diagnosis and to prescribe a course of therapy.

Accuracy in measuring intake and output is of prime importance. In the interest of accuracy, and economy of time, most health agencies have forms that facilitate keeping intake and output records. Intake forms usually indicate the capacity of the various dishes and glasses normally in use so that all personnel may record like amounts. At best, recording intake and output is subject to error, since cups, glasses and dishes may not always be filled to the same level, and substitute containers will vary in capacity. To keep the best intake record, the patient must be included in the procedure. When a patient is able to assist in keeping his own intake and understands how to do it and why, the entire procedure is more likely to be accurate.

How intake and output records are kept is an individual decision for each agency. There is no one method acceptable to all agencies, but all depend on nursing personnel being as accurate as possible.

Health agencies provide separate calibrated containers for measuring urinary output. Collecting bottles are used and carefully labeled when urine is to be saved. In many agencies, a preservative and a deodorizer are added to the contents in the bottle to prevent deterioration and odor.

Study Situation

A frequent nursing problem is met with in persons who suffer from bowel consciousness beyond the point of good reason. Misleading literature and advertisements, especially in relation to frequency of defecation, have caused people to upset habits that were completely normal. For example, some begin taking laxatives rather routinely because they have read in advertisements that bowel "sluggishness" occurs after 35 years of age.

Examine the variety of preparations available the next time you are in the drug department of a store. Read the labels for evidence of what action is supposed to be induced—where (i.e., small or large intestines), frequency of administration, and dosage. Do a count of the varieties available to the public for self-medication. Don't forget there are some that are kept refrigerated.

References

1. Davson, H., and Eggleton, M. G.: Starling's Principles of Human Physiology, ed. 13, pp. 617-646, pp. 733-739.
   Philadelphia, Lea and Febiger, 1962.
2. Hollinshead, W. H.: Embryology and anatomy of the anal canal and rectum.
   DIS. COLON RECTUM, *5*:18, January-February, 1962.
3. Stafford, N. H.: Bowel hygiene of aged patients.
   AMER. J. NURS., *63*:102, September, 1963.
4. Steigmann, F.: Are laxatives necessary?
   AMER. J. NURS., *62*:90, October, 1962.

(References in Chapters 18, 24, and 25 relate to this chapter also.)

CHAPTER

23

Providing for Rest

Chapter 20 pointed out the dangers of bed rest and discussed the needs of patients for activity even when confined to bed. Without negating the importance of activity, provision for rest also is an essential patient need.

The word "rest" has a very broad meaning: refreshing quiet of sleep; refreshing ease or inactivity after exertion; relief from anything that wearies, troubles or disturbs. In this chapter, rest connotes a condition in which the body is in a decreased state of activity with the consequent feeling of being refreshed. For some, rest occurs while leisurely enjoying a break in the day's activities. For others, rest may not come until sleep.

General Principles of Rest

The body requires periods of decreased activity in order to refresh itself. This principle, which recognizes rest as essential to well-being, becomes the basic guide to nursing practice in relation to rest.

Exactly why prolonged sleeplessness leads to ill health is not known; however, the fact remains that sleep deprivation does produce changes that can markedly alter physical and mental functioning. When in doubt, it is best that the nurse err on the side of safety and employ efforts to promote rest as a need essential to well-being.

Rest is more likely to occur under conditions of reduced stress. This principle can be stated in another way: stress and anxiety-producing situations tend to interfere with a person's ability to relax and to obtain sufficient rest for well-being. Illness and hospitalization are stress and anxiety-producing situations for nearly everyone. Hence, nursing measures should be directed toward relieving them as much as possible.

Periodicity and duration of rest vary among individuals. For no known reason, eight hours of sleep every night has been the accepted standard, despite obvious variance shown in the general population. Factors such as the person's physiologic metabolism, age, physical condition, type of work, amount and kind of exercise, and the like, can influence patterns of rest. In other words, there is no rigid formula concerning periodicity and duration of sleep. Of importance, however, is that each person follow a pattern of rest that will maintain his well-being.

Despite variations, some generalities can be stated. On the average, infants sleep from 18 to 20 hours each day. Growing children require from 12 to 14 hours of sleep. Adults average seven to nine hours. Those who are able to relax and rest easily, even while awake, often find that less sleep is needed, while others may find that more sleep is required in order to overcome fatigue. The sleep patterns of older persons vary as much as those of younger persons.

A large segment of our society is geared to working during the daytime hours and sleeping during night hours. However, night workers can sleep equally well during daytime hours once they become accustomed to this routine.

Evidence indicates that there are "larks" and "owls" among our population. The "larks" experience their greatest peaks of energy early in the morning and prefer an early bedtime hour. The opposite is true of the "owls." There is no indication that either one of these patterns is better than the other.

Persons who have excellent self-command may keep arduous schedules without fatigue. The astronauts demonstrated this ability to maintain and preserve strength by "commanding" themselves to periods of sleep whenever the opportunity was present.

Fatigue can be considered a protective mechanism of the body, nature's warning that sleep is necessary. Fatigue is normal; if ignored, it usually results in nervousness, restlessness and below-par functioning. However, chronic fatigue is abnormal and is often a symptom of illness. A person who complains of chronic fatigue should be advised to see his physician.

Sleep

The phenomenon of sleep remains a physiologic mystery. Its fundamental nature, mechanisms, and functions are as yet to be defined. That alterations in behavior occur after periods of sleeplessness is well established, even from personal experience. However, there seems to be a vital need for sleep for physiologic and psychologic well-being, even though the nature of this need has not been determined exactly.

Sleep is a state of relative unconsciousness, but the depth of unconsciousness is not uniform. During the different stages of sleep, various degrees of stimuli produce wakefulness. The depth of unconsciousness for the sensory organs also varies. For example, the depth is greatest for the sense of smell, which may explain why home fires gain headway unbeknownst to the sleeping occupants, who do not smell the smoke. The depth is least for pain and for hearing. This explains why patients often are wakeful, because pain frequently accompanies illness.

Research has indicated that there are, in effect, four stages of sleep. The first stage is light, and the subject can be awakened with relative ease. During each stage, sleep becomes deeper. During stage four, the sleeper is difficult to arouse. In the course of a prolonged sleeping period, it is believed that the individual experiences these four stages several times, going from stage four back to stage one, and so on. Following stage four, possibly as a portion of stage one again, sleepers go through a period known as REM, for a "Rapid Eye Movement" phase. This theory on stages of sleep casts into doubt the long-held opinion that the first hours of sleep are the most restful.

During REM, it has been observed that the eyes tend to dart back and forth, respirations increase, and the heart beat becomes more rapid and irregular. If persons are awakened during this phase, they almost invariably report that they have been dreaming. When persons report that they do not sleep well, even when appearing to be asleep, it is theorized that possibly sleep stages, and especially the REM phase, have been interrupted or altered for some reason. The quality of their sleep may indeed be poor. When dream deprivation occurs experimentally, that is, when persons are awakened during REM, the subjects become irritable and anxious. These same subjects, when allowed to sleep uninterrupted, experience more frequent REM periods, as if the body were trying to make up for losses. Irritability and inability to concentrate, often leading to poor judgment, usually can be observed with sleep deprivation. Relationships with other people also suffer. Depression is a common mental symptom and, in extreme cases, a person's ethical standards have been known to deteriorate. Symptoms of psychoses have appeared in rational people after prolonged sleep deprivation.

The question is often asked as to whether sleep "debts" can be repaid. Interestingly enough, it appears that a given number of hours of sleep loss can be repaid in much less time. Persons suffering from severe and prolonged sleep loss have been observed to be refreshed after as little as 10 to 15 hours of sleep.

Nursing Measures to Promote Rest

Unfortunately, a common complaint of patients is the inability to obtain sufficient rest in the hospital. Nursing will have failed unless concerted effort is expended to aid in meeting this important need.

Determining the Patient's History in Relation to Rest. Realizing that there are differences in rest patterns, the nurse can begin by determining the patient's usual routines. It can also be helpful to inquire about the patient's activities that have tended to promote sleep in the past. For the acutely ill, for children, and for the elderly, conferring with family members often is helpful.

Promoting Relaxation. To relax means to become less rigid, to slacken in effort and decrease tensions. One can relax without sleeping, but sleep rarely occurs until one is relaxed.

Relaxation is an individual matter. For some, purposeful effort may help. For example, a patient can be assisted to relax by having him take several deep breaths; on the last breath, encourage him to try to feel as limp as possible. Then, while the patient is in a comfortable position, instruct him to contract the muscles in his leg and then purposely allow the leg to go limp. Have him repeat this for the other leg, the gluteal muscles, each arm and shoulder, and the face, each time stressing that he must first purposely contract the muscles and then allow them to go limp. Gentle massage helps muscles to relax; therefore, massage of the back is often helpful in producing sleep.

Relieving monotony is in itself frequently relaxing. This is especially helpful to remember when caring for patients undergoing long convalescence. Diversional activities are discussed in Chapter 13.

Some people have a bedtime ritual that tends to aid relaxation and promote sleep. For some, having something to eat is a *must*. A cup of coffee may relax one person despite the presence of caffeine, a central nervous system stimulant. Other persons may prefer milk or tea. Reading, listening to the radio, or watching television are common before-sleep activities. Children display similar idiosyncracies. A favorite stuffed animal or blanket, or bed-rocking, are examples. Readiness for sleep is preceded by a personal hygiene routine for many persons—such as brushing the teeth, washing the hands and face, voiding, or taking a bath or shower.

There are no scientific explanations for bedtime rituals. The important thing is that they work for the persons using them. The wise nurse will be alert to the patient's bedtime rituals and make every effort to observe them as far as possible to aid in promoting relaxation and sleep.

Important for relaxation is a comfortable position in a comfortable bed. The bottom linen should be tight and clean. Upper linen, while secure, should allow freedom of movement and not exert pressure, especially over the legs and feet. Having the body in good alignment, as discussed in Chapter 20, is conducive to relaxation. For patients who must assume unusual positions because of their illness, ingenuity and skill are necessary in order to keep muscle strain and discomfort at a minimum. For example, the patient who must remain in the orthopneic position to aid breathing should be supported in a manner that relieves muscle strain, as with the use of a foot support, an armrest and possibly some support in the lumbar curve. Although most individuals relax best while lying down, other positions are not contraindicated.

Providing an Environment Conducive to Sleep. A quiet and darkened room, with privacy, is relaxing for nearly everyone. In a strange environment, unfamiliar noises—i.e., people walking or entering and leaving the room, and the closing of elevator doors—bring complaints from patients. Although some of these sources are difficult for the nurse to control, every effort should be made toward reducing disturbances to promote relaxation and sleep.

Undue stimulation of the temperature receptors also interferes with rest. The temperature of the room, the amount of ventilation, and the quantity of bed covering are a matter of individual choice, and the patient's wishes should be met whenever it is at all possible.

Alleviating Pain, Anxiety, Fear and Stress. One of the greatest detriments to relaxation and sleep is pain: often pain is a realistic complaint when illness is present. There are nursing measures, as well as pain-relieving medications, that will promote rest. Pain and measures to relieve it are discussed in Chapter 25.

The emotional reactions of anxiety, fear and stress, common when illness and hospitalization occur, were discussed in Chapter 9. The knowledge that these reactions interfere with rest is accepted as fact. Measures to alleviate them, as described in Chapter 9, are applicable to the discussion here.

Promoting Sleep in Children. The measures just described also apply to children. Approximately the same things interfere with rest in children as in adults. Emotional reactions are somewhat different to handle because most youngsters have not learned how to express fears and anxieties. Rather, they demonstrate these reactions by wakefulness, crying, irritability, and so on.

Picking up children, holding them securely, rocking them, and being readily available are measures that often appear to relieve their reactions to a strange environment and separation from parents. Also, leaving a night light near a frightened child often is helpful. A child's fears are very real to him, and respecting them will aid in helping to promote relaxation and sleep.

Insomnia. Difficulty in falling asleep, intermittent sleep, and/or early awakening from sleep describe *insomnia*. Usually, persons complaining of insomnia have been observed to sleep more than they report. But the condition can lead to such distress as to cause further wakefulness. Although there are some physical conditions that lead to wakefulness, insomnia usually results from over-stimulation by anxiety and stress. When a patient complains of being wakeful, the nurse should investigate further and take every step possible to aid in promoting relaxation and sleep. In severe cases, skilled psychological management may be necessary.

Drugs to Promote Sleep. Although drugs that promote sleep are studied more fully in pharmacology courses, the nurse's role in relation to their administration is worth mentioning at this time. Because no one enjoys restless, interrupted sleep and long periods of wakefulness, most patients accept a medication readily if they are anxious about how well they will sleep. Accepting a drug without a real need often starts patients off on habits that last long after hospitalization. Therefore, the nurse should attempt to promote sleep without the use of drugs whenever possible. If the patient is still unable to sleep, a medication should be offered. If the patient knows he can have a medication if necessary, often he will fall asleep naturally. The first Study Situation below suggests reading an article that describes how medications for sleep were reduced when other nursing measures were employed to promote relaxation and sleep.

Study Situations

1. In the following article, the author reports on several nursing studies, one involving sedation for sleep:

- Schwartz, D. R.: The value of small local nursing studies.

AMER. J. NURS., *66*:1327-1329, June, 1966. What measures did the author use to promote relaxation and sleep? What significance did she attach to the physician's bedtime visit? By what per cent was sedation reduced for these patients? While reading this article, study how the problem solving method, as described in Chapter 3, was used in this author's experiments.

2. For a more detailed description of REM, read the following article:

- Golub, S.: Rapid eye movement sleep. NURS. OUTLOOK, *15*:56-58, February, 1967.

What medical implications may REM sleep have, according to this author?

3. For the interested student of sleep, the following publication is recommended as a source of research findings in relation to sleep:

- Kety, S. S. *et al*, eds.: Sleep and Altered States of Consciousness. Research Publication of the Association for Research in Nervous and Mental Diseases, Volume 45, 591 p. Baltimore, Williams & Wilkins, 1967.

References

1. The Anatomy of Sleep. 135 p. Nutley, New Jersey, Roche Laboratories, 1966.
2. Beeson, P. B., and McDermott, W., eds., Cecil-Loeb Textbook of Medicine, ed. 12, pp. 1429-1432. Philadelphia, W. B. Saunders, 1967.
3. Dement, W. C.: Recent studies on the biological role of rapid eye movement sleep. AMER. J. PSYCHIAT., *122*:404-408, October, 1965.
4. Illingworth, R. S.: Sleep problems of the toddler. PRACTITIONER, *200*:345-350, March, 1968.
5. Narrow, B. W.: Rx rest is . . . AMER. J. NURS., *67*:1646-1649, August, 1967.
6. Snyder, F.: Progress in the new biology of dreaming. AMER. J. PSYCHIAT., *122*:377-391, October, 1965.

CHAPTER

24

Maintaining Fluid and Electrolyte Balance

Introduction

In her delightful book, *The Sea Around Us*, Rachel Carson indicated that as organisms came from the waters, they took with them a heritage from the sea that has been passed on to every succeeding generation. Interestingly enough, whatever man's origin, there are striking similarities between man's body fluid and the sea around us.

Within the last three decades or so, remarkable progress has been made in the knowledge of body fluids and their role in health and disease. We know that our very life depends on maintaining the proper amount of body fluid as well as maintaining the fluid's proper constituents and proper placement, each in relationship to the other. This balance is maintained by the process of homeostasis.

Fluid and electrolyte balance is affected by virtually all disease processes. For example, balance can be affected by conditions ranging from such common entities as vomiting, diarrhea and pyrexia to the more dramatic ones, such as diabetes mellitus, burns, surgical procedures and infectious processes. Therapeutic regimens also may upset fluid and electrolyte balance. For example, the use of diuretics and of some of the adrenal cortex hormones has been shown to upset this balance if not used judiciously. Special disease entities and their common therapeutic regimens are discussed in other texts. In this chapter, fundamental information necessary for administering intelligent nursing care to aid in the maintenance of fluid and electrolyte balance, without regard to specific clinical problems, will be presented.

If the nurse's responsibility in relation to fluid and electrolyte balance had to be spelled out in one word, the most appropriate one would no doubt be *observation*. Therefore, the nurse with a knowledge of fluid and electrolyte balance, of how imbalances occur, and of what symptoms characterize them is in a position to observe and to take action intelligently.

Definition of Terms

Fluids are present in two body spaces. There is fluid within each of our millions of body cells. This is referred to as *cellular* or *intracellular fluid.* All fluid outside of the cells is *extracellular fluid.* The extracellular fluid consists of fluid within the vascular system, called *intravascular fluid* or *plasma.* The fluid in which tissue cells are bathed is called *interstitial fluid.* All body fluid, intracellular and extracellular, contains electrolytes. However, the amount of fluid and the distribution of electrolytes differ considerably between intra- and extracellular fluid.

An *electrolyte* (sometimes called a salt or a mineral) is a substance capable of developing electrical charges when dissolved in water. *Cations* develop positive charges and include such electrolytes as calcium, sodium, potassium and magnesium. *Anions* develop negative charges and include electrolytes as chloride, bicarbonate, phosphate, sulfate, proteinate, carbonic and other organic acids. An *ion* is either a cation or an anion.

Each cell is nourished and gets rid of its wastes through the extracellular fluid. We know that the exchange of waste for nutrients, including electrolytes, is vital to life itself; but science has as yet to explain the basis for this exchange. However, it is known that the passage of water from intracellular to extracellular space, and vice versa, occurs by *osmosis.* Each cell is enclosed in a semipermeable membrane which allows easy passage of water back and forth. The membrane is more selective in allowing passage of other substances.

Water passes by osmosis from a less concentrated solution to a more concentrated one. When a body cell is placed in an isotonic solution (one having approximately the same concentration of electrolytes as the cell) the size and shape of the cell do not change because there is no gain or loss of water in the cell. If placed in a hypertonic solution (one having greater concentration than the intracellular fluid) water moves out of the cell, causing it to shrivel and become smaller. In a hypotonic solution (one having less concentration than intracellular fluid) the cell absorbs water, swells, and eventually bursts. This is called *hemolysis.* Knowledge of the osmotic process is important when, for example, the physician chooses to give intravenous fluids. Distilled water is rarely given intravenously for fear of creating hypotonicity of plasma that will cause blood cells to swell and burst.

The unit of measure to describe body fluid is the *milliliter,* abbreviated ml. Each milliliter is 1/1,000 of a liter. It is roughly equivalent to a cubic centimeter, abbreviated c.c.

The unit of measure to describe an electrolyte is a *milliequivalent,* abbreviated mEq. From chemistry one recalls that the atomic weight of an ion does not necessarily describe its chemical power. The unit of chemical power of any ion is equivalent to the chemical power of one mg. of hydrogen. For example, one sodium ion carries one positive charge while calcium carries two. In terms of chemical power, a calcium ion can be said to be twice as strong as a sodium ion, weight being no factor. A chloride ion has one negative charge; it takes two chloride ions to combine with one calcium ion to form a molecule, while it takes only one sodium ion to combine with a chloride ion. Almost any cation can unite with any anion to form a molecule, and one mEq of any cation is equivalent chemically to one mEq of any anion. The concept of milliequivalents is used to express chemical activity on an equal basis. It is like the common denominator concept in mathematics. Using milliequivalents as a unit of measure eliminates the need for calculations and conversions when electrolyte therapy is indicated.

Fluid and Electrolyte Balance

Healthy human beings maintain fluid and electrolyte balance automatically. The task is indeed a formidable one. We ingest a wide variety of materials of various quantities, often unmatched with bodily needs, and dispose of wastes and excesses as a result of intricate chemical mechanisms, to maintain a relatively small range of normality. What is normality?

The average total body fluid in adults comprises approximately 60 per cent of body weight, a little less in females than males. Approximately one-third is extracellular fluid. About one-quarter of the extracellular fluid is intravascular and three-fourths is interstitial fluid. Approximately two-thirds of the body fluid is cellular fluid.

In infants, total body fluid comprises about 75 per cent of body weight, with approximately three-fifths being intracellular and two-fifths being extracellular. Because infants have a higher basal metabolism rate, a proportionately greater body surface, and a larger percentage of body fluid than the adult, they suffer from fluid deficits more quickly than older persons. Also, infants normally require relatively greater fluid intake in proportion to body weight than do adults.

The electrolyte composition of body fluids shows marked mEq/L. variations in terms of the location of the fluid. Normal body secretions also have marked variations in terms of electrolyte content. Figure 24-1 illustrates these statements.

Fluid and electrolyte balance is maintained by mechanisms that trigger the body to rid itself of excesses and indiscretions in fluid and electrolyte ingestion and to conserve those that are essential for health. These mechanisms are homeostatic in that they function constantly and in a fantastically intricate manner to maintain a balance that is amazingly narrow in range.

The lungs are essential for homeostasis.

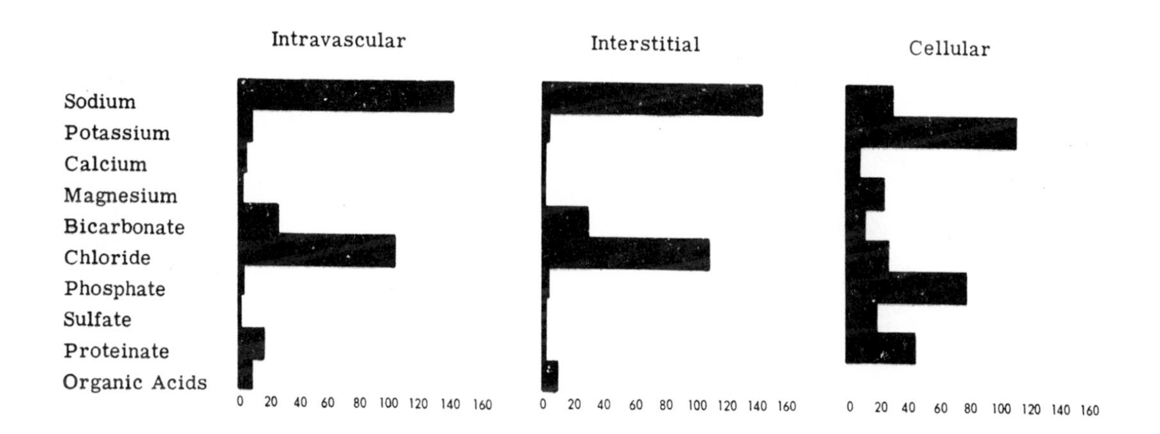

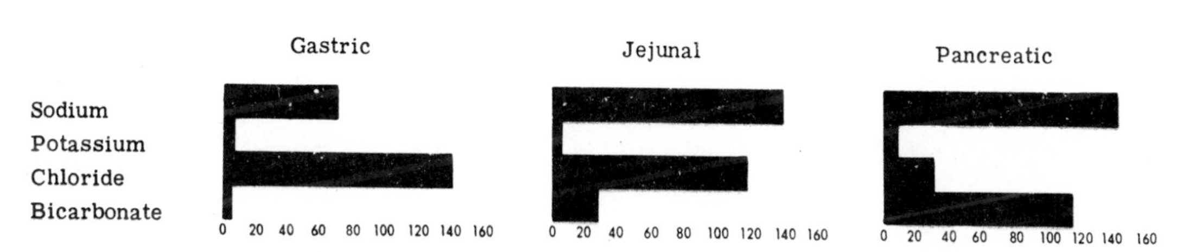

FIG. 24-1. Electrolyte composition of intravascular, interstitial, cellular and transcellular fluids. (From A Guide to Parental Fluid Therapy, Glendale, California, McGaw Laboratories, Inc., 1963.)

Table 7. Various fluid and electrolyte disturbances, common symptoms and problems likely to produce them*

Clinical Entity	Common Symptoms	Examples of Problems Likely to Lead to Disturbance
Extracellular fluid volume deficit	Dry skin and mucous membranes Scanty urine Weight loss Lassitude	Insufficient water intake Vomiting Diarrhea Pyrexia Excessive perspiration
Extracellular fluid volume excess	Puffy eyelids Shortness of breath Dyspnea Moist rales Edema Weight gain Bounding pulse Hypertension	Excessive ingestion or injection of fluids with sodium chloride or sodium bicarbonate Renal malfunction Congestive heart failure disease
Sodium deficit	Apprehension Abdominal cramps Diarrhea Rapid weak pulse Hypotension Convulsions Depressed body temperature	Excessive perspiration and drinking water Gastrointestinal suction and drinking water Repeated use of water enemas Infusions without sodium chloride Irrigation of Levin tube with distilled water
Sodium excess	Dry sticky mucous membrane Scanty urine Thirst Flushed skin Psychic excitement Firm tissue turgor Elevated body temperature	Inadequate water intake and excessive sodium chloride intake Diarrhea Pyrexia with rapid breathing
Potassium deficit	Weak and faint pulse Falling blood pressure Malaise Anorexia; vomiting Distention Soft, flabby musculature	Diarrhea Ulcerative colitis Burns Starvation diet Diuretic administration Low sodium diet
Potassium excess	Nausea Irritability General weakness Scanty to no urine Intestinal colic Diarrhea Slow pulse rate	Burns Crushing injuries Kidney disease Excessive infusion of potassium
Calcium deficit	Tingling of fingers Muscle cramps Tetany Convulsions	Sprue Hypoactive thyroid glands Excessive infusion of citrated blood Subcutaneous infections—massive Peritonitis Removal of parathyroid glands
Calcium excess	Relaxed musculature Flank pains Kidney stones Deep bone pains, as "shin splints"	Prolonged bed rest Tumor-parathyroid gland Excessive Vitamin D intake Overactivity of parathyroid glands

Table 7. Various fluid and electrolyte disturbances, common symptoms and problems likely to produce them* (Continued)

Clinical Entity	Common Symptoms	Examples of Problems Likely to Lead to Disturbance
Primary base bicarbonate deficit (metabolic acidosis)	Disorientation-stupor Shortness of breath Deep rapid breathing Unconsciousness when severe	Decreased food intake Systemic infections Renal insufficiency Diabetes mellitus
Primary base bicarbonate excess (metabolic alkalosis)	Depressed shallow respirations Hypertonic musculature Tetany	Vomiting Excessive ingestion of alkalies Gastric suction Adrenal cortex hormone administration
Primary carbonic acid deficit (respiratory alkalosis)	Unconsciousness Deep rapid breathing Tetany	Deep rapid breathing Deliberate over-breathing Oxygen lack Fever Extreme emotion Salicylate intoxication
Primary carbonic acid excess (respiratory acidosis)	Disorientation Respiratory embarrassment Coma Weakness	Pneumonia Emphysema Respiratory suppression Asthma Respiratory obstruction
Protein deficit	Depression Anorexia Fatigue Pallor Weight loss Loss of muscle tone	Hemorrhage Trauma Wounds or ulcers Burns Inadequate protein intake
Magnesium deficit	Disorientation-hallucinations Hypertension Slow pulse rate Tremors Hyperactive deep reflexes Convulsions	Chronic alcoholism Vomiting Diarrhea Impaired intestional absorption Enterostomy drainage
Plasma to interstitial fluid shift	Slow, weak to absent pulse Pallor Cold extremities Hypotension Unconsciousness	Burns Massive crushing injuries Intestinal obstruction Perforated peptic ulcer
Interstitial fluid to plasma shift	Early—hypertension Late—hypotension Air hunger Moist rales Bounding pulse Engorgement—peripheral veins Pallor Weakness	Excessive infusion of hypertonic solutions Compensation following hemorrhage Recovery phase of plasma to interstitial fluid shift

* Adapted from: Metheny, N. M., and Snively, W. G.: Nurses' Handbook of Fluid Balance. Philadelphia, J. B. Lippincott, 1967.

They are responsible for maintaining proper oxygen and carbon dioxide levels in the blood. Hence, they play an important role in balancing the acid and alkali levels of the body fluids.

The kidneys have often been referred to as the body's master chemists. Their cells eliminate a variety of undesirable or excess amounts of chemicals and preserve those chemicals for which the body has a need.

The kidneys and lungs function in harmony to preserve a very delicate acid-alkaline balance in the body. Normally the pH level of the blood serum is 7.4, slightly alkaline. To illustrate its critical nature, as well as the marked coordination of body functions, a variation of .4 of a pH unit in either direction in the blood serum can be fatal!

Certain hormones from the pituitary, parathyroid, and adrenal glands play a role in fluid and electrolyte balance. Fortunately, their malfunction is relatively rare. But should disease rob them of proper functioning, imbalance will be present. Kidney function in particular is influenced by hormones from these glands.

Normally, there is little electrolyte loss through the skin. Normal perspiration accounts for sufficiently small losses as to have little significance when proper fluid intake is maintained.

How is fluid balance upheld? The same body mechanisms maintaining electrolyte balance function in relation to water balance. Normally we ingest approximately 2,200 c.c. of fluid per day. About 1,200 c.c. derives from liquids, and about 1,000 c.c. is ingested as part of our food content. In addition, approximately 300 c.c. a day results from the process of oxidation of foodstuffs within our body. Balance is normally maintained by escape of fluids from the large intestine, the lungs, the skin and the kidneys; the loss is approximately 100 c.c., 500 c.c., 500 c.c., and 1,400 c.c., respectively, each day. Not only is the total amount of body fluid kept remarkably constant but so also is its placement, intra- and extracellularly.

The body takes in electrolytes and fluids with everything we eat and drink. Water (except distilled) contains electrolytes. Food is rich in electrolytes as well as in proteins, fats, carbohydrates, vitamins and water. As mentioned, water also becomes available through the normal chemical process of digestion.

From this discussion, this basic principle can be stated:

In health, water and electrolyte gains and losses are maintained in balance and in harmony with bodily needs.

Fluid and Electrolyte Imbalance

Imbalances in normal fluid and electrolyte needs result from abnormal differences between gains and losses of fluids and electrolytes. This basic principle aids in diagnosing fluid and electrolyte disturbances as well as in guiding the treatment of them.

One authoritative source on the subject approached the study of fluid and electrolyte imbalances through 16 clinical entities. The classification is as follows[4]:

- A deficit or an excess in volume of fluid
- A deficit or excess in sodium, potassium, calcium, base bicarbonate or carbonic acid concentration
- A deficit in magnesium or protein concentration
- Changes in the position of fluid (shift from plasma to interstitial space or from interstitial space to plasma).

Each of these has its own clinical picture, symptoms, and laboratory findings. It is more frequent to have fluid and electrolyte disturbances in combinations or in a series of successions. But an understanding of the single entities is basic.

Common Symptoms of Fluid and Electrolyte Imbalances. Table 7 describes some of the more characteristic symptoms of the various fluid and electrolyte imbalances. In addition, examples of entities that are likely to produce the disturbances are given.

Attention is called in particular to the first two entries in Table 7: fluid deficit and fluid excess. Fluid deficit presents a group of symptoms, as given in the table, that is frequently referred to as *dehydration*. This is among the most common of fluid disturbances and the nurse will want to be on the alert for its symptoms in all of her patient care. Excess fluid in interstitial spaces leads to *edema*, as Table 7 indicates. This too is a common entity and requires prompt attention. The significance and treatment of edema usually is discussed more fully in clinical courses in nursing.

Implications for Nursing

Observation. The point was made earlier that observation is an essential nursing function in helping to maintain fluid and electrolyte balance. Hopefully, the previous discussion in this chapter has given the nurse many important clues concerning balance, how the body maintains it, and signs of disturbances. Some of the suggestions in Chapter 17 concerning observation also will assist.

There is a large variety of other signs indicative of fluid and electrolyte imbalance for which the nurse will want to be on the alert. A few are given here; others are discussed in clinical texts.

When the hands are elevated, the peripheral veins in them empty quickly. In the dependent position, the opposite phenomenon occurs in a matter of a few seconds. Disturbances in the intravascular fluid volume alter these signs. Increased volume increases the amount of time needed to empty the veins and decreased volume increases the amount of time needed to distend them. Poor skin turgor and dry oral mucous membrane (when not caused by mouth breathing) are symptoms of dehydration. Speech disturbances may indicate imbalances. For example, hoarseness is one sign of extracellular fluid excess. Excess fatigue, drawn or puffy facial expressions, weakness or cramping of muscles, anorexia, unusual thirst and marked weight loss or gain (5 to 10 per cent or more) are all symptoms of the apparent presence of fluid and electrolyte disturbances.

Still another significant observation is the character and volume of urine. The patient's state of hydration can be determined by the specific gravity of the urine. If there is no renal failure present, a high specific gravity indicates water deficit; a low specific gravity indicates the possibility of over-hydration.

Normally, variations in the pH level of urine are rather wide. Also, some kinds of drug therapy can alter the pH. But certain problems of illness that predispose to fluid and electrolyte disturbances may alter the pH level of urine. For example, the pH level can be expected to be low in diabetic acidosis. Severe vomiting may lead to alkalosis and alkaline urine. Many factors influence the volume of urinary output, such as amount of fluid intake, kidney function, the body's need for fluid, age, and so on. But any marked change in relation to what might be expected to be normal under whatever circumstances exist suggests imbalance. In order to make judgments concerning volume changes, an accurate measurement of all fluid intake and output is essential. The procedure was discussed in Chapter 22.

The Patient's History. In addition to making observations, the nurse will want to be familiar with the patient's illness, the history of his illness, and the medical plan for therapy, any one, or any combination, of which may predispose to fluid and electrolyte imbalance, if symptoms are not already present. Because balance is maintained normally when compatibility exists between the intake of fluids and electrolytes on one hand and their ouput on the other, anything that upsets the scale on either side acts as a warning. For example, typical questions for which the nurse seeks answers are these: Has the patient's normal food and fluid intake been influenced by his illness? If so, for how long? Have there been restrictions for any reason on what he could eat and drink? Has there been any abnormal loss of body fluids? What particular body fluid is involved? What is the patient's intake and output of fluids? Once these questions are answered, the nurse can better judge any predisposition to fluid and electrolyte disturbances and plan nursing care accordingly.

Preventive Measures. Once the history is known, the next step concerns prevention of fluid and electrolyte imbalance. Every measure, nursing as well as medical, is ordinarily taken to aid in maintaining balance in the first place. For example, drugs are ordered to handle many infectious processes that predispose to imbalance, before trouble begins. Every effort is made to encourage patients to take adequate nourishment when lack of appetite is a problem. Nursing measures were discussed in Chapter 18. Fluid intake should be encouraged or guarded, depending on the circumstances. Efforts are taken, as described in Chapter 19, to avoid the development of decubitus ulcers, which, if allowed to develop, can result in exuding ulcers that may upset balance. The inactivity of bed rest often accompanying illness may result in such disturbances as an increased excretion of nitrogen. Hence, high protein diets often are prescribed for patients requiring prolonged bed rest. Calcium is mobilized from the matrix of bones during long periods in bed and excreted through the kidneys. Hence, nursing measures, such as were discussed in Chapter 20, are used to promote activity to the greatest extent possible. Additional measures are discussed in the next chapter, such as, for example, when pyrexia is present.

Once imbalance occurs, the nurse will observe common symptoms as described earlier. The reader's attention is called in particular to deviations in the vital signs, given in Table 7. Personnel other than nurses often assist in obtaining vital signs. When fluid and electrolyte balance is at stake, the nurse is encouraged to make her own observations.

Corrective Measures. When fluid and electrolyte disturbances are present, action must be taken to correct them. For example, an exuding decubitus ulcer may require surgery in order to prevent continued loss of essential fluid and electrolytes. A patient unable to take nourishment by mouth may need gastric gavage, to be discussed further in Chapter 33. Or patients with certain heart conditions may require medications to assist the body in eliminating excessive retained fluid. The nurse is responsible for observing the results of such therapy and assisting with its administration if necessary.

A relatively common form of therapy for handling fluid and electrolyte disturbances is the use of various solutions injected intravenously or in some cases, subcutaneously (interstitially). Although the physician is responsible for ordering the proper kind of solution and the amount to be used, the nurse is responsible for observing the therapy. Hence she is in a better position if she familiarizes herself with the solutions commonly used in the agency in which she is studying or working.

The variety of solutions on the market is almost without limit. There are maintenance solutions containing a multitude of electrolytes in the proportion normally found in the body. There are replacement solutions with electrolyte content similar to fluids being lost. Solutions with electrolyte content similar to blood plasma are available. There are isotonic, hypertonic and hypotonic solutions. In some agencies, solutions are tailor-made to meet a particular patient's requirements. Should the nurse have questions concerning the selection of a particular solution, two good sources usually are readily available. The physician in charge of the therapy generally is glad to explain his selection. The pharmaceutical companies preparing the solution have excellent literature explaining the nature and common indications of each.

There are several ways in which the amount of fluid is calculated. Although age and weight are important, either one in itself rarely gives sufficient knowledge to calculate amount. It is easy to see that a 40-year-old man weighing 200 pounds requires quite different amounts from a 40-year-old woman weighing 120 pounds. A combination of weight and age is often used as a guide.

Using the patient's weight to estimate his body surface area in square meters also is common. Charts that list estimates of surface area in relation to weight are available, although calculations still are necessary when the patient's body build deviates considerably from the average for his age.

Whatever method is used in the agency—and the nurse will want to be familiar with it—another factor influences the physician's decision always and that is the patient's clinical picture. A patient suffering from severe depletion or excess of fluids and/or electrolytes has needs different from one with moderate or mild imbalance. The amount is still different from that needed by a patient with no indication of imbalance, who is placed on maintenance dosages because a condition exists that without care may lead to disturbances.

The nurse's role in relation to assisting with the administration of parenteral fluids is discussed further in Chapter 29.

Study Situations

1. In the article given below, the author develops the idea that an understanding of the patient's situation comes with an understanding of the rationale of his illness. This understanding in turn leads to appropriate nursing action. On page 2206 of the article, note the facts about Mr. A. V. that became the basis for appropriate nursing action. Add to the plan the author gives and describe nursing care that would aid in maintaining fluid and electrolyte balance for Mr. A. V.

- Donovan, C.: Making theory work in patient care.
  AMER. J. NURS., *66*:2204-2206, October, 1966.

2. The following article is suggested for study:

- Abbey, J. C.: Nursing observations of fluid imbalance.
  NURS. CLIN. N. AMER., *3*:77-86, March, 1968.

What does this author suggest as the single most valuable observation for aiding the determination of fluid and electrolyte changes in the patient? The hazards of giving a patient ice chips when hemorrhage has occurred can change fluid balance. What substitute for ice chips does the author suggest?

References

1. Burgess, R. E.: Fluids and electrolytes. AMER. J. NURS., *65*:90-95, October, 1965.
2. DeVeber, G. A.: Fluid and electrolyte problems in the postoperative period. NURS. CLIN. N. AMER., *1*:275-284, June, 1966.
3. A Guide to Parental Fluid Therapy, 96 p. Glendale, California, McGaw Laboratories, Inc., 1963.
4. Metheny, N. M., and Snively, W. D. Jr.: Nurses' Handbook of Fluid Balance, 279 p. Philadelphia, Lippincott, 1967.
5. Potassium imbalance. Programmed Instruction. AMER. J. NURS., *67*:343-366, February, 1967.
6. Snively, W. D. Jr.: Toward a better understanding of body fluid disturbances. NURS. FORUM, *3*:60-77, #1, 1964.
7. Statland, H.: Fluid and Electrolytes in Practice. ed. 3, 329 p. Philadelphia, Lippincott, 1963.

CHAPTER 25

Managing Common Problems of Illness

COMMON DISTURBANCES OF ELIMINATION FROM THE INTESTINAL TRACT

Constipation

Constipation is defined as the passage of unduly dry, hard stools. This definition, it will be noted, makes no mention of frequency. Some persons may be constipated and yet have a daily bowel movement, while others who regularly defecate no more than three times a week are not constipated. The habits of elimination vary exceedingly among healthy persons. Therefore, defining constipation on the basis of frequency of evacuation is meaningless until careful comparisons are made with the person's usual habits.

Constipation is among the commonest and oldest of all medical complaints. It is found in all cultural, economic, and age groups. There are references to laxatives in the Bible and anthropologic investigations suggest the use of enemas even before recorded time. Interestingly enough, many ancient methods for treating constipation are very similar to those used today.

Common Causes of Constipation. Certain organic diseases cause constipation. Other factors causing it require attention once the physician has ruled out organic disease.

When no pathologic changes are involved, a common cause of constipation is the result of poor elimination habits. If the desire for defecation is ignored repeatedly, the feces become hard and dry because of increased water absorption. In addition, the colon becomes insensitive to normal chemical and mechanical stimulation, and eventually the stool in the rectum is no longer sufficient to stimulate the defecation reflex. Neglecting to observe the normal desire for defecation may result from carelessness, occupational demands, the stress of modern life, and, in children, the reluctance to interrupt play.

Many patients resort to the use of laxatives and cathartics which, by either chemical or mechanical means, increase stimulation for muscle contraction. In the habitual use of these the body needs ever larger doses before the urge to defecate becomes apparent.

Certain types of diets predispose to constipation. A diet that is low in roughage often leaves so little residue that the fecal mass is small in amount and becomes dry before sufficient quantity is present to stimulate the defecation reflex. Increasing the bulk of the diet with foods such as fresh fruits and vegetables, bran, etc., is often sufficient for relief. Lack of sufficient fluid intake is also a cause of constipation.

Investigations indicate that the colon in some individuals absorbs an unusually high percentage of water from the feces, and constipation results. For these persons, increased fluid intake often is the answer. If a bland diet is prescribed for medical reasons, the physician may recommend a medication for the patient to counteract constipation. Certain drugs, such as iron preparations, may be constipating for some persons.

Emotions, as tension, may cause the gastrointestinal tract to become spastic, and fecal content is not moved along the large intestine sufficiently well. The importance of relaxation to aid defecation has been mentioned, and relief is often obtained as the person learns to assume a way of life that allows time for relaxation. Constipation due to spasticity usually is referred to as *hypertonic* or *spastic constipation.*

Authorities differ in opinion concerning *atonic constipation* or constipation that is due to an abnormally sluggish and "lazy" colon. Some state that the condition is doubtful, since the colon and the rectum do not become too weak to propel feces. Others believe that the colon does become too weak to function, especially when debilitating chronic illness, emaciation or prolonged habitual use of laxatives is present.

In addition to the hard, dry stool, the nurse will observe that some persons who are constipated complain of headache, malaise, anorexia, foul breath, furred tongue and lethargy. It generally is agreed that these symptoms probably are reflex in nature and are due to the increased pressure in the lower colon. Relief is usually rapid following a bowel movement. These symptoms of constipation have also been produced experimentally by packing the rectum with cotton. Therefore, the general belief that poisons are being absorbed when constipation is present is unfounded.

When constipation is not due to pathologic changes, the nurse can help the patient to understand some of the ways in which the situation can be corrected, as by establishing habit patterns of elimination, increasing fluid intake, eating high-roughage foods and increasing physical activity. Also, the nurse can assist by teaching the patient the importance of establishing an evacuation habit. One suggestion is that the patient go to the bathroom regularly, an hour or so after a meal, and remain there for a while until the defecation urge appears. Distractions, such as reading, are helpful during this period to aid in reducing anxiety. It takes time to develop an evacuation habit just as it takes time to overcome the one that was present originally. But success has been observed among patients whose cooperation has been obtained.

Mr. Bartoni is an example of a person with a normal habit that was interrupted by bed rest. He was distressed about his constipation, a problem he said he had never had previously. He was sure that it was because he was in traction and could not get to the bathroom. In talking with him, the nurses learned that he arose every day at 5:30 A.M. and always had a bowel movement immediately after breakfast.

He was also awake every day in the hospital at 5:30. However, there was no breakfast until 8 or 8:15 A.M. In talking about it a bit more they suggested that he try having a glass of water and possibly some fruit when he awakened. The first morning did not yield results, but his desire to help himself gave him confidence that it would work. In a short time his former habit had been re-established.

Common Therapeutic Measures to Relieve Intestinal Tract Disturbances

In some instances, the physician asks the nurse to administer certain therapeutic measures when constipation is present.

Suppositories

A suppository is a small solid, so shaped that it is easy to insert into the rectum; it melts at body temperature. Since a certain amount of absorption can take place in the large colon, some medications for systemic effect can be given by a suppository. However, the most frequent use of the suppository is to aid in stimulating peristalsis and defecation. When effective, results are obtained usually within 15 to 30 minutes, but it could be as long as an hour.

A variety of suppositories is available. Some act as fecal softeners, others have direct action on the nerve endings in the mucosa, and some liberate carbon dioxide when moistened. Bland white soap also can be cut and shaped into the form of a suppository. The physician orders the type to be used, his selection being based to a large extent on the observations reported to him. When constipation or an impaction is present, the use of suppositories is often a prophylactic measure until the causes are acted upon.

Suppositories are helpful in a program to aid a patient in regaining good evacuation habits. A procedure which has been found to be satisfactory is to insert one or two suppositories one-half hour before a meal. Since the intake of fluids and food usually results in a peristaltic action, it is more common to have the urge to defecate after meals.

The literature indicates that suppositories having a direct stimulating effect on the rectum (such as Dulcolax) are more effective than glycerin. Carbon dioxide suppositories also have been found favorable. When moistened, these suppositories liberate about 200 cc. of the gas, and this causes distention, thus producing stimulation and the evacuation impulses.

To be most effective, the suppository should be introduced beyond the internal sphincter of the anal canal. To reduce friction, lubricate the suppository before inserting it. A finger cot or a glove is used to protect the finger when inserting the suppository. If the patient breathes through the mouth while the suppository is being inserted, the anal sphincter is said to be more relaxed.

Some patients are able to insert suppositories for themselves. The nurse should establish whether the patient has an understanding of the correct procedure since incorrect insertion will not produce the desired results.

Enemas

An enema* introduces a solution into the large intestine. A cleansing enema is frequently ordered when constipation is present for emptying the rectum and lower colon. However, there are purposes other than cleansing for giving an enema. For the sake of convenience, enemas for whatever use are discussed here because the procedure is similar, regardless of purpose.

Classification of Enemas and Solutions Used. Enemas are best classified in relation to their purpose and the following discussion will consider them accordingly.

Purgative Enema. Solution introduced into the rectum for the purpose of aiding in the expulsion of fecal contents is referred to as a purgative enema. A variety of solutions can be used, such as soap solution, physiologic saline, tap water and cottonseed, mineral or olive oil or hypertonic solutions.

Soap solution, saline and tap water enemas usually are prepared in large quantities —500 to 1,500 cc.—and a sufficient amount is given to stimulate peristalsis to help evacuate the colon. Results are expected immediately to within 15 minutes.

The oils are prepared in smaller amounts —150 to 200 cc.—so that the patient is able to retain the amount given. The oils act to soften, lubricate and distend the feces in the colon. Oil enemas vary widely in the length of time in which they are effective, since usually they are administered to severely constipated patients. It is not uncommon for an oil enema to be followed by a soap solution, tap water or saline enema after several hours if an evacuation does not result from the oil enema.

Soap solutions can be made by dissolving a small amount of a bland white soap or castile soap in the water. Bar soap that has been used previously is not recommended because it has been found that these bars often harbor organisms. A safer and more nearly accurate method of obtaining the proper soap concentration is to use the prepacked soap solution for enemas. The purpose of the soap is to aid in stimulating peristalsis by chemical irritation of the mucous membrane. Too much soap produces over-irritation of the membrane of the colon, as do strong soaps. Introducing pieces or lumps of soap into the colon should be avoided. Over-irritation causes the mucous membrane to become engorged and reddened, and the mucus is thinned to ineffectiveness. For this reason, many proctologists discourage the use of soap for enemas, particularly for patients having known or suspected rectal pathologic changes or for patients being prepared for rectal examinations.

While the soap solution enema requires caution and understanding in its preparation, tap water also must be administered cautiously to infants or to adults who have altered kidney or cardiac reserve. If a large quantity of hypotonic solution is absorbed through repeated enemas, fluid and electrolyte balance may be altered and blood volume increased. This reaction is usually called water intoxication, and symptoms include weakness, sweating, pallor, vomiting, cough or dizziness. Because of such reactions, infrequent though they may be, it is felt that saline is the solution of choice when enemas must be repeated until the return contains no formed feces.

The commercially prepared, disposable enema units contain hypertonic solution, usually four ounces, or 120 cc. This solution causes very little irritation to the mucosa of the colon, since it acts to withdraw fluid from the body by osmosis, thus creating fluid bulk in the colon. The bulk, in turn, stimulates peristalsis, and evacuation of the lower colon results. The administration is simple, results are obtained readily within two to seven minutes, and evacuation of the colon is good. In many agencies, it has become the method of choice for preparation for examination of the rectum with a proctoscope or for x-ray visualization of the rectum by the barium enema. It is less fatiguing and distressing to the patient.

Disposable units of hypertonic solution have been very successful for patients unable to retain the usual large quantity enema. For patients having anal incontinence or

* The plural of enema is enemas or enemata.

fecal impactions, this type of enema is good. It produces evacuation without oral catharsis and eliminates distressing attempts at trying to introduce large quantities of fluid into the colon. It is also effective for patients who are immobilized in casts or traction and cannot assume a sitting position.

Carminative Enema. Solution introduced into the colon for the purpose of stimulating peristalsis to aid in the expulsion of flatus is referred to as a carminative enema. Although there are many medications that can help stimulate peristalsis, solutions directly in contact with the lower colon often prove to be more effective. Solutions most commonly used are milk and molasses, turpentine solution and combinations of magnesium sulfate, glycerin and water.

Milk and molasses solutions usually are prepared in equal parts—commonly 250 cc. of each. The action of this solution results from several factors working in combination or individually. The molasses, an end product of the preparation of sugar, contains invert sugar which acts as an irritant to the intestinal mucosa. An additional benefit is derived from the fact that the molasses, held in milk as a suspension, is a viscid solution and adheres to the mucosa, thus serving to apply heat more intensely. The application of heat to the nerve plexuses in the mucosa helps to stimulate peristalsis. It is best if the patient is able to retain a milk and molasses enema for as long as possible before expelling it.

A solution of magnesium sulfate, glycerin and water frequently is referred to as a one-two-three enema, because the ingredients are prepared in those proportions: 30 cc. of 50 per cent magnesium sulfate solution, 60 cc. of glycerin and 90 cc. of water. This combination acts to irritate the mucosa and to withdraw fluid from the blood and the tissues, thereby distending the colon and aiding in stimulating peristalsis.

Turpentine may be added to soap solution to help produce a carminative effect. The usual amounts for this combination are four cc. of turpentine and 500 cc. of a soap solution. The turpentine must be mixed thoroughly in the solution since it is not soluble in water and is irritating to the mucosa when it comes in contact with it.

Anthelmintic Enema. An anthelmintic aids in the destruction of intestinal parasites. Oral medications for intestinal infestation are effective, and rectal instillations for local effect are used less frequently. However, there are still instances when anthelmintic enemas are used—for example, when the patient has liver damage or some other organic disease which would make it unsafe to administer an anthelmintic orally. Anthelmintic enemas usually are administered as retention enemas.

Emollient Enema. A solution used to protect or soothe the mucous membrane of the colon is referred to as an emollient enema. The protective agents are usually fats, oils or fat-soluble substances. Those most frequently used are the vegetable oils, such as olive or cottonseed oil. Because of the purpose, emollient enemas are to be retained.

Medicated Enema. On occasion, when it is impossible to give a patient a medication for systemic effect by any other route, instillation into the rectum offers a possibility. Some absorption does take place in the colon, but not to the same degree for all medications. Medications most likely to be administered rectally are those which produce sedation, such as paraldehyde and chloral hydrate. Since most drugs may be irritating to the mucous membrane and thus stimulate the desire to expel them, some vehicle is used to aid in the administration of the drug. Saline and oil are used commonly. It is desirable to use only enough of the vehicle to help to instill the drug so that there is the least possibility of stimulating the defecation impulse. The rapidity with which certain medications can be absorbed is demonstrated clearly by some types of anesthesia administered via this route.

Nutritive Enema. In some few instances, it may become necessary to introduce solutions into the rectum for the primary purpose of supplying nutrition to the patient. The solution most likely to be used is dextrose in varying concentrations. Because of the selective absorption that takes place in the colon, adequate nourishment via this method is impossible.

Rectal Instillations as Emergency Measures. On rare occasions patients may need to be given fluids via the rectum to help sustain them until better means can be utilized. The solutions most likely to be administered are saline or coffee. The saline is used for the patient who has suffered fluid and electrolyte loss. The coffee is more likely to be used if the patient is suffering from shock or severe depression. Instillation of such fluids may be managed so that they are administered in small amounts over a long period of time; therefore, the patient is able to retain them.

The procedure for instilling fluids via the rectum by a drip method is usually referred to as *proctoclysis.* A quantity of fluid can be prepared, using equipment similar to the can method for giving an enema (see p. 276). The rate of flow of the solution is controlled by a clamp. The rate of flow is determined by the rate of absorption. If the fluid is not being absorbed, usually the patient will expel it. Since the drug hyaluronidase, which increases the permeability of the cell membrane, has been available, administration of fluids subcutaneously has been enhanced. Administration of fluids via the recutm is less common.

Factors Guiding the Preparation of Equipment and Solution for Enemas: Size of the Rectal Tube. A rubber or pliable plastic rectal tube is the best means for introducing fluid into the colon. It is flexible, it conforms to the shape of the rectum and the colon, and, if introduced properly, there is little likelihood of damaging the mucosa.

The larger the lumen of the rectal tube, the greater the stimulation of the anal sphincters. This is to be desired if the purpose in giving the enema is to aid in emptying the colon. If the purpose is to introduce a solution which is to be retained, a smaller size rectal tube should be used.

The larger the lumen of the rectal tube, the faster the solution will flow, if the head

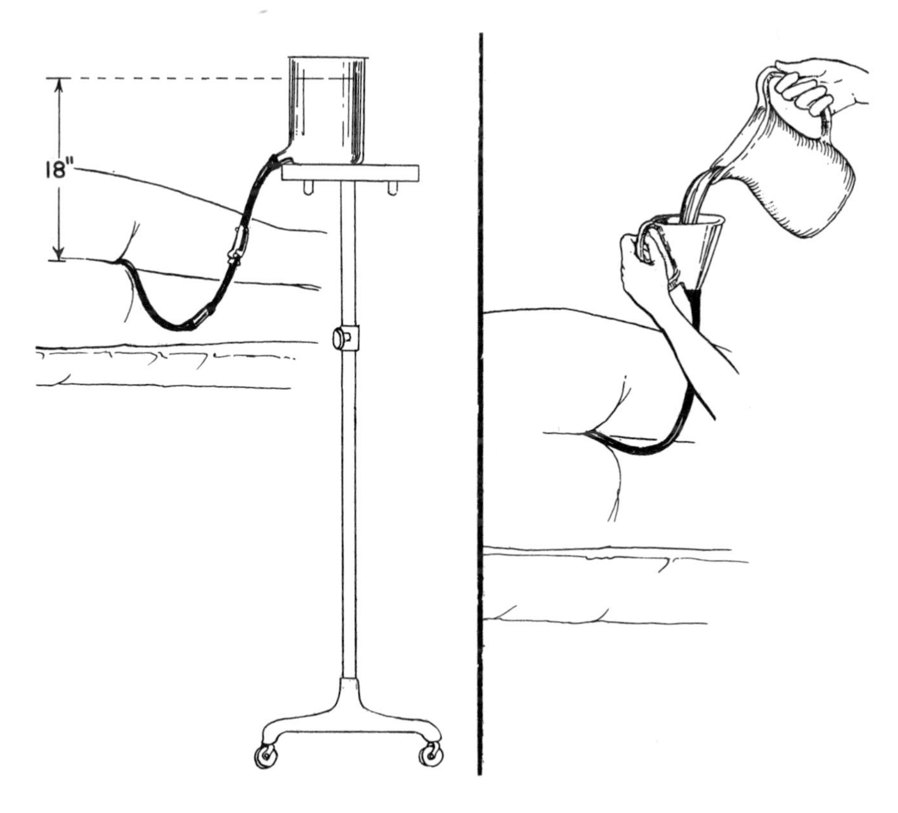

FIG. 25-1. (Left). Position of equipment for administering an enema using the can method.

FIG. 25-2. (Right). Position of equipment for administering an enema using the funnel method.

or the upper level of the fluid to be introduced is held at the same level. Since a small-sized rectal tube is used for a retention enema because it is less stimulating to the sphincters, the height of the solution to be introduced should be such that *the solution is just able to flow*. Any reduction in the height of the solution should halt its flow. In this way, it is possible to assume that there is a minimum of pressure being exerted against the mucosa and therefore less likelihood of stimulating peristalsis.

If an enema is to be expelled immediately, the most commonly used rectal tubes are between No. 26 and No. 32, Fr., and for enemas to be retained, No. 14 to No. 20, Fr. The size of the tube used for retention enemas depends on the viscosity of the solution to be administered. The larger sized tubes should be used for solutions of high viscosity because of their resistance to flow.

Equipment for the Can and the Funnel Methods. In addition to the disposable enema unit, there are two other methods commonly used for introducing solution into the colon. One provides for a direct flow of the solution from a reservoir (can or bag) into the patient and the other requires that the solution be introduced into a funnel attached to the rectal tube.

The funnel method is the safer, since it is not possible to elevate the solution to a height which could create too much pressure against the wall of the colon and cause injury to the patient. The funnel method also can prevent rapid distention of the colon, which stimulates peristalsis to the extent that some patients are unable to permit enough solution to be introduced to receive satisfactory results. In addition, the funnel method is practical and convenient for enemas of small amounts that are given to be retained.

For the can or bag method, the following pieces of equipment are basic: irrigating can or bag, connecting tubing, connecting tip, rectal tube and clamp. Figure 25-1 illustrates this equipment.

For the funnel method, the following pieces of equipment are basic: pitcher, funnel and rectal tube. A clamp is helpful but not essential. Figure 25-2 illustrates this equipment.

The lubricant for the distal end of the rectal tube should be applied and, until insertion, should be protected by a piece of toilet tissue.

While the colon is not sterile, and the equipment and the solution used need not be sterile, they should be handled so that they are kept free from contamination by pathogens. For example, the rectal tube should not be allowed to lie on work areas where used items from patient care are placed before being cleaned.

Amount of the Solution. The greatest danger of prescribing an exact amount of solution to be used for the cleansing enema lies in the fact that some persons assume that all of that amount must be introduced into the patient if it is to be effective. Since a range is necessary as a guide, from 750 to 1,000 cc. per enema is considered satisfactory for the adult. However, if the primary purpose in giving the enema is to stimulate the defecation impulse and to aid in emptying the lower colon, there may be no reason to insist on introducing any exact amount. This guide should be used with the understanding that, for some patients, quantities under this amount are sufficient for the purpose and that the patient need not be subjected to almost unbearable discomfort because a larger quantity has been prepared. On the other hand, some patients may require additional amounts before results are obtained.

Temperature of the Solution. To prevent injury to the mucosa of the colon, the temperature of the solution as it is introduced should not be too much greater than body temperature. It is difficult to offer an exact range of temperature for each type of enema, since patients present individual differences, especially those having pathologic changes in the intestines. The range of temperature most often stated as satisfactory is from 105° to 115° F. (40.5° to 49° C.). This is the temperature of the solution at the time of preparation. The other point for consideration in each instance is the method of administration. If the can method with rather long tubing is used, there is more cooling than if the solution is poured directly from a pitcher via a funnel into the rectal tube. The hypertonic solution disposable enemas usually are given at room temperature. Patients will invariably feel the coolness of the solution. Even when it is at 72° F. some patients will comment that the initial introduction of the solution makes them feel chilly. While there is no recommendation that disposable units be warmed, care should be taken to see that they are not stored or placed where they can be cooled below room temperature.

Factors Guiding the Administration of Enemas. A physician's order is necessary for an enema. When the order is for an enema to be given every other day or whenever necessary, the reason usually is that the patient is not having regular bowel movements. Either order has nursing care implications. What does the nurse do to reduce or to eliminate the need for such a measure? What help does the patient need in order to regain his normal pattern of elimination? Will fluid intake, diet, activity or other measures help? To have elimination return as a normal function, not dependent on an aid, should be a nursing care objective for the patient. It is not uncommon to find that the order for "whenever necessary" is left to the discretion of the person caring for the patient on that day, but the patient should also be included in this decision. He should be consulted about when he feels it is necessary. If a daily movement is his normal pattern, he may be distressed if permitted to go two, three or four days without one. Such a situation might also be conducive to fecal impaction formation.

Explanation of the Procedure. Since the enema is a common procedure, many patients understand its use and how it is administered. However, the procedure offers an excellent opportunity for health teaching, since many persons are not familiar with the principles underlying it. Failure to observe one or more of these principles may be responsible for their considering the procedure a disagreeable one.

Most patients believe that solutions introduced into the colon are to be expelled as soon as possible. When a solution is to be retained, care should be taken to have the patient understand this. If the procedure is explained as a small enema, the patient still may believe that it is to be expelled. It is best if the patient is helped to understand that it is an instillation which is to be retained. An additional precaution is to keep the bedpan out of sight.

Position of the Patient. The position of the descending colon on the left side of the abdomen makes it seem that the solution will flow into the colon with less resistance if the patient lies on his left side. However, some patients may not be able to lie on the left side, and it is still possible for enemas to be given. Either side seems to be satisfactory.

The hypertonic phosphate solution enemas prepared commercially recommend that the patient be in the knee-chest position. This position helps the solution to flow farther into the colon and ensures the distribution of the small amount of solution over as wide a surface area of the lower colon as possible. In this way, more fluid is drawn into the colon. The knee-chest position is difficult for some patients to assume and impossible for others. In this event, it is best if the patient is placed flat in bed on the left side so that gravity aids in the flow of the fluid into the descending colon. In addition, it is best if the patient is kept on the left side or the back-lying position for a few minutes. If the patient is permitted to sit up, the solution may pool in the lower portion of the colon and not be too effective.

A common misunderstanding about enemas is that the solution can be administered effectively while the patient is in the sitting position. The amount of pressure needed to force the solution up into the colon while sitting is far greater than that needed while lying down. In addition, solution will tend to pool and distend the lower colon since it must go against gravity in order to ascend the colon. This will cause the desire to empty the colon sooner than may be desirable for effective results.

Removing Air From the Rectal Tube and Tubing. Many procedures for enemas state that all air should be removed from the tubing before the solution is introduced into the colon. However, the amount of air that could be introduced is not harmful to the patient. The amount of air varies, depending on the size and the length of the rectal tube and tubing. It does not act as an irritant, but it may aid in stimulating peristalsis by helping to distend the intestinal wall. Hence, the practice of eliminating air from the rectal tube and tubing when administering enemata that are not to be retained does not seem to be essential. Injecting air, though, should be

PRINCIPLES GUIDING ACTION WHEN ADMINISTERING A CLEANSING ENEMA

The purpose is to introduce solution into the colon to aid in stimulating peristalsis and removing feces.

SUGGESTED ACTION	PRINCIPLE
Use rectal tube No. 28 to No. 32, Fr. for adults.	The larger the size of the rectal tube, the greater the possibility of stimulating the sphincters.
Prepare the solution ordered by the physician and mix the ingredients thoroughly.	Agents used to help stimulate peristalsis act as irritants on the mucosa; agents not dissolved or mixed thoroughly could produce harmful local irritation.
Prepare the amount of solution ordered, or 750 to 1,500 cc. for an adult.	The adult colon is estimated to hold approximately 750 to 2,000 cc.
Prepare the solution at a temperature of 105° to 110° F. (40.5° to 49° C.), depending on the equipment to be used and the length of time before administration. Use the higher temperature for the can method.	Heat is effective in stimulating nerve plexuses in intestinal mucosa. The temperature of the environment, the length of tubing and the rate of flow of the fluid will influence the temperature reduction of the solution. Solutions entering the rectum at body temperature or slightly above will not injure normal tissue.
Lubricate the end of the rectal tube for 2 to 3 inches.	Friction is reduced when a surface is lubricated.
Place the patient in position by having him lie flat in bed, preferably on the left side; the right side or back-lying, if necessary.	Gravity aids the flow of fluids into the colon.
Insert the rectal tube slowly for 4 to 5 inches (10 to 12.7 cm.).	The anal canal is approximately 1 to 1½ inches in length (2.5 to 3.8 cm.). Slow insertion of a lubricated rectal tube minimizes spasms of the intestinal wall.
Elevate the funnel or the reservoir to the point where the solution begins to flow *slowly* into the colon.	Gravity aids the flow of the solution from the reservoir into the rectum. The higher the elevation of the fluid the greater will be the rate of flow into the colon and the pressure exerted on the colon.
Stop the flow of fluid and remove the rectal tube when the patient has a strong desire to defecate.	Distention and irritation of the intestinal wall, which produce strong peristaltic action, should be sufficient to empty the lower intestinal tract.
Place the patient in a sitting position on the bedpan, or assist him to the bathroom or to a commode if permissible.	Contraction of the abdominal and the perineal muscles which aid in emptying the colon is easier when the patient is in the sitting position.
Wash all equipment thoroughly and sterilize it before reuse, if disposable equipment is not used. (See Chapter 16.)	Normally, there is an abundant growth of bacteria in the large intestine.

avoided if the solution is to be retained. This is for several reasons; the air occupies space that should contain the fluid; it distends the colon and the rectum and therefore may stimulate peristalsis. However, running a small amount of solution through the tubing to remove air does warm the tubing.

Insertion of the Rectal Tube. The rectal tube should be inserted beyond both the anal sphincters. Since the anal canal averages one to one and one-half inches in length, four to five inches brings the end of the rectal tube well into the rectum. Occasionally, the rectal tube seems to meet with some resistance as it is being inserted. In such instances, it is best to permit a small amount of solution to enter, withdraw the rectal tube slightly and then continue to insert. Sometimes the resistance may be due to kinking of the tubing. It also may be due to spasm of the colon. The solution will help to reduce the spasms, and the tube may be inserted safely to the desired distance. It is well to remember that, in introducing the tube and the solution, there is a certain element of the unknown, since the area cannot be visualized. Therefore, it is best to proceed cautiously.

When rectal tubes have been damaged by repeated sterilization and by the action of lubricants containing hydrocarbons, they become soft and are compressed easily by the sphincters. Often the person administering the enema attempts to elevate the height of the solution so that it can be forced in, thus increasing the pressure of the solution against the wall of the colon. As previously mentioned, it is not safe to administer solutions under pressure. Therefore, only good rectal tubes should be used.

Administering an Enema to a Patient Who Has

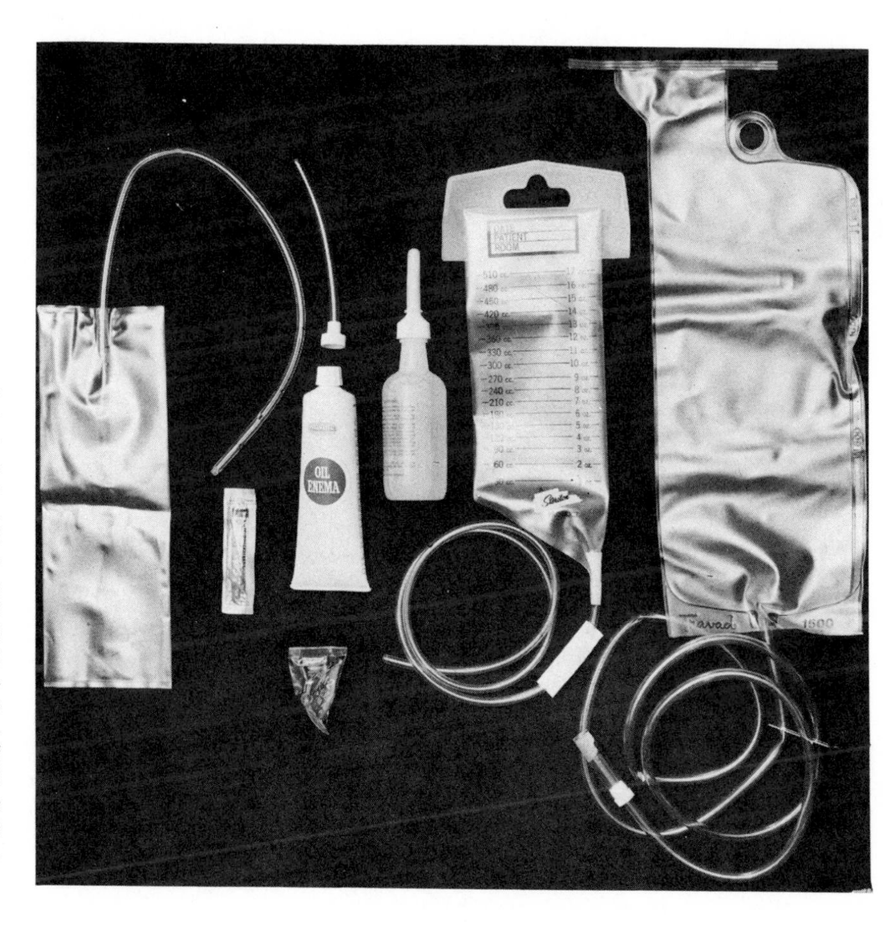

FIG. 25-3. A sampling of disposable units used in the treatment of disturbances of elimination from the large intestine. While different from the equipment diagrammed in Figures 25-1 and 25-2, correct application of principles ensures their effectiveness. From left to right: flatus bag with rectal tube; package of lubricant to be used with oil enema in squeeze tube (rectal tube is attached after cap is removed); below oil enema is a package of soap for a soap solution enema; a squeeze bottle of hypertonic solution for a small enema (usually 4 ounces); a child's enema unit, calibrated in ccs. and ounces; a 1,500 cc. adult enema unit.

Poor Sphincter Control. Occasionally it is not possible for a patient voluntarily to contract the external sphincter and assist in retaining the solution being given. Such a patient may need to have the rectal tube inserted and then be placed on the bedpan and the solution introduced. The nurse wears a glove to hold the tube in place. The head of the bed should be elevated slightly so that the patient's back is not arched. A pillow support to the lumbar region may be necessary. If the head of the bed is elevated beyond a 30° angle, there is less likelihood of the solution's entering the colon freely. Most of the solution will drain back out, and evacuation of feces in the colon may not be accomplished.

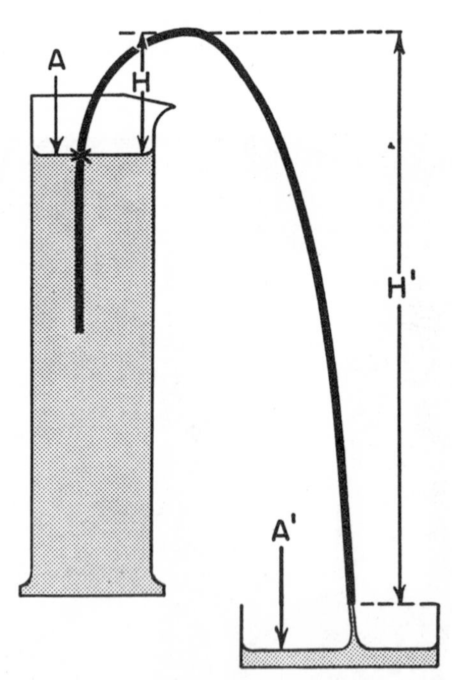

FIG. 25-4. By means of a siphon, a liquid is lifted over an obstacle to a new, lower level. The pressure at A and A' is that of the atmosphere.

The pressure downward on the surface of the liquid at X is that due to the column of liquid in the tube indicated by H. (From the surface of the liquid to the highest point in the tubing.)

The pressure downward in the tube (from the highest point to its end) is equal to a column of the liquid indicated by H'. H' is greater than H—therefore, fluid will be forced to the right and into the container.

For patients who are unable to retain large quantities of fluid for a cleansing enema, the commercially prepared hypertonic solution enemas are very satisfactory. The quantity is so small that usually there is no difficulty in retaining that amount. However, the patient should remain flat in bed following its administration unless the knee-chest position was used.

Withdrawing an Enema That Cannot Be Expelled. Sometimes, patients are unable to expel the solution administered. This most frequently happens when neuromuscular response is reduced. When it occurs, the solution should be withdrawn.

There are two methods by which this can be achieved, namely, by gravity flow or by siphonage. The former is tried first, and if not successful, then the latter. In preparing the equipment it is best to be prepared for siphonage. The following items are needed: a rectal tube, a connecting tip and connecting tubing, a funnel, lubricant and a pitcher with 250 cc. of water at the same temperature as for an enema.

The patient's bedpan should be placed on a chair alongside of the bed. If it is on the bed there may not be sufficient distance between the patient's rectum and the end of the tubing to permit the fluid to flow down. Place the patient on his left side if possible, place the end of the tubing in the bedpan, insert the lubricated rectal tube gently four to five inches. If contact is made with the solution in the patient, it will be emptied out by gravity flow. If no fluid returns, use the siphon method, which is done as follows: Withdraw the rectal tube. Attach the funnel to the end of the tubing. Fill the tubing with solution before reinserting it into the patient. After it is inserted, a small amount of solution is introduced into the patient, and then the funnel is lowered down to the bedpan. If solution continues to drain out through the funnel, contact has been made with the solution in the patient, a siphon has been established and the rectal tube should be held in position until the solution stops running. If siphonage cannot be started on the first attempt, small amounts of additional solution should be introduced and the procedure repeated until siphonage is created.

It is necessary to measure the amount of solution used to start the siphon so that the amount withdrawn also can be measured accurately. It is not expected that all of the solution given will be returned. The small amount which is retained will be absorbed.

Administering an Enema To a Child. When an enema is to be given to an infant or a child, the amount of solution to be administered is dependent on the age and the size of the child. Various amounts have been offered as guides. The amount increases with the age of the child and is rarely more than 500 cc. before the child is 14 years of age.

Small rubber-tipped bulb syringes which hold approximately 100 cc. of solution have been used satisfactorily. Being able to manage the solution with one hand is almost essential, since frequently the child requires support with the other. The solution should be introduced with a minimum of pressure.

As mentioned earlier, the hypertonic solution enemas have proved to be very satisfactory for use with children.

Colonic or Rectal Irrigations

Occasionally, the physician may order the irrigation of the colon with a large amount of fluid. This procedure is referred to as a colonic or rectal irrigation. The equipment used for such a procedure makes provision for the introduction of solution, usually isotonic, into the colon and then for the solution to be drained, as Figure 25-5 illustrates. Two methods are possible. In the single rectal tube method, a No. 32, Fr., rectal tube can be attached to two pieces of tubing by

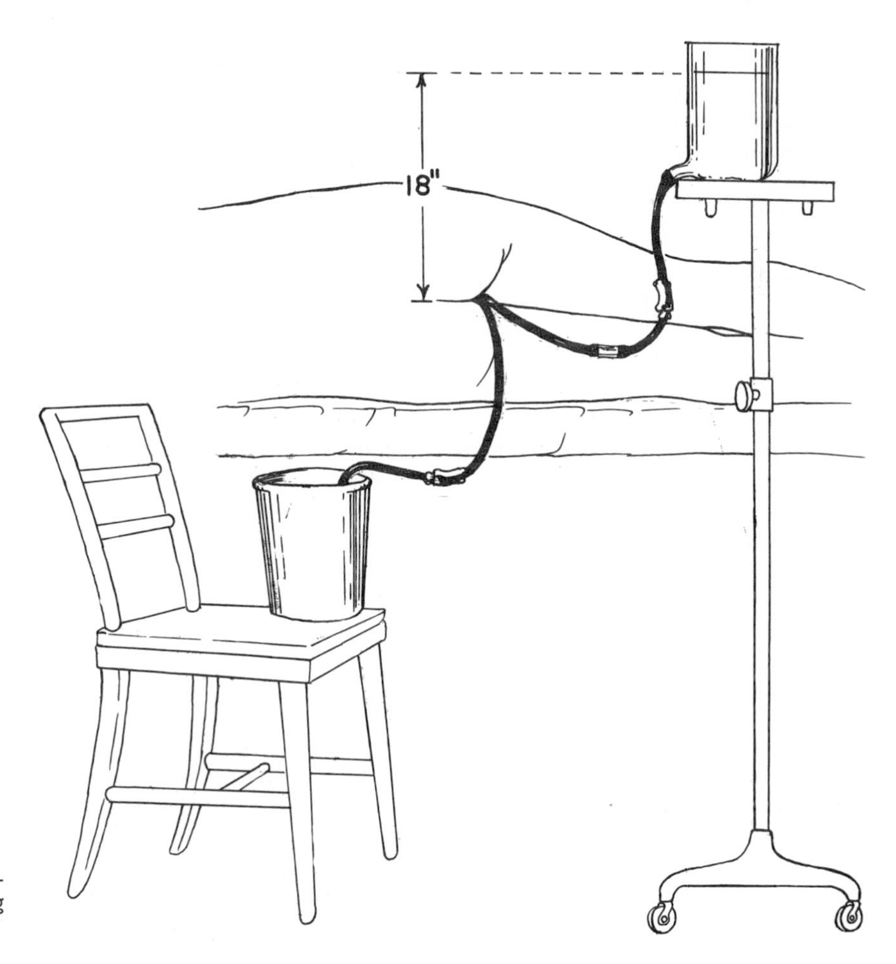

Fig. 25-5. Position of equipment for colonic irrigation using the 2-tube method.

using a Y connector. One piece goes to the reservoir of solution and the other down to a drainage container. When the solution is being introduced, the drainage tubing is clamped. When the drainage tubing is open, the solution tubing is clamped. Another method is to use two rectal tubes as Figure 25-5 illustrates. A No. 22, Fr., inserted about four or five inches (10 to 13 cm.), is used to introduce solution, and a No. 28, Fr., inserted about three inches (8 cm.), acts to drain the solution. The alternate clamping of these tubes would be the same as for the single-tube method.

Since the drainage of the solution from the colon is by gravity flow, the end of the drainage tubing should not be too far below the level of the rectum. There is danger of trauma to intestinal mucosa if the pull is too great. The container used to collect the drainage should be placed on a chair alongside the bed.

The amount of solution used depends on the purpose and the physician's order. A common amount is 3,000 to 4,000 cc.

Fecal Impaction

A fecal impaction is a prolonged retention or an accumulation of fecal material which forms a hardened mass in the rectum. It may be of sufficient size to prevent the passage of normal stools.

The medical literature describes a condition referred to as obstipation which is the accumulation of hardened feces extending well up into the colon and in some instances almost amounting to intestinal obstruction. While it is common for a fecal impaction to prevent the passage of normal stools, the situation may be misleading, because the patient has liquid fecal seepage. Small amounts of fluid present in the colon are able to go around the impacted mass. As a matter of fact, such liquid fecal seepage and no passage of normal feces are almost a confirmation of the existence of an impaction.

Fecal impactions frequently are due to constipation and poor habits of defecation. They may result when parts of a hardened, dry stool become lodged in the folds of the rectum.

Certain conditions predispose to fecal impactions, and the nurse will need to be alert to prevent their development. For example, patients who are required to maintain complete bed rest may find normal defecation difficult, and, unless some action is taken, constipation and fecal impactions may result. This may mean determining if the patient's food and fluid intake can be improved to aid the process. Or, it may mean consulting the physician about the possibility of permitting the patient to use a commode or having a mild laxative daily.

Patients who are required to take constipating drugs over a period of time are also prone to develop fecal impactions; barium enemas for x-ray examinations of the colon are likely to develop fecal impactions if care is not taken to cleanse the colon of barium following examination.

Investigations have shown that some fibrous foods, such as bran and fruit seeds have been known to cause fecal impactions, as have coated pills.

The patient with a fecal impaction may complain of constipation, uncontrolled liquid fecal seepage or both. Usually, he experiences a frequent desire to defecate but is unable to do so. Rectal pain may be present. Very careful observation is needed to prevent fecal impactions. There is no particular time span associated with their formation. Some have been known to occur within 24 hours. There have been reports in the literature of impactions removed by surgical procedures. Prevention is based on observation of the stool as to amount, consistency and frequency. If the patient is ambulatory, he will need to be instructed to make these observations. If he does not use the bathroom, nursing personnel must assume this responsibility. If the causes are not eliminated, impactions are likely to recur. As with the prevention of constipation, all efforts to help a patient should be entered on the nursing care plan. When fecal impactions are not associated with circumstances beyond the nurses' control, such as antiperistaltic drugs or other therapy, the occurrence of an impaction usually is a sign of less than satisfactory nursing care.

When the physician determines that a fecal impaction is present, he often orders oil to be instilled into the rectum in order to soften the stool. This is followed by a cleansing enema two or three hours later. This may be followed by enemas twice a day if necessary until normal stools are evacuated. If this procedure fails, often it is necessary to break up the impaction by digital manipulation. The physician may carry out this procedure, or in some situations the nurse may be asked to do so.

To remove an impaction, the patient should be placed in the Sims' position if possible, the top bedding folded down to the foot of the bed, the patient covered with a bath blanket; use protection for the bedding, such as a disposable pad or plastic sheeting, under the patient. The bedpan should be placed conveniently on the bed so that the pieces of removed feces may be deposited in it. Clean gloves should be used. Lubricate the first finger generously and insert it as gently as possible into the anal sphincter. The presence of the finger added to the mass already present causes considerable discomfort to the patient. By carefully working the finger into the hardened mass, it is possible to remove pieces of it. Use plenty of lubricant in order to avoid irritating the mucous membrane or inducing bleeding. When a severe impaction exists, part of the impaction will need to be removed at one time, possibly more oil instilled, and remaining parts removed at intervals of several hours. This will avoid extreme discomfort and possibly harm to the patient.

Distention

Excessive formation of gases in the stomach or the intestines is known as *flatulence.* When the gas is not expelled and accumulates in the intestinal tract, the condition is called *distention* or *tympanites.*

Any disturbance in the ability of the small intestine to absorb gases or in its ability to propel gas along the intestinal tract usually will result in distention. Irritating foods, such as beans and cabbage, predispose to flatulence and distention. Constipation is a frequent cause of distention. Certain drugs, morphine sulfate for example, tend to decrease peristaltic action and thus cause distention. Swallowing large amounts of air while eating and drinking can cause distention. Persons who are tense often can be observed to be swallowing large amounts of air, especially when taking fluids. This habit can be overcome by purposely training oneself to eat and drink without swallowing air. Usually, air swallowers will eructate a great deal, and much air escapes in this manner before it reaches the intestines.

Distention can be noted by the presence of a swollen abdomen. Gentle percussion with the fingers produces a drumlike sound. In addition, usually the patient will complain of cramplike pain, and, if distention is sufficient to cause pressure on the diaphragm and the thoracic cavity, shortness of breath and dyspnea may result.

Acting on the cause usually will relieve the distention. However, until the action is effective, temporary relief often can be afforded the patient by inserting a rectal tube.

Rectal Tube. The sizes of rectal tubes used most frequently for the relief of distention in adults range from No. 22 to No. 32. Smaller sizes are used for children. The tips of rectal tubes also vary—some have smoothly rounded tips with an opening on the side of the tube near the tip, others have an opening at the tip as well as on the side of the tube. The distinct advantage of the rubber or plastic tube for rectal treatments is that it is flexible, and, with good lubrication and careful insertion, it can be introduced with relative ease beyond the anal canal into the rectum.

Insertion of the Rectal Tube. After lubricating the rectal tube, it should be inserted for approximately four inches. However, since fluids are not being introduced, it is possible to insert it a bit farther if no resistance is encountered and if it is noted that no flatus is being removed.

The rectal tube may be attached to a piece of connecting tubing of sufficient length to reach well into a small collecting container which can be attached to the bed frame. Water then can be put into the collecting container to cover the end of the tubing to determine whether or not the patient is expelling flatus; air bubbles indicate that gas is being removed.

A rectal tube should be left in place for a short period of time; usually 20 minutes is sufficient. Leaving the tube in place for long periods of time reduces the responsiveness of the sphincters. There is more likelihood of stimulating the sphincters and peristalsis if the rectal tube is reinserted every two to three hours as necessary. If the tube is inserted repeatedly over a period of several hours and no gas is removed, and the patient remains distended, the observation should be reported to the physician.

Carminative enemas, described earlier in this chapter, may be prescribed for distention.

Diarrhea

Diarrhea is the passage of excessively liquid and unformed stools. Frequent bowel movements do not necessarily mean that diarrhea is present, although patients with diarrhea usually will pass stools at frequent intervals. Diarrhea often is associated with intestinal cramps. Nausea and vomiting may be present, as may be the presence of blood in the stools. Diarrhea is protective in nature when its cause is the presence of irritants in the intestinal tract.

Diarrhea may have a functional basis. The patient may have allergies to ingested food or drugs. The abuse of cathartics, and also certain dietary indiscretions, may cause diarrhea. Some persons know that, for them, certain foods and fluids, as rich pastries, coffee, or alcoholic beverages may produce temporary diarrhea. Avoidance of the factor causing it usually remedies the situation easily.

Diseases in parts of the body other than the intestinal tract may be at the root of the trouble. Examples include uremia and certain cardiac and neurological disorders.

Diarrhea may be caused by certain intrinsic conditions existing in the intestine itself. Examples include these: viral, bacteriologic, fungal, protozoan or metazoan invasion; alterations in the normal bacterial flora of the intestine; antimicrobial therapy; fistulas; inflammatory conditions such as ulcerative colitis; and tumors in the intestinal tract.

If the cause of diarrhea is psychic in nature, the nurse may be able to play an important part in assisting the patient to understand the cause. Situations in daily living may be disturbing to him. However, diarrhea may be associated with deep-seated emotional problems that require the help of the physician or a psychiatrist.

Diarrhea is often an embarrassing and usually a painful disturbance. Local irritation of the anal region and possibly even the perineum and the buttocks from frequent watery stools is not uncommon. To help to prevent irritation the nurse may need to initiate special hygienic measures, such as washing the area after each movement, drying it thoroughly and possibly using one of the medicated creams or powders. Also, it may be necessary to caution the patient to use only very soft toilet tissue.

When a person has diarrhea it is often impossible to control the urge to defecate for very long, if at all. Therefore, when it is known that a bed patient has diarrhea, a comment to this effect should appear on the nursing care plan. This will alert nursing personnel to watch for his signal light. Or, it may be necessary to place the bedpan within easy reach for the patient, but yet out of sight to prevent embarrassment.

A review of Table 7 in Chapter 24 illustrates how very frequently diarrhea leads to or is involved in fluid and electrolyte disturbances. Large amounts of fluids and electrolytes may be lost relatively quickly in the presence of diarrhea. This is especially true with infants; if neglected, such loss may easily place a baby's life in jeopardy. Parenteral fluids may be necessary when diarrhea is present. If oral intake is possible, cold fluids and rich foods, especially sweets, should be avoided.

Anal Incontinence

Anal incontinence is the inability of the anal sphincter to control the discharge of fecal and gaseous material voluntarily. Usually, the cause of incontinence is an organic disease resulting either in a mechanical condition that hinders the proper functioning of the anal sphincter or in an impairment in the nerve supply to the anal sphincter.

While anal incontinence rarely is a menace to life, incontinent patients suffer embarrassment and may become disturbed emotionally. They require much emotional support and understanding as well as special nursing care to prevent odors, skin irritation and soiling of the linen and the clothing.

Too often, incontinence is accepted as an inescapable situation. This attitude should not exist until every effort has been made to determine if continence can be achieved. While the situation itself is distressing to the patient, some of the nursing measures may be equally disturbing if not managed with tact, since they are not too different from those used with children before they gain bowel control.

Typical nursing measures follow. Note if there is a time of day when incontinence is more likely to occur, as after a meal. If so, the patient could be placed on a bedpan at such times. If there is no pattern as to when incontinence occurs, place the patient on a bedpan at frequent intervals, as every two or three hours. The patient's attempts at trying to use the pan may be successful and may lead to better muscular control. Consult with the physician about the advisability of using suppositories or a daily enema. For some patients, the problem is so severe that a diaper may be necessary in order to limit soiling of the patient and the bed clothing. Disposable diapers are available and convenient to use. For the conscious adult patient, wearing a diaper is a disheartening experience. Psychologically, it is better to refer to them as incontinent pads or protective pads. Also their use should be accompanied with the explanation that efforts to correct the situation will continue and that this is a temporary measure for the patient's comfort. Even if a patient is not lucid, efforts to minimize incontinence should be continued so that the diaper is not a permanent thing.

Anal control is dependent ultimately on proper functioning of the anal sphincter, and nursing or medical therapeutic measures depend on the cause. In certain instances, functioning of impaired anal sphincters can be improved with a planned program of bowel training. For these patients, aid in regaining bowel control becomes an important part of nursing care.

Bowel Training. The matter of planning a regimen for bowel training is certainly a mutual proposition involving the physician, the patient and the nurse. As might be expected, it has great psychological implications for the patient, since almost every lucid individual desires normal control of this body function. The physician must first determine the feasibility of initiating such a program. Is there any possibility for success? It would be a disaster to the patient if even partial success were impossible. As a plan is being developed, and once it has been established, it should be a conspicuous part of the patient's nursing care plan, since interruptions may jeopardize the progress being made.

Before beginning bowel training, the patient will need to determine what time of day is best for him to have an evacuation. This can be decided in terms of his past pattern of evacuation and after he has considered his schedule at home and the facilities available. It is also essential that the nurse review the diet, the amount of exercise permitted and the medications being administered.

Arrangements then should be made so that the patient can try to have an evacuation at the time of day selected. If possible, the patient should be on a toilet or a commode, since in this position gravity and more effective muscular contraction aid defecation.

If the patient is paralyzed, frequently the external sphincter is relaxed, but the training of the internal sphincter is possible. The patient should be encouraged to bear down as is done in normal bowel evacuation. However, straining or persistent bearing down should be discouraged because of the possibility of inducing hemorrhoids.

A time limit for trying should be set, such as 15 to 25 minutes. If the patient had any previous habits that seemed to be associated with bowel evacuation, these should be included. Frequently, patients state that hot coffee or a glass of water upon arising helped. Smoking or reading have some value in the procedure for certain patients. There is merit in taking advantage of any of the patient's suggestions and wishes in relation to his previous bowel habits.

The physician may need to be consulted about using suppositories. Inserting one or two suppositories is often a satisfactory means of helping to create stimulation and subsequent emptying of the rectum. The results from the suppositories may not be obtained until several hours later, so that, during the early training period, the patient may be having results at other than the desired evacuation time.

Because of the many discouraging aspects to such a program, especially the long-time span before any progress is evident, the patient will need much encouragement to continue. He should also receive praise for his efforts.

There is no usual span of time which can be estimated for a bowel-training program. The rapidity with which a satisfactory pattern can be established depends on the patient's condition and often on the perseverance shown by both the patient and the nurse. If the patient becomes discouraged, the nurse may need to modify the procedure from time to time so that the patient has a feeling of some gain.

COMMON DISTURBANCES OF ELIMINATION FROM THE URINARY TRACT

Definition of Terms. There are certain terms commonly used to describe urine and voiding with which the nurse will need to be familiar. *Anuria* refers to suppression of urine. When total anuria occurs, the kidneys produce no urine; therefore, the bladder remains empty. When the kidneys produce only scanty amounts of urine, the term *oliguria* is used. Anuria and oliguria are usually serious signs. *Polyuria* refers to an increased output of urine.

Hematuria refers to urine that contains blood. If present in large enough quantities, the urine becomes reddish brown in color. Pus in the urine is called *pyuria*. The urine appears cloudy. Pyuria should not be confused with the cloudiness which may occur when normal urine stands and cools. Albumin in the urine is called *albuminuria*. Albumin is sometimes present in urine that is voided following periods of standing, walking and running. This is called *orthostatic albuminuria* and is a phenomenon of the circulatory system and not necessarily a symptom of kidney disorders. *Glycosuria* refers to the presence of sugar in the urine. If glycosuria is due to an unusually large intake of sugar or to marked emotional disturbances and is temporary in nature, there is little cause for alarm. This condition is called *alimentary glycosuria*.

Dysuria refers to difficulty in voiding. It may or may not be associated with pain. A feeling of warm irritation occurring during voiding is called *burning*. *Frequency* refers to voiding at very frequent intervals. Voiding during the night when not associated with large fluid intake is called *nycturia* or *nocturia*.

Retention

Retention occurs when urine is being produced normally but is not being excreted from the bladder. The bladder continues to fill and may distend until it reaches the level of the umbilicus. The abdomen swells as the bladder rises above the level of the symphysis pubis. The height of the bladder can be determined by palpating with light pressure on the abdomen.

Retention is often temporary in nature. It is common following surgery, especially if ambulation is delayed. Any mechanical obstruction—for example, swelling at the meatus, which often occurs following childbirth—will cause retention. The cause also may be psychic in nature or be due to certain disease conditions.

While urine that is retained in the bladder can be removed by introducing a catheter, every effort should be made to help the patient void. Medical literature abounds in caution against using the catheter too freely. It is generally conceded that infections of the bladder can occur following even one insertion of a catheter, despite the most careful procedure.

Nursing measures should be instituted as soon as a patient feels that he cannot void even if the interval since the last voiding was only four to five hours. This is particularly true if the patient has been having a normal fluid intake.

There are several measures that often aid in initiating normal micturition if there is no mechanical obstruction or disease condition causing retention. Placing the patient in the normal position for voiding—that is, in the sitting position—is usually helpful if sitting is not contraindicated. Sometimes, voiding will begin if the patient sits at the edge of the bed on a bedpan and supports his feet on a chair. If the patient is allowed out of bed, the patient can sit on a bedpan placed on a chair, or a commode can be used. The male patient often can induce voiding if permitted to stand. A toilet is best if the patient can walk or be moved to one. The back-lying position has been found to be least successful in helping to initiate voiding. If the patient's condition permits, he should be provided privacy while he attempts to void. In many instances the patient may need to wait several minutes for the urge to void to appear or reappear.

Additional measures which often assist in the voiding process include offering the patient fluids, especially warm drinks; warming the bedpan before use; allowing water to run from a tap within hearing distance of the patient; or placing the patient's hands in warm water or pouring warm water over the perineum (if no specimen is desired).

Retention is painful. The patient often becomes anxious and concerned, which usually further interferes with normal voiding.

Occasionally, a patient will void but the quantity is insufficient by comparison with the fluid intake. Or, the patient may say that he feels as though he still needs to void. When almost all of the urine does not leave the bladder during a voiding, it is referred to as *residual urine*. One article[4] reports that percussion over the bladder immediately after the patient voids can help to determine the presence of retained urine. In this report, approximately 135 cc. in the bladder produced a dullness upon percussion 1 cm. (1 finger-breadth) above the symphysis. This amount of urine in the bladder immediately after voiding is considered as residual.

Common Therapeutic Measures to Relieve Urinary Retention

Catheterization

Catheterization of the urinary bladder is the introduction of a catheter through the urethra into the bladder for the purpose of withdrawing urine. In recent years, the value of catheterization, formerly unquestioned, has become increasingly dubious in view of the hazards involved.

Several physiologic facts should be recalled. The bladder is normally a sterile cavity. The external opening to the urethra can never be sterilized. The bladder has defense mechanisms, namely, the emptying of urine and intravesical antibacterial activity not dependent on an antibacterial factor in the urine. These help to maintain a sterile bladder under normal circumstances and also aid in clearing an infection if it occurs. Infections introduced into the bladder can ascend the ureters and lead to pyelonephritis. A normal bladder is not so susceptible to infection as a damaged one. A patient's lowered resistance to infection, present in many disease entities, predisposes to urinary infection. These patients are rarely catheterized unless absolutely necessary because of the danger of acquiring an infection.

The hazards of introducing an instrument or a catheter into the bladder are sepsis and trauma; the possibility of the latter to the male urethra, because of its length, is obvious. An object forced through a stricture or irregularity from the wrong angle can cause serious damage to the urethra. While the urethra in the female is shorter, it also is susceptible to damage if a catheter is forced through it.

Purposes of Catheterization. It was formerly considered essential to catheterize for a urine specimen free of contamination, but this practice has been abandoned by many physicians. Microorganisms present in the urethra can be introduced into the urine, and the patients accordingly are treated for nonexistent bladder infections. "Clean catch" is an alternative method for collecting specimens, used first with male patients and now with females as well. These specimens may be used for culture. The procedure is simple. The external meatus is cleansed thoroughly with soap and water or an antiseptic solution, such as aqueous Zephiran. Then, the patient voids about 50 to 100 cc., which is discarded. Next, he voids into a sterile specimen bottle until an adequate amount for study is obtained, usually about 100 to 200 cc. Then the remaining urine in the bladder is voided and discarded.

Catheterization may be used before surgery to empty the patient's bladder completely since tension and preoperative sedation can result in incomplete emptying of the bladder. It is used postoperatively when patients are unable to void and all nursing measures to induce voiding have failed. It is used before and after delivery for the same reasons.

Catheterization also may be used to remove urine from a greatly distended bladder. It generally is agreed by urologists that gradual decompression of the distended bladder is a safer procedure than rapid removal of all urine. Rapid emptying of the bladder has resulted in damage to the organ with severe systemic reactions, such as chills, fever and shock. Gradual decompression aids in preventing engorgement in the vessels as well as helping to improve the tone of the bladder wall by adjusting the intravesical pressure in stages.

For patients who have severe retention—for example, if as much as 2,000 cc. is suspected—a special apparatus may be used to decompress the bladder over a period of 24 hours or more. However, there are instances when the nurse will need to exercise judgment as to the amount of urine to withdraw at a single catheterization. Safe procedure for catheterization is that no more than 750 to 1,000 cc. of urine be withdrawn from a patient at any one time. The physician is notified when this amount is removed easily, and it is apparent that more urine is present. In other words, there is a full steady flow.

Equipment. Commonly used catheters are made of rubber or plastic material. For male patients, there also are silk woven catheters that are firm, yet flexible, and follow the contour of the urethra with ease.

Catheters, like rectal tubes, are graded on the French scale according to the size of the lumen. For the female patient, sizes No. 14 and No. 16, Fr., catheters usually are used. Smaller catheters are not necessary, and the size of the lumen is so small that it increases the length of time necessary for emptying the bladder. Larger catheters distend the urethra and tend to increase the discomfort of the procedure. For the male patient, sizes No. 20 and No. 22, Fr., catheters usually are used, but if this appears to be too large, a smaller caliber should be tried. Sizes No. 8 and No. 10, Fr., commonly are used for children.

In addition to the catheter, a receptacle for collecting urine and materials to cleanse the meatus and area around it are necessary.

All of the equipment used during a catheterization should be sterile and handled while using strict aseptic technic. Sterilization with steam under pressure is usually recommended.

Disposable catheterization sets are becoming more popular and for several reasons. They are sterile when purchased and are used only once, thereby decreasing the possibility of introducing infection. These sets are easy to use and economical as well. When catheterization must be done in a home, a disposable set is first choice inasmuch as it eliminates sterilization problems.

Preparation of the Patient. It is assumed that the patient will have an adequate explanation of the procedure and the reason for it beforehand. A catheter being inserted produces a sensation of pressure in the area rather than one of pain. This should be explained to the patient. In addition, the patient should be assured that every measure to avoid exposure and embarrassment will be taken. The more relaxed the patient can be, the easier it will be to insert the catheter.

The best position for the patient is the

dorsal recumbent, and preferably on a firm surface such as a treatment table. Catheterization in the bed, especially for the female patient, is not as satisfactory because the patient's pelvic area is not supported firmly, and visualization of the meatus is difficult. Also, sinking into the bed may cause the patient's bladder to be lower than the outlet of the catheter. If the patient is in bed, supporting the buttocks on a firm cushion is helpful.

For the female patient, good positioning and lighting are essential to locating the meatus quickly and easily. Artificial light is almost always necessary for this procedure. The patient should be protected adequately from unnecessary exposure of the perineal area and from drafts by proper and adequate draping. Figure 25-6 illustrates the position of the female patient for catheterization.

Cleansing the Area. Bacteria can be introduced into the urinary bladder by passing a catheter through the external meatus and the urethra into the bladder. The area around the meatus should be made as clean as possible in order to minimize contamination of the catheter.

It would seem that the best preparation of the glans penis or the labia and the introitus prior to introducing a catheter is to wash the area thoroughly with soap and warm water. Some agencies specify a thorough washing of the local area immediately before the procedure, and then cleansing with an antiseptic solution on cotton balls prior to the insertion of the catheter. If soap is used to wash the area, benzalkonium chloride should not be used until all of the soap has been rinsed away. Soap destroys the action of benzalkonium chloride. The nurse will be guided by local procedure also.

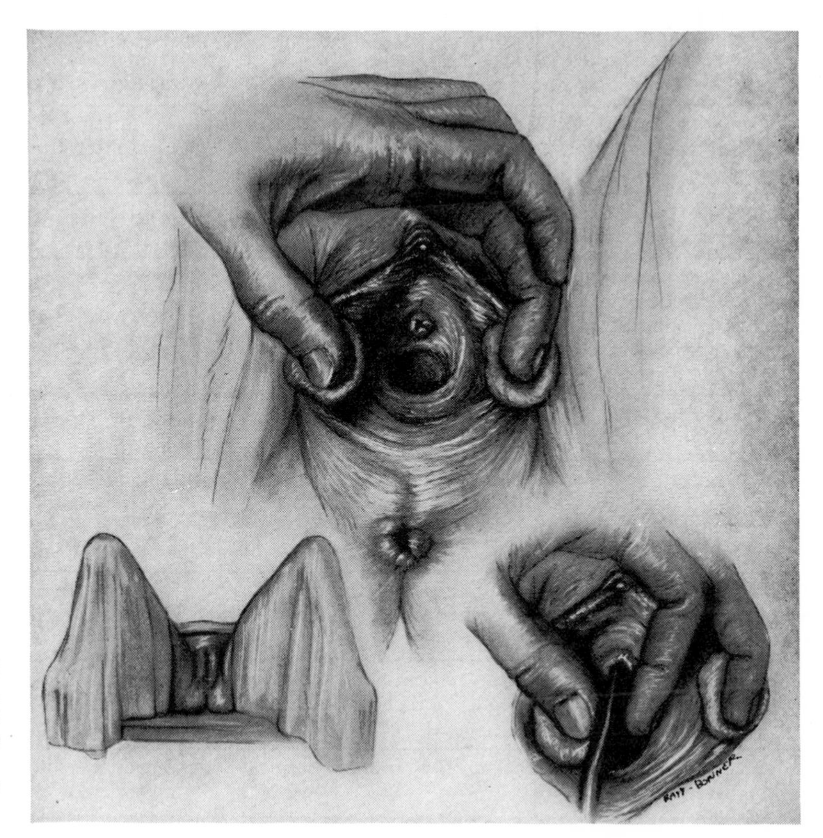

Fig. 25-6. (Bottom, left). Position of the female patient for catheterization.
Fig. 25-7. (Top). Visualization of the meatus by properly separating the labia minora.
Fig. 25-8. (Bottom, right). Fingers in position to pinch off the catheter.

PRINCIPLES GUIDING ACTION FOR CATHETERIZATION OF THE URINARY BLADDER (FEMALE)

The purpose is to remove urine from the bladder.

SUGGESTED ACTION	PRINCIPLE
Add solution(s) for cleansing the perineum and a lubricant to the tray. Use paper bag for discarded cotton balls before bringing all equipment to the unit.	Preparation of equipment where the patient can observe it may be disturbing and frightening.
After providing for privacy place the patient in the dorsal recumbent position with the hips firmly supported.	Good visualization of the meatus is essential to introduce the catheter. Gravity will aid flow of urine when bladder is higher than end of catheter.
Drape the patient's thighs and cover the chest. Use sufficient covering, depending upon patient's age, condition and environmental conditions.	Embarrassment and chilliness can cause the patient to become tense. Tension can interfere with easy introduction of the catheter.
Arrange equipment for convenience and to avoid contamination of sterile items. Place materials for cleansing the perineum so that reaching over the sterile field is avoided.	Placement of equipment in order of use increases speed of performance. Reaching over sterile items increases the risk of contamination.
After either putting on gloves or protecting the fingers with cotton balls, place the thumb and one finger between the labia minora, separate and pull up.	Smoothing the area immediately surrounding the meatus helps to make it visible.
Cleanse the area using as many cotton balls as necessary to assure absolute cleanliness. Use one cotton ball for each stroke, moving it from above the meatus downward toward the rectum.	Thorough cleansing of the meatus and the area surrounding it reduces possible introduction of microorganisms into the bladder. Contamination from rectal area can result by stroking from this area toward the meatus.
As soon as the area has been cleansed thoroughly and the meatus is visible, keep the hand in position while preparing the catheter for insertion.	Permitting the labia to close over the meatus contaminates the area just cleaned.
Lubricate the catheter for about 1½ inches, being careful not to plug the eye of the catheter.	Lubrication reduces friction.
Pick up the catheter at least 3 inches from the tip, using a sterile clamp or sterile gloves, or with the fingers if a hand-washing technic has been used and the perineum has not been touched with the fingers.	The bladder is normally a sterile cavity.
Insert the catheter for 2 to 3 inches, or until urine begins to flow.	The female urethra is approximately 1½ to 2½ inches long.
If a specimen is to be collected, pinch the catheter with the thumb and the first finger while placing the specimen container in position, as Figure 25-8 illustrates.	Urine will flow out of the catheter if the lumen is not occluded.
Rest the hand on the pubis to hold the catheter in place and to prevent pulling and pushing the catheter in the urethra.	Withdrawing the catheter and then pushing it back into the urethra increases the possibility of contaminating the urethra.
When the flow of urine begins to diminish, withdraw the catheter slowly, about ½ inch at a time until urine barely drips.	The tip of the catheter passes through urine remaining in the bladder.
Cleanse all equipment thoroughly immediately after use, if not disposable.	Secretions, lubricant and other substances are removed more easily when they are not coagulated.

A good many agencies specify the use of sterile gloves for catheterization for the female as well as the male patient. Many sets are issued with disposable gloves. Also, in instances when edema or pathologic changes of the perineum of the female distort the area, sterile gloves facilitate the procedure and make it more comfortable for the patient. If gloves are not worn, the nurse must wash her hands thoroughly under running water immediately before starting the procedure. When a sink is in the patient's unit, it is recommended that the hand wash be done after the patient has been draped, if possible. While this means that the patient must keep her knees flexed, it also eliminates the nurse's touching contaminated linens and other objects immediately before handling the catheters.

To catheterize the female, good visualization of the meatus facilitates the procedure and reduces the chance of contaminating the tip of the catheter. This can be accomplished by inserting the thumb and the first or the second finger well into the labia minora, spreading it apart and then pulling upward toward the symphysis pubis, as Figure 25-7 illustrates. This irons out the area and makes the meatus visible. In many women, it is rather difficult to find the meatus, and it may appear as a small dimple in the area. Once the meatus has been cleansed, do not allow the labia to close over it. This risks the chance of contaminating it.

The insertion of the catheter normally does not produce severe pain. If the patient seems to be experiencing unusual discomfort, discontinue the procedure and notify the physician. Some patients have strictures in the urethra, in which case it is best for the physician to introduce the catheter.

Immediately following the insertion of the catheter, some patients react by tightening the muscles in the area, and the flow of urine may be delayed for a few seconds until the patient is able to relax.

Following catheterizaiton, there are observations which are made and recorded. These include the color and the transparency of the urine and the amount obtained. Occasionally, urine has an unusual odor, and this should be recorded. Any unusual discomfort experienced by the patient should also be noted. A specimen, if desired, is handled according to agency policy.

Catheterization of the Male Patient. Although the female nurse is rarely asked to catheterize the male patient, there may be occasions, especially in the home, when female nurses may need to carry out this procedure. Principles guiding actions to maintain asepsis and to prevent trauma are identical for catheterization of the male as for the female. However, knowledge of the differences in

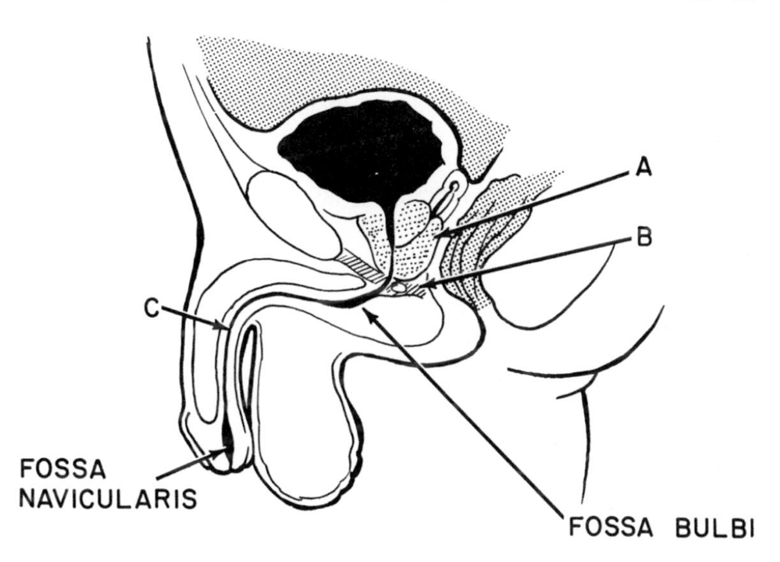

Fig. 25-9. Male anatomy. A. pars prostatica. B. pars membranosa. C pars cavernosa.

anatomy is essential to understanding the differences in technic.

The male urethra consists of three parts: the pars prostatica, situated in the pelvis; the pars membranosa, situated in the perineum, and the pars cavernosa, situated in the penis. Figure 25-9 illustrates these parts.

The upward-directed concave curvature of the subpubic curvature is fixed; the downward-directed concave curvature of the prepubic curvature can be straightened out by lifting the penis. The pars pendulosa of the penis is freely movable, and pars membranosa is firmly fixed and the other parts are slightly movable. The lumen at the external and the internal orifices and the pars membranosa are narrowed. The lumen at the pars prostatica, the fossa bulbi and the fossa navicularis is wider.

With the patient in the dorsal recumbent position, the legs are spread apart and somewhat externally rotated, and the knees are slightly bent. A urinal or a kidney basin is placed between the thighs of the patient. The orifice of the urethra is cleansed according to agency policy. The operator grasps the penis at the coronary sulcus and elevates it by a slight traction so that it becomes vertical to the long axis of the body. Slight pressure on the glans with the thumb and the index fingers causes the orifice to gape. A few drops of a sterile lubricating jelly may be inserted into the orifice. The other hand which is covered by a sterile glove picks up the sterile catheter on which a few drops of a sterile lubricating jelly have been placed near its tip (about one and one-half inches) and pushes this length of the catheter slowly into the urethra. Immediately upon its insertion the catheter may encounter a slight resistance caused by the fold of the mucosa at the upper wall of the urethra (Guerin's fold) or by the pouch of the fossa navicularis at the lower wall of the urethra. These obstacles can be overcome easily by a slight twisting of the catheter. The further insertion of the catheter is accomplished by successive grasping of the catheter a similarly short distance above the urethra and pushing it into the urethra until it reaches the bladder.

The catheter usually glides easily through the cavernous portion of the urethra up to the bulbus. The bulbus is an existing pouch in the lower wall of the urethra, and it might offer resistance if the tip of the catheter is pushing against the blind end of the pouch and has not entered the narrow membranous part of the urethra. If this occurs, pull the penis with more force, retract the catheter slightly and lower the penis and the catheter slightly. Then push the catheter forward by short shoving motions. The patient is requested to take a deep breath to avoid any reflex contraction of the perineal musculature. The appearance of urine indicates that the catheter has entered the bladder.

If sterile gloves are not available, two sterile ribbed forceps or a sterile straight clamp can be used to insert the catheter. In this case, an assistant or the patient holds the penis in the required position.

Retention Catheter

If a catheter is to remain in place for a period of 24 hours or more, a retention or indwelling catheter usually is used. The catheter used is so designed that it does not slip out of the urethra. Such catheters are used for incontinent or unconscious patients, for gradual decompression of an overly distended bladder, for intermittent bladder drainage and irrigation, or for continuous drainage of the bladder.

A retention catheter has a portion which can be inflated after the catheter is inserted into the bladder. Because the balloon is larger than the opening to the urethra, it is impossible for the catheter to slip out. There are several types of retention catheters available, but the principle on which they operate is similar. The catheter has a double lumen. One lumen is connected directly with the balloon which may be distended with either water or saline, and the other is the portion through which the urine drains. When the balloon is distended, the sidepiece through which the solution was introduced is clamped. There are also catheters which are self-sealing. Equipment for inflating the balloon is needed when a retention catheter is inserted.

The basic procedure is the same as for catheterization. As soon as the bladder has been emptied of urine, the bag of the retention catheter is distended with solution, usually normal saline or sterile water. The balloons are designed to hold from five to 30 cc. of solution. Each catheter indicates the amount of solution to be injected into the bag. The means for injecting the solution varies with the make of catheter. Some balloons must be distended by means of a syringe with an adapter, and then the inlet is clamped off. Other balloons are distended with a syringe and a No. 20 needle because the inlet is self-sealing. If the patient complains of pain or real discomfort while the balloon is being filled, stop injecting the solution, withdraw the fluid and insert the catheter farther, for it may be that the balloon is in the urethra.

After the balloon has been distended, it is best to test the catheter to see that it is secure. *Slight* tension on it will indicate whether or not it is secure in the bladder. For patients with pathologic changes of the bladder and/or the urethra, it may be necessary to irrigate the catheter after the balloon is distended. This will help to determine more definitely whether the catheter is inserted properly.

Attachment of the Retention Catheter. An advantage of the retention catheter is the fact that it remains in place without a great deal of anchoring with adhesive or cellophane tape.

It is general practice for a retention catheter to be attached to a straight drainage set if intermittent drainage is not to be started. The catheter should be connected to the drainage tubing, which is of sufficient length to reach the collecting container and still give the patient freedom to move about in bed. If the drainage tubing is too long, urine pools in the tubing, and it may interrupt the drainage from the bladder.

When the tubing is attached to the catheter, a glass or plastic connecting rod is used. This makes it possible to examine drainage from the catheter. The drainage tubing should then be secured by some means which permits movement of tubing and prevents tension and pull on the catheter. It is essential that the tubing be placed so that it cannot be compressed by the weight of the patient's buttocks or thigh.

To place the drainage tubing over the patient's thigh has a disadvantage in that urine may pool in the bladder until there is a sufficient amount of pressure to force it up the tubing. Drainage will not occur until the urine forces its way over the thigh, and then gravity suction will empty the bladder rapidly. The degree of suction will depend on the distance of the collecting container from the bladder. The greater the distance between the bladder and the container, the greater will be the pull on the bladder once siphonage has started.

If constant drainage is to be in effect, the drainage tube should be so arranged that accumulation of urine in the bladder or back flow into the bladder will not occur.

The Drainage Container. The drainage bottle or plastic disposable bag should be placed so that suction on the bladder is minimized in the event that occasional siphonage should occur. Attaching it to the bed frame is common practice. In addition, it should be inconspicuous to avoid embarrassment to the patient, yet easy to examine. Calibrated drainage containers have several advantages. Amounts of drainage can be determined readily, and measuring when emptying the bottle is eliminated.

Irrigation of the Retention Catheter. The physician usually orders irrigation of the retention catheter while it is in place to determine its patency. Catheter irrigations are done daily, and, in some instances, may need to be done several times daily because of the nature of the drainage.

Sterile equipment consisting of a bulb syringe, a basin and solution and a clean collecting basin are necessary. The catheter should be separated from the drainage tubing so that the solution is injected directly into the catheter. Varying amounts may be specified, but 30 cc. per instillation, repeated three or four times, usually is sufficient. This should be done while following strictest aseptic technic.

Care of the Drainage Tubing and Bottle. While normally the flow of urine is downward in the tubing, there is always the possibility of back flow of urine into the bladder, depending on the patient's position and activity. Therefore, drainage tubing should receive careful attention. Urine forms salt deposits in the tubing and in the container if allowed to stand for any length of time. Drainage tubing should be replaced frequently enough to avoid using tubing in which deposits have collected. The salt deposits are so difficult to remove that mere irrigation of the tubing is ineffective. Ideally, daily change is desirable, but two or three days should be the maximum length of time for one drainage tube to be attached.

It is impossible to overemphasize the importance of observing rigid asepsis when retention catheters are used, because of the high risk of bladder infections. Open drainage systems (those that terminate in an open bottle or a split plastic bag) are especially prone to lead to trouble. Organisms reach the container, ascend the tubing and catheter and cause bladder infections in many instances. Closed drainage is preferred, with the complete unit being a sterile closed circuit. The tubing terminates in a specially sealed container or in a container with cotton filters at the air outlet. Many persons recommend adding an antiseptic solution to the collecting container to aid in inhibiting the growth of organisms in the stale urine. Or a three-way catheter set-up can be used, which allows bladder rinses with antiseptics at regular intervals. Complete and at least daily cleansing of the area around the meatus is recommended for female patients, because organisms allowed to accumulate in this area can ascend and cause infection. Immaculate body hygiene is urged for all patients with retention catheters as still another effort to reduce the possibility of infection.

Unless contraindicated, the patient should be encouraged to take larger amounts of fluids than usual. Highly concentrated urine tends to promote bacterial growth. Also, a continuous discharge of urine aids in "washing" organisms away from the bladder.

Whenever the tubing is disconnected for any reason, the end of the catheter, and of the connecting tubing, should be carefully protected to prevent contaminating the set-up.

Retention catheters have increased the comfort of the ambulatory patient with bladder disturbances, whether he is in a health agency or at home. There are rubber or plastic urinals available, so designed that the catheter fits into the top. The urinal is then attached to the leg and held in place by small, soft straps. These urinals make it possible for the patient to be completely dressed without any evidence of the attachment. However, the patient should be taught that pressure on the container could force urine back into the bladder and should be avoided because of the danger of infection. Some patients are taught to use a clamp on the catheter and to release it to empty the bladder at specified intervals, such as every two or three hours. This practice makes the use of a collecting container unnecessary.

Patients who have retention catheters in place should have the benefit of full explanation on how the system is functioning and on how they can assist. Teaching points include keeping the tubing free from kinks, maintaining constant downward flow of the urine and keeping a record of the output.

When a retention catheter is in place, note any comments that the patient may make about it, such as, irritating, burning or annoying. Also note the drainage. Any signs of infection should be reported to the physician. After a retention catheter has been removed, it should be noted on the patient's nursing care plan. There is still need for observation. Frequency, burning on voiding, interference with the urinary stream, as inability to start it, and cloudy urine may be some of the aftermath of a retention catheter. Too often, patients endure the discomfort because they believe that is what is to be expected.

While a normal bladder is able to overcome these conditions, in some patients it has taken as long as four months to accomplish this. With a damaged bladder the time is much longer. Early recognition of and action on symptoms might very well have reduced this.

Urinary Incontinence

Incontinence is the inability to retain urine by voluntary effort. If the bladder is unable to store any urine and urine dribbles almost constantly, the condition is called *total incontinence.* If the bladder cannot be emptied normally, urine continues to accumulate, and, when there is sufficient pressure in the bladder, small amounts of urine may be forced out. The dribble of urine ends when the pressure has been reduced somewhat, but the bladder is not empty. This is called *overflow* or *paradoxical incontinence.* This type sometimes accompanies retention. Incontinence may be either permanent or temporary in nature, depending on the cause. It is a problem faced by many of our elderly patients.

Nursing Measures for Incontinence. As soon as a medical evaluation of the patient's problem has been made, nursing measures should be directed toward helping to restore normal function if there is a possibility of success. As with fecal incontinence, urinary incontinence should not be a situation to which everyone becomes resigned. The psychological value to the patient of knowing that effort is being made to help him cannot be underestimated. For example, suggesting a routine for taking fluids followed by periods of time to try voiding can be successful with some patients. They may not understand the relationship of fluid intake to voiding. Also voluntary efforts either to control or to induce voiding may be sufficiently stimulating to help restore function. For some patients, especially the elderly chronically ill, it may be as simple as taking them to the bathroom or offering a bedpan every two to three hours.

A quick course of action is to have a retention catheter inserted. The cost in terms of physical discomfort to the patient may be exceedingly high. Infection from an indwelling catheter is very common. One author[10] reports that the incidence is likely to be 95 per cent for those persons having a catheter in place three days or more. For some patients it will require months after the catheter is removed before the infection is cured.

In addition to efforts to help the patient to regain control of this function, other measures also must be considered, such as keeping the patient dry, clean and comfortable. Often, great skill and ingenuity are required to prevent odors and discomfort from wet clothing and linens. The ammonia of the urine and lying on wet linen quickly irritate the skin and predispose the patient to ammonia dermatitis and decubiti.

Patients with incontinence usually are embarrassed and insecure. The nurse can be of assistance by demonstrating tact and understanding while carrying out her nursing responsibilities. Offering emotional support, allowing the patient to talk of his problem and allowing him to assist with decision making about his care also are helpful. When the conscious patient is incontinent, it is best from a psychological standpoint to consult him about measures to help absorb urine, such as diapers or incontinent pads or keeping urinals in place. (Be sure to avoid the use of the word "diaper.")

In certain disease conditions, voluntary control of voiding may be impaired, but the reflex act of micturition is intact. These patients may be helped with bladder training. Drugs also are used to assist these patients.

Bladder Training. Bladder training, as with bowel training, should be instituted with the consent of the physician, since a complete evaluation of the patient's physical condition is essential. To start a patient on such a program when there is little or no possibility of his achieving results would be psychologically disastrous for him. Even if a patient is considered eligible for bladder training, he must be helped to understand that it will be a slow process and that the gains may be slight and very gradual. As in any situation, it is poor policy to permit a patient to set unrealistic goals for himself.

A primary factor in bladder training is the management of the patient's fluid intake. In addition to liquids such as milk, tea, broth, water and soup, foods of high liquid content also must be considered. Because of the time relationship between drinking and the occurrence of urine in the bladder, it is best to plan a drinking schedule that will permit convenient occasions for attempting to empty the bladder. For example, most persons urinate shortly after awakening, and this is usually the first and the best time for the patient to attempt to empty the bladder. Having some water immediately on waking is helpful. Other fluids can be spaced throughout the day according to the patient's wishes. Fluids should be limited in the late evening hours, thus limiting the risk of being incontinent during the night.

Position of the Patient. When the patient attempts to start bladder training, it is essential that conditions conducive to the process be provided. For example, the patient should be comfortable and relaxed, and adjustments should be made so that a good sitting position may be maintained. If the patient is not able to get out of bed and is going to use the bedpan, the head of the bed should be raised and the patient well supported by pillows. It is also best if the patient's knees are flexed during the period of time that an attempt to void is being made.

The position found to be most helpful is the normal sitting position. This position can be simulated by some patients if they are permitted to have their feet over the edge of the bed while sitting on a bedpan. In addition, they should have a foot support and a chair or overbed table on which to lean. A toilet or a commode is best if the patient is able to be out of bed.

Time. A regular schedule is also essential for helping the patient to establish a pattern. If there has been any regularity to the patient's incontinence of urine, these times should be considered in the scheduling. For example, if the patient notes that a frequent "wetting time" is 10:30 A.M., then provision for attempting to void should be made at 10:00 A.M.

The times selected for attempting to empty the bladder need not be spaced regularly, such as every four hours. However, they should be at the same time each day. The intervals between each voiding will be dependent on the patient's fluid intake and success in initiating the stimulus to void.

The Stimulus or Call. Any sensation which precedes the act of micturition is referred to as the *stimulus* or *call.* The patient should be informed that this may not be the usual kind of stimulus produced by a full bladder, but it may include other reactions, such as sensations in the abdomen, chilliness, sweating, muscular twitching, etc. It is important that the patient understand these signs as a part of the process, so as not to become apprehensive. Fear will interrupt the attempt.

Methods for Assisting the Process. While the patient is in the sitting position, it is helpful if he bends forward in a slow, rhythmic fashion. This creates pressure on the bladder. It also helps if the patient applies light pressure with the hands over the bladder. The pressure should be directed toward the urethra.

Other measures, such as those which are used to help patients void, also should be used if necessary. These include drinking fluids to the extent allowed, listening to running water, and smoking (if the patient enjoys it).

It is possible for the patient to void during the attempt without any knowledge of it or without any specific stimulus or control. This is still considered as involuntary voiding. Not until the patient is able to use a specific method to stimulate and empty the bladder is the bladder training program considered successful.

For those patients with severe neuromuscular involvement, the best method for inducing the stimulus and emptying the bladder may require considerable exploration; 15 to 20 minutes for each attempt is sufficient. Unsuccessful attempts are discouraging, and the patient should be helped to maintain a positive and hopeful attitude toward the process.

As a means of gauging the success of the attempts, examination for residual urine often is included as a part of the process. Percussion directly over the symphysis is one method. In some programs of rehabilitation, tests for residual urine are made by inserting a catheter. As the amount of residual urine diminishes and the success of emptying the entire bladder increases, the frequency of examination is reduced.

PAIN

Pain has intrigued the curiosity of science and has led to a huge array of pain-relieving technics since time immemorial. Yet despite its universality and eternal presence among mankind, the nature of pain remains an enigma.

Pain has been defined, and occasionally still is, on a philosophical and religious basis as punishment for wrongdoing. Aristotle defined pain as well as anyone when he wrote that it is the "antithesis of pleasure . . . the epitome of unpleasantness."

Pain is interpreted as a threat to the organism's integrity. The body has no mechanism for sensory adaptation to pain. As a matter of fact, we tend to become more sensitive as pain continues. Possibly this is caused by the physical and psychologic depletion that so often accompanies prolonged pain.

Pain is an imperative sensation. It has a preoccupying characteristic that tends to make us negate other sensations in its presence. Although pain warns of tissue injury or disease, the degree of pain is not necessarily in direct proportion to the amount of tissue damage.

From these introductory statements a basic principle concerning pain can be stated thus: *Sensations of physical discomfort may indicate injury or its threat to the body.*

There are two facets to pain—perception and reaction or response. Perception is concerned with the sensory processes when a stimulus for pain is present. The reaction or response to pain is concerned with the organism's method of coping with the sensation. Although this distinction is made, the reader's attention is called to the fact that not all literature on the subject makes this same differentiation.

Perception of Pain

The threshold of perception is the lowest intensity of a stimulus that causes the subject to recognize pain. This threshold is remarkably similar for everyone.

Pain sensations are conducted along a pathway which has been rather clearly defined in certain areas, although it is still somewhat questionable in others. There are no specific pain organs or cells in the body. Rather, an interlacing network of undifferentiated nerve endings receive painful stimuli. Sensation is carried to the dorsal grey horn cells of the spinal cord, then to the spinothalamic tract and eventually to the cerebral cortex. Although the autonomic nervous system is an efferent system—that is, it carries impulses *from* the central nervous system—pain sensations from the viscera apparently course along the autonomic system. Through that system, these sensations from deep-lying structures reach the spinal cord by way of the dorsal roots and then continue along the same pathways as sensations from the skin and superficial body structures. Pain impulses are also carried by the cranial nerves to the central nervous system. There is integration (perception as well as reaction) of the sensory impulses of pain along its entire central nervous system route, but the highest level of integration occurs in the cortex.

Stimulants for Pain. When the threshold of perception for pain has been reached, the injured tissue releases chemicals that modify pain receptors by increasing their sensitivity. Receptors in the skin and superficial organs, although incapable of responding selectively, are stimulated by mechanical, thermal, chemical and electrical agents. Friction from bed clothing and pressure from a cast are examples of mechanical stimulants. Sunburn and cold water on a tooth with caries are examples of thermal stimulants. An acid burn is the result of a chemical stimulant. The jolt of a static charge illustrates an electrical stimulant.

Stretching of the hollow viscera and pulling on the omentum result in pain. Some investigators believe that at least some of the deep-lying organs have their own individual pain receptors, the uterus being an example.

When tissue injury results in pain in an area removed from that in which stimulation has its origin, it is called *referred pain.* Very often, for example, patients with diseases of the gall bladder complain of pain in the upper back or shoulder areas. Several theories have been advanced concerning the phenomenon of referred pain, but none has widespread acceptance.

Responses to Pain

There are three responses the body makes to pain: voluntary, involuntary, and emotional or psychic.

Voluntary Responses. Voluntary responses are muscle reactions that trigger efforts to remove the painful stimulus. It is a kind of fight-or-flight reaction that spells protection or defense. One example is removing the hand hurriedly from a hot object. Grimacing and pacing the floor are examples also. Another person reacts by placing the injured part in a position that tends to relieve pain and by keeping the muscles rigid to maintain that position in efforts to avoid further injury. An example is to pull the knees up to the abdomen when abdominal pain is severe. These voluntary responses are protective in nature; also, through cognizance of pain, one remembers its causes and makes voluntary and purposeful attempts to avoid them in the future.

Involuntary Responses. Involuntary responses, often called autonomic responses, also are protective in nature, in that they increase the body's alertness to pain and promote organic homeostasis. In other words, the body prepares for emergency action. Examples include increases in perspiration, blood pressure, pulse and respiratory rates, pupil dilatation and an increase in the output of adrenalin. The physiology of these involuntary responses, discussed in other courses, teaches how each one prepares the body for necessary action when a threat to its integrity exists.

Emotional or Psychic Responses. *The emotional or psychic responses to pain have a wide and varying threshold among individuals.* The basis for this principle has been observed many times. A person's previous experience with pain and his racial, cultural and religious backgrounds all play a part. As one example, in certain cultures, weeping, crying loudly and other overt expressions of distress are part of the pain phenomenon. In other cultures, this behavior may be considered unacceptable. Personality characteristics also influence pain responses. Highstrung, neurotic persons in general have a low threshold of reaction, while stoic individuals appear to have a high threshold.

Preoccupation with other things has been observed to lower or raise the threshold. For example, soldiers severely wounded while under fire often indicate that they felt little pain until the excitement of battle subsided. Players injured during the exciting moments in a competitive game may be unaware of injury and pain until the game is completed.

Pain is almost always accompanied by anxiety and fear, sometimes anger too. These emotional reactions tend to intensify the emotional reactions to pain. Under these conditions, a vicious circle forms that may be difficult to break. Increased irritability, depression, feelings of loneliness, fatigue due to poor resting, and anorexia often add to the problem of relieving pain.

Experienced nurses have observed that patients tend to complain of pain more commonly during the night hours. The question has been asked as to whether pain is more persistent or severe during night hours. The answer is probably no. During the night, patients do seem to experience more anxiety and loneliness, which possibly in turn aggravate pain.

As pointed out earlier, although the perception threshold of pain seems fairly constant in nature, it has been observed that it can be altered to some extent for most people. In turn, reaction thresholds also are influenced. A loud noise, gripping an object (as the dentist's chair), clenching the jaws or experiencing pain elsewhere can alter perception thresholds. Also, hypnosis, alcohol and anesthesia alter perception thresholds and responses to pain.

Nursing Implications

Pain is a very personal, subjective experience and difficult to describe to another. It is a complicated phenomenon as well as an invisible process. It rarely responds to any one single approach. However, experience and research have shown that many nursing measures are helpful in promoting patient comfort when pain is present. These measures also have been demonstrated to enhance the effectiveness of more drastic measures when they must be used also.

Understanding the Patient. Inasmuch as a patient's background is very likely to influence his reaction to pain, it is well to start learning something about the patient who is complaining of pain by taking a nursing history. How much does the patient know about his present illness and of the pain he is experiencing? What types of pain has the patient experienced in the past? How did he react then? What environmental and personality factors may be influencing his reactions to pain? Can the family assist in attempting to understand the patient's reaction to pain? Answers to questions such as these will help the nurse in selecting measures that are likely to promote the patient's comfort.

In addition, the nurse will want to familiarize herself with the patient's medical history, his diagnosis, and the physician's plan of therapy.

Understanding the Nature of the Pain. Observing and reporting on the nature of pain was discussed in Chapter 17. It was pointed out that the quality, the intensity and the location are important. In addition, the nurse will want to know which factors tend to provoke pain and which ones tend to relieve it. What was its mode of onset? What has been its duration? If the patient has had previous experiences with similar pain, what measures tended to relieve pain at that time?

Removing the Source of Pain and Decreasing Pain Stimuli. Although the source of pain is often illusive, in some situations it can be determined rather readily. Removing the source of pain is ideal and sometimes possible. Here are a few examples: removing or loosening a tight binder if permissible; seeing to it that a distended bladder is emptied; taking steps to relieve constipation and/or flatus; changing the patient's position in bed, and giving him a back rub if muscles have become tense and sore; and changing soiled linen that may be irritating the skin. Although some of these measures may require the physician's consent, depending on agency policies, it is often the nurse who identifies a source of pain that can be remedied with relative ease.

There are factors that may be contributing to discomfort and removing their source often promotes comfort. For example, although the factors given in the previous paragraph are not the actual or only sources of pain for certain patients, they may be contributing to discomfort. Hence, the suggested nursing measures given above apply also in helping to decrease painful stimuli. The hungry or thirsty patient may need a snack or a drink to feel more comfortable. Fatigue tends to increase sensitivity to pain, and promoting rest with measures as discussed in Chapter 23 is helpful. If the source of pain is an exuding wound, a soiled wet dressing may be the source of trouble and changing it will promote comfort. For the patient uncomfortable with a cast after the fracture of an extremity, elevating the extremity may relieve pressure sufficiently to promote comfort. The patient in pain usually feels more comfortable when the environment is quiet and comfortable. Taking steps to eliminate unnecessary noise and glaring lights is helpful. Sometimes the nurse may want to speak with visitors who may be tiring the patient in pain.

These are just a few examples of nursing measures that experience has shown can aid in promoting patient comfort. Almost every chapter in this text offers still more additional suggestions for alleviating discomfort. The ingenious and resourceful nurse who has observed her patient with care is armed with a host of measures that, when used with skill, aid in assisting the patient suffering with pain.

Offering Emotional Support. Experience and research on controlling pain have shown that nursing measures offering emotional support to the patient are essential aids in relieving pain. The reader is encouraged to review Chapter 9, which offered suggestions in helping patients who are anxious and fearful, emotional responses often accompanying pain.

One study found that reduction of a patient's pain occurred following certain nurse/patient interactions. After introductions to initiate the interaction, the process included discussing pain with the patient, suggesting various pain-relieving measures other than medications, and allowing the patient to decide on the method of relief. In the experimental group of adult patients with moderate pain, most of them experienced relief with this type of nursing care.[14]

In another reference at the end of this chapter, the authors describe discussing pain with the patient, remaining with the patient and providing touch as important tools for providing comfort.[12]

Experience has demonstrated to many physicians and nurses that patients who feel confidence in health personnel caring for them do not require as much therapy for the relief of pain as those who are less confident. Without confidence, nothing seems to work. With it, often amazing results have been obtained using measures that ordinarily are only modestly effective.

Medically Prescribed Measures. There are times when medically prescribed measures become important. There is available a wide variety of analgesic drugs that certainly play an important role in pain control. When medication is required and is used judiciously, its administration is indeed desirable. However, using drugs as a substitute for good nursing care is an act indefensible for nurses interested in holding to high standards of patient care.

In certain instances, when pain is intractable, the physician may find it necessary to use procedures that obliterate or sever pathways for pain impulses. Even when such are indicated, they do not replace the patient's need for high caliber and individualized care which includes physical as well as emotional support.

ABNORMAL BODY TEMPERATURE

The body's mechanism for maintaining normal body temperature was discussed in Chapter 17. As was pointed out, pyrexia accompanies many clinical entities; hence, care of a patient with pyrexia is a common nursing experience. Although lowered body temperature is less common, it too can become cause for concern in certain situations.

There is a definite temperature range for efficient cellular functioning and proper enzymatic activity. This basic physiologic principle indicates that abnormal body temperature interferes with proper functioning and activity. Hence, there is need for concern when body temperatures fluctuate outside of normal range.

Common Symptoms of Abnormal Body Temperature

Common symptoms of elevated and lowered body temperatures are given here.

Table 8. Common symptoms of abnormal body temperature

Elevated Body Temperature	Lowered Body Temperature
Oral temperature above 99°F. (37.2°C.)	Oral temperature below 95°F. (35°C.)
Rapid full pulse, eventually weakens	Pulse varies, rapid or slow
Rapid respirations, sometimes with panting	Slow respirations
Flushed, hot, dry skin	Cool skin with gooseflesh, shivering, pallor
Feeling of warmth	Feeling of chilliness
Excessive perspiration	Numbness and loss of skin sensation
Malaise, restlessness, irritability	
Eventual delirium and loss of consciousness	
Convulsions, especially in children	

A *chill* is an involuntary muscular twitch, which occurs as the body tries to achieve homeostasis by raising the temperature through a form of muscular activity. Chills often accompany fever (for instance, with a urinary infection) and are reflex in nature. Nursing care of a patient experiencing a chill includes provision of warmth, giving antipyretic medications as ordered by the physician, and keeping a check on the blood pressure and pulse rate, because patients having a chill may go into a state of shock.

When hypothermia (lowered body temperature) is prescribed and desirable, a chill, which raises body temperature, is contraindicated. Drugs usually are given to counteract the effects of a chill in such instances.

Nursing Implications When Pyrexia is Present

Of vital importance is observation and assessment of the severity of the condition. An elevated temperature is a protective mechanism. But if it is not kept under control, the mechanism becomes destructive in nature. For example, a temperature rising above 106° F. (41.1° C.) could be fatal because of its destructive effect on body cells. Prolonged elevated temperatures of lesser degrees may become so debilitating to the body that life is threatened. Hence, keeping close watch on patients with pyrexia is an essential nursing function.

Heat leaves the body by way of conduction, radiation and convection currents. The body keeps cool, to a degree, through evaporation of normal perspiration. Heat from the body is utilized to cause evaporation of moisture, which conducts heat away. When the atmospheric humidity is high, evaporation is slower because of the already moisture-laden air. When humidity is low, evaporation occurs more rapidly. Ice caps also help to reduce temperature by conducting body heat away to the ice.

Radiation transfers heat in the form of waves. Radiation is responsible for the feeling of warmth when one places his hand near a light bulb. In the same manner, the body loses heat by radiation. The convection principle is in operation when currents of air are present; the air, which absorbs heat, becomes lighter, rises, and is replaced by cooler air. This explains why body cooling results when one is in a draft, near a fan, or in an air-conditioned room.

These basic facts of physics help to guide nursing practice when the body temperature is abnormal. Here are examples of measures that are useful when pyrexia is present: tepid sponges reduce body temperature by evaporation and conduction. If alcohol is added to the water, the cooling process is increased since alcohol evaporates more readily than water. Removing extra bed linen and clothing allows for additional heat loss through evaporation and radiation; the use of a fan increases loss of heat by convection currents.

There are nursing measures that aid in decreasing the body's heat production also. Activity increases the rate of metabolism and, hence, heat production. Therefore, keeping the patient quiet is important. Serving easily digested fluids and food aids in reducing the heat production of digestion. During rest heat production is decreased. Hence, extra rest periods are encouraged for patients with pyrexia.

Excessive perspiration and increased respirations account for increased fluid and electrolyte losses when pyrexia is present. Disturbances are further aggravated when there is an inadequate intake of fluids and food. Nursing measures to promote fluid and electrolyte balance, discussed in Chapter 24, apply here. Of special importance are encouraging fluid intake (within medical orders) and keeping a close account of the patient's intake and output. In many instances parenteral fluids will be ordered by the physician.

Because of the effects of pyrexia on the body, needs for certain additional nursing measures become evident. A pyrexic patient usually is restless, thus stimulating even more heat production. Assisting to position the patient comfortably aids in promoting rest. When perspiration is present, keeping bed linens and clothing dry is important. Many patients with elevated temperatures need extra oral hygiene measures in order to keep the teeth, mucous membrane, tongue and lips clean and moist. Although easily digested food is indicated, an adequate-to-surplus intake of protein is desirable to aid in tissue repair. The skin requires extra attention to prevent irritation that can easily lead to decubiti in a debilitated patient when pyrexia is present.

There are drugs, aspirin being a common example, that the physician may order to aid in controlling body temperature. These drugs are called *antipyretics*.

Patients with pyrexia need psychologic comfort as well as physical support. A plea is made here, as has been done on previous occasions in this text, to recognize emotional components and to make concerted efforts to assist patients in coping with them.

Nursing Implications When Lowered Body Temperature is Present

The same underlying principle and facts of physics as used in the care of patients with pyrexia apply here. However, instead of measures to increase heat loss and decrease heat production, measures that promote the opposite are used. Here are a few examples: use additional bed linen and clothing as indicated; keep the environmental temperature warmer than usual; apply external heat; offer warm or hot fluids and food; and keep movement of air at a minimum. If the patient's condition warrants it, body activity and sturdier meals are desirable.

The same comments made in relation to the emotional support of patients with pyrexia apply here.

NAUSEA, VOMITING AND ANOREXIA

When nausea and vomiting are present, the body is placed in jeopardy by disturbances of two essential bodily needs: adequate nourishment and fluid and electrolyte balance. The basic principles in relation to these two needs were given in Chapters 18 and 24, and the reader is encouraged to review them.

Nausea

Nausea is a feeling of sickness with a desire to vomit. It is felt in the back of the throat or the pit of the stomach. Perspiring, vasomotor disturbances resulting in pallor, and excessive salivation commonly accompany nausea. Retching also is often present.

It is believed that increased tension, stretching, and pressure on the walls of the stomach and duodenum are responsible for the sensation of nausea. Also, distention of the lower portion of the esophagus produces nausea. If for any reason the stomach descends, tension on this general area of the gastrointestinal tract is present and nausea follows. This last phenomenon is believed responsible when such things as offensive odors and rapid changes in the speed of an elevator bring on waves of nausea. The nausea associated with motion sickness seems to result from semicircular canal stimulation.

Nausea usually precedes vomiting but either one may be present without the other.

Vomiting

Vomiting is a common and complex symptom associated with numerous clinical entities. It is a reflex act that relieves the upper gastrointestinal tract of its contents. The contents are referred to as *emesis* or *vomitus.* Vomiting is a protective mechanism that enables the body to rid itself of irritating contents.

Projectile vomiting refers to the expulsion of vomitus with great force, often without the presence of nausea. Persistent and intractable vomiting is called *pernicious vomiting.* Bringing stomach contents to the throat and mouth without vomiting effort is *regurgitation.* It occurs commonly among infants when, it is believed, the infant spits up excess food. *Eructation* or *belching* is a discharge of gas from the stomach through the mouth.

The part of the gastrointestinal tract most sensitive to stimulants producing vomiting is the first part of the duodenum. However, sufficient stimulus in almost any section of the tract can produce vomiting. For example, mechanical irritation of the pharynx and fauces produces vomiting in most people. The irritation of an obstruction anywhere along the intestinal tract often produces violent vomiting. When abnormal stimulation of other organs in the body exists, vomiting is often present also. This can be observed when injury or disease affects the uterus, kidneys, heart, semicircular canals, or the brain. Cranial pressure generally produces violent vomiting, projectile in nature. It is a significant sign of deterioration and the physician should be notified when it occurs.

Psychic stimuli for vomiting include nauseating odors, sights, tastes, thoughts, and the like.

The Vomiting Mechanism. It has been demonstrated that a vomiting center is located in the medulla oblongata. Near the center is a trigger zone that apparently collects impulses of chemical irritants (drugs being an example) that in turn produce the vomiting. Other impulses eventually reach the center from the cortex and from other areas in the body, the exact pathways being largely undetermined. Some authorities believe that the vomiting center is not stimulated directly except by chemical irritants. Efferent pathways from the central nervous system carry impulses that influence the mechanical act of vomiting.

The most generally accepted theory concerning the mechanism of vomiting is that antiperistalsis occurs to expel gastrointestinal contents through the mouth (however, investigation continues—which may eventually throw the antiperistalsis theory into doubt). Abdominal and diaphragmatic muscular contractions aid in forcing food from the tract. Breathing ceases temporarily and the glottis closes, both mechanisms helping to prevent the aspiration of vomitus into the respiratory tract. In the unconscious patient, the glottis does not close, thus adding to the vomiting problem the danger of respiratory aspiration of vomitus.

Anorexia

Anorexia is defined as a lack or a loss of appetite or a marked aversion to food. The causes include those having a physiologic basis (as a gastric irritation) or a psychic basis (as any factor that makes eating distasteful) or both. Many times nursing measures such as were discussed in Chapter 18 will assist in overcoming anorexia. In some instances, persistence of the symptom may require medical attention to supplying necessary bodily nutrients by routes other than normal eating and drinking.

Anorexia is commonly associated with nausea and vomiting. One has only to recall a personal experience or two with nausea and vomiting to remember the accompanying distress of anorexia.

Nursing Implications

Attention has been called to the basic principles that indicate every person's need for an adequate intake of food and fluids. When nausea, vomiting and anorexia are persent, nursing measures are directed toward eliminating them as much as possible, so as to avoid placing the body in jeopardy from lack of food and fluids.

When the cause can be identified and removed, the problem may be largely solved. For example, when a patient is experiencing nausea and vomiting from unsightly odors and sights, removing them may be an easy solution. When the cause has a physiologic basis, nausea and vomiting may be present until therapy begins to make amends. For example, when cranial pressure is relieved, vomiting usually ceases. When gastritis is relieved, so also is nausea.

In some instances, drugs called *antiemetics*, which act to allay vomiting, may be prescribed by the physician. There are drugs too that aid in reducing the nausea and vomiting associated with motion sickness. Some of them have been used effectively with other conditions as well, the nausea and vomiting of early pregnancy being an example. In some cases, certain preparations also assist in stimulating the appetite and help in overcoming anorexia.

The patient who is vomiting needs protection and comfort. The danger of aspirating vomitus is often present and is a serious hazard, especially with the semi-conscious and unconscious patient, or with infants and small children. Suction may become necessary for these patients to clear the upper gastrointestinal and respiratory tracts. Turning the patient's head to one side aids in ridding the mouth of its contents. Gravity helps if the patient's head can safely be lowered slightly. Marked Trendelenburg positions are to be avoided as gravity may then be strong enough to produce more vomiting.

For patients with abdominal wounds, supporting the area with binders, a pillow splint, or with the nurse's hand is helpful. These procedures offer comfort to the patient and help to prevent opening of a wound, although this is an uncommon complication.

Comforting the patient includes special mouth care. This should be instituted as soon as possible after vomiting ceases, because the taste and odor of vomitus often is sufficient to produce more. Soiled linen and clothes are changed and emesis basins are emptied promptly.

The tension often associated with vomiting may be relieved by giving the patient a back rub. A clean, quiet and comfortable environment also helps.

Additional measures that assist the patient with nausea and vomiting include these: limit the patient's activities as much as possible, especially if motion has brought on the symptoms; assist the patient to assume a comfortable position; take steps to alleviate pain if present; limit the patient's intake until the symptoms subside. Then offer fluids and food separately; offer bland and nonfatty foods; assist infants to bring up air bubbles by burping them; be prepared to offer emotional support when emotional components are present.

Observations and recording concerning emesis were discussed in Chapter 17.

Study Situations

1. The following article deals with the subject of pain:

- Jarratt, V.: The keeper of the keys.
  AMER. J. NURS., *65*:68-70, July, 1965.

Consider the author's suggestion that routinized patterns followed by many nurses in handling a patient in pain are the result of their inability to deal effectively with the patient suffering discomforts. Do you believe nurses sometimes choose a "flight response" in order to avoid involvement with the patient in pain? Explain your answer. List various nursing measures that often can relieve pain without using drugs, discussed in the last six paragraphs of this article.

2. The two references below are programmed instruction on pain. The reader is urged to go through both of these programs carefully as an excellent supplement to the discussion of pain presented in this chapter.

- Pain. Part 1. Basic concepts and assessment.
  AMER. J. NURS., *66*:1085-1108, May, 1966.
- Pain. Part 2. Rationale for intervention.
  AMER. J. NURS., *66*:1345-1368, June, 1966.

3. The following article describes how reflex responses can be conditioned to aid in controlling certain involuntary behavior:

- Elizabeth, Sister R.: Sensory stimulation techniques.
  AMER. J. NURS., *66*:281-286, February, 1966.

What technics does the author suggest to stimulate voiding? What technics, does she say, promote retention when incontinence is a problem? Note also that a similar method is suggested for bowel control.

4. In the April, 1967, issue of the American Journal of Nursing, (*67*:780-797), there are seven articles under the title, "The Hazards of Immobility." Note the following two in particular, which deal with content discussed in this chapter:

- McCarthy, J. A.: Effects on gastrointestinal function.

List the deterring factors for hospitalized patients that tend to cause ignoring of the defecation act. What nursing measures does the author suggest as aids to prevent constipation?

- Schroeder, L. M.: The effects on urinary function.

According to this author, what dangers exist when retention is allowed to continue? What is the primary danger when retention or indwelling catheters must be used? Note the electrolyte disturbances the author describes when bed rest is prolonged and the danger of "stones of recumbency" exists.

5. The following article supplements material on vomiting presented in this chapter:

- Downs, H. S.: The control of vomiting.
  AMER. J. NURS., *66*:76-82, January, 1966.

Note the diagram on page 78, which describes stimuli that initiate vomiting.

6. Reducing the number of persons to a team of "experts" who may insert and irrigate catheters is one means of reducing the high incidence of bladder infections. How did this agency devise such a system and why? Note the technic used for "urethral toilette."

- Lindan, R., and Keane, A. T.: The catheter team.
  AMER. J. NURS., *64*:128-132, September, 1964.

7. In case the reader has considered the use of the problem solving process as an approach to nursing problems only, it should be understood that the process is helpful for patients as well. Some patients can benefit from being taught how to use it. No patient going home from the hospital, or even one managing health problems at home, always has someone available to him, giving him pat answers each time he has a problem or a question. Teaching the patient how to handle such situations is as valuable as any other health teaching that may be necessary.

- Collins, R. D.: Problem solving, a tool for patients too.
  AMER. J. NURS., *68*:1483-1485, July, 1968.

References

1. Barnard, J.: Understanding and treating the patient in pain.
   R.N., 73-78, May, 1967.
2. Barnhill, S. E. *et al*: Cleansing the perineum.
   AMER. J. NURS., *66*:566, March, 1966.
3. Beeson, P. B., and McDermott, W., eds.: Cecel-Loeb Textbook of Medicine. ed. 12., pp. 846; 848-850; 1468-1473.
   Philadelphia, W. B. Saunders, 1967.
4. Boyarsky, S., and Goldenberg, J.: Detection of bladder distention by suprapubic percussion.
   NEW YORK J. MED., *62*:1804, June 1, 1962.
5. Cox, C. E., and Hinman, F., Jr.: Retention catheterization and the bladder defense mechanisms.
   J.A.M.A., *191*:171-174, January 18, 1965.
6. Dembicki, E. L.: The two sides of pain—(Part I).
   J. PSYCHIAT. NURS. MENTAL HEALTH SERVICES, *5*:183-186, March-April, 1967.
7. Downs, H. S.: The control of vomiting.
   AMER. J. NURS., *66*:76-82, January, 1966.
8. Eckenhoff, J. E., (Guest Editor): Pain and its clinical management.
   MED. CLIN. N. AMER., *52*:228, January, 1968.
9. Hanken, A. F.: Pain and systems analysis.
   NURS. RES., *15*:139-143, Spring, 1966.
10. Kaye, M.: The initiation of urinary tract infection following a single bladder catheterization.
    CANAD. M.A.J., *86*:9, January 6, 1962.
11. Mackinnon, H. A.: Urinary drainage: The problem of asepsis.
    AMER. J. NURS., *65*:112, August, 1965.
12. McCaffery, M., and Moss, F.: Nursing intervention for bodily pain.
    AMER. J. NURS., *67*:1224-1227, June, 1967.
13. McCarthy, R. T.: Vomiting.
    NURS. FORUM, *3*:48-59, #1, 1964.
14. Moss, F. T., and Meyer, B.: The effects of nursing interaction upon pain relief in patients.
    NURS. RES., *15*:303-306, Fall, 1966.
15. Rogers, A.: Pain and the cancer patient.
    NURS. CLIN. N. AMER., *2*:671-682, December, 1967.
16. Santora, D.: Preventing hospital-acquired urinary infection.
    AMER. J. NURS., *66*:790-794, April, 1966.
17. Saxon, J.: Techniques for bowel and bladder training.
    AM. J. NURS., *62*:69, September, 1962.
18. Stafford, N. H.: Bowel hygiene of aged patients.
    AM. J. NURS., *63*:102, September, 1963.
19. Thompson, S. M.: Managing the problems of elimination.
    NURS. OUTLOOK, *14*:58-61, November, 1966.
20. Tillery, B., and Bates, B.: Enemas.
    AMER. J. NURS., *66*:534-537, March, 1966.
21. Webb, C.: Tactics to reduce a child's fear of pain.
    AMER. J. NURS., *66*:2698-2699, December, 1966.
22. Whitehead, J. A.: Urinary incontinence in the aged: Propantheline bromide as an adjunct to treatment.
    GERIATRICS, *22*:154-158, January, 1967.
23. Zborowski, M.: Cultural components in response to pain.
    J. SOC. ISSUES, *8*:16-30, #4, 1952.

CHAPTER 26

Special Considerations When Death Appears Imminent

Introduction

A terminal illness is one from which recovery is beyond reasonable expectation. The illness may be due to a disease condition or the result of accident or injury. Errors of judgment concerning recovery sometimes are made, and some readers may recall from personal experiences patients whose illnesses were considered as being terminal, but they survived and lived for many years. Because errors of judgment can occur, and during the course of an illness medical progress may bring forth a means of saving a life, there is good reason to remain hopeful while caring for terminally ill patients. The patient and his family often find courage and support in knowing that everything possible is being done and that hope for recovery is not abandoned.

The inevitability of death is nowhere better expressed than in Ecclesiastes 3:1-2—"To everything there is a season, and a time to every purpose under the heaven; A time to be born, and a time to die; . . ." Everyone has the privilege of and the right to meet death serenely and comfortably, and the nurse can do much to make this experience less fraught with sorrow, fear and discomfort for all concerned.

Although there is an increase in the amount of literature concerning the terminally ill, systematic investigation still is sadly lacking. Health personnel are constantly on the look-out for ways to control and combat disease—a fact that may well stand in the way of studying death per se. As a result, our actions are guided primarily by observations of persons who, while terminally ill, expressed their feelings, or by those who have cared for them. Although research is scarce, still these observations can do much to assist the nurse who is caring for terminally ill patients.

The Nurse's Attitude Toward Terminal Illness

Understanding others through understanding oneself is an oft-repeated psychological principle the importance of which probably would be argued by few. Since impending death is accompanied by fear of the unknown and the natural instinct of all creatures to cling to life, it becomes particularly important for the nurse to understand her own feelings toward terminal illness, death and its usual accompanying grief in order to help to meet the needs of patients for whom she is caring. One author expressed this thought in the following way[17]:

> . . . I would like first to emphasize that the part of life experience concerned with death is one of the most difficult for people to think about and take part in . . . This may be true because in our culture we put tremendous value on youth and to a considerable extent ignore aging and dying as important experiences in the life process. If nurses are to be useful to patients in these experiences, they must give some consideration to what death means to them as individuals and to others. They have to consider the meaning of fear, of crying, of anxiety and panic. They also have to consider the nursing skills they must develop if they are to be able to work with patients on these problems.

The nurse who neglects to think how she feels concerning terminal illness and death is in a questionable position to be able to analyze and consider the needs of patients who are facing death. Therefore, one's own personality, feelings and attitudes play a major role in determining how one cares for a patient with a terminal illness. Everyone—not only nurses—has emotional problems when death is pending. The easy way to react is to ignore the problems. Sadly enough, as a result, the dying person is often emotionally abandoned and left to travel his lonesome road.

Helping the Patient Who Has a Terminal Illness

Helping to Meet Emotional Needs. Discussion in Chapter 7 pointed out the importance of helping patients to feel secure. The importance of helping a patient to maintain self-identity, his sense of worth and his feeling of belonging were stressed. These factors in helping patients face death are especially important. Even when it is known that nothing available to medical science can prolong a patient's life, hope continues and the patient benefits when helped to feel secure.

How can the nurse help patients meet the emotional need for security? Although the content in Unit Two offers many clues, there is no magic formula. However, there are two general guides: being available and present as much as possible and offering whatever assistance can be given. The nurse's judgment and advice are not sought; her understanding, respect for the patient, and support are needed.

The manner in which patients face death depends on several factors. Philosophies of life and death differ. Most patients are afraid, while others may look forward to death as a relief from earthly suffering and sorrow. Some patients—often those having strong religious beliefs—have been observed to be spiritually exalted and ready to enter another life to which they look forward with joy. Other patients may treat death as an avenger and feel so depressed and desperate that they have suicidal tendencies. Also, the patient's attitudes toward and philosophy about death may be the result of his cultural background.

The age of the patient often influences the manner in which terminal illness and death are accepted. Children usually approach death with little fear or sorrow. Teenagers and adults through middle age often consider death as an injustice for they yearn to continue the experience of life and are sad about leaving their loved ones. This earnestness to live almost always subsides as death approaches, but in some cases it may not. Older people more often face death as a friend. They may have little desire to live and often are lonesome and tired of life, especially when loved ones have died before them.

A patient's reaction to approaching death

may change from day to day. A discouraged person may feel more so one day and less so another. The nurse must often develop great sensitivity in order to detect the patient's responses if she is to find clues for guiding her action.

Sometimes, a patient may mask his true feelings about death or may not really want to face the truth. The patient may claim to be unafraid and prepared for death when he really is fearful and just trying to appear brave. Patience, careful observation and listening in order to learn true feelings are a prerequisite if the nurse desires to give sincere comfort and support to the dying patient.

It is often said that the so-called "strong" personality faces death with courage and composure. However, it seems more likely that this type of person simply does a better job than most of concealing his depression from others. Possibly, death is faced better when there seems to be little to lose. On the other hand, the "strong" person has much more to lose (many friends, usually success in his work, family, etc.) ; thus, death is not easy to face.

Observations of dying patients suggest that often patients are most afraid and anxious when they first realize that they are terminally ill, but, as death approaches, fear and sorrow often seem to subside. Possibly at this point, the patient no longer needs to deny the truth about approaching death.

Knowing the patient's attitudes and feelings helps the nurse to care for him intelligently. The behavior of a patient facing death may not conform to what the nurse believes to be correct. But her actions must be guided by the patient's feelings and attitudes, not hers. Comfort, support and encouragement are essential, but the manner in which they are offered depends on individual circumstances. In some instances, the nurse may find that it is best to say nothing and just listen. The patient may find comfort in having someone with whom he can talk out his feelings. The lonely patient may experience support and understanding by a simple handclasp. Offering pity and displaying signs of grief are least helpful.

The question usually arises concerning what to tell the terminally ill patient about his prognosis. It is the physican who is responsible for deciding what and how the patient shall be told. Usually he makes this decision after discussing the problem with the patient's family and after assessing the patient individually.

In some situations, the physician may prefer to deny the patient the truth about his prognosis. He may feel that the experience of knowing may precipitate a psychological state of depression leading possibly to suicide. In some instances, this argument may be valid. The knowledge of impending death may be too much for some to tolerate. Other times, there may be neither a desire nor a need for the patient to know the truth. For example, a son or a daughter of an elderly patient who is terminally ill may be taking the responsibility for the patient. The patient may be content and reveal no real interest in his condition.

In other situations, the patient does have an interest and a desire to know. It is unkind and unfair to permit such a patient to die without his having known the seriousness of his condition. For example, by not knowing, he may have had the time denied him to arrange important business affairs, papers, finances and the like. Many people, especially those who have responsibilities to others, such as their children, find comfort in the fact that, should they die, "their house is in order."

Most people now seem to feel that withholding the truth from the patient is undesirable and often even harmful. From many observations, it has been seen that most patients realize without being told that they are suffering from an incurable illness. They feel even more isolated, lonely and rejected when the truth is withheld, especially when falsehoods are told them. After the prognosis has been discussed in an open and frank manner, health personnel must be prepared to offer the patient support. But usually the patient finds solace eventually in knowing and realizing that he will not be left to meet death alone.

The important thing for the nurse is to determine what the physician's wishes are in relation to what the patient and family are told. Patients and families often direct questions to the nurse concerning prognosis. Unless the nurse is aware of the physician's decision, the nurse and physician may be working at cross-purposes. It is up to the nurse to take the initiative to discuss the problem with the physician in circumstances in which uncertainty exists.

Helping To Meet Spiritual Needs. Most terminally ill patients find great comfort in the support that they receive from their religious faiths. It is important to aid in obtaining the services of a clergyman as each situation indicates. In some instances, the nurse may offer to call a clergyman when the patient has not expressed a desire to see one, but this must be handled tactfully and in good judgment so that the patient is not frightened by the suggestion. However, it must be remembered that a religious faith is not an insurance policy guaranteeing security from the tragedy and the loneliness of death. The chaplain's visit does not replace the kind words and the gentle touch of the nurse. Rather, he should be considered as one of the team assisting the patient to face terminal illness.

Helping To Meet Physical Needs. Unless death occurs suddenly, there are certain nursing problems concerning the patient's physical needs that the nurse usually can expect to encounter.

Nutrition. The patient who is terminally ill usually has little interest in food and fluids. His appetite fails, and often the physical effort to eat or drink is too great for him. Meeting nutritional needs may in itself help to prolong life, and it also often helps to make the patient more comfortable. Dehydration and cachexia predispose to exhaustion, infection and other complications, as the development of decubiti. Therefore, maintaining the nutritional state of the patient plays an important part in sustaining energy and preventing additional discomfort. When the patient is unable to take fluids and food by mouth, the physician very often orders intravenous therapy.

When death is pending, the normal activities of the gastrointestinal tract decrease. Therefore, offering the patient large quantities of food may only predispose to distention and added discomfort.

If the swallowing reflex is intact, offering sips of water at frequent intervals is helpful. As swallowing becomes difficult, aspiration may occur when fluids are given. The patient can suck on gauze soaked in water or on ice chips wrapped in gauze without difficulty since sucking is one of the last reflexes to disappear as death approaches.

Care of the Mouth, the Nose and the Eyes. If the patient is taking foods and fluids without difficulty, oral hygiene is similar to that offered other patients. However, as death approaches, the mouth usually needs additional care. Mucus that cannot be swallowed or expectorated accumulates in the mouth and the throat and may be aspirated. The mouth can be wiped out with gauze, or, if indicated, suctioning may be necessary to remove mucus. Positioning the patient on his side and placing a gauze wick in his mouth to keep it open, if necessary, very often aid in keeping the mouth and the throat free of accumulated mucus.

The mucous membrane should be kept free of dried secretions. Lubricating the mouth and the lips is helpful as well as comfortable for the patient.

The nostrils should be kept clean also and lubricated as necessary.

Sometimes, secretions from the eyes accumulate. The eyes may be wiped clean with wipes or cotton balls moistened in normal saline. If the eyes are dry, they tend to stay open. The instillation of a lubricant in the conjunctival sac may be indicated to prevent friction and possible ulceration of the cornea.

Care of the Skin. As death approaches, the patient's temperature usually is elevated above normal. But, as peripheral circulation fails, the skin feels cold, and the patient often perspires profusely. It is important to keep the bed linens and the bed clothing dry by bathing the patient and changing linens as necessary. Using light bed clothing and supporting it so that it does not rest on the patient's body usually give additional comfort.

The patient often is restless and may be observed to pick at his bed clothing. This may be due to the fact that he feels too warm; sponging him and keeping him dry often promote relaxation and quiet sleeping.

If the patient is incontinent of urine and feces, care of the skin becomes particularly important to prevent odors and decubiti. If a diaper is used, it is important for the nurse to explain to the patient that she is helping to protect his skin. Using a diaper can be psychologically upsetting to the patient, even when dying.

Problems of Elimination. Some patients may be incontinent while others may need to be observed for retention of urine and for constipation, both of which are uncomfortable for the patient. Cleansing enemas may be ordered for relieving and preventing constipation and distention, but it should be remembered that, if the patient is taking little nourishment, there may be only small amounts of fecal material in the intestine.

Some physicians order retention catheters or catheterization at regular intervals when problems of urinary elimination are present.

Positioning the Patient. The dorsal recumbent position often is associated with the dying patient. However, good nursing care provides for good positioning with frequent changes in position. The patient may not be able to express a desire to have his position changed, or he may feel that the effort is too great. Even though the patient appears to be unconscious, proper positioning is important. Poor positioning without adequate support is fatiguing as well as uncomfortable.

When dyspnea is present, the patient will be more comfortable when supported in the semi-sitting position. Stertorous or noisy breathing frequently is relieved when the patient is placed on his side. This position helps to keep the tongue from obstructing the respiratory passageway in the oropharynx. Proper positioning has been discussed earlier in this text, and the same principles that were discussed then guide action in positioning the terminally ill patient.

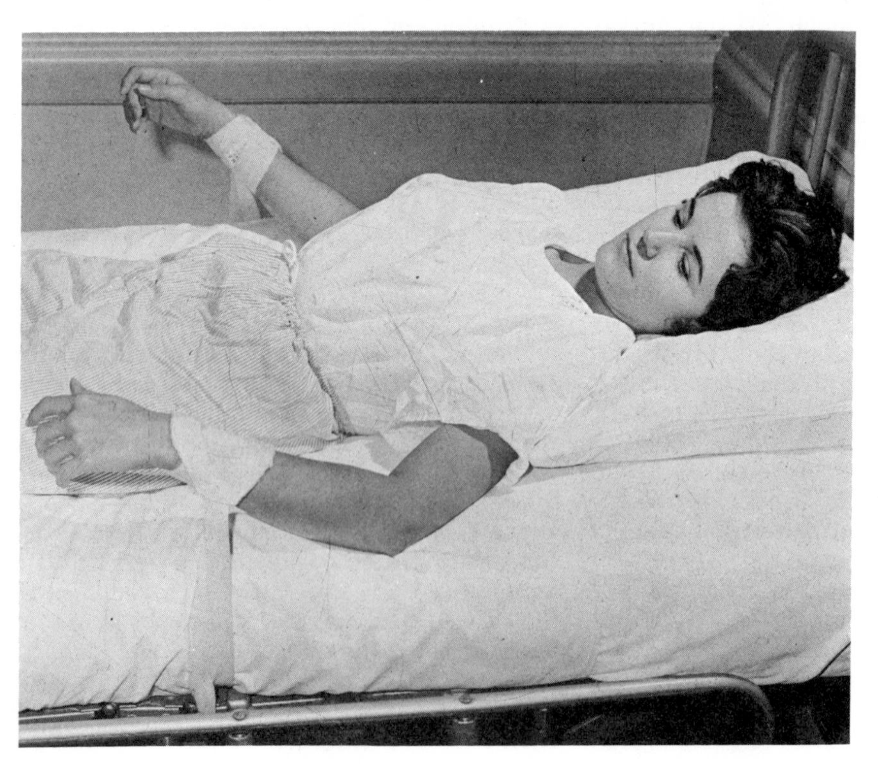

Fig. 26-1. Hand restraints should not immobilize the patient's arms. If they are needed to prevent the patient from pulling out a catheter, a nasal tube, an infusion, or from touching a dressing, they should be applied to serve this purpose. These restraints allow the patient to turn his arms and to lift his arms to some extent.

Protecting the Patient From Harm. The terminally ill patient is often restless. In these instances, special precautions are necessary to protect the patient from harm. The use of bedrails may be indicated. Restraining the patient usually is undesirable but may be necessary in extreme cases. Figures 26-1 and 26-2 illustrate several types of restraints. If relatives ask to watch and remain with the patient so that he does not injure himself, the nurse must explain the responsibility carefully and use good judgment, since it still is her responsibility to protect the patient from harm.

Care of the Environment. It is economical of nursing time to place the patient in a unit that is convenient for giving nursing care and for observing him at frequent intervals. Very often, the patient is placed in a private room to avoid distressing other patients. However, this experience in itself may be upsetting to the patient, as the case of Mr. Edd, related later in this chapter, illustrates. Social deprivation can be distressing to the patient, even if he cannot express this.

Normal lighting should be used in the patient's room. Terminally ill patients often complain of loneliness, fear and poor vision,

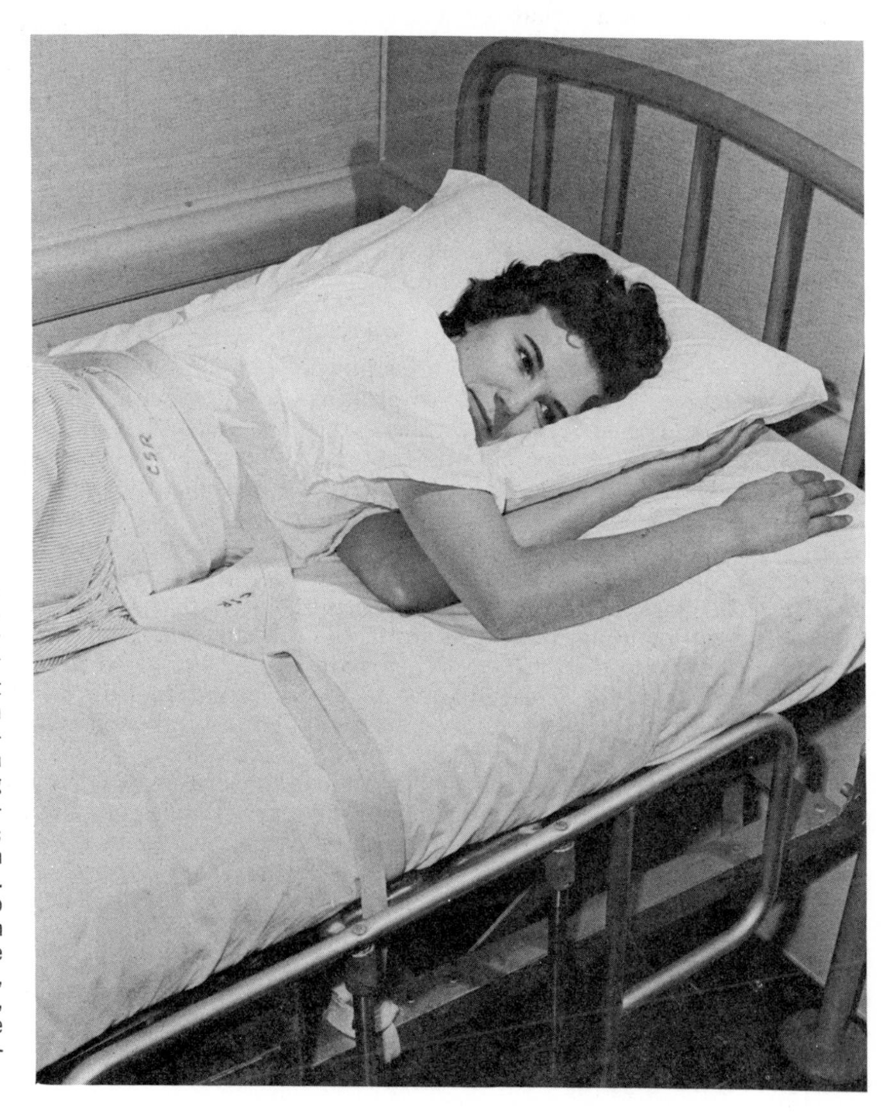

FIG. 26-2. Restraints which can be adjusted to the specific activity limitation desired are more likely to be accepted by the patient and his family. For example, preventing a patient from sitting up, but allowing him to turn from side to side; permitting him to sit up and to turn from side to side, but preventing him from climbing over the siderails or from getting out of bed; or preventing a patient from turning on one side or the other. The purpose of restraints is to help to prevent the patient from harm. They should not interfere with physiologic functioning, such as impairing circulation, limiting muscular activity to the point of immobilization or interfering with respiration.

all of which are exaggerated by darkening the room. The room should be well ventilated, and the patient protected from drafts.

While conversing near the patient's bedside, it is preferable to speak in a normal tone of voice. Whispering can be annoying to the patient and may make him feel that secrets are being kept from him. It generally is believed that the sense of hearing is the last sense to leave the body, and many patients retain a sense of hearing almost to the moment of death. Therefore, care should be exercised concerning topics of conversation. Even when the patient appears to be unconscious, he may hear what is being said in his presence. It generally is comforting to the patient for others to say things which he may like to hear. Even when he cannot respond, it is kind and thoughtful to speak to him. It also remains important for the nurse to explain to the patient what she is going to do when giving nursing care or working in the unit so that the patient does not misunderstand her actions or become fearful.

Keeping the Patient Comfortable. Efforts to meet the physical needs of a terminally ill patient may still fall short of keeping him comfortable, and then it becomes necessary to consider the use of medications that relieve pain and restlessness. In most instances, the physician will order a narcotic to aid in relieving pain. Although such medications should be administered with the usual precautions, there appears to be little excuse for withholding their use until the patient suffers from discomfort. When pain is intense, analgesia is more difficult to attain. Therefore, it is better to keep pain in remission. The problem of drug addiction is present when it is expected that the patient may live with a terminal illness for a long period of time, but this problem decreases as death draws near.

It has been observed that complaints of pain sometimes are a camouflage for fear. In such instances, the pain may appear to be disproportionate to the patient's pathology. However, pain is less likely to be over-rated when the nurse has gained the patient's confidence. Persons working with the terminally ill have noted that patients experiencing good emotional support require less analgesic drugs.

Drugs are indicated also for very anxious patients. Sedatives, and narcotics in particular, aid in clouding mental alertness and their use may be the kindest therapy one has to offer. It is best to plan nursing care for these patients when drugs have reached peak action.

As peripheral circulation fails, the absorption of drugs given subcutaneously is impaired, and other routes of administering the drug may become necessary.

Signs of Approaching Death

Death is a progressive process—the body does not die suddenly. During this process, there are signs that usually indicate rather clearly that death is imminent.

Motion and sensation are lost gradually; this usually begins in the extremities, particularly the feet and the legs. The normal activities of the gastrointestinal tract begin to decrease, and reflexes gradually disappear.

Although the patient's temperature usually is elevated, he feels cold and clammy, beginning with his extremities and the tip of his nose. His skin is cyanosed, gray or pale. The pulse becomes irregular, weak and fast.

Respirations may be noisy, and the "death rattle" may be heard. This is due to an accumulation of mucus in the respiratory tract which the patient is no longer able to raise and expectorate. Cheyne-Stokes respirations occur commonly.

As the blood pressure falls, the peripheral circulation fails. Pain, if it has been present, usually subsides, and there is mental cloudiness. The patient may or may not lose consciousness—the amount of mental alertness varies among patients, which is important to remember when giving care to the patient who appears to be dying. It has been noted by some observers that some patients see visions just prior to death.

The jaw and the facial muscles relax and the patient's expression, which may have appeared anxious, becomes one of peacefulness. The eyes may remain partly open.

Consider Mr. Edd's experience with death.

Mr. Edd was having a difficult postoperative recovery; one complication followed another. His condition grew progressively worse, and it was considered opinion that he perhaps was not going to recover. As is usual in most such instances, he was moved to a single room, since he was receiving intensive therapy, and there was the need for constant attendance.

He grew weaker and became unresponsive, his pulse became thready, his respirations shallow, and he began to have diaphoresis. To all, it seemed like a matter of hours. His wife had been close by constantly for two days, leaving for only short periods of time to go home to the children who were being cared for by a neighbor. His parents and brothers also were in almost constant attendance. It was apparent that there was some conflict between Mrs. Edd and her husband's family. Rarely were they together, and never did they come and go together. In some instances, Mr. Edd's brothers made requests which rightfully should have been channeled through the patient's wife, and these situations required the utmost in tact, understanding and diplomacy on the part of the nursing staff.

Somehow, and wonderfully so, Mr. Edd seemed to gain in strength, his pulse became stronger, his other symptoms subsided, and in 36 hours he was fully responsive. There was every indication that he was on his way to recovery. It was a wonderful and satisfying experience to see this man "come back to life," and it was an example to all who participated in it that there is always hope. But the greatest lesson was yet to come. After several days Mr. Edd was feeling well enough to talk about his experience. These are some of the things he told.

When he was moved into the room by himself, he knew it was because he was dying, for that was what happened to others who were moved to single rooms. But when he was in the room, one of the nurses who had helped to move him brought her head close to his and explained in a calm reassuring way that it would be better for the staff and the other patients if they were able to care for him in an individual room; that as soon as he did not require such intensive therapy he could return to his former unit; and that since he and the other patients in his unit were such good friends, the nurses would let them know when they could visit with him. Even though he could not reply, he could not help but feel that maybe things really weren't so bad. But then he heard many other things said at his bedside and in his room, and he knew that the nurse's explanation for his being in this room was a "white lie." He became fearful that they would think he was dead when he was not. However, there was one thing that caused him to think that maybe all was not over. That was during the night when there was evidence of real concern on the part of all who came to see him. He tried hard to determine what time it was by staring through very hazy eyes at the watch on the interne's arm while the interne listened to his chest. As far as he could make out, it was 3 A.M. Mr. Edd consoled himself with the thought that if he were dying, he was sure that his wife would be there by his side. Since she was not, he must be all right.

What Mr. Edd did not know was that his wife was there. She was on the porch barely 50 feet away, and this is where she had been for two days almost constantly. Throughout those days, she entered his room and visited with him only during the regular afternoon and evening visiting hours. In discussing this with her after Mr. Edd's recovery, she said that she really did not know why she did this except that perhaps it was just for the reason Mr. Edd chose to believe.

Signs of Death

The patient is considered dead when no pulse and respirations can be determined for a period of several minutes, even with auscultation. The pupils remain dilated and fixed. The physician is notified if he is not present. It is he who is responsible for pronouncing the patient dead.

Recently after approximately 30 heart transplants had been performed, surgeons met to discuss various problems including determining the death of a donor. On at least three criteria there was general agreement:

the donor must no longer have any heartbeat, respirations or reflexes. Also, the donor must have no brain wave activity—which is reflected as a "flat" electroencephalogram. But consensus was not reached on the length of time brain wave activity must be absent. Research continues concerning absolute signs of death. It is possible that with the era of human organ transplants upon us, legislative and judicial bodies may well become involved in attempts to define death more precisely than has been true in the past.

The World Medical Assembly meeting in Australia in 1968, although making no attempt to define death, discussed a code of ethics for human transplants. In general, representatives to the meeting agreed that death is a gradual process, its progress depending on the varying ability of tissues to live without oxygen. Certainty of death is present when the process of death becomes irreversible by whatever technics of resuscitation may be employed. The electroencephalograph currently is the most helpful diagnostic aid to support clinical judgment in determining death.

Care must be observed to avoid confusing death with *suspended animation*. Suspended animation sometimes occurs when a patient has been submerged in water for a period of time or when he has received an electric shock. Although he may appear to be dead, the patient may recover if artificial respiration is continued for a period of time.

Helping the Patient's Family

As was true in regard to the patient, the nurse will be able to offer comfort and support to the patient's relatives if she can understand their position. The family is about to lose a loved one. Kindness and respect for their feelings expressed in dignified and tactful actions and words are important.

Words of comfort usually are hard to find. Again, it may be best to say nothing and to be a listener if the relatives wish to express their thoughts. Relatives find comfort in feeling that everything possible is being done for the patient and in knowing that he is being kept comfortable. They, too, need to be offered hope. They derive little comfort from efforts to cheer them and suggestions that they try to forget and think of something else.

The considerate nurse will remember that relatives often become tired and "edgy" while waiting at the bedside of the dying patient for long periods of time. They may need reminding to get sleep, rest and regular meals. In some situations, it may be possible for the nurse to prepare a cup of coffee or tea for them while they are with the patient.

Too many visitors may tire the patient, and, when explanations are offered, relatives usually understand this readily. When they wish to remain at the hospital, it is desirable to direct them to a place where it is quiet and they may relax.

The nurse often can help relatives to overcome signs of grief prior to their visit with the patient. Frequently, it is helpful to suggest that they prepare themselves before entering the room by considering themselves as helpers and supporters rather than as grievers and mourners. Sometimes, allowing a willing member of the family to assist with aspects of nursing care is comforting to the patient as well as to the relative.

The grief expressed at time of death depends on many factors. Often, it is due to the fact that the loss is a great personal one, and so, in a sense, one is feeling sorry for oneself. In other instances, the customs of a cultural group require that proper bereavement be shown for one who has died. In other instances, it may be feelings of guilt that cause the family to show great emotion. The nurse will want to recognize that there is no *one* approach to either the patient or his family. The nurse will need to proceed carefully in the direction in which she feels she can serve both and keep her own feelings from interfering with her effectiveness.

It is the physician's responsibility to obtain permission for an autopsy when one is desired. Sometimes, the patient may grant this permission before he dies. When permission is being sought from relatives of the patient, the nurse often can assist the physician by helping to explain the reasons for an autopsy. This requires tact and good judgment, but many relatives will find comfort when they are told that an autopsy may help to further the development of medical science as well as establish proof of the exact cause of death.

Home Care of the Terminally Ill Patient. In some cases, the terminally ill patient may be taken home, and the family becomes responsible for his care until death occurs. However, the family may want or need assistance, and some health agencies now offer services for the care of the terminally ill at home. The nurse in the hospital may anticipate this need and assist the family in obtaining such care.

Certain hospitals, usually voluntary agencies, have a policy of not being able to admit or re-admit a terminally ill patient as death approaches. These policies are determined carefully and with reason, and it may become part of the nurse's responsibility to explain such policies to the family members.

Relatives rarely forget the understanding, sincere and tactful nurse and generally receive comfort and support during the trying days when they find her to be a kind and sympathetic person whose help is readily available.

Study Situations

1. The following article describes how a patient avoided discussion of her serious condition and how the nurse handled the situation when the floodgates opened:

- Magill, K. A.: How one patient handled fear.
  AMER. J. NURS., *67*:1248-1249, June, 1967.

What technics did the patient use to avoid speaking of her conditon? What did the nurse do to attempt to establish rapport with this patient? Note the last paragraph concerning the author's observations in relation to reserve strengths that aid to tide many patients over during periods of great physical and emotional shock.

2. The following article reports on a study of perceptions of mothers concerning care given to dying children:

- Geis, D. P.: Mothers' perceptions of care given their dying children.
  AMER. J. NURS., *65*:104-107, February, 1965.

What does the author give as a possible reason when mothers complained that nurses appeared to avoid their children? What was the most common answer mothers gave when they were asked for suggestions concerning care given their children? As you read, keep in mind the steps in problem solving as discussed in Chapter 3. Can you identify each of the steps in this study?

3. For a brief, but meaningful account of a student's first encounter with death see:

- Hingley, S.: Today I saw death.
  AMER. J. NURS., *67*:825, April, 1967.

4. The following article discusses the practical problems as well as the theory of grief:

- Engel, G. L.: Grief and grieving.
  AMER. J. NURS., *64*:93-98, September, 1964.

Note in particular the practical considerations given on pages 97 and 98. Note too the suggestion given nurses with the sketch on page 93 concerning the relative of a dead patient.

5. Problem solving in nursing practice can be used very effectively when a patient becomes confused or delirious, especially when we cannot be sure whether we are "getting through" to him. Understanding what restraints and isolation can do both to the patient and to his family should guide nursing personnel into seeking all other possible sources of therapeutic action first. For a further understanding of this nursing problem, read the following article:

- Gerdes, L.: The confused or delirious patient.
  AMER. J. NURS., *68*:1228-1233, June, 1968.

References

1. Anonymous: A Way of Dying. Skipper, J. K. Jr., and Leonard, R. C., eds.: Social Interaction and Patient Care, p. 179-184. Philadelphia, Lippincott, 1965.
2. Barckley, V.: The crises in cancer. AMER. J. NURS., *67*:278-280, February, 1967.
3. Baxter, C. R.: Three days with Mrs. M. AMER. J. NURS., *67*:774-778, April, 1967.
4. Bonine, G. N.: Students' reactions to children's deaths. AMER. J. NURS., *67*:1439-1440, July, 1967.
5. Breen, P.: Who is to say? AMER. J. NURS., *67*:1689-1690, August, 1967.

6. Bridgeman, J.: From joy to grief to acceptance.
NURS. OUTLOOK, *14*:45, September, 1966.
7. Bright, F., and France, Sister M. L.: The nurse and the terminally ill child.
NURS. OUTLOOK, *15*:39-42, September, 1967.
8. Davidson, R. P.: Let's talk about death—to give care in terminal illness.
AMER. J. NURS., *66*:74-75, January, 1966.
9. Fox, J. E.: Reflections on cancer nursing.
AMER. J. NURS., *66*:1317-1319, June, 1966.
10. Glaser, B. G., and Straus, A.: Awareness of Dying. 305 p.
Chicago, Aldine Publishing, 1965.
11. ———: Time for Dying. 270 p.
Chicago, Aldine Publishing, 1968.
12. Kneisl, C. R.: Thoughtful care for the dying.
AMER. J. NURS., *68*:550-553, March, 1968.
13. Knipe, M. L.: Serenity for a terminally ill patient.
AMER. J. NURS., *66*:2252-2254, October, 1966.
14. Lewis, W. R.: A time to die.
NURS. FORUM, *4*:7-27, #1, 1965.
15. McVay, L.: An interaction study involving a patient with a guarded diagnosis.
AMER. J. NURS., *66*:1071-1073, May, 1966.
16. Meinhart, N. T.: The cancer patient: Living in the here and now.
NURS. OUTLOOK, *16*:64-69, May, 1968.
17. Norris, C. M.: The nurse and dying patient.
AMER. J. NURS., *55*:1214, October, 1955.
18. Nover, R. A.: The burden of responsibility. (Editorial)
J.A.M.A., *200*:153, May 22, 1967.
19. Patrick, M. L.: Care of the confused elderly patient.
AMER. J. NURS., *67*:2536-2539, December, 1967.
20. Quint, J. C. *et al*: Improving nursing care of the dying.
NURS. FORUM, *6*:369-378, #4, 1967.
21. Quint, J. C.: Obstacles to helping the dying.
AMER. J. NURS., *66*:1568-1571, July, 1966.
22. ———: The Nurse and the Dying Patient. 307 p.
New York, Macmillan, 1967.
23. Saunders, C.: The last stages of life.
AMER. J. NURS., *65*:70-75, March, 1965.
24. Sharp, D.: Lessons from a dying patient.
AMER. J. NURS., *68*:1517-1520, July, 1968.
25. Vernick, J., and Lunceford, J. L.: Milieu design for adolescents with leukemia.
AMER. J. NURS., *67*:559-561, March, 1967.
26. Verwoerdt, A., and Wilson, R.: Communication with fatally ill patients. Tacit or explicit?
AMER. J. NURS., *67*:2307-2309, November, 1967.
27. Watson, M. J.: Death—a necessary concern for nurses.
NURS. OUTLOOK, *16*:47-48, February, 1968.
28. Wygant, W. E. Jr.: Dying, but not alone.
AMER. J. NURS., *67*:574-577, March, 1967.

CHAPTER

27

Care of the Body After Death

The care the nurse administers to the body after death has two primary objectives: to meet legal requirements accurately and with dispatch; and to aid in keeping the body tissues in the best possible condition so that problems in preparing the body for viewing are minimized.

Preparing the Body for Discharge

After the physician has pronounced the patient dead, the nurse is responsible for preparing the body for discharge from the health agency. The nurse will be guided in this responsibility by local procedure. Although these procedures vary from agency to agency, there are certain commonalities.

Inasmuch as the body is washed by the mortician, a complete bath is unnecessary except as individual situations indicate. A shampoo is unnecessary, but hairpins should be removed to avoid scratching the face. Most procedures now specify that dentures *not* be replaced. It generally is considered better for the mortician to place the teeth in position in order to minimize possible trauma, should they become situated oddly in the mouth. The nurse should see to it that dentures, properly identified, are given to the mortician when he calls for the body. Most morticians prefer that the jaw *not* be tied, since tying it may result in tissue damage and distortion of the face.

Double identification of the body is advised. One tag should be fastened securely to the shroud or garment in which the body is wrapped. The second one should be tied to the ankle. If it is tied to the wrist, the wrist should be padded first and the tag tied loosely around the padding to avoid damaging tissue from a tight band. *The importance of proper and complete identification of the body cannot be overstressed.* Mistakes which have occurred can cause embarrassment and added sorrow for all concerned.

Many morticians prefer that the rectum and vagina not be packed because of the pressure packing can cause on tissue, which, in turn, can interfere with the embalming process. If drainage is present, padding held in place loosely with a diaper is preferable. Draining wounds should be well covered with clean dressings.

It is best to place the arms over the abdomen. Tying them in place may result in tissue damage. The legs may be tied together at the ankles. With the body lying straight in the horizontal position, the head should be in line with the body—that is, not turned to either side. The body is then wrapped in a shroud, discard sheet, or other garment provided by the agency. To facilitate moving the body from the bed, placing a full sheet around the body and tucking it securely in place prevent the extremities and head from falling out of place and minimize tissue damage.

When death occurs following certain communicable diseases, the body requires special handling to aid in preventing the spread of the disease. The requirements are specified by local law and policy. The measures taken will depend on the causative organism, the mode of transmission, the viability and other characteristics.

Coroner's Case

If death is caused by accident, suicide, homicide or illegal therapeutic practice, the coroner must be notified according to law. The coroner may decide that an autopsy is advisable and can order that one be performed even though the family of the patient has refused to consent. In many cases, a death occurring within 24 hours of admission to the hospital is reportable to the coroner.

The Death Certificate

The laws of this country require that a death certificate be prepared for each patient who has died. The laws specify the information that is needed. Death certificates are sent to local health departments, which compile many statistics from the information that become important in identifying needs and problems in the fields of health and medicine.

The mortician assumes responsibility for handling and filing the death certificate with proper authorities. However, the physician's signature is required on the certificate, as well as that of the pathologist, the coroner, and others in special cases. The death certificate also carries the mortician's signature, and, in some states, his license number as well.

The death certificate indicates the cause of death as specified by the physician. However, the nurse can assist the mortician by giving him information, not readily available on the certificate, that will assist him in handling the body with greater ease.

Care of Valuables

Each agency has policies concerning the care of valuables when patients are admitted to the institution. Those which the patient has chosen to keep with him—usually rings, a wristwatch, money and the like—require careful handling after death. Occasionally, the patient's family may take the valuables home when death becomes imminent, and this should be noted on the form sheet which the agency specifies. If valuables are still with the patient at the time of death, they should be identified, accounted for and sent to the appropriate department for safekeeping until the family claims them. If it is impossible to remove jewelry, such as a wedding ring, the fact that it remained on the body should be noted, and, as a further safeguard, the article should be secured with adhesive so that it becomes impossible for it to slip off and be lost. Loss of valuables is serious and can result in a legal suit against the hospital. The nurse owes it to the patient's family as well as to the agency in which she works to use every precaution to prevent loss and misplacement of valuables.

Tissue and Organ Transplants

It is no longer rare for permission to be granted to take skin, bone and corneal tissue for transplants or to remove certain organs for medical research or study. Prior to death, patients may grant such permission. However, in many states, after death the next of kin still must sign a permit and have it properly witnessed before tissue or organs can be removed from the body. The nurse will want to acquaint herself with local laws in relation to transplant permits, to aid in avoiding the unpleasantness of possible legal action.

Although the nurse will want to keep herself informed, should an organ such as the heart be used for transplant immediately upon death, responsibility for permission remains with the physician.

Nursing Responsibilities in Relation to Other Commonly Prescribed Therapeutic Agents and Measures

Unit 5

CHAPTER 28

Principles and Practices Guiding the Preparation and Administration of Therapeutic Agents

General Principles of the Preparation and the Administration of Therapeutic Agents
The Physician's Order
Safeguarding Drugs
Preparing Therapeutic Agents for Administration
Administering Therapeutic Agents
The Nurse's Role in Case of Error
Omitted or Refused Therapeutic Agents
Study Situations

General Principles of the Preparation and the Administration of Therapeutic Agents

Appropriate precautionary measures avoid errors and accidents in the preparation and the administration of therapeutic agents.

Physiologic activities of the body can be maintained, improved, or, in some instances, restored by the administration of appropriate therapeutic agents and measures.

Persons vary in the way they metabolize injected or ingested agents, or react to agents applied externally.

Therapeutic measures are such only if the patient benefits from them. The physician orders such measures—but the nurse is expected to be knowledgeable concerning them.

The Physician's Order

A physician's order is required before a nurse administers any therapeutic agent. Safe practice is to follow only a *written* order. A written order by the physician is least likely to result in error or misunderstanding. In some situations and under certain circumstances, a verbal order from the physician may be given to a registered nurse. The legal consequences of administering therapeutic agents without a written order can be serious.

Each health agency has a policy specifying the manner in which the physician writes his order. In most cases, orders are written on a form specifically intended for the physician's orders. This becomes part of the patient's permanent record.

Types of Orders. There are several types of orders that the physician may prescribe. One type is called a *standing order* and is to be carried out as specified until it is canceled by another order. Occasionally, the physician writes a standing order and its cancellation simultaneously—that is, the physician specifies that a certain order is to be carried out for a stated number of days or times. After that number of days or times has passed, the order is canceled automatically. A second type of order is called a *single order*—that is, the order is carried out only once, either at early convenience or at a time specified by the physician. A *stat order* is also a single order, but it is one which is to be carried out at once. When a patient has an operation or when he is transferred to another clinical service, it is general practice that all orders related to therapeutic agents are discontinued, and new orders are written. To keep physicians aware of orders in effect, some agencies specify a day of the week when orders are to be rewritten or they will be automatically discontinued.

It is usual hospital policy that when a patient is admitted, all therapeutic agents which the physician may have ordered while the patient was at home are discontinued. This sometimes may prove to be a problem when a patient brings his medications to the hospital. To avoid the possibility of having the patient continue taking his medications while receiving the same ones or others under new orders, all medications should be sent home with the family or removed from the patient's unit and placed in safekeeping. Of course, this will require an explanation of how the physician's orders will be followed while the patient is in the hospital.

In some health agencies, policy permits a patient to keep a medication at his bedside if the physician wishes him to do so. In this case, best practice would be for the physician to write an order to this effect so that nursing personnel are aware of the medication that the patient is taking and can observe him for effects.

The Parts of the Order. The physician's order consists of seven parts: (1) the name of the patient; (2) the date and the time when the order is written; (3) the name of the therapeutic agent to be administered; (4) dosage, concentration, and so on of the agent; (5) the time and the frequency to administer; (6) the route by which it is to be administered and (7) the physician's signature.

Name of the Patient. The patient's full name usually is used. The middle name or initial is included if there are patients on the unit with the same or a similar name.

Date and Time the Order Is Written. The date and the time when the order is written are indicated for several reasons. This avoids confusion over when the order is to begin. Since the nursing staffs change several times during each 24-hour period, the date and the time help to prevent errors of oversight as different nurses take charge of a unit. When an order is to be followed for a specified number of days, the date and the time are important in order that the discontinuation date and time can be determined accurately. Law indicates the period of time that an order for a narcotic remains valid, usually 24 or 48 hours. Therefore, the date and the time when the order was written are essential to determine when the order for a narcotic becomes invalid.

Name of Therapeutic Agents. The name of the agent is stated in the order after the physician has indicated the patient for whom it is intended. Most agencies require that the physician use generic nomenclature. Certain trade-marked names are well known, but the practice of using the official name is the safest one. If the nurse is unfamiliar with a drug she can investigate by referring to certain standard references. In this country they include *The United States Pharmacopeia* (U.S.P.), the *National Formulary* (N.F.) and the *Homeopathic Pharmacopeia.* Most other countries have similar texts which describe official therapeutic agents. Many agencies also provide their own book listing the official drugs commonly used by the agency. Another commonly used reference is *The Physician's Desk Reference,* commonly called P.D.R.

The nurse caring for a patient at home often will be asked to administer a drug for which the physician has written a prescription. Unless the physician indicates otherwise, the pharmacist who fills the prescription omits the ingredients on the label. However, this practice does not excuse the nurse from learning the contents of the medication before administering it. It is expected that she will inquire of the physician before administering the medication. Without such knowledge she would have no idea of how to judge its effect, good or bad, on the patient.

The Council on Drugs of the American Medical Association has gone on record as favoring labeling of prescriptions. While it is agreed that at times, for some drugs and for some patients, the drug should be nameless, in most cases labeling seems to be desirable for several reasons. With labeling there may be less likelihood of taking incorrect medications, especially when several persons in a home may have prescribed drugs on hand. In case of accident, emergency treatment could be facilitated when the exact content of the drug is known. With the trend in teaching patients concerning their therapy, the patient usually is told what drugs he is receiving.

Amount or Concentration of the Therapeutic Agent. The dosage of a drug is stated in either the apothecary or the metric system, depending on the agency's policy. Most agencies post a table of common equivalent dosages for persons who have learned to use one system and find that the agency in which they work uses the other system. Although these tables are convenient and useful, the nurse should be prepared to convert from one system to the other, since such tables are not available in every situation (see Table 9). The nurse also should be familiar with common equivalent measurements when using household equipment, such as teaspoons, tablespoons and the like, since usually the home is not equipped with special measuring equipment.

Certain standard abbreviations are used commonly. Before a nurse can administer therapeutic agents, she will be required to acquaint herself with these common abbreviations (see Table 10).

The nurse also should be aware of common factors that influence dosage calculation; for example, a child's dose for a drug is smaller than an adult's dose. Various formulae have been devised to calculate children's dosage by reducing adult dosages in proportion to the age or the weight of the child. One common formula is Clark's Rule, based on the assumption that the average adult weighs 150 pounds:

$$\text{Usual adult dose} \times \frac{\text{weight of child in pounds}}{150} = \text{child's dose.}$$

Weight may be a factor in dosage calculation. In general, the heavier the person, the larger the dosage of drugs he can tolerate.

The route of administration influences dosage calculations. Drugs given by mouth are absorbed more slowly and less completely than those given intravenously. Hence, the dosage of a drug given intravenously generally is smaller than when the same drug is given orally.

The general condition of the patient, his

Table 9. Approximate equivalents for fluid and weight measures

Metric	Apothecary	Household
1 gram	15 or 16 grains	
0.065 gram	1 grain	
0.032 gram	½ grain	
0.016 gram	¼ grain	
0.010 gram	1/6 grain	
0.0011 gram	1/60 grain	
0.0006 gram	1/100 grain	
4 cc.	1 dram	1 teaspoonful
15 or 16 cc.	4 drams	1 tablespoonful
240 cc.	½ pint	1 glass or cup
0.06 cc.	1 minim	1 drop
1 cc.	15 or 16 minims	
30 cc.	1 ounce (8 drams)	
1,000 cc.	34 ounces	
950 cc.	1 quart	

Table 10. Common abbreviations for measures

Abbreviation	Unabbreviated Form
mg. or mgm.	milligram
Gm.	gram
cc.	cubic centimeter
gr.	grain
ʒ	dram
℥	ounce
♏	minim
tbsp.	tablespoon
tsp.	teaspoon

idiosyncracies, drug intolerance—are factors that may influence dosage calculation.

Time and Frequency. The time and the frequency with which a therapeutic agent is to be administered usually are stated in standard abbreviations in the physician's order. The most common abbreviations are listed in Table 11.

The nursing service department of each health agency usually determines the hours at which routine drugs are given. For example, if the physician wishes certain drugs to be given every four hours, policy set by nursing service indicates the times. One agency may use the hours 4 A.M., 8 A.M., 12 NOON, 4 P.M., 8 P.M. and 12 MIDNIGHT. Another agency may use the hours 5 A.M., 9 A.M., 1 P.M., 5 P.M., 9 P.M. and 1 A.M. If a drug is ordered to be given before or after meals, the time will depend on the hours at which meals are served.

If a drug is to be given only once or twice a day, the decision as to which hours to use will depend on the nature of the drug and the patient's plan of care. Whenever possible, there should be consideration for the patient's choice of time unless there is a need to maintain a constant level of drugs in the blood, such as those controlling cardiac arrhythmia. Not infrequently, patients will ask to have medications left at the bedside. Those patients who have become accustomed to taking prescribed drugs at home may find hospital policy inconvenient or unsatisfactory for personal reasons. When it is possible and safe to make adjustments for the patient, usually it is desirable to do so, and such adaptations should be indicated on the patient's nursing care plan.

Table 11. Common abbreviations used in prescribing drugs

Abbreviation	Unabbreviated Form	Meaning
a.a.	ana	of each
a.c.	ante cibum	before meals
ad lib.	ad libitum	freely
b.i.d.	bis in die	twice each day
c.	cum	with
gtt.	gutta	a drop
p.c.	post cibum	after meals
p.r.n.	pro re nata	according to necessity
q.d.	quaque die	every day
q.h.	quaque hora	every hour
q.i.d.	quater in die	4 times each day
s.	sine	without
s.o.s.	si opus sit	if necessary
ss.	semis	a half
stat.	statim	at once
t.i.d.	ter in die	3 times each day

Route. If an agent can be given in more than one way, the route by which it is to be administered should be stated clearly. Abbreviations usually are used, such as I.M. for intramuscular administration and P.O. for oral administration. When a therapeutic agent can be administered in more than one way, the nurse must recognize the legal implications if she elects to use one method and untoward results occur.

As in the case of calculating dosages, there are several factors that influence the choice of route. These include the desired action of the therapeutic agent, the speed of absorption, the nature of the therapeutic agent and the condition of the patient.

The action of agents is either systemic or local. A systemic action occurs when the agent is absorbed by the blood stream and is distributed throughout the tissues and the fluids of the body. For example, an antibiotic given by injection is absorbed by the blood and acts upon certain organisms wherever they may be harboring in body tissues or fluid. Oxygen also is given for its systemic effects.

A local action occurs when the agent is placed directly in contact with tissue and it is intended to act upon that specific tissue only. An example is applying a drug for athlete's foot where the drug acts directly upon the diseased tissue and the causative organism. Other examples include eye drops containing drugs which can, when instilled, either dilate or contract the pupil, and heat applied to an abscess or cold to a sprain.

Table 12 illustrates common routes by which therapeutic agents are administered.

The Physician's Signature. The physician's signature follows the order. The signature is of importance for legal reasons when it is important to know which physician prescribed. Also, an unsigned order should raise a question in the mind of the nurse. It may have been an oversight on the part of the physician, but possibly the physician was called away before having completed his order. In addition, should there be a question concerning the order, having the signature indicates which physician should be contacted.

Questioning the Physician's Order. The nurse is responsible for questioning an order if in her judgment the order is in error. The suspected error may be in the name of the patient, the agent or measure prescribed, dosage, the time or the frequency with which it is to be administered, or the route by which it is to be given. The legal implications are serious when there is an error in the physician's order and when the nurse involved could be expected, from her knowledge and experience, to have noted the error. On occasion, the nurse may not feel that there is an error in the order, but she may not understand why the physician has prescribed it as written. In such an instance, the nurse should also ask the physician so that she may understand how his order relates to the patient's plan of care.

While the physician is responsible for his orders, the nurse still can be legally charged with negligence when errors in an order occur. Occasionally, a nurse may have difficulty reading the physician's order. Guessing is gross carelessness, and rechecking with the physician is the only safe procedure.

Safeguarding Drugs

On each patient-care unit, there is an area where drugs are stocked and kept in readiness for dispensing to patients. The cabinet or room is locked, and only authorized nursing personnel have access to the key.

Handling of Narcotics. Narcotics are kept in a locked drawer, box or room. This precaution is observed as an additional safety measure. Narcotics may be ordered only by physicians registered under the Harrison Narcotic Act, which is a Federal law governing the use of opium and coca leaves and their derivatives. According to Federal law, a record must be kept for each narcotic that is administered. Health agencies provide forms for keeping such records, and these forms are kept with the narcotics. Although the forms differ, the following information generally is required: (1) the name of the patient receiving the narcotic; (2) the amount of the narcotic used; (3) the hour

Table 12. Routes for administering therapeutic agents

Route	How Therapeutic Agent is Administered	Term Used to Describe Route
Given by mouth	Having patient swallow therapeutic agent	Oral Administration
Given via respiratory tract	Having patient inhale therapeutic agent	Inhalation
Given by injection	Injecting therapeutic agent into 1. Subcutaneous tissue 2. Muscle tissue 3. Corium (under epidermis) 4. Vein	Parenteral Administration 1. Hypodermic or subcutaneous injection 2. Intramuscular injection 3. Intracutaneous injection 4. Intravenous injection
Given by placing on skin or mucous membrane	Inserting therapeutic agent into 1. Vagina 2. Rectum Placing therapeutic agent under tongue Rubbing therapeutic agent into skin Placing therapeutic agent in direct contact with mucous membrane Flushing mucous membrane with therapeutic agent	 1. Vaginal administration 2. Rectal administration Sublingual administration Inunction Instillation Irrigation

the narcotic was given; (4) the name of the physician prescribing the narcotic and (5) the name of the nurse administering the narcotic. It is common practice to check narcotics with each change of shift; i.e., morning, evening, and night. The amount of narcotics on hand is counted, and each used narcotic must be accounted for on the narcotic record. A narcotic count which does not check must be reported immediately. The law requires these special precautions in the use of narcotics in order to aid in the control of narcotic drug addiction. The nurse administering narcotics has a responsibility to see that the Federal law is observed.

Preparing Therapeutic Agents for Administration

When the nurse is to give a therapeutic agent, her first step is to follow the agency's policy specifying the manner in which the physician's order is checked. Most agencies use a card system.

For some therapeutic agents, drugs given by mouth or by injection particularly, it is usual procedure to transfer the physician's order to a card. This is for the convenience of the nurse and the safety of the patient. The cards can be used at the place where the medications are prepared, and then they are kept with the prepared drugs. Considering the large number of medications prepared at any one time, it would be virtually impossible for a nurse to prepare them accurately and quickly without such a system.

When an agent such as oxygen is being given continuously, it would not require such a measure. However, other agents, even if administered only once or twice a day, should in the interest of safety and accuracy have cards also. Examples would be eye ointments, rectal and vaginal suppositories, rectal or vaginal irrigations or skin ointments.

For each drug to be administered, a card is made out on which the patient's name, the name of the drug, the route, the dosage, the time and the frequency of administration are indicated. This information is identical with the physician's order. Some health agencies use colored cards to indicate the time of day and the frequency with which the drug is to be given.

It is common practice to provide a check system in order to be certain that the cards follow the physician's order accurately. Very often the physician's order is copied onto a nursing service form, such as a Kardex, a treatment sheet or a medication chart. Prior to preparing the drugs, the nurse checks each order as it appears on the nursing service form with the appropriate medication card. This practice provides for checking accuracy each time a drug is given.

Safe practice calls for checking the physician's order first and then finding the corresponding card. This can be done quickly and accurately when the physician's order has been transferred to a nursing service device, such as a Kardex, a treatment sheet or a medication chart. Finding the physician's order first avoids the possibility of having medications omitted or administered beyond the prescribed period because cards are missing or have *not* been destroyed.

The procedure of preparing a medication card and writing the order on a nursing service form frequently is referred to as *posting the order.*

Automation is beginning a revolution in the method of posting and preparing drugs. Although only in use on a limited basis, drug orders can be forwarded to the pharmacy, prepared there, delivered to the unit, and through other safety features of the system recorded as "taken" or "refused" or "omitted."

Knowledge of the Patient and the Drug. The patient's diagnosis and disease process are essential for the nurse to understand in order to administer therapeutic agents intelligently. Understanding the physician's plan of therapy is equally important. Without such knowledge, the nurse cannot report observations that have meaning to the physician who will plan and adjust therapy according to changes in the patient.

The nurse should know the desired action, both local and systemic, of the agents she administers; their toxic manifestations and side actions.

Safety Measures in Preparing Drugs. It is important that good lighting be available. Also, while the nurse is preparing drugs, she should work alone. This practice helps prevent distractions and interruptions, which may lead to errors.

Read the label on the medication bottle and check it with the medication card *three times:* (1) when reaching for the container of medication, (2) immediately prior to pouring the medication and (3) when replacing the container on the shelf. The importance of this checking three times cannot be overemphasized. The safe nurse does not allow automatic habits of preparing drugs to replace *constant thinking, purposeful action* and *repeated checking* for accuracy.

When liquids are being poured from a stock bottle, the liquid should be poured from the side of the bottle opposite the label. This prevents drops from running onto the label and making it difficult to read. Hold the container and the stock bottle at eye level and place the thumb nail on the line on the container which indicates the proper dosage. Because of surface tension, a meniscus forms on the liquid in the measuring container. The liquid should be measured at the *bottom* of this meniscus.

When tablets or capsules are ordered, the correct number is poured into the cover or the cap of the container and then emptied into the container to carry to the patient's bedside. Pouring tablets or capsules into the hand is not good practice for obvious reasons.

If a label on a bottle becomes difficult to read or accidentally comes off the bottle, the bottle should be returned to the pharmacy. A medication never should be given from a bottle without a label or with a label that cannot be read with accuracy. Because of the danger of error, medications should not be

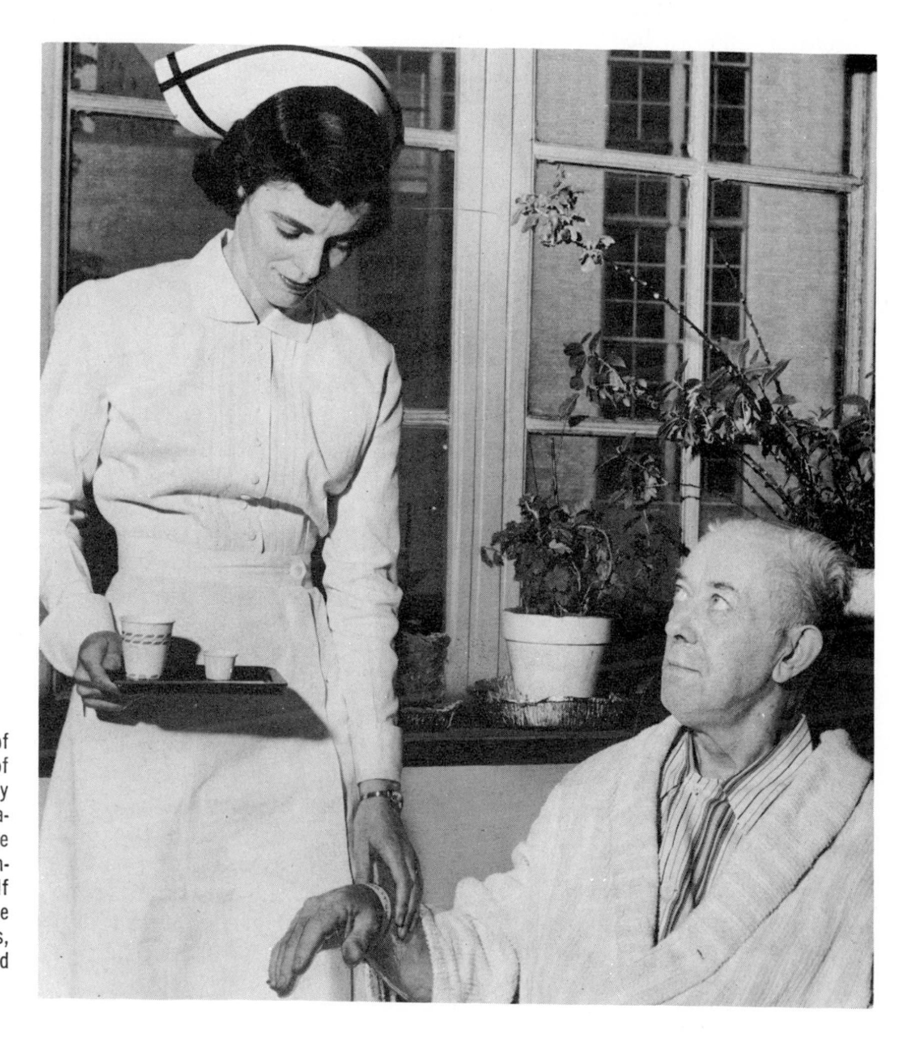

Fig. 28-1. A cardinal rule of safety in the administration of medications is that of properly identifying the patient. Ambulatory patients who have language handicaps or are likely to be confused should be identified. If commercially prepared bands are not available, improvised ones, such as this patient has, should be prepared.

returned to their container. Therefore, care should be exercised to pour carefully to prevent unnecessary loss. Medications should not be transferred from one container to another. Most medication bottles now have a "control" number on them. If similar medications were mixed and a patient had a "reaction" it would be difficult to identify which drug was responsible. A medication with an unexpected precipitate should not be used, nor one which has changed color.

If a patient receives several medications at one time, it is safe practice to use separate containers for each one so that each can be identified individually. Once the nurse begins to prepare drugs for administration, she should not leave them. If interruption is imperative, requiring her to leave for a short period of time, the drugs which have been prepared should be placed carefully in a locked area until her return.

Safety in Transporting Drugs. Special trays or carts on which to carry medications to the patient's bedside are provided. These trays are designed for individual or group use. They usually provide a means by which the medication card and the medication container can be held together safely. Because of the large number of medications given by injection, it is safer as well as convenient to have medication trays or carts which also hold syringes securely. During the time the nurse is administering the medications to the patients, the tray or cart should never be out of her sight. This is to prevent persons from taking medications not intended for them and accidental dislodging of cards or spilling of drugs.

When medications are to be given to more than one patient, it is efficient to arrange the medications in order of administration. This may be according to location of the patients or problems associated with the administration of drugs to certain patients. If a patient requires a great deal of assistance, it seems safer if all other medications are given first and only his medications remain on the tray.

Administering Therapeutic Agents

Identifying the Patient. When the nurse reaches the patient's bedside to administer the drug, she checks carefully to see that she is giving the drug to the right patient. The patient's name, usually posted on the patient's bed, is checked with the name of the patient on the medication card. Then the patient is called by his name. When calling the patient by name, accuracy and clear diction are important so that the nurse can be sure of proper identification. When the patient is unknown to the nurse, he should be asked to *give his name.* This is particularly important when the patient has a language handicap or is confused.

Administering a Drug. The nurse who prepares a medication should also administer it. To give a medication that has been prepared by another person is unsafe. If there is an error in the preparation, both the preparer and the giver may be legally held liable.

The nurse should remain at the bedside while the patient takes the drug and see that he swallows it before she leaves. If the patient receives several drugs, offer them separately so that if one is refused, or dropped, positive identification can be made and thus recorded or replaced. Leaving medications at the bedside for the patient to take later, or allowing one patient to give a medication to another, is unsafe practice. The patient may not take the drug after the nurse leaves. Also, the nurse should not record a drug as given unless the patient has actually swallowed it. If the drug is harmful in large doses and the patient has intentions to harm himself, he may save a sufficient quantity to do so, as with sleeping pills.

Preparing Drugs for the Physician to Administer. Policy in an agency dictates whether the physician or the nurse administers certain drugs by certain routes. For example, in most agencies, drugs injected directly into the vein are administered by the physician.

In an emergency, a physician may ask for a drug to be prepared which he will administer. The nurse prepares it and, as she gives it to the physician, repeats the name of the drug and the dosage. When possible, it is even safer practice to show him the label on the container from which the drug was taken. Even if it is a single dose and time permits, it is safe practice to prepare a medication card and give that to the physician, with the prepared medication. When a drug is given daily by the physician, a card is made out for it.

The Nurse's Role in Case of Error

It is certainly necessary to have the greatest respect for the responsibilites involved in the administration of therapeutic agents. Errors rarely occur until carelessness and habit replace care and thoughtful action.

Whenever an error occurs, the patient's welfare is at stake. The physician is notified, and remedial measures are begun as necessary. The physician is notified as soon as the error is noted, and the error also is described on the patient's permanent record.

Most agencies require that the nurse responsible for an error fill out a special form for reporting errors. These are frequently called accident or error reports. The forms usually require a full explanation of the situation and the steps that were taken following its commission. For legal reasons, it is essential that errors be described fully and accurately.

Omitted or Refused Therapeutic Agents

Inadvertently omitting a therapeutic agent that has been ordered for a patient constitutes an error and is handled as described above.

If a therapeutic agent is omitted for a legitimate reason, the omission and the reason for it are indicated on the patient's chart. For example, if a patient is to have a treatment and is to have nothing by mouth prior to the treatment, oral drugs usually are omitted or their administration is delayed, depending on the physician's wishes. Another example occurs when the physician has ordered a laxative for a patient who is constipated; if the patient has a bowel movement and the laxative is no longer needed, the laxative may be omitted. Omitting any therapeutic agent requires judgment and an understanding of the physician's plan of therapy for the patient.

If a patient refuses a therapeutic agent which is considered essential to his therapeutic regimen, the physician will want to be informed promptly. In many instances, the nurse can play an important role in determining the reason for the refusal and in convincing the patient of the importance of accepting therapeutic agents. However, if reasonable efforts fail to accomplish this, it is unwise to continue urging a patient who adamantly refuses a therapeutic agent. The responsibility for handling the situation then is more appropriately taken care of by the physician. Refusals to take prescribed therapeutic agents and the way in which the situation was managed should be described on the patient's chart.

Study Situations

1. The following article describes a court case involving a medication error:

- Hershey, N.: Question that drug order . . . the court lays down the law.
  AMER. J. NURS., *63*:96-97, January, 1963.

Review why the court held that the physician was negligent. What parts of his written order were unclear or omitted? Note how the court indicated that poor communications existed between the physician and the nurse. What action on the part of the nurse clearly violated the first general principle described early in this chapter?

2. Automatic drug-dispensing systems have been introduced into some health agencies which reportedly have advantages over conventional systems for dispensing and safeguarding drugs. The following two articles describe such systems:

- Using a new drug dispensing system.
  AMER. J. NURS., *62*:94-95, April, 1962.
- Hosford, R. F.: Automatic drug dispensing.
  HOSPITALS, *37*:96 passim, January 16, 1963.

3. After considering all the precautions mentioned in this chapter, how many have you seen violated by your family, friends, or yourself? How often is your home medicine closet emptied of drugs that have been in it for a year or more? How many medication containers have expiration dates on them? How accessible are medications to children in a home? How would you provide for an elderly person to take his own medication safely?

CHAPTER 29

Suggested Methods for Administering Therapeutic Agents

ORAL ADMINISTRATION

While many drugs are administered by mouth, there are certain disadvantages to this route. One is that the amount of drug absorbed cannot always be determined with accuracy. Absorption can be affected also by certain disease conditions, such as diarrhea, and, in such cases absorption is even more uncertain.

Drugs which are destroyed by digestive juices and those that are very irritating to the mucous membrane of the gastrointestinal tract often are given by another route. Some irritating drugs can be prepared with a coating that will not dissolve in the stomach. Action from the drug is delayed until the coating is acted upon by the secretions in the intestinal tract. Coated medications require close observation of the patient, since there is the possibility that the patient may expel them without having received any benefit. If the patient is constipated, coated tab-

PRINCIPLES GUIDING ACTION IN THE ADMINISTRATION OF ORAL MEDICATIONS

The purpose is to prepare and administer oral medications safely and accurately so that the patient may derive maximum therapeutic effectiveness from them.

SUGGESTED ACTION	PRINCIPLE
Begin by checking the physician's orders or posted orders and then find the corresponding medication card.	The source of the order is more reliable than the medication cards, which are only a device for convenience.
Arrange the cards purposefully, either by the location of the patients or by some other factors. Keep all medications for one patient together.	Organization and planning result in economy of time and effort and minimize confusion.
Read the labels 3 times while preparing the drugs.	Frequent checking helps to ensure accuracy and to prevent errors.
Place each medication in a separate container.	If drugs are spilled or refused, positive identification as to type or amount can be made.
Keep medication card and drug together at all times.	Keeping drugs identified ensures proper administration of the correct drug to the correct patient.
Transport medications to the patient's bedside carefully and keep the medications in sight at all times.	Careful handling and close observation prevent accidental or deliberate disarrangement of medications.
Identify the patient carefully, using all precautions: check the bed card, look at identification band, call the patient by name or ask the patient to state his name.	Illness and strange surroundings often cause patients to be confused.
If more than one drug is to be given at one time, administer each one separately.	Individual administration ensures accuracy.
Remain with the patient until each medication is swallowed. Unless the nurse has seen the patient swallow the drug, it cannot be recorded that the drug was administered.	The patient's chart is a legal record.
Offer the patient additional fluids as necessary.	Fluids help to dissolve and dilute solid drugs.
Immediately record the medications given, refused or omitted.	Immediate recording avoids the possibility of accidentally repeating the administration of the drug.
File the medicine cards promptly.	Careful management of the medicine cards reduces the possibility of error.

lets have been known to contribute to the formation of a fecal impaction. If an irritating drug is to be given orally, gastric irritation can be decreased when the drug is dissolved and diluted before administration. Also irritation is often decreased if the drug is given with food, as a cracker or a piece of bread, or immediately after a meal.

Certain drugs given orally discolor the teeth or tend to damage the enamel. Such medications usually are mixed well with water or some other liquid vehicle; the patient takes it through a drinking tube, and water is taken following administration. This practice reduces the strength of the drug that comes in contact with the teeth. Dilute hydrochloric acid is an example of a drug that damages the enamel of the teeth and should be given well diluted and with a drinking tube.

Many patients object to the taste of certain medications. Their taste can be disguised or masked. For example, if the patient is allowed to suck on a small piece of ice for a few minutes, the taste buds become somewhat numb, and objectionable tastes are less discernible. Oily medications are often stored in a refrigerator, since oil is less aromatic when cold than when given at room temperature. Pouring a medication over crushed ice and serving it with a straw makes it less distasteful.

Various vehicles also are used to disguise the taste of a drug. These include fruit juices, milk, applesauce and bread. The disadvantage of using food for disguising distasteful medications is that the patient may learn to dislike the food which he associates with the objectionable-tasting medication. This is particularly true with children.

The oral route is contraindicated for patients who have nausea and vomiting or are unable to take medications by mouth because of disease conditions. Oral medications also are contraindicated for unconscious or irrational patients and for infants because of the danger of aspirating the drug.

Also, make appropriate observation of the patient to determine if there is any contraindication to administering the medication: e.g., pulse, rate and rhythm, level of sedation if the patient is on routine sedation, and signs of allergic reactions.

Most of the absorption of drugs administered orally occurs in the mucosa of the small intestine. There is little if any absorption from the large intestine. Certain drugs are absorbed from the mucosa of the stomach; alcohol, for example, is absorbed quite rapidly in this area. Absorption is quicker when the stomach and the small intestine are empty. Therefore, drugs taken before and between meals are absorbed more rapidly. Powders and tablets must first enter into solution before they can be absorbed; and when they are in solution before taken, absorption can commence more rapidly.

Where medication carts and newer systems for preparing and issuing drugs are used, the procedure suggested on page 333 will have modifications. However, the principles still apply.

PARENTERAL ADMINISTRATION

Introduction

The term *parenteral* refers to routes other than the oral. However, the term is used more commonly to indicate the injection routes, and it is used in that context in this book.

Absorption occurs more rapidly in the injection method than it does when other routes are used. Absorption is also more nearly complete; therefore, the results are more predictable, and the desired dosage can be determined with greater accuracy. Giving drugs by injection is particularly desirable for patients who are irrational, unconscious or having gastric disturbances. This method of administering drugs is also good in emergencies, since absorption occurs rapidly.

For patients who will need to administer their own medications at home, parenteral administration presents a more involved teaching problem than do most other routes. However, many patients have learned to give themselves injections skillfully and safely when the teaching has been well planned and the patient is able and willing to learn.

Minimizing the Discomfort of Injections. The discomfort associated with injections sometimes is considered to be a disadvantage of the injection route. However, skill in giving injections can greatly reduce discomfort. Several practices aid in decreasing pain.

The pain of an injection is usually the result of the needle's passing through a cutaneous pain receptor. For the very sensitive or anxious patient, this discomfort can be minimized by applying cold compresses or by placing an ice cube on the area of injection for a short time immediately prior to the injection. Some physicians may also recommend spraying a volatile solution such as ethyl chloride on the site of injection. The use of cold and of volatile sprays numbs sensory receptors and therefore decreases pain.

Subcutaneous tissue is relatively insensitive, but if the needle pulls fascia of underlying muscle tissue, pain will result. The injection of nonirritating drugs in an isotonic solution is usually painless. A small amount of anesthesia, such as procaine hydrochloride, is often added to irritating drugs.

It is of prime importance to use a sharp needle, free of burrs, and to select one of the smallest gauge that is appropriate for the site and for the solution to be injected. Pain is minimized by inserting and removing the needle without hesitation and by injecting solutions slowly so that they may be dispersed into the surrounding tissues. Select a site where the skin appears free of irritation and danger of infection.

Following an injection, firm rubbing of the injection site hastens absorption of the drug and relieves discomfort. If injections are being given often to a patient, rotating the site also aids in decreasing the discomfort of inserting the needle into an area recently injected.

Preparing Drugs for Parenteral Administration

Drugs for parenteral administration are marketed in several ways. Those that deteriorate in solution usually are dispensed as tablets or powders and placed in solution immediately prior to injection. If drugs remain stable in solution, usually they are dispensed in ampules, bottles or vials in an aqueous or oily solution or suspension.

Removing Drugs From Ampules and Vials. The most commonly used dispensing units are the single-dose glass ampule, the single-dose rubber-capped vial and the multiple-dose rubber-capped vial. They are illustrated in Figures 29-1, 29-2, and 29-3.

Single-Dose Glass Ampule. Most single-dose glass ampules have a constriction in the stem of the ampule which facilitates opening it. Before preparing to open the ampule, make certain that all of the drug is in the ampule proper and not in the stem. The drug tends to be trapped in the stem, and it may be necessary to tap the stem several times to help bring the drug down. Ampules without a constriction do not present this problem.

A practice in some agencies is to wipe the outside of the ampule with an antiseptic solu-

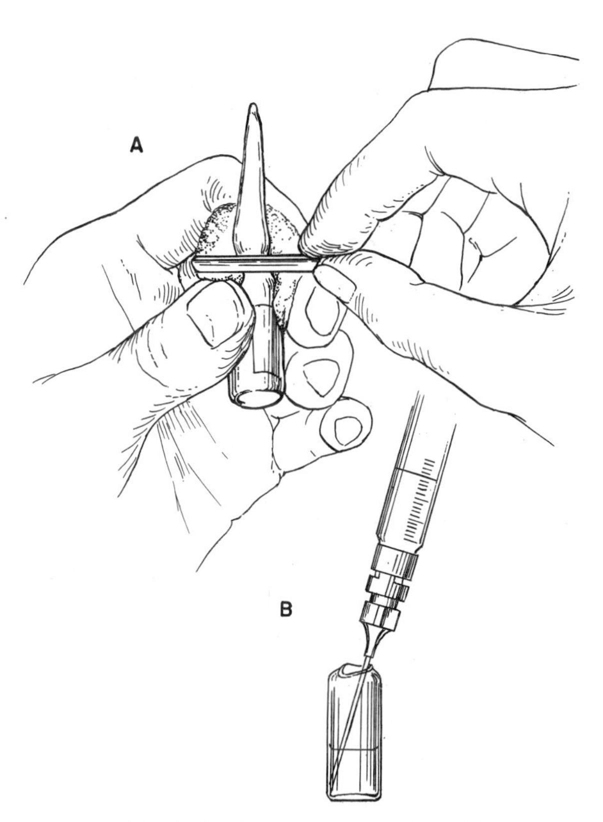

FIG. 29-1. (A) The fingers are protected by cotton when the stem of the closed glass ampule is scored with a file and then broken off. (B) When the stem of the glass ampule is removed, the drug is drawn up into the syringe easily because air displaces the fluid. The sterile needle should not touch the rim of the ampule.

tion before it is opened. This practice has never been justified scientifically. Considering that the antiseptic is merely passed over the glass briefly, and that immediately thereafter it will be scored by an unsterile file, it would appear that this gesture adds nothing to the safety of the procedure.

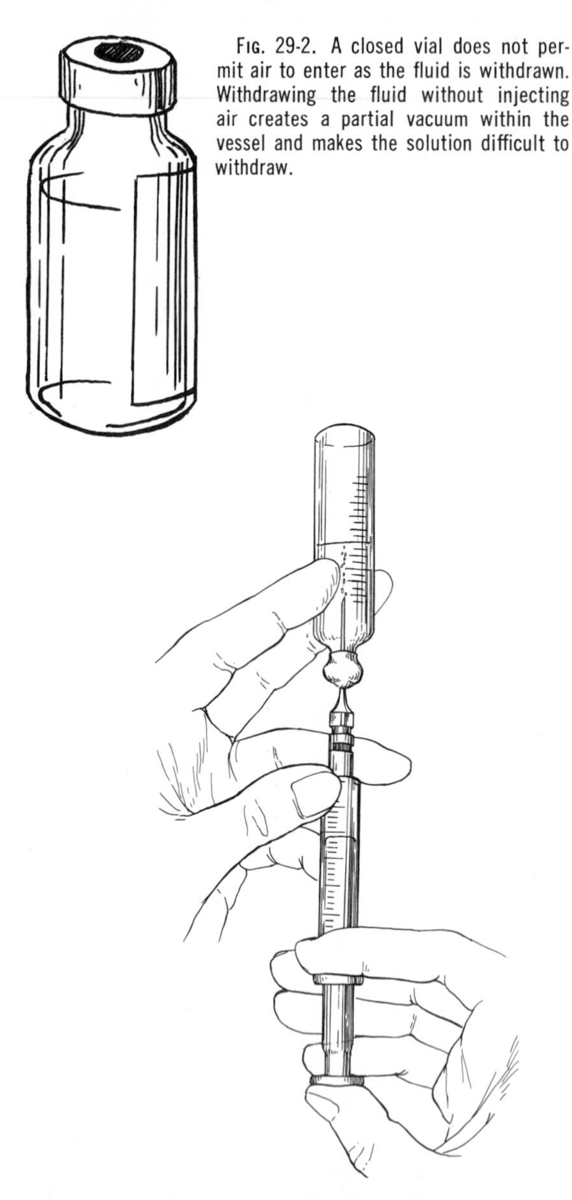

FIG. 29-2. A closed vial does not permit air to enter as the fluid is withdrawn. Withdrawing the fluid without injecting air creates a partial vacuum within the vessel and makes the solution difficult to withdraw.

FIG. 29-3. An amount of air equal to the amount of solution to be withdrawn is injected. Pressure within the vial is increased and the drug is removed easily and accurately.

When all the drug has been brought to the bottom of the ampule, gauze is used to hold the ampule firmly and to protect the nurse's fingers. Sterile material is considered safe practice because it will be in close proximity to the opening into the ampule when the stem is removed. A saw-tooth file is used to scratch the glass gently on the stem, well above the level of the medication. Scratching it on opposite sides helps to ensure a quick, even break. After the scratch marks have been made, the ampule is held in one hand, and the other is used to break off the stem. Many single-dose ampules are prescored and do not require filing. These are identified by a colored marking at the neck of the ampule. However, there is still need to protect the fingers.

The medication in the ampule is now in an open vessel. To remove it, insert the needle into the ampule and withdraw the solution. Be careful not to touch the edge of the glass with the needle in order to minimize all chances of contamination. The fluid in the ampule is immediately displaced by air; therefore, there is no resistance to its withdrawal. With additional skill, it will be possible to pick up the ampule and hold it between two fingers of one hand and the syringe in the other hand. When removing the drug in this fashion, the trick lies in keeping the needle in the solution at all times, even as the ampule is inverted.

Single-Dose Rubber-Capped Vial. For safety in transporting and storing, the single-dose rubber-capped vial usually is covered with a soft metal cap which can be removed easily. The rubber part which then is exposed is the means of entrance into the vial. At the time of preparation, this rubber portion of the seal was sterilized, but many agencies specify that the cap be cleansed with an antiseptic before the needle is inserted. Use friction when cleansing.

To facilitate the removal of the drug from the closed container, it is best to inject an amount of air comparable with the amount of solution to be withdrawn. This increases the pressure within the vial, and then the drug can be withdrawn easily, since fluids move from an area of greater pressure to an area of lesser pressure. If air is not injected first, an area of lesser pressure (a partial vacuum) is created in the vial as fluid is withdrawn, because air cannot displace the fluid being removed. This area of lesser pressure exerts pull on the fluid, making it difficult to withdraw.

Multiple-Dose Rubber-Capped Vial. Some drugs are dispensed in vials containing several or multiple doses. An example is an insulin vial. These are managed in the same manner as the single-dose sealed vial. The cap is cleansed by thorough rubbing with a cotton ball or a gauze pledget soaked in an antiseptic solution. An amount of air equivalent to the amount of solution to be withdrawn is injected. The air should be injected accurately, since not enough air will make withdrawal of the drug difficult, and increasing the pressure in the vial by adding too much air will interfere with the ease of preparing the correct dose by pushing solution into the syringe.

If the amount of fluid to be removed from a vial is rather large or several doses are to be removed in succession, a simple method is to insert a separate sterile needle through the cap. This will allow air to enter and replace the fluid as it is being withdrawn.

Surgical and Medical Asepsis in Parenteral Therapy

While details of methods for administering injections may vary from one agency to another, there is one basic principle which underlies all—strict asepsis minimizes the danger of injecting organisms into the patient's tissues or blood stream.

All objects coming in contact with the drug and the patient's tissues should be sterilized prior to use by the most reliable means available. Findings in relation to homologous serum jaundice leave little doubt that it is transmitted easily via parenteral therapy. Most agencies are taking extra precaution by using disposable items, including syringes, needles and single dose cartridges for medications, such as narcotics.

If a drug must be prepared and then transported to the patient's unit, the needle must be kept sterile. Using the holder which protected the needle offers the greatest amount of safety.

Cleansing the Skin for Parenteral Injections. The choice of an antiseptic agent for cleansing the skin prior to parenteral therapy is of periodic concern to every health agency. However, as was pointed out, sterilization of the skin cannot be expected.

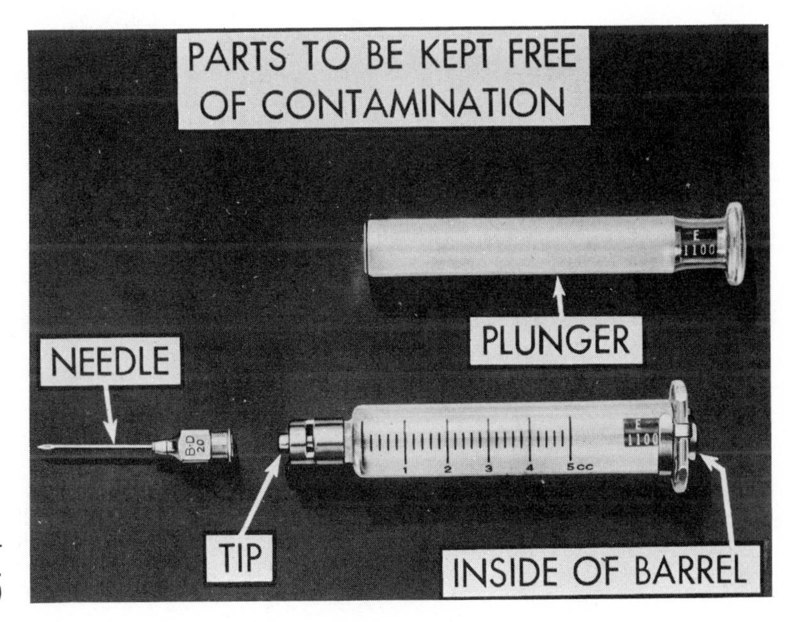

FIG. 29-4. Hypodermic syringe and needle-parts to be kept free of contamination. (Becton, Dickinson and Co., Rutherford, N.J.)

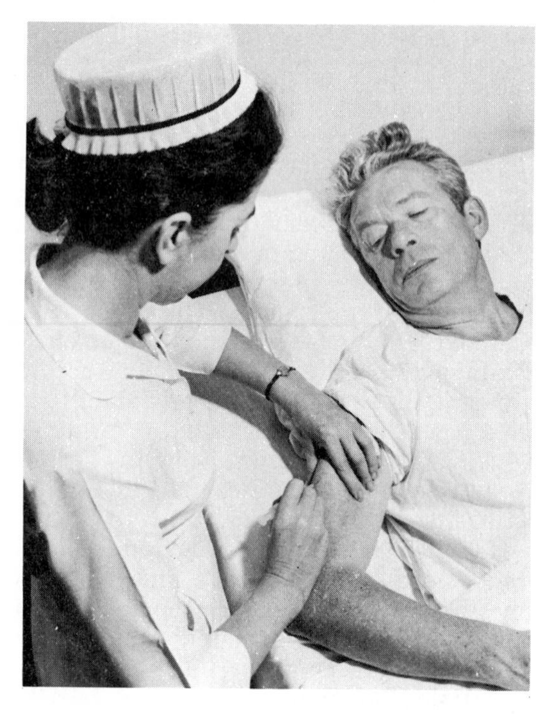

Fig. 29-5. For a subcutaneous injection into the upper arm, the tissue is picked up and held firmly. Then the needle is held at an angle which will help it enter subcutaneous tissue—usually a 45° angle for the average adult.

Since sterilizing the skin is not possible, the purpose of cleansing the area is to make certain that it is free from gross contamination and dried skin cells. In cleaning the area, a circular motion is used, beginning at the point of injection and moving outward and away from it. This carries material away from the critical site. Haphazard up-and-down movements should be avoided, since they bring the material right back again. The correct action is accompanied by firm pressure so that mechanical cleansing is also accomplished. Individually packaged gauze moistened with an antiseptic is now in common use.

In those instances when the patient's skin is soiled from drainage or discharges, thorough cleansing with soap and water is to be preferred to reliance on a brief contact with an antiseptic. This is especially true for incontinent patients who may need to have intramuscular injections. This point cannot be stressed too much, namely, that the nurse exercise careful judgment in the preparation of any body site for injection and not rely on the conscience-salving procedure of a

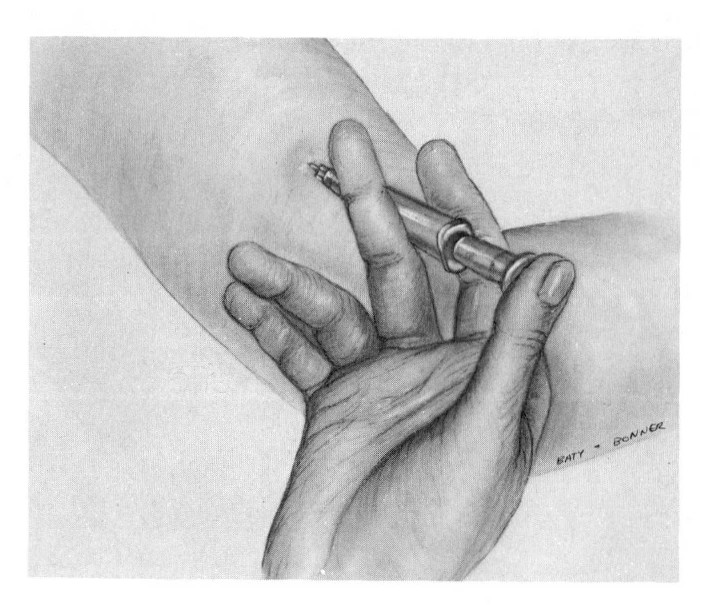

Fig. 29-6. Once the needle has pierced the skin quickly, the tissue is released so that the fluid need not be injected under pressure. Releasing the tissue facilitates the distribution of the drug.

superficial swipe with an antiseptic-soaked pledget.

Surgical Asepsis for Parenteral Therapy in the Home. Since many patients and their families are learning to administer injections, the problem of sterilization at home will arise. A patient's home equipment is purchased for him and used only for him. Therefore, the possibility of cross-contamination between patients is eliminated. Boiling of syringes and needles in the home has been recommended for years and found to be safe, as long as the equipment is not shared.

For home technic, cotton used to cleanse the skin need not be sterile as long as the patient is instructed not to cover the needle with it. Since the patient will not have a needle protector, he will need to be shown how to keep the needle sterile. Usually, the patient is advised to keep it off the edge of the table or surface on which he will place the syringe while preparing the skin. It should be directed so that the patient cannot touch it accidentally.

The cost of disposable equipment has been reduced, therefore more patients are using such items for injections that are given at home.

Subcutaneous Administration

While there is subcutaneous tissue (areolar connective) all over the body, for convenience, a site on the upper arm or on the thigh usually is selected. Patients who give themselves hypodermic injections generally find the thigh the most convenient site.

If a patient is to receive frequent injections, it is best to alternate the sites, which helps to prevent irritation and permits complete absorption of the solution. It is not uncommon for patients who receive injections repeatedly in one site to note induration from unabsorbed drug or to complain of itching in that site. For alternating sites, it is necessary for the routine to be incorporated in the patient's nursing care plan so that succeeding nurses will know which arm or leg to use. It is fruitless to rely on mem-

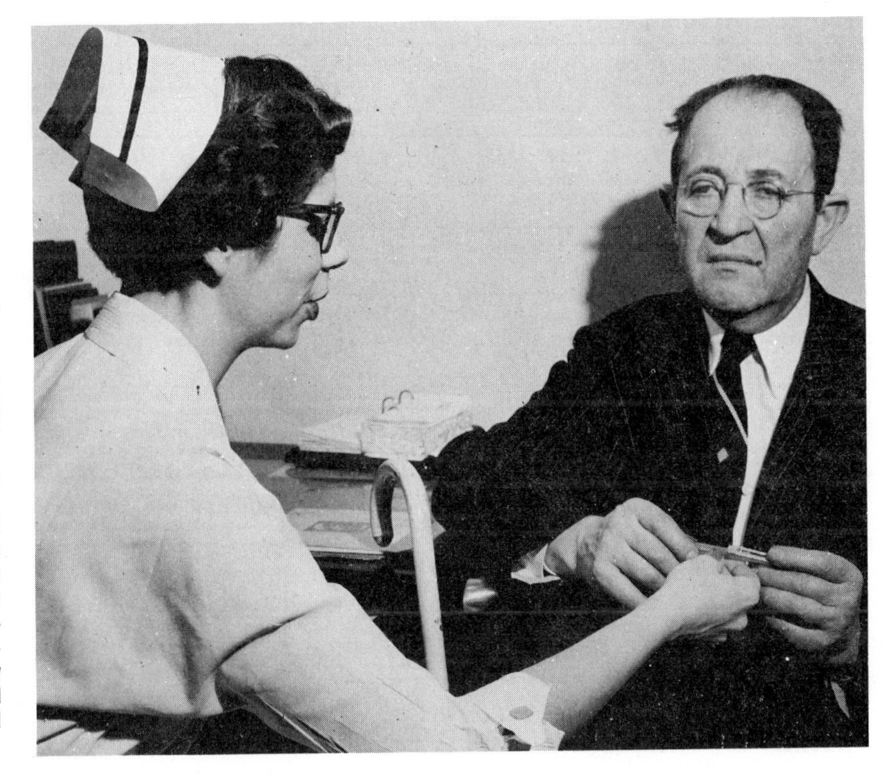

Fig. 29-7. Teaching patients to prepare and administer their own insulin is a common nursing activity. To teach a patient who is sightless, the procedure is a real challenge. Here the nurse is beginning to instruct the patient by allowing him to feel the metal adaptor which will make it possible for him to draw up his own dose. Often family members or friends insist that they give blind patients their injections. While it is important that someone close to the patient also know how to give the insulin, the patient should be offered the opportunity to learn so that he may have the feeling of security and independence such knowledge and skill will bring him.

ory; not even the patient will always be able to recall where he had the previous injection.

The amount of subcutaneous tissue underlying the skin is not a constant factor in all individuals. Some persons may have very little, and others a great deal. For the average adult it generally is recommended that the needle be injected at a 45° angle. However, for an obese patient, a needle injected at this angle may not reach subcutaneous tissue, while muscular tissue may be reached in a very thin and dehydrated patient. Drugs may be absorbed poorly in fat tissue, although usually there is no harm to the fat tissue, since drugs given subcutaneously rarely are irritating (see Figs. 29-5 and 29-6).

Equipment Commonly Used for Subcutaneous Injections: *Needles.* The needle most commonly used for injecting into subcutaneous tissue is a 25-gauge, five-eighths-inch needle. However, there are variations in this, and some physicians prefer using a shorter needle of three-eighths inch or one-half inch.

The needle must be in perfect condition and free from burrs on the point. Once a needle has been bent, it should not be forced

PRINCIPLES GUIDING ACTION IN THE ADMINISTRATION OF A SUBCUTANEOUS INJECTION

The purpose is to inject a medication into subcutaneous tissue.

SUGGESTED ACTION	PRINCIPLE
Obtain equipment and drug. Assemble syringe and needle according to agency procedure. Keep drug and sterile items in sight.	Sterile items that are out of sight are in danger of being contaminated accidentally.
Draw the drug into the syringe and protect the needle with a sterile holder or a sterile dry cotton ball until ready for injection.	Prolonged exposure to the air and/or contact with moist surfaces will contaminate the needle.
Carry to the patient on a tray or a medication carrier.	Keeping the prepared syringe on a flat, steady surface reduces the possibility of moving the plunger and thus possibly losing the drug.
Cleanse the area of the skin to be injected by using firm, circular motion while moving out from the center of the area with each stroke.	Friction aids in cleansing the skin. A clean area is contaminated when a soiled object is rubbed over its surface.
Grasp the area surrounding the site of injection and hold in a cushion fashion.	Cushioning the subcutaneous tissue helps to ensure having the needle enter areolar connective tissue.
Inject the needle quickly at an angle of 30° to 60°, depending on the amount and the turgor of the tissue.	Subcutaneous tissue is abundant in well-nourished, hydrated persons and sparse in emaciated, dehydrated ones.
Once the needle is in situ, release the grasp on the tissue.	Injecting the solution into compressed tissues results in pressure against nerve fibers and creates discomfort.
Pull back gently on the plunger of the syringe to determine whether the needle is in a blood vessel.	Substances injected directly into the blood stream are absorbed immediately.
If no blood appears, inject the solution slowly.	Rapid injection of the solution creates pressure in the tissues, resulting in discomfort.
Withdraw the needle quickly.	Slow withdrawal of the needle pulls the tissues and may cause discomfort.
Rub the area gently with the sponge.	Rubbing aids in the distribution and the absorption of the solution.

straight for re-use. Because a needle is a delicately constructed item having a lumen, the shaft is weakened if the needle is bent and then bent back into place again. Weakening the shaft of the needle increases the possibility of its breaking in the patient's tissues if the patient moves or other strain is placed on it.

Patients who are being taught to take their injections at home should be shown how to test the point of the needle for burrs. This is done easily by running the point of the needle, both sides, over a piece of cotton or along the back of the hand before sterilizing it. If the point of the needle picks up cotton or scratches the hand, it requires sharpening. A needle with a burr on its point results in a painful injection.

More and more agencies are using disposable needles for all types of parenteral therapy. The multiple advantages to both the patients and the agency are self-evident. However, public health officials have cautioned all who use such needles to destroy them before discarding them. The needle should be bent off the hilt. This will prevent needles from getting into the hands of addicts.

Syringes. Since numerous substances can be given subcutaneously, there is a variety of syringes to facilitate their measurement and injection.

Syringes for hypodermic injections are calibrated in both minims and cubic centimeters. They are available in two, two and one-half and three cc. sizes.

When a very small dose of a therapeutic agent must be measured, as when giving an allergen extract or a vaccine, a one-cc. syringe calibrated in tenths and hundredths of a cc. and in minims is used. Such syringes provide for more accuracy that cannot be obtained from the usual syringe.

For the administration of insulin, there is a variety of syringes available that are calibrated according to the unit strength of the insulin being used. For example, if a patient is taking 60 units of U 80 insulin, it is best for the patient to have a U 80 insulin syringe. Insulin syringes also come in long- and short-barrel designs. The patient may have some preference either from the standpoint of handling the syringe or reading the markings. Since the markings are spread out farther on the long-barrel syringe, some patients find this easier to read.

Hypodermic needles and syringes are dispensed in a variety of ways, some already assembled and others unassembled. If the needle is to be attached to the syringe, it should be held by the hilt. A small sterile forceps can be used both to attach and to tighten the needle. However, the fingers can be used, provided that the hilt does not come in contact with a sterile surface following this, i.e., a needle protector or a sterile cotton ball.

When completely disposable injectables are used, the procedure suggested on page 340 will have modifications, but the principles still apply.

Intramuscular Administration

The intramuscular route often is used for drugs that are irritating, since there are few nerve endings in deep muscle tissue. If a sore or inflamed muscle is entered, the muscle may act as a trigger area, and severe referred pain often results. It is best to palpate a muscle prior to injection. Select a site that does not feel tender to the patient and where the tissue does not contract and become firm and tense.

Absorption occurs as in subcutaneous administration but more rapidly because of the greater vascularity of muscle tissue. Approximately two to five cc. of solution usually is given via this method. However, when as much as five cc. of a solution is ordered to be given intramuscularly, some judgment should be used as to whether the dose should be divided and half given into one site and half into another. The pressure created by the introduction of such a quantity usually creates discomfort for the patient. If divided doses are not possible because of the frequency of subsequent ones, the injection should be given very slowly to allow for dispersal of the solution in the tissues.

Because of the widespread use of intramuscular injections, it is not too surprising that complications have occurred, possibly

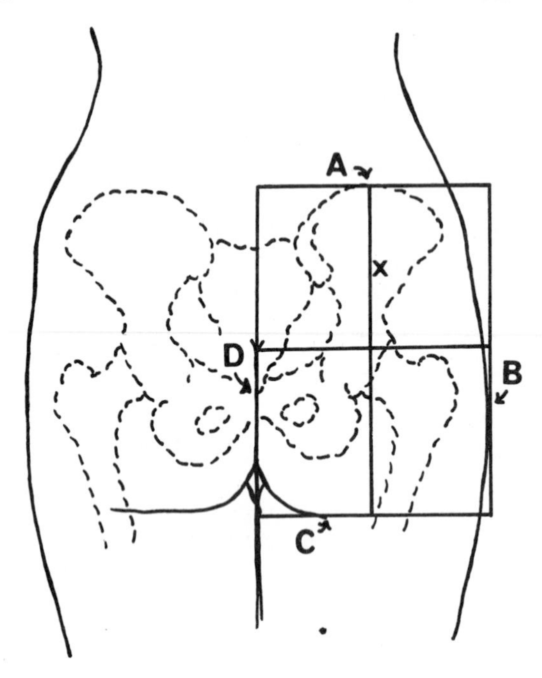

FIG. 29-8. One site for an intramuscular injection is the inner angle of the upper outer quadrant. This area is obtained by using the following guides. The upper line is determined by the iliac crest, A; the outer lines by the division of the buttocks and the outer surface of patient's body, D and B. The lower line is determined by the lower edge of the buttock, C. This area is then divided into equal parts vertically and horizontally. The injection is given two to three inches below the top of the iliac crest in the upper outer quadrant.

even more frequently than the literature reports. Common complications have included abscesses, necrosis and skin slough, nerve injuries, lingering pain and periostitis.

A crucial point in the administration of an intramuscular injection is the selection of a safe site, one that is away from large nerves and the large blood vessels.

Dorsogluteal Site (Gluteus Maximus Muscle). The dorsogluteal site, located on the buttock has been a common site for giving intramuscular injections. The classic method is to inject about two to three inches below the crest of the ilium in the upper outer quadrant of the buttock. Figure 29-8 illustrates how the area is located.

Another method for locating a site on the buttock is illustrated in Figure 29-9. Locate a line from the posterosuperior iliac spine to the greater trochanter of the femur; an in-

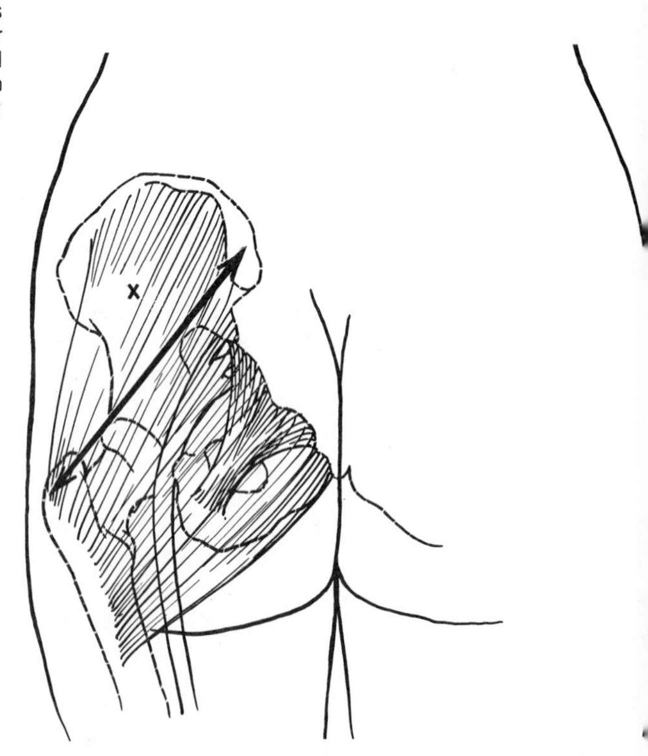

FIG. 29-9. Another method for mapping out the gluteus maximum is to draw an imaginary line from the ridge on the ileum to the head of the femur. The needle is injected outside and above the midline.

jection lateral and slightly superior to the midpoint of the line will also avoid the dangerous area.

A common error in locating a site is improper mapping of the area. Many people believe that the fleshy part of the buttock should certainly be the safest spot. Nothing could be more incorrect. Also, many incorrectly include the fleshy portion of the upper thigh, especially in obese patients, as a part of the buttock. The site is so important that no injection into the buttock should be given without good visualization of the entire area and careful mapping to locate the proper site.

Ventrogluteal Site (Gluteus Medius and Gluteus Minimus Muscles). This is preferred to the dorsogluteal site in children, and it is recommended also by many physicians for adults as well. There are no large nerves or blood vessels in this area; there is less fat here than in the buttocks; the area is cleaner, since fecal contamination is rare on the thigh, and the patient can be on his back for the injection.

The correct site, illustrated in Figure 29-13, is located as follows: place the tip of the index finger on the anterosuperior iliac spine; abduct the adjacent finger (to form a V), place it on the crest of the ilium and then slide the finger just below it; rest the palm of the hand on the thigh; an injection into the V will fall within the region of the gluteal muscles.

Vastus Lateralis Muscle. This muscle is not used commonly but is being recommended more frequently. It is a thick muscle and there is little or no danger of serious injury. There are no large nerves or vessels in close proximity, and it does not cover a joint. The muscle covers the anterolateral aspect of the thigh. It is bounded by the mid-anterior thigh on the front of the leg and the mid-lateral thigh on the side. The middle third of the

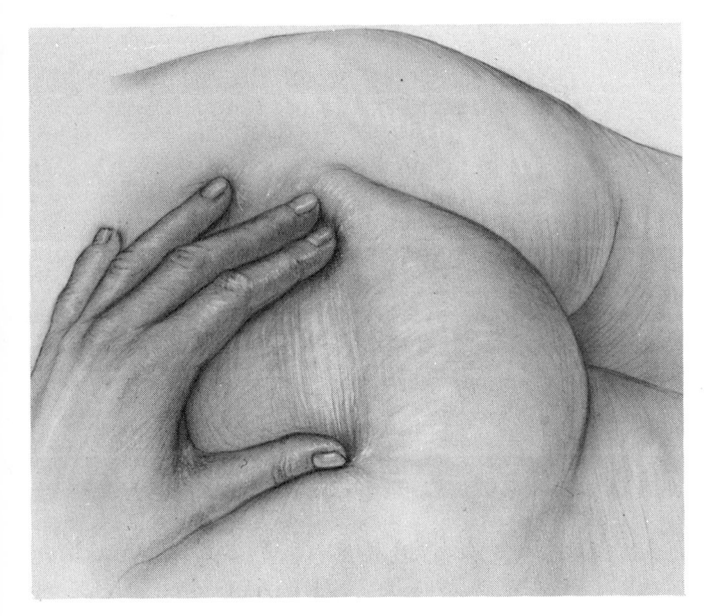

FIG. 29-10. After mapping out the area carefully, press down the tissue and hold it taut.

muscle, measuring up from just above the knee and down from the greater trochanter, is recommended for injections. This provides space for a large number of injections. (Fig. 29-12).

Deltoid and Posterior Triceps Muscles. These muscles also may be used. However, in general, they rarely are used, since they are small, and a misplaced needle may injure the radial nerve. Also, many patients experience more pain and tenderness in this area than in others.

Rectus Femoris Muscle. This muscle is on the anterior part of the thigh. The site is used only when others are contraindicated, since many patients find it uncomfortable. However, some patients who must inject themselves at home use this site.

Preparation of the Drug for Intramuscular Injection. As mentioned previously in the discussion of subcutaneous injections, the length of the needle to reach the desired tissue varies with each individual. The most commonly used needle for intramuscular injection is a 22-gauge, one and one-half-inch needle. However, for drugs of an oily nature, a larger gauge, such as a 20 gauge, is indicated. The length of the needle for an intramuscular injection should be based on the site to be used and the condition of the patient. This is especially important if the patient is obese and the drug is irritating; three-inch needles cause no more discomfort than one and one-half-inch needles, and, with proper injection, there is a greater likelihood of the drug's being introduced into muscle. For children, a shorter needle is necessary, such as a three-quarter-inch or a one-inch needle. In many instances, it is possible to use a hypodermic needle to give an intramuscular injection to an infant.

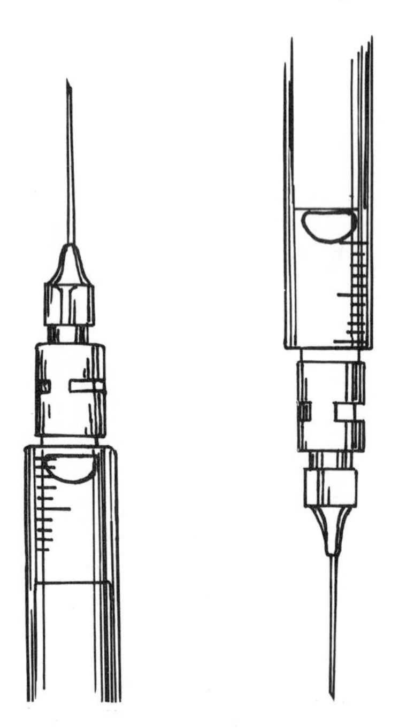

Fig. 29-11. A small amount of air, 0.2 to 0.3 cc., is drawn into the syringe as final preparation for intramuscular injection. When the syringe and the needle are inverted, as during injection, the bubble rises in the syringe. The air serves to push the solution trapped in the shaft of the needle into the tissues.

The age, the weight, the condition and the tissue turgor of the patient should be taken into consideration rather than relying on a standard needle gauge for each type of injection.

The points of caution observed for the preparation of equipment for a subcutaneous or any other parenteral injection are employed also when preparing an intramuscular injection. There is an exception in the procedure: just prior to injection, a small air bubble, approximately 0.2 to 0.3 cc., is included in the syringe with the solution. This is measured when the syringe is held in the upright position. When the needle is injected, this air bubble will rise to the top of the solution in the syringe (see Fig. 29-11). After the solution is injected, this air bubble will aid in expelling the remaining solution that is trapped in the shaft of the needle. Solution which remains in the shaft of the needle is in danger of being pulled up through the tissues as the needle is withdrawn. If the drug is a particularly irritating one, this causes real discomfort to the patient and may result in tissue damage.

Only the points of difference between subcutaneous and intramuscular injections are given in the following method for intramuscular injection into the gluteus maximus muscle.

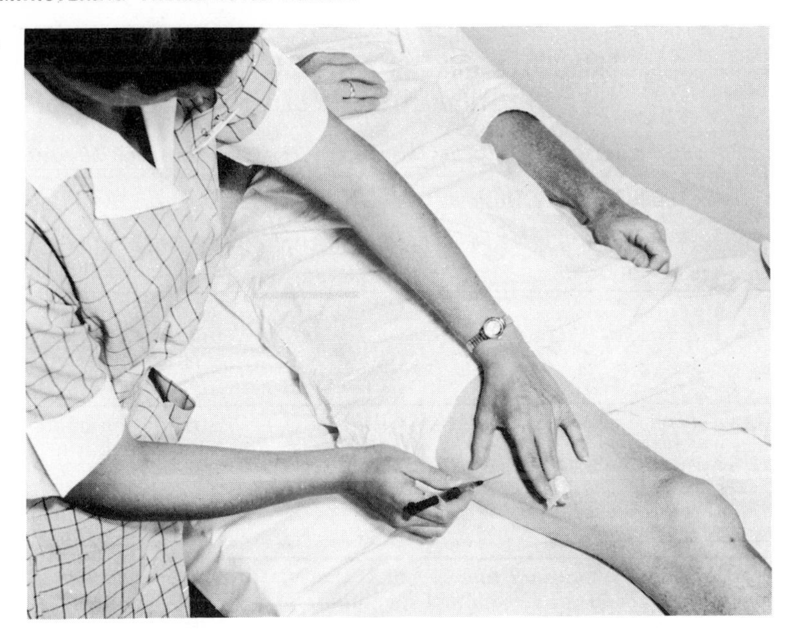

Fig. 29-12. Lateral thigh injection.

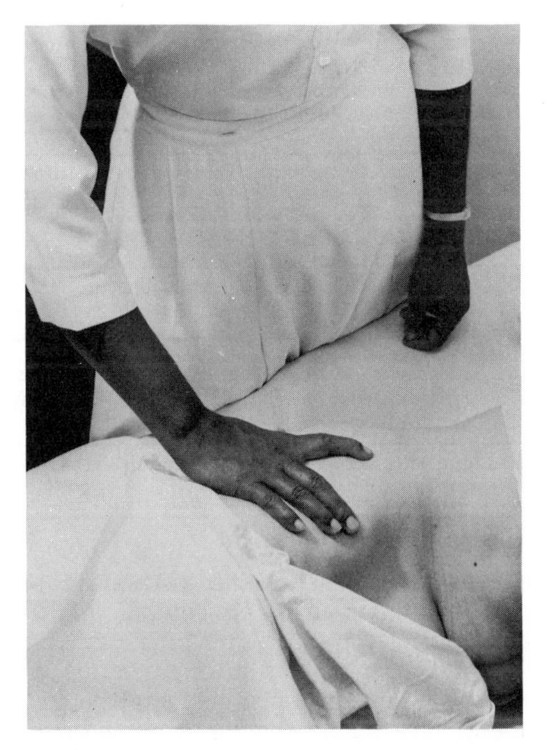

Fig. 29-13. Ventral site intramuscular injection with the patient in the side-lying position. The nurse palpates for the anterosuperior iliac spine. When she locates it she will hold her finger on it and move her second finger along the bony prominence to form a V, as illustrated.

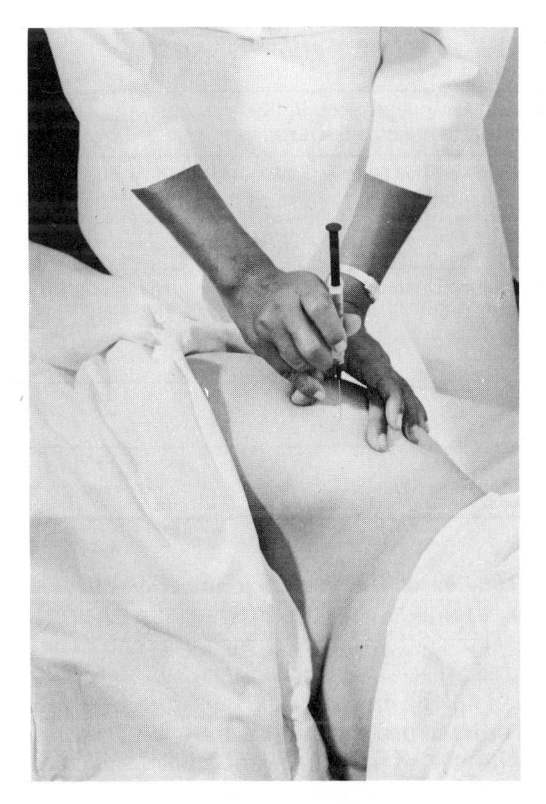

Fig. 29-14. Having located the site, the nurse puts her hand in position, presses down the tissues, and injects needle.

PRINCIPLES GUIDING ACTION IN THE ADMINISTRATION OF AN INJECTION INTO THE GLUTEUS MAXIMUS MUSCLE

The purpose is to inject a medication into the gluteus maximus muscle.

SUGGESTED ACTION	PRINCIPLE
Have the patient assume a comfortable side-lying or face down position.	Injection into tense muscle causes pain. Good visualization of the buttock aids correct location of site.
Locate the site.	The area about 2 to 3 inches below the top of the iliac crest in the upper outer quadrant avoids the sciatic nerve and large blood vessels and is still over the gluteus maximus.
Gently tap the selected site of injection with the fingers several times.	Stimulation of the peripheral nerves helps to minimize the initial reaction when the needle is inserted.
Cleanse the area thoroughly, using friction.	Pathogens present on the skin can be forced into the tissues by the needle.
Using the thumb and the first 2 fingers, press the tissue down firmly and in the direction of the thigh.	Compression of the subcutaneous tissue helps to ensure having the needle enter muscle. Moving the tissue downward will help to disperse the solution and seal the needle track when the tissue is permitted to return to normal position.
Hold the syringe in a horizontal position until ready to inject.	The pull of gravity may alter the position of the plunger, causing loss of drug.
When ready to inject, quickly thrust the needle into the tissue at a 90° angle.	Quick injection minimizes pain. Thrust helps to insert needle.
As soon as the needle is in place, slowly pull back on the plunger to determine whether the needle is in a blood vessel. If blood is noted, pull the needle back slightly and test again.	Muscle tissue is vascular. Drugs injected into the blood stream are absorbed immediately.
If no blood comes up into syringe, inject solution slowly, followed by air bubble into the needle.	The air bubble will force the solution through the shaft of the needle and prevent dribbling of the solution in the muscle and the subcutaneous tissues as the needle is withdrawn.
Remove the needle quickly.	Slow removal of the needle pulls the tissues and may cause discomfort.
Rub the area.	Rubbing aids in the distribution and the absorption of the solution.

Rotation of Intramuscular Injection Sites. Because many drugs are given via the intramuscular route and therapy often calls for repeated injections, consideration should be given to the rotation of the sites used. The sites described earlier all may be used.

The use of the different muscle groups is almost essential for patients receiving injections every four hours. The slight discomfort created by the use of other areas does not seem to outweigh the discomfort produced in the gluteals following multiple piercings or the induration which may result.

When a pattern of rotating sites is used for a patient, a comment should appear in the nursing care plan. The time and the site to be used should be indicated.

Intravenous Administration

Intravenous administration refers to the

introduction of solutions or drugs directly into a vein. Giving a large quantity of solution is referred to as an *infusion.*

In some health agencies, nurses assume responsibility for certain types of intravenous administration. There has been considerable discussion of the legal implications of this, the problem being whether or not intravenous administration is legally a medical responsibility. If local policy permits, it is assumed that the agency's policies will be observed and that the nurse will acquire the appropriate knowledge and practice in the technic under the supervision of a qualified person.

Since certain types of intravenous therapy are being assumed by nurses, a discussion of the procedure for intravenous infusion is presented here.

Solutions are given intravenously for a variety of purposes but most commonly to restore or to maintain fluid and electrolyte balance and as a vehicle to give medications.

Fluid and electrolyte balance was discussed in Chapter 24. Other common problems of illness for which intravenous infusions are prescribed were discussed in Chapter 25—i.e., nausea, vomiting and abnormal temperature.

Selection of a Vein for Intravenous Therapy. Veins of the cubital fossa (inner aspect of the elbow) are first choice. These veins are convenient to get at, tend to be quite superficial, are fairly large and are well supported by muscular and connective tissue. The most commonly used vein is the median cephalic, although any other in the area is satisfactory.

Veins on the back of the hand and at the ankle are sometimes used but they are more difficult to enter and tend to roll easily. In infants, it is not uncommon to use scalp veins or a jugular vein. When veins in the cubital fossa cannot be used, a cut-down to a vein may be necessary in which case the physician assumes responsibility for introducing the needle. Local policy must be observed when the cubital fossa is not used, since in most instances nurses do not give intravenous therapy when veins at the elbow are contraindicated.

Either arm may be used for intravenous therapy. If the patient is right-handed and both arms appear to be equally usable, usually the left arm is selected so that the right arm is then free for the patient's use.

Equipment Commonly Used for Intravenous Infusions. Since a vein is being entered, sterile technic is observed. Most health agencies use disposable infusion tubing and needles, thus eliminating possible sources of contamination and reducing the cost of the aftercare of the equipment.

For most intravenous infusions for adults, an 18-, 20- or 22-gauge needle, one and one-half to two inches in length, is used. Smaller gauge needles impede the flow of the solution. If an infusion needle is to remain in place for a prolonged period of time, a plastic cannula may be threaded through the needle into the vein.

Normally, the pressure in the patient's vein is greater than atmospheric pressure. Therefore, if a solution is to be injected into

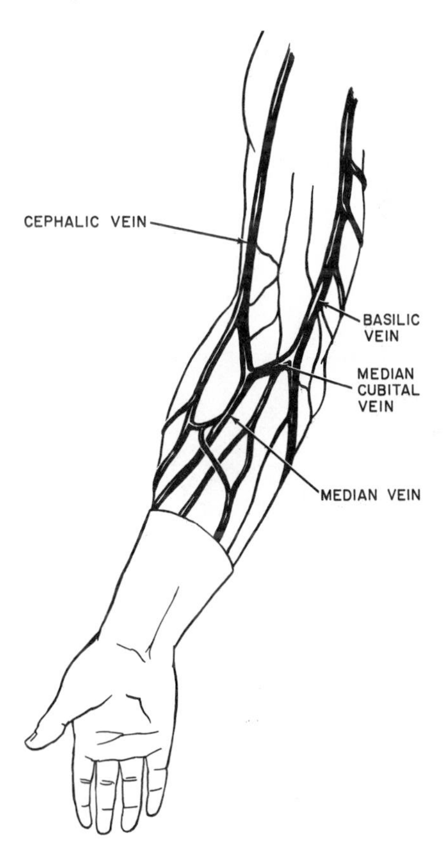

FIG. 29-15. Sites for intravenous therapy.

the vein, pressure must be great enough to overcome the pressure in the vein. One of two methods is used. For small amounts, such as a drug, the drug is drawn into a syringe, and the plunger is used to force the solution into the vein. When large amounts of solution are administered, the gravity method is used. The solution is placed at a level approximately 18 to 24 inches above the level of the vein or at a height where gravity is sufficient to overcome the venous pressure and to allow the solution to enter the vein. When the gravity method is used, the bottle of solution is suspended on a pole, and the solution flows through the attached tubing and the needle directly into the patient.

The rate of flow of the solution is controlled by a clamp or constricting device on the tubing. A device known as a dripmeter is included in the tubing. This makes it possible to count the drops being administered per minute. Where extreme accuracy in the administration of a drug by intravenous infusion is essential, a microdripmeter is used. The standard dripmeter usually delivers about 20 drops per one cc. The microdrip is 60 drops per one cc.

Solution for Intravenous Infusions. The kind of solution and the amount are specifically ordered by the physician. Also, the physician orders the addition of vitamins, antibiotics or salts to the solution if he so desires. When anything is added to the solution to be administered the same principles for assuring accuracy and safety are in effect.

Extreme caution is essential when adding

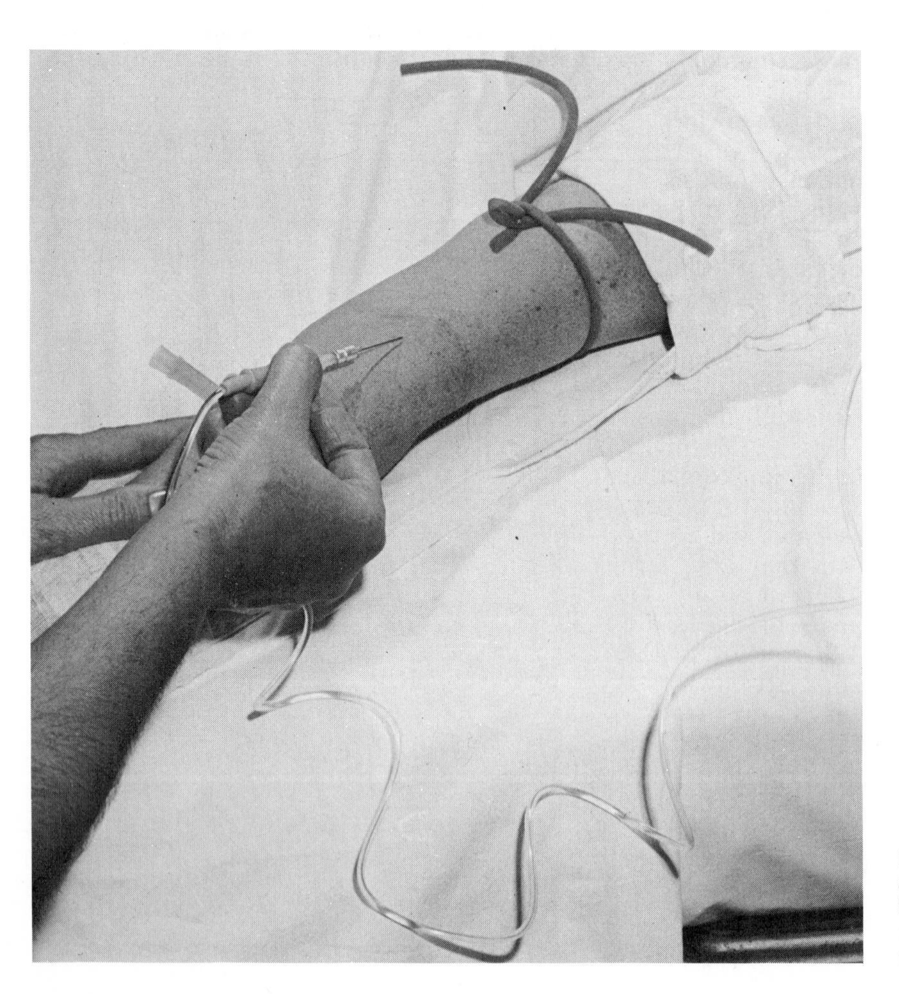

Fig. 29-16. The tourniquet is in place, the vein was located and the area cleansed. With one hand holding the skin taut, the physician is about to insert the needle to start the infusion.

any form of therapeutic agent to an intravenous infusion. Nurses should add only those agents which are clearly spelled out by agency policy. When a medication is added to any infusion solution, the agent and dosage must appear on the bottle also. In many agencies the time of adding the therapeutic agent and the name of the nurse preparing the solution must also be indicated.

Preparation of the Patient for Intravenous Infusion. Since an infusion usually takes several hours to complete, the patient should be made comfortable. If the procedure is unusually long, the patient's position should be changed frequently if he is to remain in bed. If allowed to walk, proper precautions are taken to prevent the needle from slipping out of place.

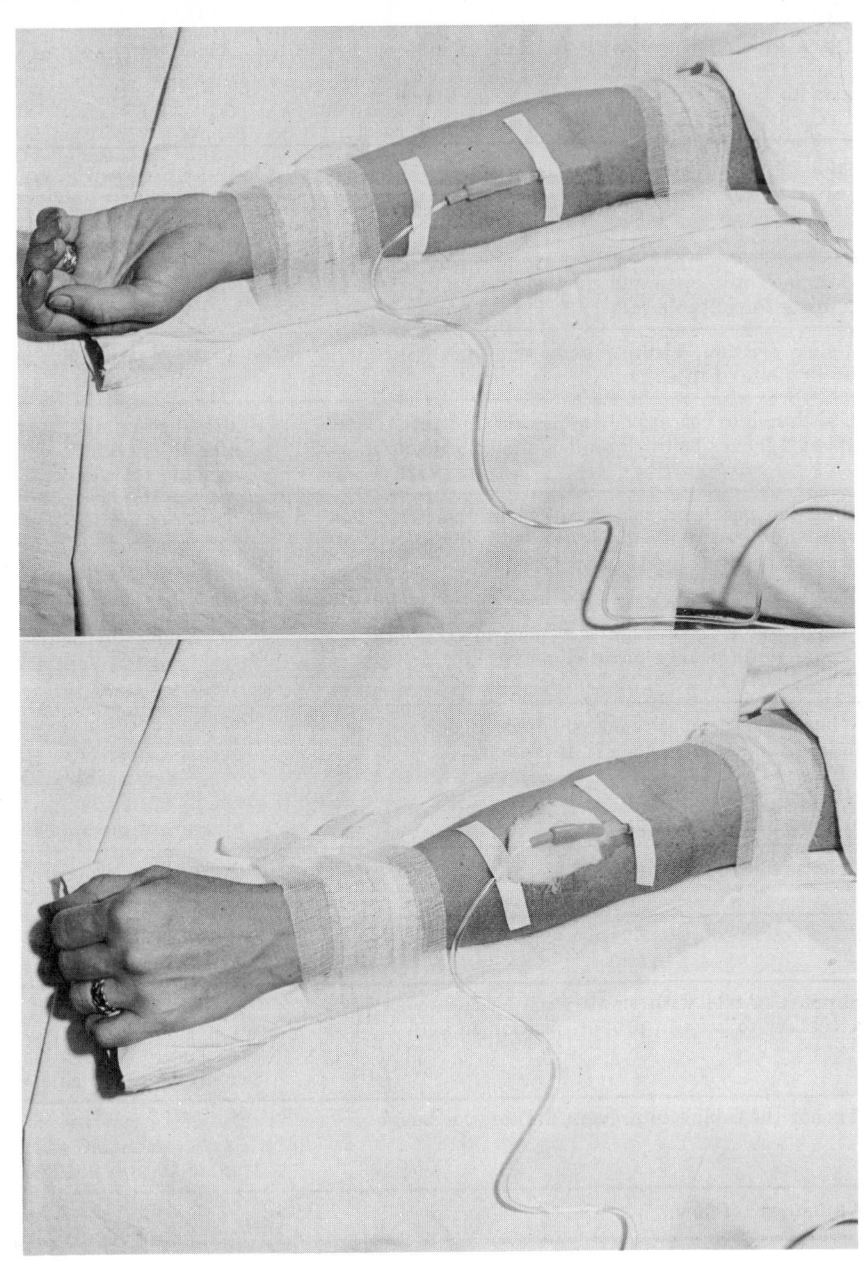

FIG. 29-17. (Top). Support under the needle to keep it from hitting the wall of the vein depends on the location of the needle and the contour of the surrounding tissues. When the patient held her arm with the palm upward, no support was needed under the needle.

FIG. 29-18. (Bottom). The needle had to be supported with cotton if the patient wished to pronate the hand. Since having the hand pronated is normal body alignment, it is less fatiguing.

PRINCIPLES GUIDING ACTION IN THE ADMINISTRATION OF AN INTRAVENOUS INFUSION USING A VEIN IN THE CUBITAL FOSSA

The purpose is to inject a relatively large amount of solution into a vein.

SUGGESTED ACTION	PRINCIPLE
Have patient in back-lying position and the bed in semi-Fowler's position.	The back-lying position when infusion is to be started permits either arm to be used while in good alignment.
Place arm on board with tourniquet under arm, about 1½ inch above intended site of entry. Secure arm to board with bandage or arm board tapes. Fix only snug enough to hold arm securely.	Arm motion will move vein, causing change in position of needle. Circulation of blood can be impaired by constricting objects.
Apply tourniquet; direct ends away from site of injection.	Interrupting blood flow back to heart causes veins to distend. Distended veins are easy to see, palpate and enter. Ends of tourniquet could contaminate the area of injection.
Ask patient to open and close his fist. Observe and palpate for suitable vein.	Contraction of muscles of lower arm forces blood along in veins, thereby distending them further.
Using friction, cleanse skin thoroughly at and around site of injection.	Pathogens present on the skin can be introduced into the tissues or the blood with the needle.
Use thumb to retract down on vein and soft tissue about 2 inches below intended site of injection.	Pressure on the vein and the surrounding tissues aids in preventing movement of the vein as needle is being introduced.
Hold the needle at a 45° angle, in line with the vein and directly alongside the wall of the vein at a point about ½ inch away from intended site of venipuncture.	Pressure needed to pierce the skin can be sufficient to force the needle into vein at improper angle and possibly through opposite wall.
When needle is through the skin, lower angle of needle until nearly parallel with skin, following same course as vein, and insert into vein.	Following the course of the vein prevents needle from leaving vein at another site.
When blood comes back through needle, insert needle farther into vein ¾ to 1 inch.	Structure of vein does not offer any resistance to needle movement. Having needle placed well into vein helps to prevent easy dislodgment of needle. "Riding" needle into vein while it is distended helps to prevent pushing it through the wall.
Release tourniquet.	Occluded vessel prevents solution from entering circulation.
Start flow of solution by releasing clamp.	Blood can clot readily in needle if not in motion with other blood or solution.
Support needle with small wipe or cotton ball if necessary to keep in proper position in vein.	Pressure of the wall of the vein against the opening of the needle will interrupt the rate of flow of solution. The wall of the vein can be punctured easily by the needle.
Anchor the tubing to prevent pull on the needle.	Smooth structure of vein does not offer resistance to movement of needle. Weight of tubing is sufficient to pull needle out of vein.
Adjust rate of flow.	

The arm to be used is abducted slightly from the body and placed on an arm board, if necessary. When the arm is secured to an arm board, attention should be given to keeping it in good position. Very often it is possible to have the forearm pronated and the palm of the hand downward and in the grasping position over the edge of the arm board. This position more nearly resembles the normal position of the arm and is therefore more comfortable for the patient. Hyperextension of the elbow causes fatigue for the patient, often to the point where it may be impossible for him to move his forearm voluntarily after an infusion is discontinued. It takes assistance in flexing and extending the elbow passively to help regain "feeling" in the arm. If the area is hairy, such as a man's arm, it would be best to shave the area involving the needle site and adhesive.

A tourniquet is applied to aid in distending the vein. The tourniquet is placed under the arm above the elbow and ready to tie. The arm is secured to the board with bandage or ties. Do not obstruct circulation or cause discomfort to the patient, but make it snug enough to hold the arm securely. The skin over the vein where the needle will be introduced is cleansed thoroughly with antiseptic solution.

The equipment is assembled, with care being taken to avoid contaminating the ends of the tubing and the solution. After the tubing has been connected to the bottle of solution, it is clamped shut, and the bottle is hung on the pole approximately 18 to 24

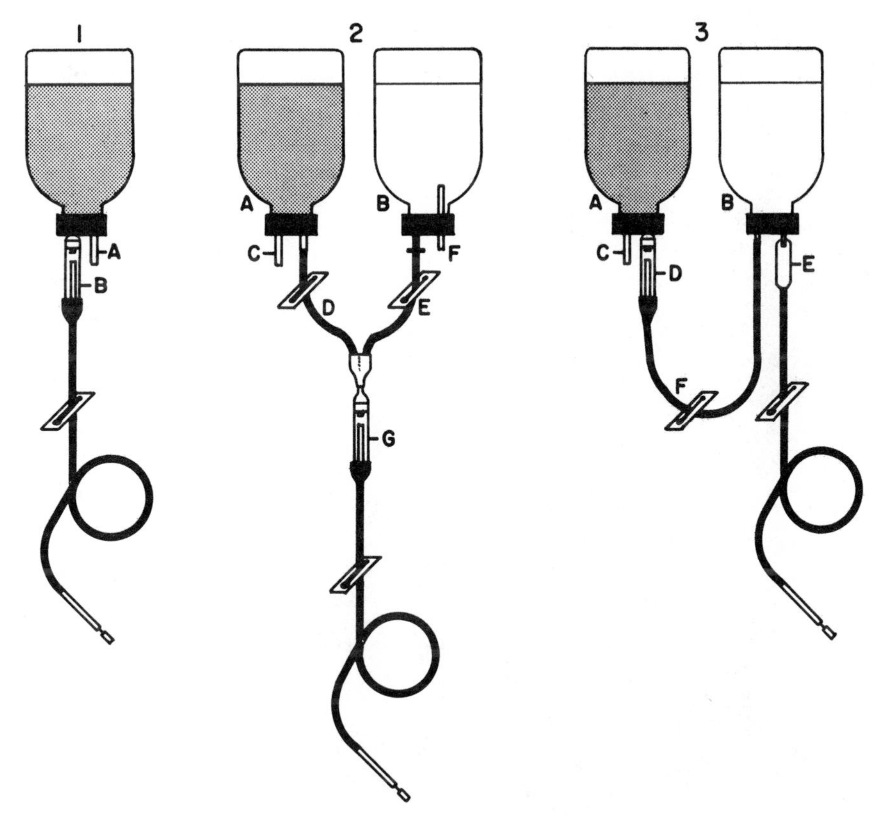

Fig. 29-19. Various means by which intravenous substances can be given by the gravity method.

(1) The solution flows through the drip-meter B (which also may be a filter if blood is given) at a rate that can be controlled by a clamp on the tubing. A provides an air inlet so that air may enter the bottle to displace the fluid that leaves. It has a one-way valve which prevents the fluid from running out.

(2) Solution may leave either bottle, depending on the regulation of the clamps D and E. In this set-up, A is blood and B is normal saline. If D stops the flow of blood from bottle A, the saline will flow from bottle B if clamp E and the clamp below the filter are opened. The reverse also can be made to happen. Therefore, both bottles must have an air inlet, C and F, so that air can enter to displace the fluid as it leaves. In this set-up, G is a filter as well as a drip-meter.

(3) This is referred to as a tandem set-up. Fluid will leave bottle B if the clamp F is open. As fluid leaves bottle B, an area of lesser pressure is created in bottle B. This lesser pressure exerts its influence on bottle A and draws fluid from it. The system will operate only if C, the air vent, is open and permits air to displace the fluid that leaves bottle A. D is a drip-meter and filter. E is a drip-meter. In this set-up, A always will empty before B. If F is clamped off, no fluid will be able to leave bottle B.

inches above the level of the vein. Air is forced out of the tubing by releasing the clamp slightly and slowly permitting the solution to fill the tubing. When all of the air is out of the tubing, it is clamped shut. The tip of the tubing to be attached to the needle is kept sterile.

Rate of Flow. Usually the nurse is responsible for maintaining an even rate of flow while the solution is entering the vein; 40 to 60 drops of solution per minute is the usual rate. The physician may order the solution given more or less rapidly, depending on the patient's condition and the kind of solution being given. Very rapid infusion usually is contraindicated because of the danger of causing too great a load on the circulatory system.

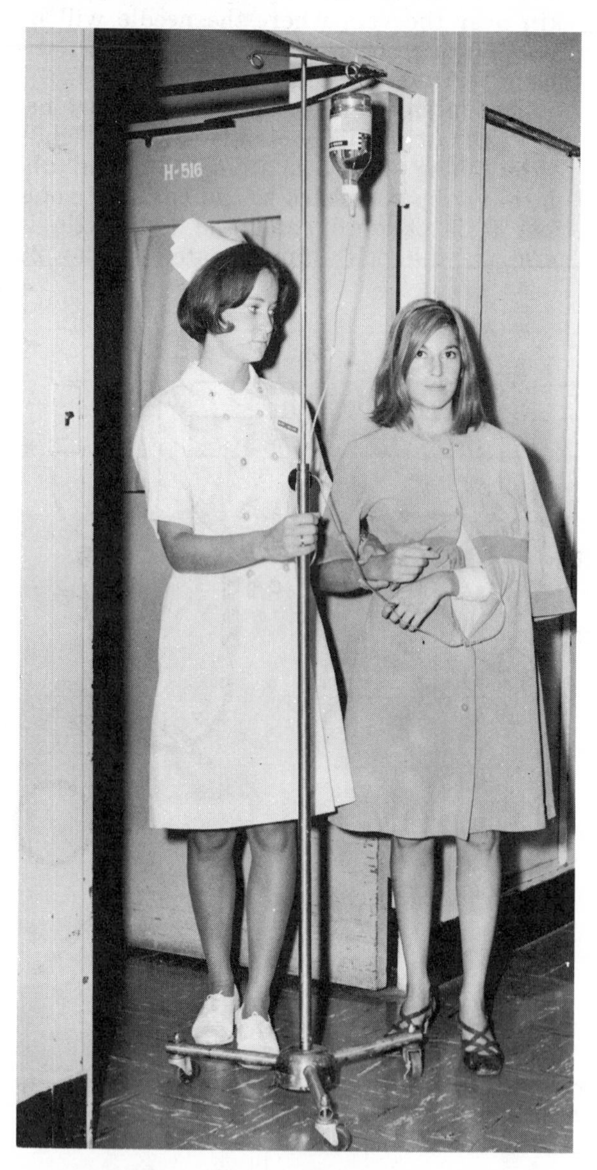

FIG. 29-20. The patient's infusion solution is hung on a pole that is easily pushed ahead of the nurse as she supports the patient.

The nurse is responsible for observing that the solution continues to flow into the vein. If the needle slips out of the vein, the solution will flow into the subcutaneous tissue, and the tissue around the needle will become swollen as fluid collects. This is referred to as *infiltration.* The rate of flow may decrease or stop altogether. The clamp on the tubing should be fastened. If there is question about whether the needle is still in the vein, the bottle of solution can be lowered below the level of the vein. If blood runs into the tubing, the needle is still placed properly. If the needle is not in the vein, usual procedure is to remove the needle, which may be clogged with blood. No attempt should be made to force the clot into the patient's circulation.

The nurse is also responsible for observing the site of injection and the path of the vein for signs of redness. This might be the beginning of phlebitis (inflammation of the vein). Observation should also be made for tenderness or pain.

If more than one bottle of solution is ordered for the patient, the nurse attaches the additional bottles. The method by which this is done will depend on the procedure of the agency. Some intravenous equipment is designed to simplify the procedure by making it possible to attach additional bottles with a tandemlike arrangement, as Figure 29-19 illustrates.

One method is to prepare all the solution, for example, two or three bottles as the case may be, at one time, and keep them in a safe place. If in addition to the labels for medications, each bottle is numbered, 1—2—3, etc., everyone concerned with the patient is in a better position to know exactly what has been given and what still must be given.

It is good practice to agree on one safe

method for managing infusions of this nature and provide for all who practice in the agency to observe it. Without such uniformity, serious errors can occur, or valuable time is lost in checking and rechecking.

Discontinuing the Infusion. When the amount of solution the physician has ordered has been absorbed, the nurse assumes responsibility for discontinuing the infusion. The adhesive strips are removed, the needle is removed quickly, and pressure is applied immediately to the site. If the patient is able to do so, he may be asked to hold the pressure dressing on for a minute or more.

If the patient's arm or leg has been immobilized for several hours or longer, the nurse should manipulate it carefully in an attempt to put the joint through range of motion and passively move the muscles of the area.

Charting the Administration of an Intravenous Injection. The following information is charted: the date and the time the infusion was started and completed; the kind and the amount of solution injected; the name and the amount of the drug added and the name of the person starting the infusion.

Symptoms of reaction are charted as well as any treatment which the physician may prescribe for it. Symptoms of desired effects are charted also.

Intracutaneous Administration

Solutions injected into the corium of the skin are referred to as intracutaneous or intradermal injections. Solutions are absorbed slowly via the capillaries. Small amounts of solution are used—usually no more than several minims. A common site for injection is the inner aspect of the arm, although other areas are also satisfactory. Intracutaneous injections generally are used for diagnostic purposes; examples are the tuberculin test, and tests to determine sensitivity to various substances. The advantage of the intracutaneous route for these tests is that reaction of the body to these substances is easily visible, and, by means of comparative studies, degrees of reaction are discernible. Vaccination for smallpox is an example of a therapeutic intradermal injection, although this also may be done by multiple skin punctures and scratches.

INHALATION THERAPY

Gases and certain drugs are administered by inhalation. Most of the absorption occurs on the very vascular surfaces of the alveoli, and, because of the large surface area in the lungs, absorption after inhalation generally is rapid.

Administration of Drugs by Inhalation

Before drugs can be inhaled, they must be vaporized to permit their entry into the body with inspiration. A few drugs are volatile and vaporize when exposed to air. Nonvolatile drugs are added to a vehicle, which, when vaporized, carries the drug into the respiratory tract.

Administration of a Volatile Drug. Ammonia is an example of a volatile drug. The gas vaporizes from ammonia water, frequently called smelling salts, and, when inhaled, acts systemically to stimulate the heart and respiration. The ammonia water is poured onto a small piece of absorbent cotton or gauze and held near the nose so that the vapors are inhaled. The gas is very irritating and should be used cautiously for only short periods of time. The patient's eyes should be protected or kept closed.

Administration of a Nonvolatile Drug. *Steam Inhalation.* A way to vaporize a drug so that it may be inhaled is to add it to water which, when heated, produces steam that is laden with the drug to be inhaled. This drug acts locally to soothe irritated, inflammed and congested mucous membrane and to loosen secretions in the respiratory tract. In addition to the action of the drug, the steam soothes the respiratory membrane. The inhaled air, carrying warm minute droplets of water, carries heat to the area and produces the same results as when heat is applied locally to other parts of the body.

Nebulizing. A mistlike spray is another common means of administering nonvolatile drugs for inhalation. A device called a nebulizer is used to separate a drug in solution into minute particles for inhalation.

Atomization usually refers to the production of rather large droplets, while nebulization is the production of a fine mist or fog. The finer the particles, the farther they will travel into the respiratory tract. If the inhalation is intended to produce effects in the nasal passage as well as in the remainder of the respiratory tract, the patient closes his mouth while he breathes and inhales through his nose. Otherwise, the mist is inhaled through the mouth. The vapor produced by this method is often referred to as *cold steam.*

There are several ways in which a spray may be produced. The hand nebulizer uses a bulb attachment which, when compressed, forces air through the container holding the drug in solution. The increased pressure in the unit forces solution into a specially constructed strictured device. The force with which the solution is made to move through this stricture and to leave the container is sufficient to break the large droplets of fluid into a fine mist.

The same effect may be accomplished by using the force of an oxygen stream or compressed air to be passed through the fluid in a nebulizer. This method is valuable for patients who require 10 to 15 minutes of inhalations of a special drug several times a day. The hand nebulizer would prove to be quite fatiguing. The oxygen stream is also useful in the production of vapors when high humidity is needed continuously for long periods of time.

Only one medication should be nebulized at a time if more than one is prescribed. Safe

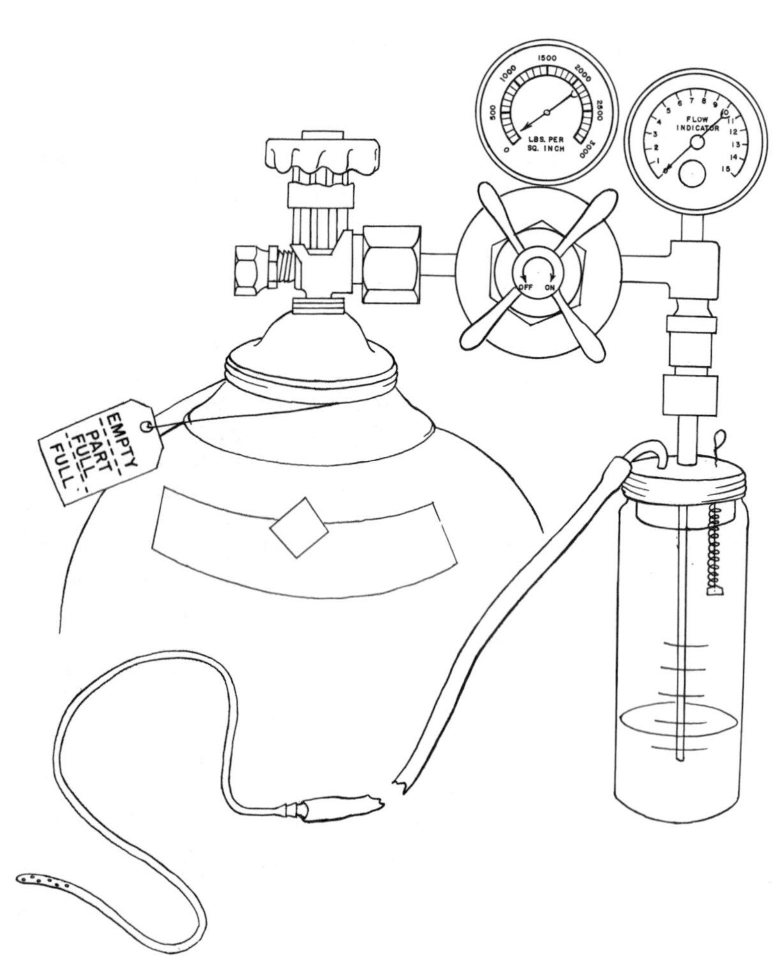

FIG. 29-21. Oxygen tank with regulator. The regulator is fastened to the tank valve and tightened with a wrench. The valve atop the tank admits oxygen to the regulator. When this valve is opened, the left-hand gauge will indicate the tank pressure. The regulator valve (below the tank gauge) then is turned; it releases the oxygen and then is adjusted for the correct rate (shown on the right-hand gauge). A humidifier attached to the apparatus is used when oxygen is administered via nasal catheter.

practice is not to mix them in the event that one causes undesirable effects.

Commercially prepared aerosol containers with medications, such as bronchodilators or mucolytic agents are available. These are helpful for home use.

Administration of Oxygen

Oxygen is essential for life, and the body has no reserve of it. Therefore, when there is insufficient oxygenation of the blood, oxygen must be added to inhaled air in order to sustain life. *Anoxia* is the term for oxygen deprivation, regardless of its cause. Whenever anoxia occurs, it presents an emergency; therefore, it is essential that the nurse fully understand how to manage oxygen equipment and the means for administering therapeutic concentrations.

Numerous conditions result in poor oxygenation of blood when normal air is inhaled. For example, when congestion of the lungs from an infection such as pneumonia is present, the total functional lung surface is reduced. Oxygen is added to the inhaled air so that the blood can be oxygenated more easily. In this example, there is inadequate oxygenation because of an abnormality of the lungs. The need for adding oxygen to inhaled air at high altitudes is an example of aiding oxygenation occurring in normal lungs. When circulation of blood in the lungs is impaired by congestion, as often occurs with certain heart conditions, increasing the intake of oxygen relieves anoxia. Occasionally, when strict rest is essential in a disease condition, oxygen may be given so that the least amount of energy is used by the body in the act of respiration.

Oxygen therapy must often be instituted with such speed that there is little time for explaining to the patient. However, depending on the device used to administer it, some concurrent instructions may be necessary. As soon as the patient is out of danger and is breathing easily, he should be told about the device and the essentials necessary to serve him effectively. It is a terrifying experience to be unable to breathe, and the patient deserves the support and comfort of feeling that all possible is being done for him.

There are patients who must become proficient in administering oxygen to themselves. They may have asthma or chronic lung ailments or impaired cardiac functioning and have oxygen at home for self-administration.

Special Consideration in Handling Oxygen. Oxygen, which constitutes approximately 20 per cent of normal air, is a tasteless, odorless and colorless gas. In addition to its vital importance in sustaining life, it has a chemical characteristic which requires careful consideration. Oxygen supports combustion. Therefore, open flames and sparks must be kept away from the unit where oxygen is being administered. This precaution cannot be emphasized enough since periodically tragic accidents occur as a result of this hazard. "No Smoking" signs should be placed in many prominent places in the unit and the patient and his visitors taught the necessity of observing this regulation.

All electric devices such as heating pads, stoves, electric bell cords, razors and radios, should be removed from the unit. The greatest care should be taken also in the management of linens, since many fabrics—including wool, silk, rayon and nylon—generate static electricity and sparks from such sources are equally dangerous.

In most hospitals, oxygen is piped into each patient unit and is immediately available from an outlet in the wall. This piped-in oxygen is a valuable asset: it increases the patient's safety by eliminating the delay in transporting oxygen in tanks and the constant vigil on the gauge to check on the amount of oxygen remaining in the tank. Some hospitals do not have it in all units, but are providing for it in delivery, operating and recovery rooms. When oxygen is not available from a wall outlet, it is obtained in portable cylinders.

The Tank of Oxygen. Oxygen usually is compressed and dispensed in steel cylinders (tanks). The tank is delivered with a protective cap to prevent accidental force against the cylinder outlet. When a standard, large-size cylinder is full, its contents are under more than 2,000 pounds per square inch of pressure. Such force behind an accidentally partially opened outlet could cause the tank to take off like an uncontrolled, jet-propelled monster.

To release the oxygen safely and at a desirable rate, a regulator is used. The regulator valve controls the rate of oxygen output. On the regulator are two gauges. The one nearest the tank shows the pressure (hence the amount) of oxygen in the tank. The other indicates the number of liters per minute of oxygen being released.

Because of the nature of oxygen, caution must be used in handling the oxygen cylinder and the regulator. The oxygen cylinder should be transported carefully, preferably strapped onto a wheeled carrier to avoid possible falling and breaking of the outlet. No oil should be used near the gauge or the outlet because of the danger of the oil being ignited.

"Cracking" the Tank of Oxygen. Because of the possibility of dust or other particles becoming lodged in the outlet of the tank and being forced into the regulator, the tank is "cracked" before a regulator is applied. This calls for slightly turning the handle on the tank which releases the oxygen so that a small amount of oxygen may be released, thus "flushing out" the outlet. The force with which the oxygen is released from this opening causes a loud hissing sound which usually startles anyone who is not aware of what it is. For this reason, it is recommended that oxygen tanks be "cracked" away from the patient's bedside. If this is not possible, the patient should be prepared for the noise by proper explanation. The oxygen can be released slowly and the sound reduced if both hands are placed on the handle. One hand helps control the movement of the other.

The Oxygen Tent. An oxygen tent is a light, portable structure made of clear plastic and attached to a motor-driven unit. The motor aids in circulating and cooling the air in the tent. The cooling device functions on the same principles as an electric refrigeration unit. A thermostat in the unit keeps the temperature in the tent at the degree considered most comfortable by the patient.

An oxygen tent fits over the top part of the bed so that the patient's head and thorax are in the tent. Usually, there is sufficient covering to extend the tent further if necessary. If the tent is well sealed by tucking the sides under the mattress and by wrapping the front flap into a piece of bed linen, a concentration of 40 to 50 per cent of oxygen can be maintained relatively easily. This can be accomplished by flooding the tent with oxygen at 15 liters per minute for about two minutes before starting the tent and after opening it for nursing care. Between floodings, approximately 10 to 12 liters of oxygen per minute usually is given. Local policy, the physician's order or the patient's condition will determine the desired rate of flow of oxygen for a tent.

Patients may be frightened by the appearance of an oxygen tent, since it frequently is

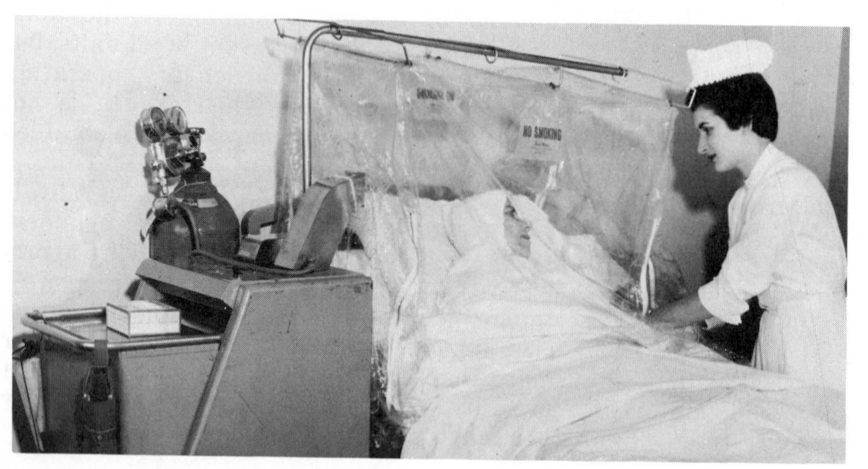

Fig. 29-22. Many nursing activities are carried out easily through the zippered openings provided in the oxygen tent. Because of the air circulation in the tent, protection for the patient's head may be necessary. Care should be taken also to avoid restricting the patient's activity by tucking the draw sheet which helps seal the bottom part of tent too tightly under the mattress.

associated with critical illness. If the patient is prepared adequately as to its advantages, few object to its use.

When a patient is prepared for surgery where there is a very good chance that he may be placed in an oxygen tent immediately following surgery, this should be explained to him. If the patient knows that he may wake up in a tent, considerable anxiety can be avoided. This is important for parents to know also if their child will be in a tent following surgery.

Special Consideration for the Patient Receiving Oxygen Via the Tent Method: *Avoid Drafts.* The tent affords the patient a great amount of freedom and comfort. One of the disadvantages of which the nurse should be aware is the possibility of too great air movement in the tent. Many tents are constructed so that there is a complete exchange of air in the tent every few seconds, in order to prevent an increase in carbon dioxide content. The air movement may create a draft on the patient to the point of real discomfort. The discomfort can be avoided by protecting the patient's head, neck and shoulders with a combination flannel hood and shawl specially designed for use in a tent, as in Fig. 29-22, or an improvised covering made with a towel or other available linen.

Watch the Temperature. While the temperature within an oxygen tent can be regulated within a desired range, there seems to be no justification for keeping the temperature much below 70° F. The combination of rather rapid air movement and low temperature makes the patient uncomfortably chilly. Physicians usually are agreed that the oxygen concentration is of prime importance and must be maintained at a level which affords the patient respiratory relief. The temperature should be maintained at a level which is comfortable for the patient. No one temperature is satisfactory for all patients. Therefore, ask the patient if he is comfortable.

The Tent Is Not Soundproof. A word of caution is necessary as a reminder that the tent is not soundproof. Usually, the patient is able to hear normal conversation outside of the tent. Speak to the patient in normal conversational tones unless he indicates that he cannot hear. It is distressing to the patient to have people outside of the tent shouting at him.

This caution also should be kept in mind when the patient's condition, progress or plan of therapy is being discussed in the immediate vicinity of the bedside. Nothing should be discussed within the patient's hearing which may be disturbing to him.

Special Considerations When Giving Nursing Care to a Patient in a Tent. Oxygen tents are so designed that the nurse may slip her arms into the tent at various places in the hood without lifting it up over the patient's head. This convenience facilitates administering medications, foods and fluids, and carrying out other aspects of nursing care.

When giving care to a patient in an oxygen tent, it is essential that there be careful planning and preparation of all needed items in order to reduce oxygen loss through prolonged and unnecessary opening of the tent.

When it becomes necessary to manipulate the hood so that care which involves turning the patient or adjusting the bed linen may be given, the oxygen concentration must be maintained. This may be accomplished best by moving the hood up to the patient's upper chest or neck and tucking the sides securely under the pillow. The oxygen flow should be increased as much as necessary to compensate for leakage from those points where the hood cannot be sealed.

A signal cord that does not have an electric button on it should be used in the tent. If one is not available, a small hand bell, such as a dinner bell, should be provided.

A non-oily lotion, such as some baby lotions, is preferred for back care. Lotion on the hands of the nurse is a hazard because of the nurse's need to touch the oxygen regulator. The nurse's hands should be washed after back care is given and before she handles the oxygen equipment. The patient's hair should be combed when the tent is not in use. In other words, when the patient's head is not in direct contact with the oxygen flow.

An oxygen tent should be washed thoroughly after use on each patient. While the plastic is easy to clean, the size and the shape of the canopy make it a rather cumber-

PRINCIPLES GUIDING ACTION IN THE USE OF AN OXYGEN TENT

The purpose is to prepare, place and manage an oxygen tent so that the patient receives a therapeutic concentration of oxygen.

SUGGESTED ACTION	PRINCIPLE
Remove all electric appliances from the unit, including the electric signal bell.	Electric appliances may produce sparks and oxygen supports combustion.
Place "No Smoking" signs in several prominent places.	Caution signs warn of the presence of oxygen in the unit.
"Crack" the oxygen tank before bringing it to the unit and attach the gauge.*	Dust particles lodged in the outlet may be forced into the regulator, thus interfering with its proper functioning.
Wheel the oxygen to the bedside on a carrier.*	Rolling an oxygen tank is a hazard because of the danger of its falling and releasing the oxygen at an uncontrolled rate.
Bring oxygen unit to bedside, plug in motor and start unit. Turn on oxygen flow. Check oxygen flow inlet in tent and exhaust outlet. Set temperature control.	Testing the mechanical aspects of the tent reduces the possibility of causing further respiratory distress for the patient in the event of mechanical defect.
Close all openings of the hood. Seal the bottom opening of the hood by bringing the sides together and folding over several times, or by tying, so that the upper half of the hood is flooded with oxygen at 15 liters per minute.	For immediate benefit for the patient, the air in the tent should contain an oxygen content of at least 30 to 40 per cent. Oxygen is heavier than air; therefore, flood the area which is to be over the patient's head.
Flood the tent for 2 to 5 minutes while the hood is closed.	A therapeutic concentration usually is established in this length of time.
Move the unit directly into position near the bed before opening the hood.	Having the unit in place prevents oxygen loss when the hood is placed over the patient.
Open bottom of hood and place over patient. Leaving some slack, tuck part at the head of the bed well under the mattress as far as it will go.	Sufficient length of hood is necessary to lower head of bed if desired.
Tuck the sides of the hood well under the mattress as far as they will go.	A tightly closed hood prevents oxygen seepage.
Enclose the part of the hood which goes over the patient's thighs in a piece of linen and arrange so that open spaces between the hood and the bedding are closed. Tuck the ends under the mattress to hold them securely. Avoid binding down the patient's legs.	Oxygen, being heavier than air, will escape through open areas at the edge of the hood. Linen, being more pliable than the hood, facilitates sealing the openings and in addition keeps the edge of the hood in place.
Test inside the tent for drafts by placing the hand in various locations near the patient's head. Protect the patient's head with a hood or other suitable object.	Forced entrance of the oxygen and provision for withdrawal of air in the tent produce air motion in the tent.
Check the oxygen gauge and reduce flow to 10 to 12 liters per minute.	Ten to 12 liters per minute usually maintains a 40 to 60 per cent concentration in the tent.
Check the temperature indicator frequently until the temperature in the tent is stabilized. Adjust to the temperature most comfortable for the patient.	A temperature of 68° to 72° F. usually is comfortable for a person who is sufficiently covered and protected from the effects of the air movement.
Empty the drainage spigot near the base of the motor unit as often as recommended, usually once every 24 hours.**	Moisture in the air which has been withdrawn from the tent condenses. There is also some condensation from the refrigeration unit.

* If wall oxygen is used, these steps are not observed.
** If this is not done by inhalation technicians.

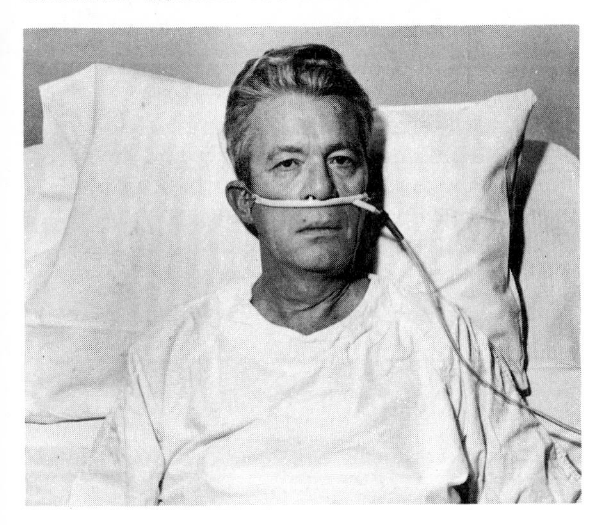

FIG. 29-23. Patient wearing nasal speculi for oxygen-taking.

some chore. Disposable oxygen canopies are coming into use, and if they prove to be adequate to the purpose and expense, they are a desirable safety measure for patients.

Oxygen Administered by Nasal Catheter. Often, oropharyngeal catheters are used for administering oxygen. The oxygen is passed through a bottle of water to humidify it before entering the catheter, in order to minimize the dehydrating effect on the mucous membrane. The catheter is inserted into the nostril and passed until it is in full view at the back of the tongue. It should be in the oropharynx. The horizontal distance from the nasal opening to the ear lobe may be used as a guide for determining the length of catheter to be inserted. If the catheter is inserted too far, there is danger of insufflating the gastrointestinal tract; if it is not inserted far enough, much of the oxygen will escape before it is inhaled.

Irritation of the mucous membrane by the catheter is minimized when the catheter is lubricated prior to insertion, preferably with water. (An oily substance may be harmful if aspirated.) Nasal catheters should be removed for cleansing at least once every eight hours.

Nasal specula, which are also disposable, are more comfortable for most patients. See Fig. 29-23. Watch areas where there may be pressure on the face.

Local policy or the physician's order indicates the desired rate of flow of oxygen. It

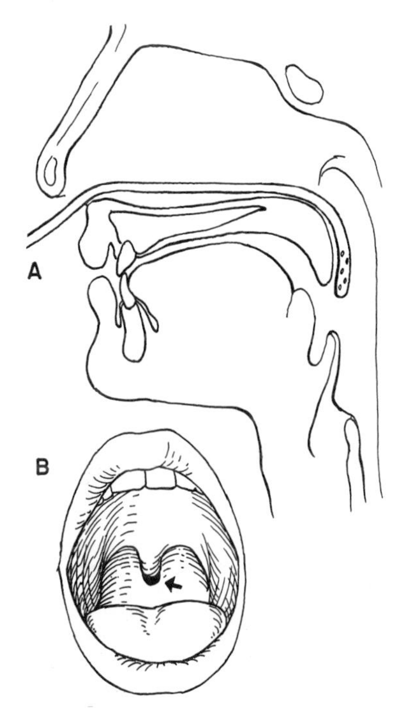

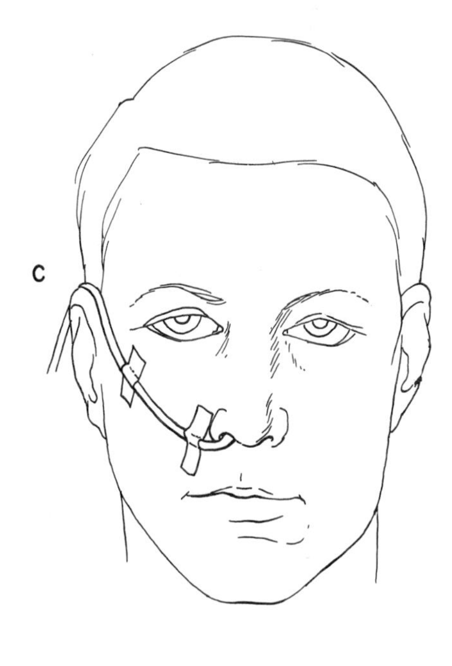

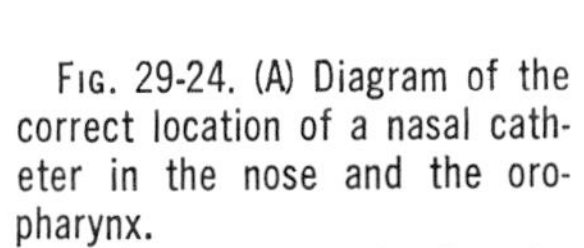

FIG. 29-24. (A) Diagram of the correct location of a nasal catheter in the nose and the oropharynx.

(B) To make certain that the catheter is placed properly, it is necessary to ask the patient to open his mouth. The tip of the catheter should be located just below the uvula (see arrow).

(C) The catheter should be taped close to the nares and on the cheek, and then draped over the ear. This provides freedom of movement of the lips and reduces pull on the catheter.

has been found that, when oxygen is administered at six liters per minute, the patient will inhale a concentration of approximately 42 per cent oxygen. A flow of seven liters per minute yields a 45 to 50 per cent concentration. Increasing the flow of oxygen will dry the mucous membrane, and the patient may complain of a sore throat.

The Oxygen Mask. Various types of face masks have been devised for administering oxygen. For most patients, a mask is more comfortable than the nasal catheter.

The oronasal mask is designed to cover both the nose and the mouth and is necessary if the patient is a mouth breather. It presents problems in feeding, giving fluids and administering oral medications.

The nasal mask covers only the nose and

PRINCIPLES GUIDING ACTION IN THE ADMINISTRATION OF OXYGEN BY MEANS OF A CATHETER

The purpose is to administer a therapeutic concentration of oxygen to a patient by direct admission of oxygen into the oropharynx.

SUGGESTED ACTION	PRINCIPLE
Observe precautions to prevent fire, such as removing electric appliances and posting "No Smoking" signs.	Oxygen supports combustion.
Attach a bottle of water to the regulator (see Fig. 29-21).	Oxygen forced through a water reservoir is humidified before it is delivered to the patient, preventing dehydration of the mucous membranes.
Attach a nasal catheter, No. 8 to No. 10, Fr., to the connecting tube on the water reservoir.	A small catheter passes through the nose easily and causes minimum discomfort to the patient.
Measure the catheter by holding it in a horizontal line from the tip of the nose to the ear lobe. Mark it with a narrow strip of tape.	The distance from the tip of the nose to the ear lobe usually places the tip of the catheter in the oropharynx when inserted.
Moisten the tip of the catheter with water.	Friction irritates the mucous membrane. Water is absorbed by the tissues and does not act as a foreign body.
Hold the tip of the patient's nose up and insert the tip of the nasal catheter into the nares downward. Move the catheter along the floor of the nose until the marking on the catheter is reached.	Direct connection from the nares to the oropharynx is made most easily by passing the catheter beneath the concha inferior.
Check the position of the tip of the catheter by depressing the tongue carefully with a tongue blade.	If the catheter has been inserted too far, it may stimulate the gag reflex.
Adjust the catheter as necessary so that the tip is visible behind the uvula.	The oxygen stream can be inspired easily at this point.
Adjust the liter flow to the rate specified by the physician, or 6 to 7 liters per minute.	High rates of oxygen flow produce a forceful stream against the mucous membrane which is both irritating and drying.
Secure the catheter with slight upward pull to the side of the patient's face and drape it over his ear.	The weight of the catheter and the moist surface of the mucous membrane will cause the catheter to slip out if not anchored.
Insert a clean catheter in alternate nostrils as often as necessary and at least every 8 hours, to prevent irritation and to keep the nares clean.	Mucous membrane is irritated by continued presence of a foreign object. Prolonged irritation of mucous membrane can cause ulceration.

permits the patient's mouth to be exposed. If it is possible for the patient to use it, this mask is more comfortable and convenient.

When a mask is used to administer oxygen, it must be fitted carefully to the patient's face to avoid leakage. If foam rubber is available it is satisfactory. The mask should be comfortably snug but not tight against the patient's face. Frequent care of the face, including washing and powdering, will help to prevent irritation from the mask. In addition, the mask should be kept clean. Frequent washing helps to reduce the odors absorbed by the rubber. Disposable masks are available and eliminate many of the problems of the rubber ones.

The face mask has a rubber bag suspended from it. Two sponge rubber disks on either side of the mask serve as valves during inspiration and expiration. The bag is distended with oxygen, and during inspiration oxygen is withdrawn from the bag, and air is drawn through the sponge rubber disks, completing the tidal volume.

A therapeutic concentration by this method usually is determined by rhythmical, easy breathing, during which time the bag almost collapses during inspiration. Depending on

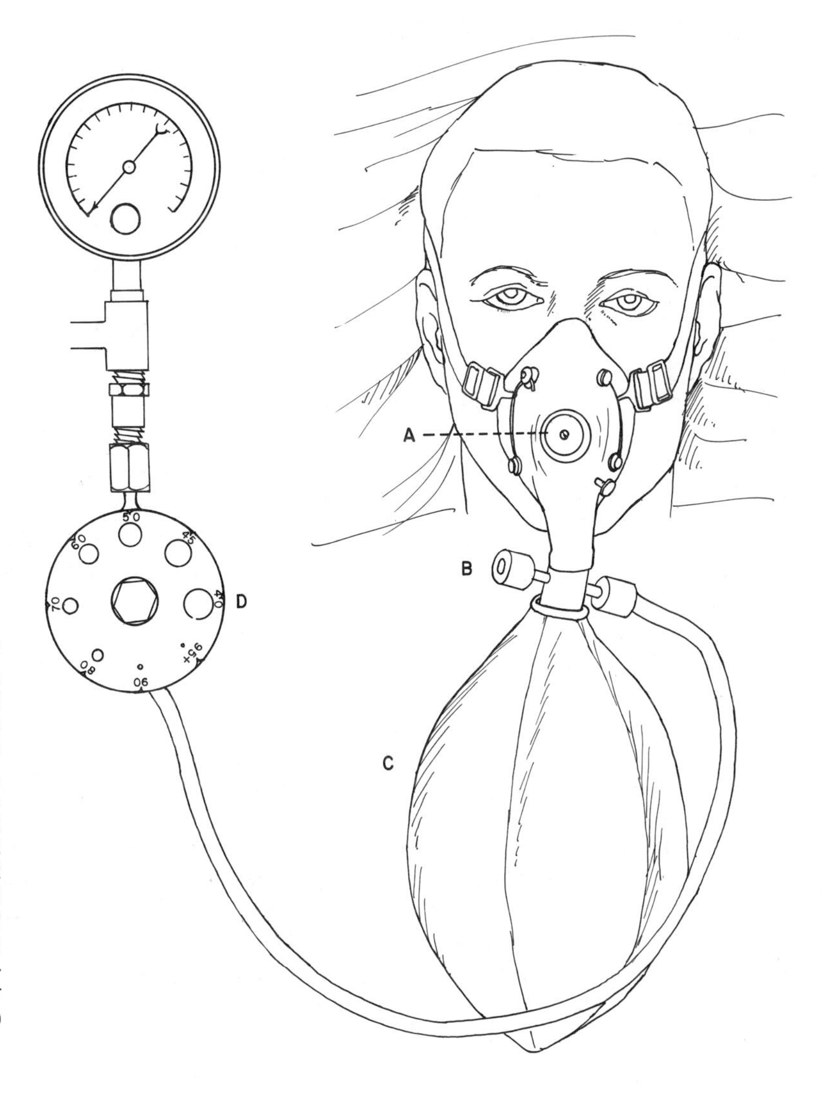

Fig. 29-25. There are many types of face masks, but almost all provide for an oxygen reservoir, a means for the expired carbon dioxide to be removed and a means for mixing air with the oxygen. (A) The flutter valve on the oronasal face mask, which provides an outlet for expired air. Pressure of the expired air forces the soft rubber disk away from the mask. (B) A safety valve that provides for an air inlet in the event of an emergency or increased depth of respirations. (C) The reservoir which contains the air and oxygen mixture inhaled by the patient. (D) The meter calibrated from 40 to 95 plus per cent, for adjusting the concentration of oxygen to be delivered to the bag.

the patient's needs, a range of six to eight liters per minute usually produces a therapeutic concentration. However, if a high concentration of oxygen is indicated, the rate of oxygen flow should be increased so that the bag does not collapse during inspiration.

Humidity with the oxygen is generally recommended. One oxygen supply service recommends injecting some water into the meter (D) in Fig. 29-25.

There are masks now available that are designed to deliver an exact amount of oxygen—e.g., 28 per cent. These masks are used for certain patients, such as those having chronic lung diseases.

ADMINISTRATION OF THERAPEUTIC AGENTS BY DIRECT APPLICATION

Introduction

When a therapeutic agent is applied directly to a body site, it is referred to as a *topical application.*

Topical applications usually are intended for direct action on the particular site. The action is dependent on the type of tissue and the nature of the agent. For example, there are agents for making the skin secrete more or less or for causing vasodilatation or vasoconstriction.

In times past, the skin was rubbed with ointments intended for systemic effect, but this is not a practice now. The only other site that is used currently for obtaining a systemic effect via topical application is the rectum, and this is not often. There are few medications that can be administered via this route, such as aspirin or some tranquilizers.

If the site of application is readily accessible, such as the skin, an agent can be placed on it easily. If it is in the nature of a cavity, such as the nose, or enclosed as the eye is, it is necessary to provide an appropriate method for introducing the agent.

This text considers the cleansing of tissues by means of irrigations as local therapeutic action, since tissues cannot serve their function well if covered with foreign matter. Moreover, the action of an irrigation often is enhanced by using a warm solution, providing still another therapeutic action, vasodilatation, which increases blood supply to the area.

The student should remember that all principles and precautionary measures discussed so far in this text apply equally well to topical applications. There are several additional points that can guide action in relation to the use of therapeutic agents on a specific body site: (1) What is the specific function or functions of the site? (2) What is the tissue structure? (3) What is the physical structure (such as its size and its shape)? (4) What is its status of asepsis?

The Skin

The skin is a mechanical and chemical barrier protecting the underlying tissues. It is a sense organ, having receptors which respond to touch, pain, pressure and temperature. It aids in excretion, regulation of body temperature and the storage of such body essentials as water, salts and glucose.

The skin is composed of two main layers: the epidermis and the derma. The epidermis is composed of stratified squamous keratinizing epithelium. It has no blood vessels; its cells receive their nourishment from tissue fluid from the capillaries in the derma. The epidermis is not equally thick all over the body. It is thickest over the palms of the hands and the soles of the feet. The derma is composed of dense connective tissue. The skin also has three types of glands: sebaceous, sweat and ceruminous. The sebaceous glands are found on the entire surface of the body except the palms and the soles. They are located in the derma, and their ducts open into the necks of hair follicles.

That some absorption into the body can take place via the skin has been proved. However, this is selective; therefore, only a few agents can be absorbed. Examples are lead and aniline dyes, both poisonous (and a hazard in some industries).

Therapeutic Agents Applied to the Skin. When a drug is incorporated in a vehicle, such as powder, oil, lotion, ointment, etc., and rubbed into the skin for absorption, the procedure is referred to as an *inunction.*

On normal skin, drugs are absorbed into the lining of the sebaceous glands. Absorption is hindered because of the protective outer layer of the skin, which makes penetration difficult, and because of the fatty substances that protect the lining of the glands. Absorption can be enhanced by cleansing the skin well with soap or detergent and water prior to administration and then rubbing the medicated preparation into the skin. Absorption also can be improved by using the drug in a vehicle such as an ointment, or a volatile vehicle as used in many of the liniments, that will mix with the fat in the gland lining. The application of local heat also helps absorption by improving blood circulation in the area.

Examples of agents applied to the skin are as follows: oils, ointments and creams to keep it soft; alcohol and other drying agents to reduce excessive secretions; antiperspirants to inhibit perspiration; oil of wintergreen (methylsalicylate) to alleviate the pain of rheumatism.

Oily substances, such as back lotion or oil for dry feet, should not be applied so heavily to the skin that they fail to be absorbed.

The Eye

The receptors for the sense of sight are located in the eye. The outer layer of the eyeball is called the *sclera*. The *cornea* is the transparent part of the sclera in the front of the eyeball. The sclera is fibrous and tough, but the cornea is injured easily by trauma. For this reason, applications to the eye are rarely placed directly onto the eyeball.

The eyelids are two movable structures located in front of the eyeball. They offer protection to the front of the eye and aid in keeping the eye bathed in the secretion of the lacrimal gland. The eyelids meet near the nose at the *inner canthus* and near the temple at the *outer canthus*. The margins of the eyelids are fringed with eyelashes which aid in keeping foreign materials out of the eye.

The eyelids are lined with mucous membrane which form two conjunctival sacs, one under the upper eyelid and the other under the lower eyelid. The conjunctival sac, a potential space, generally is described as being the space between the eyelids and the surface of the eyeball.

The lacrimal glands, which secrete tears, are situated on either side of the nose in the frontal bone. The glands empty into ducts that open in the conjunctival sacs. A lacrimal duct conveys excess fluid into the nose beneath the inferior concha.

Since direct application cannot be made onto the sensitive cornea, applications intended to act upon the eye, or the lids are placed onto, instilled or irrigated onto the lower conjunctival sac.

The eye is a delicate organ, highly susceptible to infection and injury. Although the eye is never free of microorganisms, the secretions of the conjunctiva have a protective action against many pathogens. For maximum safety for the patient, equipment used and solutions and ointments introduced into the conjunctival sac should be sterile. If this is not possible, the most careful measures of medical asepsis should be followed.

Exposing the Lower Conjunctival Sac. Exposing the conjunctival sacs is necessary for removing foreign bodies imbedded on or under the lids, for irrigations, or for the application of therapeutic agents to the eyeball or to the conjunctiva. When either conjunctival sac is exposed, it is important to work carefully and gently to prevent traumatizing the conjunctiva and the eyeball. This is of particular importance when the lids are swollen, inflamed and tender.

To expose the conjunctiva of the lower lid, the patient should look up while the nurse places her thumb near the margin of the lower lid immediately below the eyelashes and exerts pressure downward over the bony prominence of the cheek. As the lower lid is pulled down and away from the eyeball, the conjunctival sac is exposed.

Exposing the Upper Conjunctival Sac. Exposing the upper conjunctival sac requires practice to develop skill. It is referred to as *everting the eyelid*.

The patient is instructed to look down. The nurse grasps the lashes near the center of the upper lid with the thumb and the index finger of one hand and draws the lid downward and away from the eyeball. With the other hand, an applicator is placed horizontally along the upper part of the eyelid; while pressing downward on the applicator, the lid is turned up over the applicator very quickly. The index finger may be substituted for the applicator. Once the lid is everted, it may be held in place by shifting and pressing the thumb of the hand that held the applicator against the margin of the everted lid while the fingers rest on the patient's forehead. The patient continues to look downward during the entire procedure to prevent the lid from returning to its normal position. Eversion of the lid should be done with *gentleness*—never with force—to avoid injury to the eyeball and the conjunctiva.

Conjunctival Irrigation. A conjunctival irrigation, frequently called an eye irrigation, usually is done for cleansing purposes to remove secretions from the conjunctival sacs. Mild antiseptic solutions may be prescribed if an infection is present.

For cleansing purposes, physiologic saline usually is prescribed. The solution is administered at body temperature unless the physician specifies otherwise. The amount of solution will depend on the situation—as little as one ounce or as much as eight or more ounces may be necessary to accomplish the purpose of the irrigation.

Several methods may be used for irrigating the conjunctival sacs. An eye dropper is satisfactory when small amounts of solution are used. For larger amounts, a soft rubber bulb syringe is appropriate. For home use, an eyecup, washed scrupulously after each use, usually is convenient. In an emergency situation, squeezing the solution from

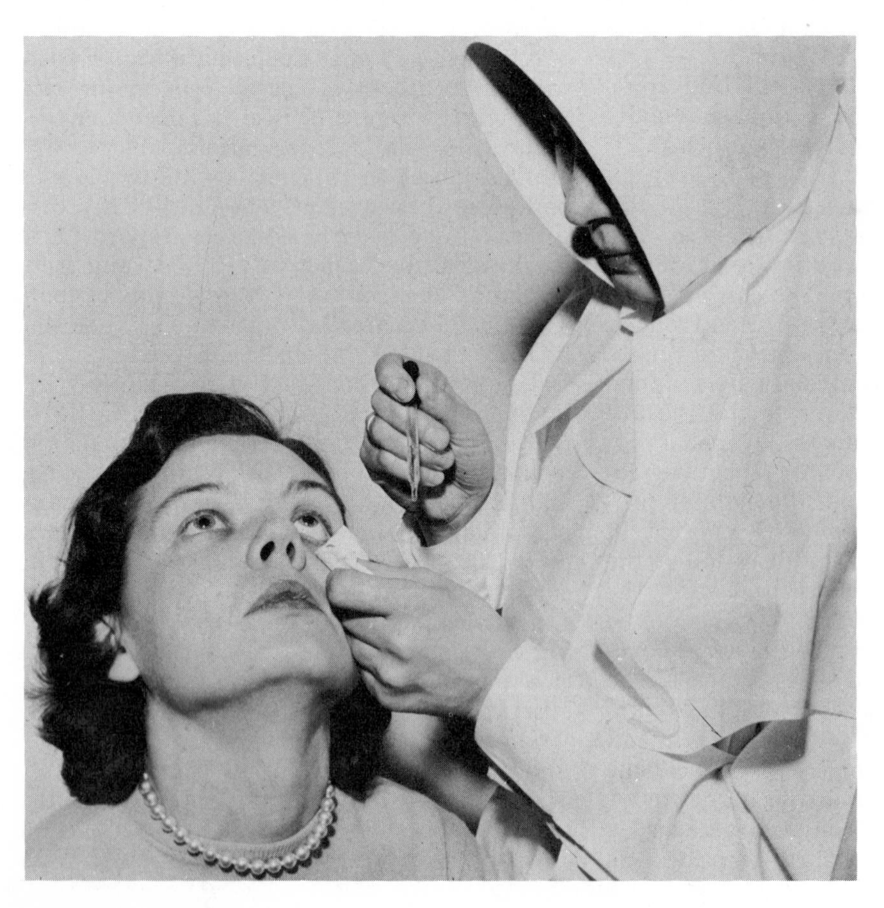

FIG. 29-26. The nurse uses a wipe to protect her finger from slipping while instilling eyedrops.

a soaked cotton ball offers a satisfactory method. The operator's hands should be washed thoroughly first.

Make certain to identify the correct eye. When eye treatments are frequent the abbreviations O.D. for right eye (oculus dexter) and O.L. or O.S. for left eye (oculus laevus—oculus sinister) may be used. It is safer practice to avoid abbreviations.

Following the irrigation, the patient should be asked to close the lids, and the excess fluid is wiped off gently from the inner canthus to the outer canthus. Any additional solution in the area around the eye is also wiped away gently with a cotton ball.

Instillations of Eyedrops. Eyedrops are instilled for local effects, such as for dilatation or contraction of the pupil for examining the eye or treating an infection. The type and the amount of solution are specified in the physician's order and will depend on the purpose of the instillation.

An eye dropper is used to instill drops of solution. No more solution than is needed should be drawn into the eye dropper, because it is unsafe practice to return unused solution to the stock bottle. Once the solution has been drawn into the dropper, the dropper is held with the bulb uppermost. Allowing the solution to enter the rubber bulb by holding the bulb lower than the dropper may result in contaminating the solution with fine particles of rubber.

The patient should be given an absorbent tissue so that he may have it in readiness when drops are instilled. The lids and the lashes are wiped clean prior to the instillation. Hold the dropper close to the eye but

PRINCIPLES GUIDING ACTION WHEN ADMINISTERING AN IRRIGATION OF THE EYE

The purpose is to cleanse the lower conjunctival sac.

SUGGESTED ACTION	PRINCIPLE
Have the patient sit or lie with his head tilted toward the side of the affected eye so that solution will flow from the inner canthus of the affected eye toward the outer canthus.	Gravity will aid the flow of solution away from the unaffected eye.
Cleanse the lids and the lashes with normal saline or the solution ordered for the irrigation.	Materials lodged on the lids or in the lashes may be washed into the eye.
Place a curved basin at the cheek on the side of the affected eye to receive the irrigating solution.	Gravity will aid the flow of solution.
Expose the lower conjunctival sac.	The conjunctival sac is less sensitive than the cornea.
Direct the flow of the irrigating solution from the inner canthus to the outer canthus along the conjunctival sac.	Solution directed toward the outer canthus aids in preventing the spread of contamination from the eye to the lacrimal sac, the lacrimal duct and the nose.
Irrigate. Use only sufficient force to remove secretions from the conjunctiva gently.	Directing solutions with force may cause injury to the tissues of the eye, as well as the conjunctiva.
Avoid touching any part of the eye with the irrigating tip.	The eye is injured easily. Touching the eye is uncomfortable for the patient.
Have the patient close his eye periodically during the procedure.	Movement of the eye when the lids are closed helps to move secretions from the upper conjunctival sac to the lower.
Continue irrigating the lower conjunctival sac.	Irrigation of the lower conjunctival sac is more comfortable for the patient.

avoid touching the eyelids or the eyelashes. This prevents injury should the patient become startled by the sensation of the dropper touching him. The lower conjunctival sac is exposed, and the prescribed number of drops of solution are allowed to fall into the center of the exposed sac. Drops should not be allowed to fall directly onto the cornea because of the danger of injuring it and because of the unpleasant sensation it creates for the patient. The patient should be asked to close his eyelids and move the eye. This helps to distribute the solution over the conjunctival surfaces and the anterior eyeball.

Application of Ointment to the Eye. Various types of drugs in an ointment base may be prescribed for the eyelids or the conjunctiva.

The eyelids and the eyelashes should be cleansed of secretions and crusts before applying the ointment. Eye ointments usually are dispensed in a tube. A small amount of the ointment is distributed along the conjunctival sac after everting the lower lid. The ointment is squeezed from the tube, but care should be taken to avoid touching the eye or the conjunctiva. Following the application, the eyelids should be closed. The warmth will help to liquefy the ointment. The patient should also be instructed to move his eye. This will aid in spreading the ointment under the lids and over the surface of the eyeball.

The Ear

The ear contains the receptors for hearing and for equilibrium. It consists of the external ear, the middle ear and the inner ear.

The external ear consists of the *auricle* or *pinna* and the *exterior auditory canal.* The auricle has very little function in man. The auditory canal serves as a passageway for sound waves. Therapeutic agents or irrigations are instilled into the auditory canal.

In adults, the auditory canal is directed inward, forward and downward. The outer portion is cartilaginous, and the inner portion consists of osseous tissue. In an infant, the canal is chiefly cartilaginous and is almost straight, but the floor of the auditory canal rests on the tympanic membrane. The direction of the canal is important to consider when administering treatments to the ear. In order for solution to reach all parts of the canal, the pinna should be pulled downward and backward for infants; for adults, upward and backward. The ear is grasped on the cartilaginous portion of the pinna when straightening the canal.

The lining of the auditory canal consists of modified epithelium. It contains ceruminous glands, which secrete the wax found in the ear, and the hair follicles.

The tympanic membrane separates the external ear from the middle ear. Normally, it is intact and closes the entrance to the middle ear completely. If it is ruptured or has been opened by surgical intervention, the middle ear and the inner ear have a direct passage to the external ear. When this occurs, instillations and irrigations should be done with great care to prevent forcing materials from the outer ear into the middle ear and the inner ear, which may result in serious infection.

Normally, the ear is not a sterile cavity. However, if the tympanic membrane is not intact, surgical asepsis should be observed.

Irrigation of the External Auditory Canal. Irrigation of the auditory canal generally is done for cleansing purposes. Antiseptic solutions sometimes are used for their local action. Irrigations may be used also for applying heat to the ear. Applying cold to the ear by irrigation is uncommon except for the Caloric ear function test.

Normal saline usually is prescribed for cleansing. However, any number of antiseptic solutions may be used. The amount of solution needed depends on the purpose of the irrigation, but approximately 500 cc. usually is adequate. The solution is prepared so that it is approximately body temperature when it enters the ear. Colder or hotter solutions are uncomfortable for the patient, since the endolymph is set in motion, and dizziness and nausea may result.

An irrigating can with tubing and an ear tip generally is used. The height of the can should be just enough to have the solution flow gently. The glass ear tip fits easily into the external canal and has two extensions projecting from it: one for the solution to enter the canal and the other for it to leave the canal and drain into a receiving basin. A soft rubber bulb syringe may be used, but it is not as comfortable for the patient, since the flow of solution must be interrupted during the irrigation while the syringe is refilled.

Instillations of Eardrops. Drugs in solution are placed in the auditory canal for their local effect. They are used to soften wax, relieve pain, apply local anesthesia, destroy organisms or destroy an insect lodged in the canal which can cause almost intolerable discomfort.

It is more comfortable for the patient if the solution is warmed to approximately body temperature. A dropper is used to instill the solution. The ear canal is straightened, and the drops are allowed to fall on the side of the canal. The patient lies on his side with the ear to be treated uppermost and remains in this position following instillation to prevent the drops from escaping from the canal. Occasionally, a loose cotton wick is inserted into the canal in order to maintain a continuous application of the solution instilled. A wick is never packed into the ear because it interferes with outward movement of normal secretions and could create pressure.

The Nose

Besides serving as the olfactory organ, the nose also functions as an airway to the lower respiratory tract and protects the tract by cleansing and warming the air that is taken in by inspiration. Small hairs, called *cilia*, project on most of the surface of the nasal mucous membrane and are important to aid in removing particles of dirt and dust from the inspired air. The nose also serves as a resonator when speaking and singing.

The nose is divided into the right and the left chambers by the nasal septum. There are four pairs of nasal sinuses that communicate with the nasal fossa: the frontal, the

PRINCIPLES GUIDING ACTION WHEN ADMINISTERING AN IRRIGATION OF THE EXTERNAL AUDITORY CANAL

The purpose is to cleanse the external auditory canal.

SUGGESTED ACTION	PRINCIPLE
Have patient sit up or lie with his head tilted toward the side of the affected ear. Have patient support a basin under his ear to receive the irrigating solution.	Gravity causes irrigating solution to flow from the ear to the basin.
Cleanse the pinna and the meatus at the auditory canal as necessary with normal saline or the irrigating solution.	Materials lodged on the pinna and at the meatus may be washed into the ear.
Fill the bulb syringe with solution. If an irrigating can is used, allow air to escape from the tubing.	Air forced into the ear canal is noisy, therefore unpleasant.
Straighten the auditory canal by pulling the pinna downward and backward for an infant and upward and backward for an adult.	Straightening the ear canal aids in allowing solution to reach all areas of the canal easily.
Direct a steady slow stream of solution against the roof of the auditory canal, using only sufficient force to remove secretions.	Solution directed at the roof of the canal aids in preventing injury to the tympanic membrane.
Do not occlude the auditory canal with the irrigating nozzle.	Continuous in-and-out flow of the irrigating solution aids in preventing pressure in the canal.
At completion of treatment have patient lie on the side of the affected ear.	Gravity allows the remaining solution in the canal to escape from the ear.

ethmoid, the maxillary and the sphenoid sinuses. Normally, these are filled with air and lined with mucous membrane similar to that which lines the nose.

Because of the position of the nose, secretions from it drain out easily when the person is in the upright position. Because of its connection with the upper respiratory tract and the mouth, secretions drain back into that area when the person is reclining.

Normally, the nose is not a sterile cavity. However, because of its connection with the sinuses, utmost caution should be taken when introducing anything into it.

Instillations of Nosedrops. Medications instilled into the nares are used primarily for the relief of nasal congestion. Most physicians prefer using a drug in normal saline solution, since oily solutions tend to interfere with the normal ciliary action in the nose and, if aspirated, may result in a pneumonitis. Anesthetics and antiseptics also may be instilled into the nose for their local effects.

Paper wipes should be provided for the patient. The patient is assisted to a sitting position with his head tilted back, or he lies in bed with his head tilted back. This position allows the solution to flow back into the nares. Sufficient solution for both nares is drawn into a dropper. The dropper is placed just inside the nares, approximately one-third inch, and the number of drops prescribed is instilled. Touching the dropper to the nares may create a desire to sneeze. The patient should be instructed to keep his head tilted back for several minutes to prevent the escape of solution from the anterior nares. The patient usually will wish to expectorate solution that runs down into the oropharynx and the mouth.

When instilling drops into the nares of an infant or an irrational patient, the tip of the dropper should be protected with a piece of soft rubber tubing to minimize the danger of injuring the nasal mucous membrane.

Nasal Spray. Solutions that are instilled by drops also may be applied to the nasal mucous membrane by using a spray. A small atomizer generally is used.

The end of the nose is held up, and the tip of the nozzle is placed just inside the nares and directed backward. Only sufficient force is used to bring the spray into contact with the membrane. Too much force may drive the solution and the contamination into the sinuses and the eustachian tubes.

The Throat

The throat, more properly called the *pharynx,* is divided into three portions: nasal, oral and laryngeal. The pharynx communicates with the nasal cavity anteriorly, with the oral cavity below this, and with the laryngeal cavity below the oral phraynx. The eustachian tubes open into the nasopharynx. The pharynx is a muscular passageway and is lined with modified epithelium.

The pharynx is a passageway for air. The oral and the laryngeal portions also serve as a passageway for food.

The adenoids or *pharyngeal tonsils* are located in the nasopharynx. The *palatine tonsils* are in the oral pharynx. The tonsils and the adenoids are composed of lymphoid tissue and often become the seat of infections.

The throat obviously is not a sterile area. However, practices of medical asepsis are observed, especially in caring for the equipment after use. The mouth harbors micro-organisms that could be harmful to others.

Throat Irrigations. Throat irrigations are used primarily for loosening and removing secretions in the throat and for applying heat to the area. Mild antiseptics and normal saline are used most frequently. Sodium bicarbonate solution also is effective, especially when the secretions are tenacious.

Usually, the solution is used as hot as the patient can tolerate it, but a temperature above approximately 120° F. is likely to cause tissue damage. If the irrigation is done primarily for applying heat, it is necessary to prepare sufficient solution so that the irrigation will continue over a period of time. Approximately 1,500 to 2,000 cc. given slowly generally is sufficient. The total amount should not be used if the patient becomes fatigued during the procedure. An irrigating can with a clamp on the tubing and an irrigating nozzle are used. It is convenient to use a pole on which to hang the irrigating can.

It is best if the patient assists during a throat irrigation by handling the nozzle himself and directing the flow of solution to various areas of the throat. The nurse should make certain that all areas in the throat are being irrigated. She shows the patient how to discontinue the flow of solution.

Throat Gargles. Gargles sometimes are used for the same purposes as throat irrigations. However, a gargle may be more uncomfortable, since gargling places strain and tension on an area that usually is already swollen, irritated and painful. Also, a gargle generally is unsatisfactory for reaching all parts of the throat tissues; therefore, an irrigation is preferred by many physicians. A gargle generally is satisfactory for cleansing the mouth and the oral pharynx.

Many persons believe that gargling with a strong antiseptic is an almost sure way of preventing sore throats and upper respiratory infections. If done often enough and with full-strength antiseptic solutions, the normal defenses in the mouth and the oropharynx may be destroyed, and more harm than good is done.

Throat Sprays and Paints. Antiseptics and anesthetics may be applied to the throat by spraying and by painting the area. The patient's head is tilted back, and his tongue is held down with a tongue depressor. The solution either is sprayed or painted onto the tissues. A cotton applicator is effective for painting. When a spray is used, more force is necessary to reach tissues in the throat than is necessary when using a nasal spray.

Lozenges may contain drugs that are used for the local treatment of the mouth and the throat. Cough drops are an example. When sucked, the lozenge liberates the active ingredient, and, when the solution is swallowed, the mouth and the throat are bathed in it. The use of lozenges is unsatisfactory for reaching all parts of the throat. The patient should be instructed to suck the lozenge since chewing or swallowing it shortens the period of contact with the tissues and decreases its effectiveness.

The Vagina

The vagina is a musculomembranous canal extending from the outside of the body at the vulva to the cervix uteri. It lies between the bladder and the rectum. The size and the shape vary, but it is capable of distending greatly as during childbirth. The anterior

PRINCIPLES GUIDING ACTION WHEN ADMINISTERING A THROAT IRRIGATION

The purpose is to cleanse the throat and/or to apply heat.

SUGGESTED ACTION	PRINCIPLE
Arrange the irrigating can containing the solution on a pole at the bedside so that the base is only slightly above the level of the patient's mouth.	The gag reflex can be stimulated by a forceful stream of water into the throat. Keeping the "head" of the solution low minimizes pressure. Gravity will cause the solution to flow as long as the irrigating tip is below the base of the fluid.
Place the patient in a sitting position with his head tilted directly over a basin placed in front of him.	Gravity causes the solution to flow back out into the basin.
Instruct the patient to hold his breath while the solution is flowing.	Breathing while the solution is flowing into and out of the mouth may result in aspirating some of the solution.
Insert the nozzle into the mouth, being careful not to touch the base of the tongue or the uvula. Direct the flow so that all parts of the throat are irrigated.	Gag reflex can be stimulated by touching the uvula or the tongue.
Clamp the tubing to interrupt the irrigation at regular intervals to permit patient to breathe and rest.	Holding the breath interrupts normal physiologic functions of respiration.

wall usually is about three to six inches long, while the posterior wall is five to seven inches long. Normally, the walls of the vagina are in contact with each other.

Normally, the vagina contains few pathogens but many nonpathogenic organisms. The nonpathogens are important, since they protect the vagina from the invasion of pathogens. The normal secretions in the vagina are acid in reaction and further serve to protect the vagina from microbial invasion. Therefore, the normal mucous membrane is its own best protection.

Vaginal irrigations should be used only under a physician's directions. Irrigations may wash out nonpathogenic organisms and normal secretions that protect the vagina and thereby invite infection. Many practicing gynecologists have recognized that frequent irrigation of the vagina as a part of hygienic care has resulted in minor or secondary infections.

Vaginal Irrigation (Douche). A vaginal irrigation often is referred to as a *douche*. The irrigation usually is done for cleansing purposes and for applying heat or an antiseptic to the area. The solution of choice is normal saline or tap water when the purpose of the irrigation is for cleansing or for applying heat. Any number of antiseptic solutions may be used, but for cleansing purposes they are actually not necessary.

Usually, a quantity of about 1,500 cc. of solution is prepared, but smaller or larger amounts may be indicated, depending on the purposes of the irrigation. The vagina tolerates relatively high temperature, but the membranes and the skin around the meatus do not. Therefore, solutions are prepared so that they are introduced at approximately 100° F., or approximately 110° F. if the effect of heat is desired.

An irrigating can or bag connected with tubing to an irrigating nozzle is used. Irri-

PRINCIPLES GUIDING ACTION WHEN ADMINISTERING A VAGINAL IRRIGATION

The purpose is to cleanse the vagina.

SUGGESTED ACTION	PRINCIPLE
Have the patient void before beginning the treatment.	A full bladder interferes with distention of the vagina by the nozzle and the solution.
Have the patient in the dorsal recumbent position. Remove all but one pillow from under the patient's head and place her on a bedpan.	Gravity will cause the solution to flow into the distal portion of the vagina.
Arrange the irrigating can or bag at a level just above the patient's hips so that the solution flows easily yet gently.	The greater the distance between the head of the fluid and the outlet in the tubing, the greater will be the force of the solution as it leaves. Undue force could drive solution and contamination into the cervical os.
Cleanse the vulva by separating the labia and allowing the solution to flow over the area. If this does not seem to be sufficient, wash it with a soap or detergent solution.	Materials lodged around the vaginal meatus can be introduced into the vagina.
Permit some solution to run through the tubing and out over the end of the nozzle to lubricate it.	Moist surfaces have less friction when moved against each other.
Insert the nozzle gently into the vagina while directing it downward and backward.	In the dorsal recumbent position, normally the vagina is directed downward and backward.
Gently rotate the nozzle in the vagina during the treatment.	Movement of the nozzle aids in directing the solution against all surfaces of the vagina.

gating nozzles are curved to fit the normal contour of the vagina and may be made of glass or plastic. The nozzle should be handled carefully and examined before use to prevent injury should the nozzle be cracked or chipped.

At home a vaginal irrigation may be done by lying in a bathtub; have the irrigating can suspended at the proper height on a towel rack or on a chair at the side of the tub. Some patients may prefer using a douche pan or a bedpan when carrying out this procedure in the tub at home.

Study Situations

1. Increase your awareness of how much self-medication advertising is done by looking for advertisements concerning the following items: eye drops to relieve eye fatigue or to beautify the eyes, nose drops to stop hay fever or to relieve colds, antiseptics for feminine hygiene and throat gargles to avoid colds. Look carefully at the wording of these advertisements. Examine the labels and determine if it is possible for the products to produce the results they claim.

2. For an account of one nurse's experience in teaching a 15-year-old girl to give herself insulin read the following article. Identify the *problem*, the nurse's approach to solving it, and the principles of teaching used:

- Zitnik, R.: First, you take a grapefruit. AMER. J. NURS., *68*:1285-1286, June, 1968.

3. For appreciation of how even one science course in the curriculum—i.e., microbiology—can improve nursing practice, see:

- Student Page: Questioning a procedure. AMER. J. NURS., *63*:126, October, 1963.

References

1. Baer, M. H., *et al*: Are organisms introduced into vials containing medication when air is injected? NURS. RES., *2*:23, June, 1953.
2. Barker, K. N., and McConnell, W. E.: How to detect medication errors. MOD. HOSP., *99*:95 passim, July, 1962.
3. Burgess, A. M.: A comparison of common methods of oxygen therapy for bed patients. AMER. J. NURS., *65*:96-99, December, 1965.
4. Dineen, P.: The exchange of skin bacteria between patients and hospital personnel. SURG. GYNEC. OBS., *125*:979-982, November, 1967.
5. Flatter, P. A.: Hazards of oxygen therapy. AMER. J. NURS., *68*:80-84, January, 1968.
6. Gilles, F. H., and French, J. H.: Postinjection sciatic nerve palsies in infants and children. J. PEDIAT., *58*:195, February, 1961.
7. Hershey, N.: The apparently erroneous order. AMER. J. NURS., *64*:111-112, January, 1964.
8. Kohan, S., Carlin, H., and Whitehead, R.: A study of contamination of multiple-dose medication vials. HOSPITALS, *36*:78 passim, July 16, 1962.
9. Kutscher, A. H. *et al*: A comparative evaluation of the jet injection technique (Hypospray) and the hypodermic needle for the parenteral administration of drugs. AM. J. MED. SCI., *244*:418, October, 1962.
10. Nordmark, M. T., and Rohweder, A. W.: Scientific Foundations of Nursing, ed. 2, Chapter 2, "Adequate Supply of Oxygen." Philadelphia, Lippincott, 1967.
11. Pitel, M., and Wemett, M.: The intramuscular injection. AMER. J. NURS., *64*:104-109, April, 1964.
12. Segal, M. S.: The use of therapeutic aerosols. G.P., *26*:108, September, 1962.
13. Travell, J.: Factors affecting pain of injection. J.A.M.A., *158*:368-371, June 4, 1955.

CHAPTER 30

Caring for Wounds and the Use of Dressings and Bandages

Introduction

There is a wide variety of commercially prepared materials which aid the professional person as well as the layman to dress wounds with ease and efficiency. Some health agencies stock many of these materials, while others may use fewer types but adapt them for many uses. In either case, basic principles guide one's action when caring for wounds.

The physician specifies the type of wound care that is to be given and whether dressings are to be applied. In some instances, the nurse acts as an assistant to the physician and applies a dressing. In other situations, the nurse is responsible for the prescribed care of the wound and for the application of a dressing. The physician may leave an order concerning the care of the wound, while, in certain other situations, he may allow the nurse considerable latitude in making judgments in its care. The nature of the nurse's responsibilities will depend on the physician's preferences, the condition of the patient, the nature of the wound and the policies of the health agency.

Before caring for wounds, the nurse washes her hands thoroughly. All the sterile dressings and instruments the agency may own may be worthless if the practitioners are not careful to wash their hands thoroughly before and after dressing wounds.

General Principles of Care for Wounds

Practices concerned with the care of wounds are guided by a basic principle that has been mentioned before: *Unbroken and healthy skin and mucous membrane serve as first lines of defense against harmful agents.* When the skin or the mucous membrane are not intact, the body is vulnerable to invasion by harmful agents, primarily pathogens. Therefore, keeping the wound as clean as possible is essential. The ultimate in safety is strict medical asepsis if the wound is sealed, and surgical asepsis if the wound is open.

If in addition to having a break in the skin or the mucous membrane, the person is in poor nutritional state, there is need for additional concern stemming from another basic principle: *The body is able to produce cellular elements and specific chemical substances which serve to protect it against harmful agents.* The nurse recognizes this when she observes the formation of a scab (eschar) on a wound, a pink appearance around the edge of the wound which is additional blood supply and, depending on the extent of the wound, a slight elevation in body temperature. When a person is in poor nutritional state, physical defenses are unable to perform to their optimum potential. He needs care of the broken skin or the mucous membrane and strengthening of the body's defenses.

Wounds and How They Heal

Types of Wounds. A wound may be *open* or *closed.* An open wound is characterized by a break in the continuity of the skin. When there is no break in the skin the wound is said to be closed. A contusion is an example of the latter type.

Wounds may be classified as either *accidental* or *intentional.* Accidental wounds are injuries due to mishaps, while intentional wounds are those purposely created by the surgeon for therapeutic purposes.

Wounds may be classified also according to the nature of the break in the continuity of normal tissue. An *incision* is a wound made with a sharp cutting instrument. It is the kind of wound that is made by the surgeon when he cuts tissue to enter the field of operation. Incised wounds also may occur by accident, as when one is cut with a knife, a sharp piece of glass or a razor.

An *abrasion* is a wound that results from scraping or rubbing off skin or mucous membrane. A "floor burn" is a typical abrasive wound.

A *puncture* or *stab* wound is caused by an object that penetrates into tissue. Injuries from nails and bullets result in puncture wounds. A surgeon may make a puncture wound to promote drainage.

A *laceration* is a wound caused by a blunt instrument or object that tears tissue. Falls against angular surfaces or cuts with irregular edges of broken glass frequently result in lacerated wounds.

Any combination of these last four types of wounds may also occur. For example, falling on broken glass may result in a wound that has lacerations as well as punctures.

The Process of Wound Healing. Wound healing is described usually in three phases. The *lag phase* occurs first, when blood and serum and red blood cells form a fibrin network in the wound. The edges of the wound are glued together by this network, or scab, as it usually is called.

The *fibroplasia phase* is characterized by the growth of fibroblasts along and in the fibrin network. As this occurs, the fibrin network is gradually absorbed. These fibroblasts and accompanying small blood vessels are called *granulation tissue,* which grows to restore the continuity of the injured tissue. It is very friable, soft and pinkish red in color. Epithelial cells then commence to grow from the edges to cover the wound. This becomes the *scar* and is considerably stronger than the granulation tissue.

The *phase of contraction* is characterized by the disappearance of the small blood vessels in the new tissue and by a shrinkage of the scar. This phase may last indefinitely.

The strength of the wound is slight until it has progressed well into the fibroplasia phase. Scar tissue is strong but not so capable of withstanding tension as normal tissue. Therefore, it is desirable that healing occur with a minimum of scar formation, especially in an area where tension and pressure normally are present.

If a large area has been denuded (i.e., when a large area of skin has been removed) as a result of either an accident or surgery, it may be difficult or even impossible to approximate the edges of a wound. It has been observed that epithelium from the periphery of a wound continues to grow for only a certain distance and then stops. When the process of repairing a wound halts, a chronic ulcer or unhealed area develops on the denuded surface. This often becomes the site of infection, and tissue debris accumulates. Cleaning an area of this sort is called *débridement*. It is done primarily to remove necrotic tissue and foreign material and to improve drainage from the wound in order to promote further wound healing. If healing still does not occur following débridement, it may be necessary to close the wound by using skin grafts.

Healing by First Intention. This process occurs when no infection is present and when the edges of the wound are well approximated. Sutures keep the edges of the wound together. Pressure may be used also by the proper application of materials that will secure the dressings in place, to aid approximation of the wound edges. Another way to maintain alignment of wound edges is to use *butterflies*. These are strips of adhesive cut so that the part of the strip that will cross the wound is folded upon itself in order to prevent applying adhesive directly on the wound. As a further caution, the area of folded adhesive that crosses the wound usually is passed through an open flame several times in an attempt to assure thorough cleanliness. One end of the butterfly is applied to the skin on one side of the wound, and the edges of the wound are approximated and held together tightly while the other end of the butterfly is applied to the opposite side of the wound.

Few accidental wounds heal by first intention. Surgeons strive for and usually attain healing of an incision by first intention.

Healing by Second Intention. The process of healing is the same as for first intention, but healing is prolonged. There is usually greater injury to tissue present, and approximation of the edges of the wound is difficult or even impossible. Sutures, pressure and butterflies may be used to aid in approximating wound edges. Infection usually is present when healing occurs by second intention. Pus, consisting of organisms, tissue debris, cell exudate and leukocytes, usually is formed.

Factors Influencing Wound Healing. The ultimate purpose of wound care is to promote healing. It is agreed generally that there is no stimulant for wound healing outside the human body, although some agents applied to a wound or to the skin prior to surgery are credited with assisting in wound healing. Healing is promoted best by good physiologic functioning of the body. Wounds will heal most readily when the patient enjoys fluid and electrolyte balance, good nourishment and adequate rest.

Factors at the site of the wound also influence healing. Examples of such that retard the process of healing include inadequate drainage of purulent materials, foreign bodies, continued trauma, poor circulation at the site of the wound and infection.

The Undressed Wound

Many physicians subscribe to the practice of leaving a wound undressed if it has sealed itself and can be protected from trauma and irritation. This is true even of wounds that have been surgically induced and sutured. Or, there may be occasions when a wound may be undressed for most of the day and then covered at bedtime. Many small cuts and abrasions are healed more quickly if left undressed.

There are several reasons for leaving some wounds undressed, all based on the principles mentioned earlier, namely: the body has resources for healing itself; friction and irritation destroy epithelial cells; and dark, warm, moist areas are suitable for the growth of microorganisms. Therefore, a dressing applied to skin in such a fashion that it produces friction can break the scab which has formed. In addition, the normal flora on the skin can be rubbed into the wound, and if the area is moist and dark, bacterial growth can take place.

A reason some physicians have offered for leaving an incision undressed after surgery is that the skin in the area has already been traumatized by the preoperative shave. Often, the skin is nicked, even though it is barely visible, and infection is already present. This then is a threat to the surgical wound.

The woman who has just delivered a baby almost always has some areas of broken mucous membrane, and her care includes prevention of contamination of the area and fortifying her own normal defenses. This is another example of an undressed wound.

The Dressed Wound

Dressings serve several purposes. If used properly, dressings and the materials used for securing them aid in preventing infection from entering the wound, absorb secretions, protect the area from trauma and restrict motion that tends to disrupt the approximation of the wounded edges. They also may be applied with pressure to promote hemostasis and to aid in approximating wound edges. For esthetic reasons, a dressing serves to cover an area of disfigurement.

Preparation of the Patient. From their own past experiences, patients usually understand the nature and the purposes of wound care. However, the nurse assumes responsibility for preparing the patient by explaining and teaching as the situation indicates.

Many health agencies use treatment rooms for applying dressings and giving wound care. If the patient is unable to be taken to a treatment room, or if the wound can be cared for conveniently with the patient in bed, a working unit is set up at the patient's bedside. Most agencies have a dressing cart on which the basic equipment for wound care can be transported easily to the patient's room. Or a tray may be used to carry the necessary equipment to the bedside, and a working unit is arranged on the overbed table.

While the care of wounds can become a rather commonplace event for nursing and medical personnel, this may not be true for the patient. Consideration should be given to providing privacy for the patient and to the probability that he may be very disturbed by the sight of the wound. In some instances, patients do not wish to look at their wounds, and they should not be encouraged to do so nor chided about it. This is particularly true of patients whose wounds involve change in their bodily functions or appearance, such as the removal of a breast, the amputation of a foot or a leg or the placement of a tube in the abdominal wall.

The patient should be helped to assume a comfortable position that affords working convenience for the physician or the nurse. If the procedure is likely to produce considerable discomfort, the physician may order a medication given before beginning the procedure.

Necessary Equipment. When preparing to change a dressing, it is necessary to have a means for removing the old dressing without contaminating the wound or the fingers of the person removing it and also equipment for cleansing the wound, dressing it adequately and securing it.

Sterile instruments are used to remove the dressings adhering to a wound and for treating it. In some instances where there is need to hold the area near the wound, as with an amputation, sterile gloves can be worn. When the instruments are removed after use, they should be handled so that they do not contaminate otherwise clean objects or surfaces, such as overbed tables, utility room counters and carts.

A safe method should be used for disposing of the old dressing and the gauze or the cotton used to clean the wound. The best practice is to discard them in a waterproof bag which can be closed and discarded for burning.

The antiseptic to clean the wound is a matter of agency policy or the physician's preference. If the wound is to be irrigated, the prescribed solution, a sterile irrigating syringe and a basin to collect returns will also be needed.

Dressing materials usually are made of gauze folded into various sizes and shapes. Some gauze sponges are filled with absorbent cotton. The size, the number and the types of dressings used depend on the nature of the wound. Cotton balls are useful for cleansing purposes, but generally they are not used as a dressing on a wound, for the cotton tends to stick to the wound and becomes difficult to remove.

Individual instrument and dressing packs afford the ultimate in safety for the patient. Surgical dressings and instruments kept in common containers cannot be counted on to be sterile after the container is opened.

Items for securing the dressings in place also are needed.

Care of Draining Wounds

If a drain is in a wound, care must be exercised so that it is not dislodged while dressings are changed. The physician may order the drain to be shortened each day. This can be done by grasping the end of the drain with sterile forceps, pulling it out a short distance while using a twisting motion and cutting off the end of the drain with sterile scissors. If the drain is in the abdominal cavity, a large sterile safety pin often is placed at the end of the drain so that it cannot slip down out of sight.

The skin around a draining wound quickly becomes irritated and excoriated unless precautions are taken. Keeping the skin clean is of prime importance. This requires that dressings be changed often enough so that drainage-soaked dressings are not left on the skin for long periods of time. The skin surrounding the wound is washed, preferably with a warm soap or detergent solution, and rinsed thoroughly with water or normal saline. A thorough cleansing is accomplished by the emulsifying and mechanical actions involved in this method. An antiseptic solution may be used on the skin after foreign materials have been washed off thoroughly and the skin dried properly. Some antiseptics are not effective if used on moist skin surfaces. Even if antiseptics are not used, the skin should be dry.

In order to prevent skin irritation and excoriation, a protective ointment or paste may be applied so that drainage cannot contact the skin. In some institutions a physician's order is necessary before a protective preparation may be applied. In other situations the nurse may use one without a physician's order if it seems to be necessary for the patient's welfare.

When a protective ointment or paste has been used on the skin, it is important to remove it at regular intervals (at least daily) and cleanse the skin under it. Ointments prepared in a water-soluble base may be removed with a soap-and-water or detergent solution. Care must be exercised when ointments and pastes are removed so that the friction created by rubbing is kept at a minimum. Friction may destroy epithelial cells, causing skin irritation.

Principles Basic to Applying Dressings to Draining Wounds

Principles Basic to Applying Dressings to Draining Wounds. A dressing placed on a draining wound is more effective and comfortable when several basic principles are observed.

The property of surface tension exhibited by liquids and the forces of cohesion and adhesion cause a column of liquid to rise in a fine tube or on a hair. This is called capillary action or capillarity. For example, absorbent cotton allows for greater capillarity than untreated cotton; therefore, sponges lined with the former material soak up more liquid. Loosely packed gauze, the threads of which act as numerous wicks, enhances capillarity and will allow for drainage to be directed upward and away from its source. Fluffed and loosely packed dressings, then, are more absorbent than flatly packed dressings and will carry drainage up and away from the wound.

Evaporation occurs more readily when there is circulation of air. Prolonged heat and moisture on the skin deteriorate epithelial cells. These principles are utilized when the nurse applies dressings and secures them so that circulation of air is possible. Loosely packed dressings secured with materials that allow for air circulation promote evaporation of moisture and dissipation of heat to the environment, both of which help to protect the skin. To protect the patient's clothing and the bed linen, waterproof material, such as a plastic, can be used over dressings on a wound that is draining profusely. This practice should be used judiciously; it cannot replace the need for frequent dressing changes. Plastic reduces the circulation of air through the dressings, and the skin and the wound may be injured due to an accumulation of heat and moisture.

Gravity causes liquids to flow from a high to a low level. Dressings on a draining wound should be arranged according to the patient's position and the expected direction of flow. For example, when a patient with a draining abdominal wound is ambulatory, a heavy application of dressings should be placed at the base of the wound and secured so that the drainage does not escape under the dressings and onto the patient.

When objects in contact move in opposition to each other, friction is produced. Friction will destroy epithelial cells. These principles are in effect when dressings are secured in a manner which causes friction on the skin and the wound, which may result in injury to tissue. A device used to prevent dressings from touching an area of the wound will also decrease friction on the wound. One such device is called a *doughnut.* It is made of gauze, wound in the shape of a doughnut and fitted to the size and the shape of the wound. This is placed so that it surrounds the wound; then dressings are placed on top of it, thereby preventing the dressing from touching the wound. The doughnut also acts to absorb drainage from the wound.

Securing the Dressing. This responsibility often demands considerable ingenuity and resourcefulness on the part of the nurse. It requires consideration of such factors as the size of the wound, its location, whether drainage is present, the nature of the drainage, the frequency with which the dressing needs changing and the activities of the patient.

For securing a very small dressing on a wound with little or no drainage, liquid adhesive or collodion may be used effectively. The edges of the outer piece of gauze that is cut to fit over the dressing are painted with the liquid adhesive or collodion and then glued to the skin.

Strips of adhesive probably are used most frequently for securing dressings. Adhesive is dispensed in various widths, and the length is determined according to the need. Elasticized adhesive allows for more movement of a body part without pull on adjacent tissues. Because adhesive often causes skin irritation, especially when dressings must be changed frequently, it is good practice to apply a protective coating to the skin before applying adhesive. A preparation most frequently used is compound benzoin tincture, which is painted onto the skin immediately before the adhesive is applied.

Some patients are allergic to adhesive mixtures; therefore, the nurse should investigate any complaint of discomfort associated with adhesive tape. Patients who have endured the discomforts of the adhesive for a period of days have been known to need treatment for months following its removal.

When dressings must be changed frequently, it is advisable to consider the use of straps for securing the dressing, since they do not require changing with each dressing as adhesive strips do. Figure 30-1 illustrates a type of strap. These can be made easily. The adhesive end of the strap is placed on the skin well away from the wound. The end of the strap near the wound remains free, since the sticky side of the adhesive is covered. Tapes passed through the eyelets are tied over the wound to secure the dressing. When the dressing is changed, the tapes are untied and turned back to allow for wound care. The skin of the patient should be protected with compound benzoin tincture before applying the straps. When adhesive is removed, some of the gummy substance will

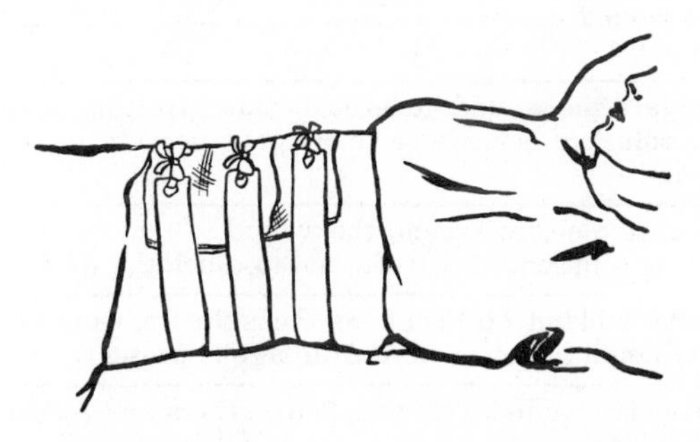

FIG. 30-1. A means for securing dressings that must be changed frequently.

remain on the skin. This should be removed. Agency policies vary as to the solution to be used for this purpose. The nurse will need to follow agency procedure.

When adhesive cannot be used safely and effectively, various types of binders and bandages may be used for securing dressings. A description of various types of binders, bandages and their application follows.

When a dressing is being secured, pressure on the wound should be exerted from the edges toward the center. This practice helps to approximate the wound edges and hence promotes healing. The dressing should be secured well enough so that it does not slip out of place as the patient moves.

Frequency of Changing Dressings. The frequency with which dressings should be changed cannot be stated categorically; it will depend on the physician's order, the nature of the wound and whether drainage is present. A surgeon may wish to leave a clean wound untouched for several days, in which case dressings are left unchanged.

PRINCIPLES GUIDING ACTION IN THE CARE OF A DRESSED WOUND

The purpose is to remove a soiled dressing, cleanse the wound and apply a sterile dressing.

SUGGESTED ACTION	PRINCIPLE
Undo materials securing the dressing. Lift dressing off by touching outside portion only. If it is soiled, use individual forceps.	Microorganisms can be transferred by direct contact.
If dressing adheres to wound, moisten with physiologic saline or peroxide. Remove when completely loose.	An intact scab is a body defense mechanism.
Drop the soiled dressing into a waterproof bag for later burning.	Burning destroys microorganisms. Confined microorganisms cannot be transmitted by air currents or by contact.
Cleanse the wound carefully with an antiseptic of the physician's or the agency's choice.	Cleansing aids in removing organisms, tissue debris and drainage.
Start from either directly on or adjacent to the wound and work away from it.	Microorganisms are normally present on the skin.
Discard the gauze or the cotton used for cleansing after each stroke over the wound.	Microorganisms removed from one area can be applied to another by direct contact.
If a wound irrigation is ordered, place the patient in such a position that the solution will flow from the wound down to a clean basin held below the wound.	Gravity causes the flow of liquids.
Irrigate the wound generously but carefully with the solution, being sure to irrigate pockets in the wound.	The solution washes away organisms, tissue debris and drainage.
Cleanse the skin around the wound to remove irrigating solution. Be careful not to touch the wound.	Microorganisms are normally present on the skin.
Place a bland ointment on the skin immediately surrounding the wound if drainage is present.	An emollient on the skin prevents drainage from irritating the epithelium.
Cover the wound with sterile dressings and secure it in place.	Well-secured sterile dressings protect the wound from trauma, minimize the danger of organisms entering the wound and absorb secretions.

Most surgeons generally believe that a frequent change of dressings on a clean, nondraining wound is a possible source of contamination. In their opinion, it is best if the wound's own protective seal is left undisturbed.

Recording the Care of the Wound. The nurse caring for a wound is responsible for observing it and for noting factors that may be interfering with the process of healing. She is expected to call the physician's attention to anything unusual in the process of healing as well as to its progress.

On the patient's permanent record the nurse records each time wound care is given, the nature of the care given and the condition of the wound. If the patient has a rather complicated dressing, details for caring for the wound should be described on the patient's nursing care plan. Often, the patient who has an extensive wound has preferences as to the time the dressings are changed and how they can be arranged best. Also, patients can become distressed if one nurse uses one method and another nurse a different one, even if both employ proper technic.

Teaching the Patient to Care for His Wound

Patients return to their homes earlier than they once did. This means that frequently a patient will still need care for his wound after discharge from the hospital. The patient may return to his physician's office or to a clinic, or a public health nurse may be asked to visit the patient in his home. In other instances, the patient or a member of his family is taught to care for the wound at home. The patient may report to his physician or a clinic at regular intervals for inspection of the wound and for supervision of its care.

Preparing the patient to care for his wound prior to discharge from a health agency is a nursing responsibility. The nature and the amount of the teaching will depend on individual circumstances. Nurses have observed that patients usually are concerned about odor from dressings besides discomfort and fear of soiling clothing when drainage is present. Other disturbing factors include fear that the dressings will slip out of place and cause infection, concern for the reaction of friends and family to the appearance of the dressings and the cost of the dressings.

While it remains important to use appropriate materials for wound care, the nurse also should assist the patient so that the cost of materials does not become unreasonable. Occasionally, the patient may need financial assistance, and an appropriate agency may be asked to help. Or, the patient may be referred to a local health organization that distributes dressings at a nominal cost or free of charge. The nurse who uses ingenuity based on appropriate principles can help the patient to keep the cost within a reasonable range and still carry out the procedure effectively.

Uses of Bandages and Binders. A bandage is a length of material applied in a manner to fit a part of the body. Usually, bandages are dispensed in rolls of various widths. A binder is a type of bandage. The term "binder" generally is used when the material is specifically designed to fit a large body area as, for example, the abdomen, the chest or the breasts. Some texts use the terms synonymously, although in the strictest sense they are not.

Bandages and binders are used for several purposes: to create pressure over an area, to immobilize a part of the body to restrict its motion, to support a part of the body, to prevent or reduce swelling, to correct a deformity and to secure a limb to a splint. They are used also to hold dressings in place.

Materials Used for Bandages and Binders. Usually, gauze fabric is used for bandages. It is light and soft and can be adjusted readily to fit a body part comfortably. Because it is porous, it is cool and allows for circulation of air. Gauze bandage is relatively inexpensive. It rarely can be reclaimed for repeated use because it frays very easily.

Muslin and flannel are materials also used for bandages. Being strong and firm, they are useful when pressure and immobilization are desired. Flannel is more absorbent than muslin and molds easily to fit the contours of the body. Flannel also helps to keep the area warm, which may be an advantage or a disadvantage depending on individual circumstances. Most binders are made of muslin or flannel. Muslin or flannel bandages are suited to home use because they can be washed and reused.

Various types of elastic webbing can be purchased which are particularly effective when bandaging is needed for firm support and immobilization and for preventing swelling in extremities. The webbing is strong and molds well because of its elastic quality. It can be washed and used repeatedly.

One type of elastic webbing has an adhesive surface on one side. This can be used like adhesive and has the advantage of molding well to body contours. It does not withstand washing and therefore cannot be reclaimed for repeated use.

Ribbed cotton material dispensed as stockinet is used for bandaging. It has an elastic quality, is inexpensive and can be reclaimed for repeated use, but it is not as sturdy and strong as elastic webbing.

General Principles Used in the Application of Bandages and Binders

A bandage or a binder well applied will promote healing, prevent damage to wounds and skin and offer the patient comfort and security. Certain general principles guide action in the application of bandages and binders and aid in attaining these objectives.

Unclean bandages and binders may cause infection if applied over a wound or a skin abrasion. This fact guides what may seem like rather obvious action, that is, that bandages and binders should be kept clean and free of contamination. Medical asepsis is observed when applying bandages and binders. Skin abrasions and wounds are first covered with sterile dressings before clean bandages and binders are applied in order to aid in protecting the wound from trauma and contamination. Certain bandages and binders may be used repeatedly, but only after they have been washed and sterilized.

When objects in contact move in opposition to each other, friction opposes motion, and friction will destroy or damage epithelial cells. Applying a small amount of fine talcum powder to the unbroken skin helps to keep it dry and decreases friction, but care must be exercised to prevent powder from entering the wound, if one is present. No two skin surfaces should be allowed to touch each other. This is another measure to decrease friction on the skin and prevent moisture from accumulating in body crevices. Use absorbent cotton between fingers and toes, in the axilla, under the breast, etc., to absorb moisture and to prevent surfaces of skin from contacting each other. A bandage or a binder should be applied securely so that it will not move about when the patient moves, causing friction that may result in chafing and skin abrasions.

Prolonged heat and moisture on the skin cause its epithelial cells to deteriorate. It will be recalled that this principle is observed when dressings are applied to a wound. When bandages and binders are used, it indicates to the nurse that the area to be covered should be cleansed and dried thoroughly before applying a bandage or a binder. An unnecessarily thick or extensive bandage should be avoided so that the part being covered does not become excessively warm. Porous materials are preferable to nonporous in order to allow air to circulate so that perspiration can evaporate.

Placing and supporting the part to be bandaged in the normal functioning position prevents deformities and discomfort and enhances the circulation of blood in the part involved. This principle has been used as a guide for action throughout this text in the discussions of the importance of proper body mechanics and body alignment. It is equally important when bandages and binders are being used. Since bandages and binders usually restrict some motion and often are intended to immobilize a part of the body, it is important that the part involved first be placed at rest and comfortably in the position of normal functioning so that deformities and impaired circulation will not result. For example, when the foot is bandaged, it should be supported so that the bandage will not force it into plantar flexion.

Blood flow through the tissues is decreased by applying pressure on blood vessels. The healing process is impaired, and tissue cells may die if the blood supply is inadequate to remove wastes and bring nourishment to the part involved. These are well-known physiologic facts that guide action in several ways. The bandage or the binder is applied with sufficient pressure to attain the amount of immobilization desired, to remain in place and to secure a dressing if one is present. However, pressure should not be great enough to prevent circulation of blood in the part involved. Tension of each bandage turn should be equal, and unnecessary and uneven overlapping of turns should be avoided to prevent undue and uneven pressure. Bony prominences over which bandages and binders must be placed are padded. Hollows in the body contour may be filled with padding to provide comfort and to aid in maintaining equal pressure from the bandage or binder. An extremity is bandaged *toward the trunk* to avoid congestion and impaired circulation in the distal part. After a bandage or a binder has been applied, the part is observed frequently for signs of impaired circulation. For example, when an extremity is bandaged, the toes and the fingers are left exposed, if possible, so that circulation in the nail beds and signs of beginning swelling, which often indicate that circulation has been impaired, can be observed. Bandage placed over a wet dressing or a draining wound is applied less tightly since shrinkage of the material may cause the bandage to become too tight to allow for adequate circulation when it dries. In addition to being dangerous, a bandage or a binder applied too tightly is usually very uncomfortable for the patient.

Pins and knots, often used to secure a bandage or a binder, are placed well away from a wound or a tender and inflamed area. Care is observed so that pins, knots and seams will not cause undue pressure or cause the patient discomfort.

A well-applied bandage or binder will be comfortable for the patient, durable, neat and clean. This is important for the patient's mental security as well as for promoting the best possible physiologic functioning of the body.

Application of Common Types of Bandages and Binders

Triangular Binders. These are triangular pieces of material usually made of muslin. The sizes of these binders vary, but, for most adults, a 36- to 40-inch square cut in half diagonally to form two triangles is a common size.

Triangular binders are used for support as slings. Figure 30-2 illustrates a sling used as an arm support and shows the method of

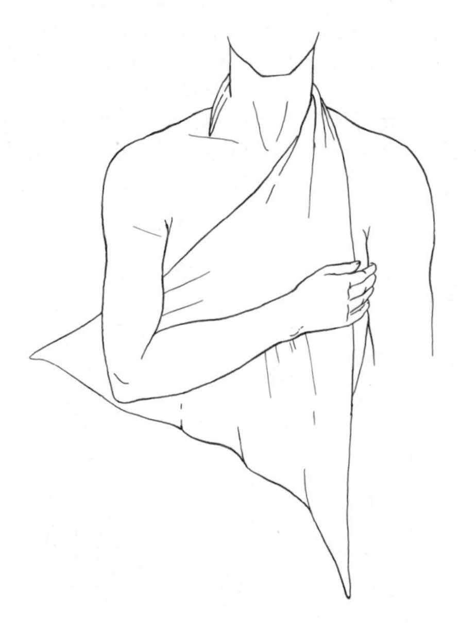

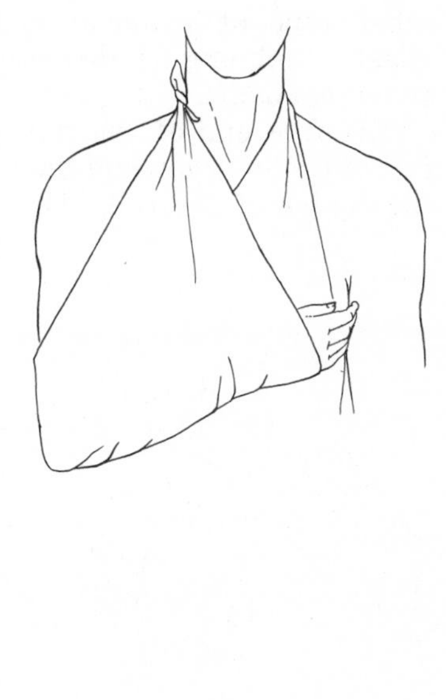

FIG. 30-2. Triangular binder used as a sling to support the arm.

applying it. The open sling or triangle is placed on the chest, and then the affected arm is placed across the sling. One end of the sling is placed around the neck on the side of the unaffected arm. The other end is placed over the affected arm, and the ends are tied off to the side of the neck so that the knot does not rub over the cervical vertebrae. The material at the elbow is folded neatly and may be secured with a pin placed behind the sling so that it will be out of sight.

Triangular binders may be made into mittens for covering foot-and-hand dressings. They are useful also for bandaging the head, the shoulders and the hips. Occasionally, two triangular binders may be used if the area is large.

Cravat Bandages. A cravat bandage is made by folding a triangular binder upon itself, from the apex of the triangle to the base and then over and over again until the desired width for the bandage is obtained. A cravat may be used as a small sling. It is used also on limbs and on the head. It is useful as a tourniquet and as a temporary measure to support a sprained joint.

Roller Bandages. A roller bandage is a continuous strip of material wound on itself to form a cylinder or roll. Roller bandages are made in various widths and lengths. They are the most commonly used type of bandage and usually are made of gauze, although any other type of material may be used also. Elastic webbing is dispensed usually as a roller bandage.

The free end of the roller bandage is the *initial extremity*, while the *terminal end* is in the center of the roll. The rolled portion is called the *body*. The *outer surface* of the bandage is the surface toward the outside of the body of the bandage. The *inner surface* is toward the inside or the center of the body. The outer surface is placed next to the patient's skin and dressing. When the bandage is begun, the initial end is held in place with one hand while the other hand passes the roll around the part. Once the bandage is anchored, usually with two circular turns, the body may be passed from hand to hand, being careful that equal tension is being exerted with each turn around the part. It is easier to keep tension equal by unwinding the bandage gradually and only as it is required. Several basic turns are used to apply bandages, the selection of the turn depending on the part to be bandaged.

Circular Turn. When using the circular turn, the bandage is wrapped around the part with complete overlapping of the previous bandage turn. It is used primarily for anchoring a bandage when it is begun and when it is terminated. Figures 30-3 and 30-4 illustrate this turn to anchor a bandage before beginning a spiral turn.

Spiral Turn. When using the spiral turn, the bandage ascends in spiral fashion so that each turn overlaps the preceding one by one-half or two-thirds the width of the bandage. The spiral turn is useful when the part being bandaged is cylindrical, such as the area around the wrist, the fingers and the trunk. Figure 30-5 illustrates this turn.

Spiral-Reverse Turn. A spiral-reverse turn is a spiral turn in which reverses are made halfway through each turn. Spiral-reverse turns are particularly effective for bandag-

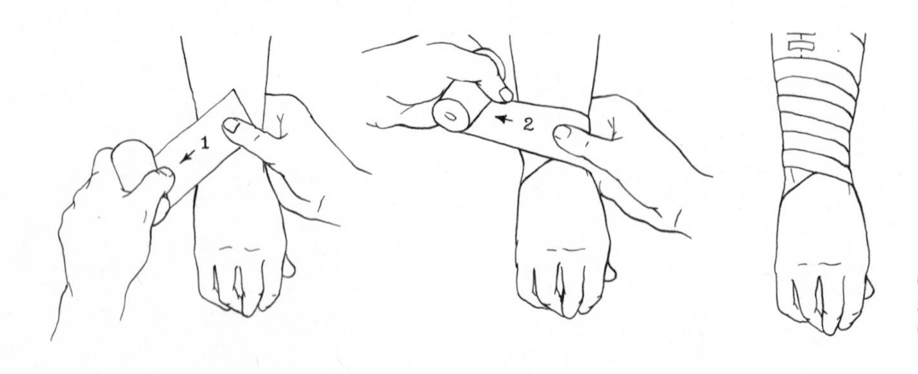

FIG. 30-3. (left) and FIG. 30-4. (center). The circular turn to anchor the bandage. FIG. 30-5. (right). The spiral turn.

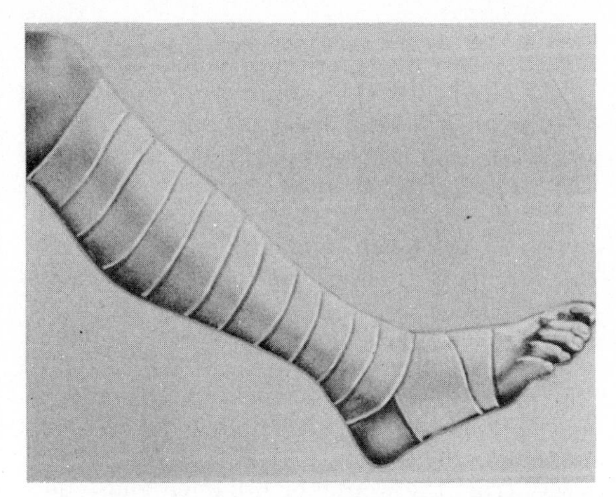

FIG. 30-6. Elastic roller bandage applied to the leg, using spiral turns. (Becton, Dickinson & Co., Rutherford, N. J.)

ing a cone-shaped part, such as the thigh, the leg or the forearm. Figure 30-7 illustrates the spiral-reverse turn. The position of the nurse's thumb on the bandage on the patient's arm shows the manner in which the reverse is made.

Figure-of-Eight Turn. This consists of making oblique overlapping turns that ascend and descend alternately. Each turn crosses the one preceding it so that it appears like the number eight. Figure 30-8 illustrates how this turn is made. It is effective for use around joints, such as the knee, the elbow, the ankle and the wrist. It provides for a snug bandage and therefore is used often for immobilization.

Spica. The spica consists of ascending and descending turns with all turns overlapping and crossing each other to form an angle. It is particularly useful for bandaging the thumb, the breast, the shoulder, the groin and the hip. Figure 30-10 illustrates its application.

Recurrent Bandage. Sometimes this type is called a *stump bandage.* It is used for fingers and for the stump of an amputated limb. After a few circular turns to anchor the bandage, the initial end of the bandage is placed in the center of the part being bandaged, well back from the tip to be covered. The body is passed back and forth over the

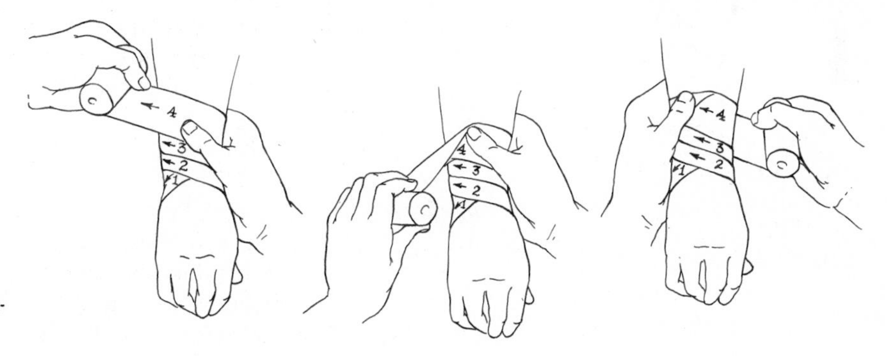

FIG. 30.7. Procedure for making the spiral-reverse turn.

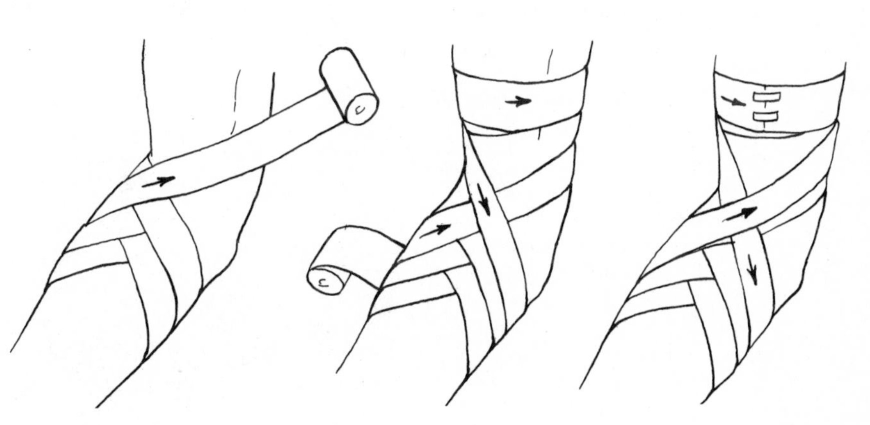

FIG. 30-8. Procedure for making the figure-of-eight turn.

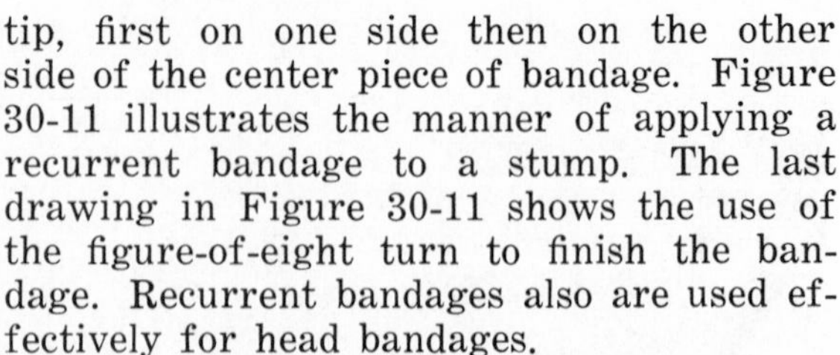
tip, first on one side then on the other side of the center piece of bandage. Figure 30-11 illustrates the manner of applying a recurrent bandage to a stump. The last drawing in Figure 30-11 shows the use of the figure-of-eight turn to finish the bandage. Recurrent bandages also are used effectively for head bandages.

Whichever turn is being used, care should be taken to provide even overlapping of one-half to two-thirds the width of each bandage, except for the circular turn. All skin should be covered by the finished bandage to prevent pinching the skin between turns of the bandage. The bandage is completed well away from the wound or inflamed and tender areas. The terminal end of the bandage may be secured with adhesive, by tying a knot or with a safety pin, being careful to avoid undue pressure.

Removing Roller Bandages. In order to prevent too much movement, it is best to cut a roller bandage with a bandage scissors. Cutting should be done on the side opposite the injury or the wound, from one end to the other, so that the bandage can be folded open for its entire length. If it is an elastic bandage and is to be reused, it may be unwound by keeping the loose end together and passing it as a ball from one hand to the other while unwinding.

T Binders. A T binder is so named because it looks like the letter T. A single T binder has a tail attached at right angles to a belt. A double T binder has two tails attached to the belt. T binders are particularly effective for securing dressings on the perineum and in the groin. The single T is used for females, and the dou-

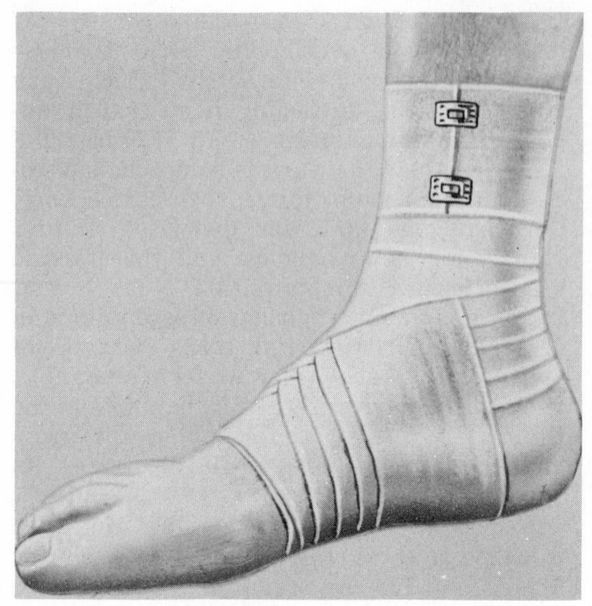

FIG. 30-9. The figure-of-eight turn used to apply elastic bandage to the ankle. (Becton, Dickinson & Co., Rutherford, N. J.)

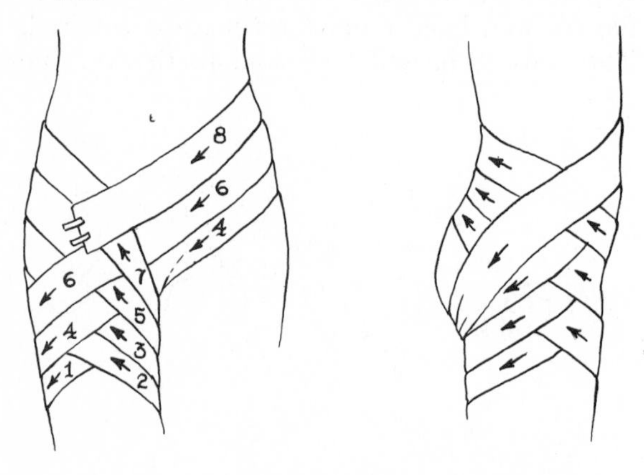

FIG. 30-10. Procedure for making the spica bandage.

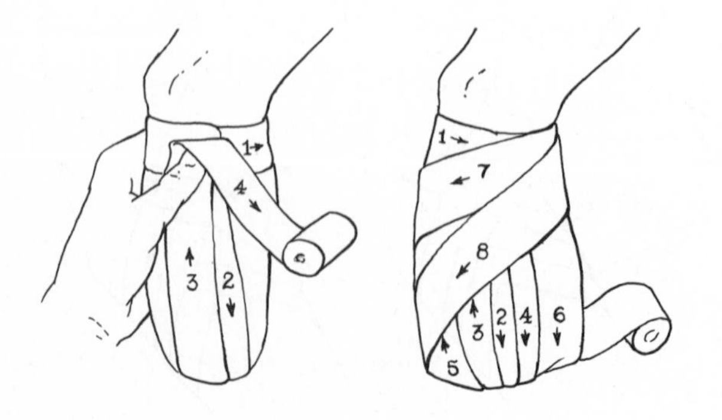

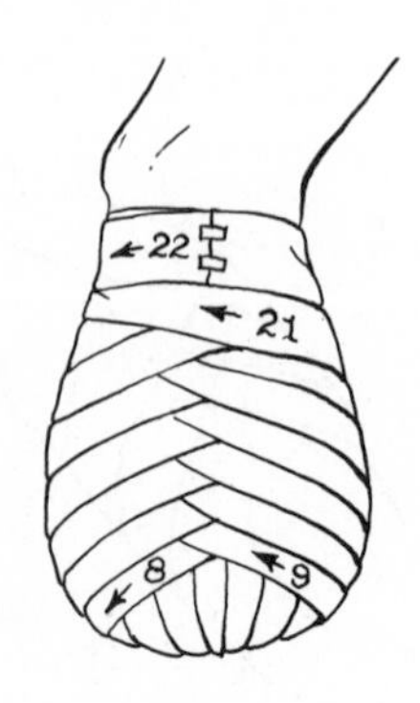

FIG. 30-11. Procedure for making a recurrent bandage to cover a stump.

ble T for males. The belt is passed around the waist and secured with safety pins. The single or the double tails are passed between the legs and pinned to the belt.

Tailed Binders. A tailed binder consists of a rectangular piece of material which has vertical tails, each about two inches wide, attached to each side of the rectangular piece. A four-tailed binder has four tails, two on each side of the binder. It is useful for securing dressings on the nose and the chin and is illustrated in Figure 30-13.

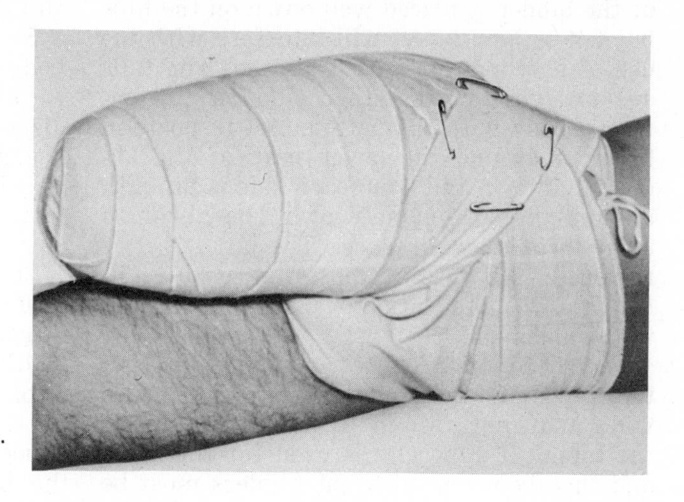

Fig. 30-12. Elastic bandage used to dress a stump. (Becton, Dickinson & Co., Rutherford, N. J.)

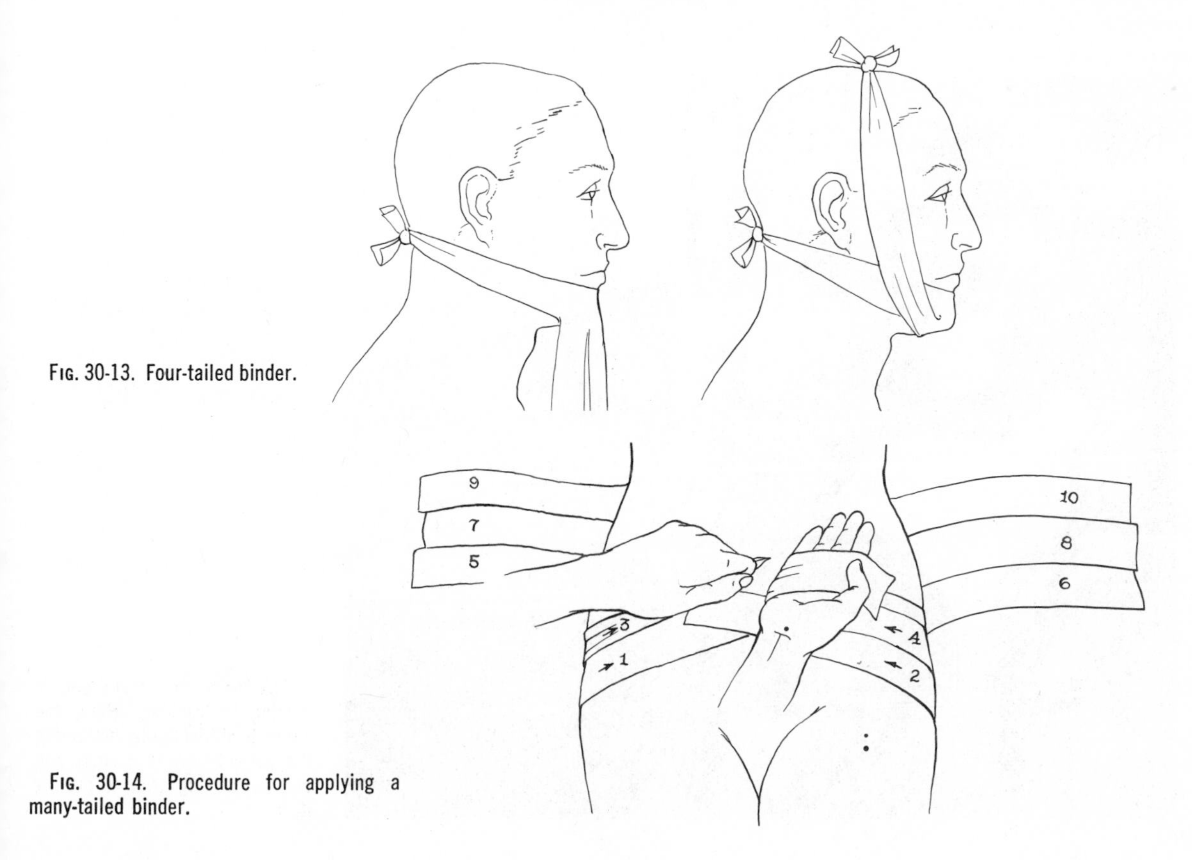

Fig. 30-13. Four-tailed binder.

Fig. 30-14. Procedure for applying a many-tailed binder.

Many-tailed binders are called *scultetus binders.* They are used to support the abdomen or hold dressings on it and on the chest. When a scultetus binder is applied to the abdomen, the patient lies on his back and on the center of the binder. The lower end of the binder is placed well down on the hips but not so low that it will interfere with the use of a bedpan or with walking. The tails are brought out to either side on the patient's body with the bottom tail in position to wrap around the lower part of the abdomen first. A tail from each side is brought up and placed obliquely over the abdomen until all tails are in place. The last tails are fastened with safety pins. Figure 30-14 illustrates the application of a scultetus binder to the abdomen.

Straight Binders. This straight piece of material usually is about six to eight inches wide and long enough to more than circle the torso. It generally is used for the chest and the abdomen. Straight binders must be applied so as to fit the contours of the body. This usually is done by making small tucks in the binder as necessary. In some instances, these tucks can be secured with safety pins. A straight binder for the chest often is provided with shoulder straps so that it will not slip down on the trunk.

Stockinet is dispensed as a tube so that a body part may be inserted into it, such as, for example, a finger, a foot or an arm. It is dispensed in various widths (diameters). It has advantages over the roller bandage in that it remains in place better, applies a uniform pressure and is extremely simple and quick to use.

Stockinet is useful for making caps for securing dressings on the head. The desired length is cut from a roll of an appropriate width, usually six inches wide. The stockinet is placed over the head and folded back on itself at the forehead for extra security. The opposite end is tied or pinned at the top of the head. Stockinet as a bandage on the

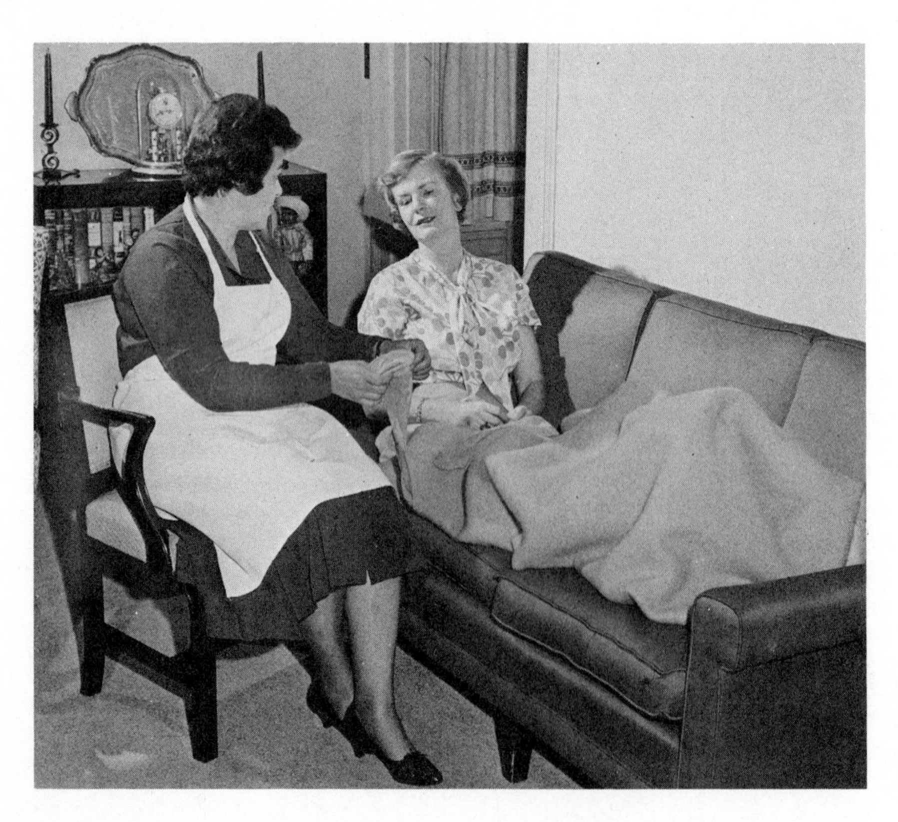

Fig. 30-15. An integral part of nursing is teaching. Here, the public health nurse is instructing the patient how to prepare the elastic stocking prior to putting it on.

head seems to offer more security than other types; therefore, it is also more comfortable for the patient.

A product that is effective for finger bandages is *Surgitube*. It is made like stockinet in a narrow width that is appropriate for finger bandages. An applicator is dispensed with the Surgitube so that it can be slipped over the finger with ease.

Elasticized Stockings. Some persons may need to have pressure applied to their legs, such as those with varicose veins or circulatory impairment of the legs, or women during pregnancy. Several manufacturers produce women's hose which are capable of applying pressure to the leg from the foot to the mid-thigh. Some apply mild pressure, while others are capable of applying pressure equivalent to an elastic bandage. Both types look like dress hose; hence, another stocking is not required underneath or over them. From a comfort and cosmetic standpoint, these hose have much to offer the woman in addition to their therapeutic effects. They are more expensive than regular nylon hose, possibly making them prohibitive for some patients. However, they wear well, and many women who are on their feet a great deal, e.g., homemakers, nurses and saleswomen, find them very useful. The mild sustained pressure aids in preventing the accumulation of tissue fluid in the feet and the lower leg. Many patients can benefit from such stockings, and the nurse should be prepared to advise about their correct use. A main point is that they should be applied immediately upon arising.

Study Situations

1. The reference below reports on a study in relation to surgical dressings. It may be of interest to you to learn what problems are commonly associated with dressings and to learn how a study of this nature was carried out:

- Wolff, L.: Identifying surgical dressing problems helps solve them.
  HOSP., J. AMER. HOSP. ASSOC., *31*:48-52, February 16, 1957.

What was the purpose of the study? What tool or method was used to obtain the data? Who supplied the data? What were the major findings in the study?

2. What has been your personal experience with undressed wounds, such as cuts, deep scratches and denuded skin areas? Have you always placed a bandage on them? If so, why? If not, why? How effective is a "Band-Aid" on a finger cut if it must become soiled and wet because of the nature of the wearer's activities?

3. Note the extreme cautions recommended in this text when caring for wounds:
   pp. 32-45 "Guide for Dressing Wounds" and "Guide for Hand Washing"

- LeRiche, W. H.: The Control of Infections in Hospitals.
  Springfield, Ill., Charles C Thomas, 1966.

References

1. Abbott, E.: Improving dressing technique. AMER. J. NURS., *60*:1263, September, 1960.
2. Cole, W. H., and Puestow, C. B.: First Aid and Diagnosis. ed. 6, pp. 69-93. New York, Appleton-Century-Crofts, 1965.
3. Moyer, C. A. *et al*: Surgery, Principles and Practices, ed. 3, pp. 7-16. Philadelphia, Lippincott, 1965.
4. Nealon, T. F.: Fundamental Skills in Surgery, ed. 2, pp. 52-69. Philadelphia, W. B. Saunders, 1962.
5. Ochsner, A., and DeBakey, M. E. (eds.): Christopher's Minor Surgery, ed. 8, pp. 19-29. Philadelphia, W. B. Saunders, 1962.
6. Suddarth, D. S.: Individual dressing packs. AMER. J. NURS., *60*:991-992, July, 1960.
7. Williams, R. E. O. *et al*: Hospital Infection Causes and Prevention. ed. 2, pp. 77-115. London, Lloyd-Luke (Medical Books) Ltd., 1966.
8. Wolff, L.: Problems with surgical dressings. AMER. J. NURS., *57*:1463-1464, November, 1957.

CHAPTER

31

Applying Heat or Cold

Introduction

Certain disease conditions are treated with the aid of physical agents. The branch of medicine that specializes in the use of physical agents is called *physical therapy*. Heat and cold are physical agents, and their application, especially when used locally, usually is a nursing responsibility. Their use for comfort or therapy can be traced back through the ages. The so-called healthy person makes use of their effects frequently. Ice caps for headaches, heating pads for menstrual cramps, hot baths for respiratory infections and for muscular aches are a part of self-treatment of minor ills and are used commonly even though the principles involved are not understood by most people.

Local applications of heat or cold may be either dry or moist. When the effect desired is dependent on the immediate reaction of the affected tissues to the temperature of the application, it is referred to as an *intrinsic effect*. However, the body also reacts as a whole to local thermal applications, and this effect is referred to as *reactionary*. If the immediate local or intrinsic effect is desired, the application should be continued for a long enough period of time to overcome the immediate reactionary effect produced in the body. The opposite of this is also true. If a reactionary effect is desired, the application should be of short duration.

General Principles Governing the Use of Heat or Cold

The blood serves as a means for transporting substances to and from body cells. Under normal conditions, the exchange of blood is maintained within certain limits to provide for changing demands of body cells. During illness, there may be times when it becomes desirable either to increase or decrease the exchange of blood in certain parts of the body.

The discernment of temperature gives the body information about its external environment. This principle is based on knowledge of how temperature sensations are received by the body, how they are interpreted by the cerebral cortex, and how they are reacted upon by the body. The principle becomes important in observing and interpreting the results of therapy and adapting therapy accordingly.

Intact skin and mucous membrane serve as first lines of defense against harmful agents. When heat or cold is used, a physical agent is being applied to the body. Unless precautionary measures are taken, these physical agents can produce irritation or injury to the skin and the mucous membrane, thereby weakening one of the body's defenses.

The Body's Reaction to Temperature Stimulation

It will be recalled that cells in the hypothalamus act as a "Thermostat" to regulate body temperature. The anterior cells of the hypothalamus are vasodilating and heat-dissipating while the posterior or caudal cells are vasoconstricting and heat-conserving. These cells receive impulses through somatic and visceral neurons in the brain and the spinal cord. The skin plays an important role in maintaining body temperature through the activity of its sweat glands and its pilomotor muscles. When one is exposed to warm surroundings, the sweat glands secrete perspiration. The body cools when the perspiration changes from liquid to vapor. Evaporation requires heat; hence, heat is released. When exposed to cold surroundings, the pilomotor muscles contract and make the hair stand on end in animals and cause "gooseflesh" in man. This phenomenon is the body's attempt to conserve internal body heat. Shivering, also under hypothalamus regulation (lateral cells), generates considerable body heat by agitating the muscles.

The caliber of the cutaneous blood vessels also plays an important role in maintaining body temperature. The smaller the caliber, the smaller will be the quantity of heat brought by the blood to the surface of the skin and lost to the environment. The larger the caliber, the larger the quantity of heat brought to the surface and lost. This phenomenon can be observed when the skin appears flushed as the body becomes too warm, and pale as the body becomes too cool. The blood vessels in the skin are capable of containing large or small quantities of blood, and their caliber increases or decreases as the local and the general needs of the body change. The change in caliber of the blood vessels is regulated by the vasomotor centers (dilator and constrictor) in the medulla oblongata of the brain stem, under hypothalmic influence.

Temperature Receptors in the Skin. When receptors for heat and cold are stimulated, they set up impulses that are carried to the hypothalamus and the cerebral cortex via the somatic afferent fibers. The conscious sensation of temperature is aroused in the cerebral cortex, while the hypothalamus serves as a reflex center to integrate somatic and visceral motor responses to maintain a normal temperature.

Receptors for cold lie superficially, while those for heat are located deeper in the skin. The density of receptors varies; in some parts of the body they are more numerous than in others. The cold receptors, for example, are particularly numerous on the thorax and the upper limbs. The cold receptors are estimated to be approximately 8 to 10 times more numerous than receptors for heat.

There is difference of opinion concerning receptors for high temperatures. It is more generally agreed that, when hot stimuli are received by the skin, the pain receptors are also stimulated, and the sensation of burning is the result of this double stimulation of receptors. A less widely accepted theory is that a second type of heat receptor in the skin with a very high threshold is stimulated when hot objects touch the skin.

An important characteristic of heat and cold receptors is that they adjust readily if the stimulus is not extreme. For example, if the arm is placed in warm water, the sensation of warmth soon diminishes because of the adaptability of the heat receptors. The same phenomenon occurs if cool water is used. This is unlike the pain receptors, which do not adapt to painful stimuli. It is important to remember the ability of receptors to adapt to heat and cold when using hot and cold applications. Once the receptors adapt, the patient may become unaware of temperature extremes until tissue damage occurs.

Tolerance of the Skin Temperature. The temperature that the skin can tolerate varies with individuals. Some can tolerate warmer and colder applications more safely than can others. Certain areas of the skin are also more tolerant of temperature than are other areas. Those parts of the body where the skin is somewhat thinner generally are more sensitive to temperature than exposed areas where the skin is often thicker. Therefore, it is important to apply warm and cold applications well within the generally known safe limits of temperature. But, in addition, the skin should be observed so that persons who are more sensitive to temperature will not receive tissue damage, even though applications have been applied within recommended temperature range.

Water is a better conductor of heat than air. This fact is used in guiding action whenever heat or cold is applied to the skin, since the skin will tolerate greater extremes of temperature if the heat or the cold is dry rather than moist. For example, a moist hot dressing should be applied at a lower temperature than a flannel-covered hot water bottle in order to prevent burning the skin. This is because the air between flannel fibers acts as an insulator.

The body tolerates greater extremes in temperature when the duration of exposure is short. When duration is lengthy, the temperature range that the body can tolerate safely is narrower. The area involved is also important. In general, the larger the area to which heat or cold is applied, the less tolerant is the skin to extremes in temperature.

The condition of the patient is an important factor to consider when heat and cold are being applied to the body. Certain patients are sensitive to physical agents and tolerate heat and cold poorly. Special care also is indicated for patients who are debilitated, unconscious or insensitive to cutaneous stimulation. Patients who have disturbances in circulation are more sensitive to heat and cold. Broken skin areas are also more subject to tissue damage, since the subcutaneous tissue is less tolerant of heat and cold, and the temperature and pain senses may be impaired and unable to heed warning stimuli.

General Considerations Concerning Heat and Cold

Definitions of Heat and Cold. Until late in the 18th century, heat was believed to be a kind of fluid that could flow from one substance to another. This theory was refuted when it was found that heat was related to motion. Heat is defined as the average kinetic energy (energy of motion) of the molecules of the material.

Cold is a relative term. It is used to mean that a material has a relatively low temperature; that is, little or no warmth. In other words, as motion of the molecules decreases, the heat is less, and the material is said to be cool or cold. Absolute zero is the temperature at which molecular motion ceases. Theoretically, this occurs at a hypothetical point 273° below zero on the centigrade scale. The important thing to realize is that for all practical purposes, heat is present in all material, therefore, discussions concerning the nature of heat apply also to those of cold. However, the *effects* of applying something warm to the human body are different from the effects of applying something cool, as will be later illustrated.

Transfer of Heat. Heat is transferred by radiation, convection and conduction.

The transfer of heat in the form of waves is called radiation. For example, heat can be felt by placing the hand near a light bulb. The heat has been transferred to the hand by radiation.

Heat transferred by convection travels in currents. Air expands and rises as it warms; cold air acts oppositely. Convection explains the phenomenon of wind, since the unequal heating of the earth's surfaces produces air currents.

When heat is transferred directly from one substance to another, it is called conduction. Local applications of heat and cold transfer heat to and from the body by conduction. A poor conductor is called an *insulator.* Many of the actions that nurses take when applying heat or cold to the body are guided by a knowledge of the transmission of heat by conduction. These are some examples:

If hot water bottles were made of metal, they would conduct heat so rapidly that the patient would be burned, since metals are good conductors of heat. Even rubber is a fairly good conductor; therefore, hot water bottles are covered with flannel before applying to the patient. Flannel is a good insulator because of its many air traps, air being a rather poor conductor of heat.

Before hot wet packs are applied to an area, the skin is lubricated with petrolatum, which acts as an insulator, since it slows down the transmission of heat.

Metal bedpans should be warmed before offering them to patients. The metal, a good conductor, removes heat from the body so rapidly that the area of the bedpan in contact with the patient will feel uncomfortably cold.

Effects of Local Application of Heat

The first visible effect of moderate heat applied to the skin is vasodilatation—that is, the caliber of the cutaneous vessels increases. The skin becomes warm and pink. The skin receptors for heat are stimulated, the impulses are carried to the hypothalamus and the cerebral cortex, and the body's reaction is to rid itself of heat that may threaten the stability of body temperature. The dilatation of cutaneous vessels allows for increased blood circulation in the skin in order that heat may be lost to the environment.

In addition to vasodilatation, other reactions are taking place simultaneously. Heat lessens the viscosity of blood, thereby increasing the rate of flow. Tissue metabolism improves as the increased blood supply furnishes more oxygen and carries away wastes more rapidly. There is a greater amount of fluid in the tissue spaces, and the flow of lymph is increased.

Local application of heat usually relieves pain, although the exact phenomenon is not understood clearly. Pain caused by muscle spasm is relieved as the muscle relaxes. Pain caused by the pressure of congestion often is relieved as circulation improves. Some authorities suggest that possibly a chemical derived from accumulated waste products in the body causes pain and that therefore the increased circulation aids in removing the chemical and thus the pain.

Heat usually is applied for its local effects. Local applications of heat are used very often for the relief of pain, congestion, inflammation, swelling and muscle spasms. Healing is promoted as tissue metabolism improves. Local heat also is often applied for comfort when patients feel cool and chilly.

Heat may also be applied locally for its more remote effects. If heat is applied to one area of the body, the amount of blood in other parts of the body decreases as the supply increases in the area being heated. For example, if the feet are placed in a basin of warm water, congestion of blood in abdominal organs is relieved as blood is diverted to the legs and the feet.

Studies have determined the depth to which heat penetrates the body when applied to a local area. One such study demonstrated that, when a hot water bag is applied to the calf of the leg, the temperature within the muscle of the leg rises. The following summary illustrates the findings:

Interior of hot water bag	133° F.
Outside of towel covering hot water bag	122° F.
Cutaneous temperature rose from . .	90° F. to 110° F. (in about 30 minutes)
Subcutaneous temperature rose from	91.2° F. to 105.5° F. (in about 40 minutes)
Intramuscular temperature rose from	94.2° F. to 99.6° F. (in about 50 minutes)

Similar studies were conducted when heat was applied to the abdomen. No marked change of temperature within the stomach and the peritoneal cavity was demonstrated when heat was applied.

It has been found that blood flow decreases when the application of heat to a local area continues beyond approximately one hour. The reason for this reaction is not understood clearly, but probably reflex vasoconstriction results from the body's efforts at homeostasis through the autonomic nervous system. If the hot application is removed for a period of time and then reapplied, vasodilatation and the concomitant results occur again. It also should be remembered that prolonged application of heat weakens cutaneous cells; therefore, the skin becomes more subject to injury.

Temperature for Hot Applications. The desired temperature for applying local hot applications cannot be stated arbitrarily. As has been pointed out, the condition of the skin, the size of the area being covered, the duration of the application, the method of applying heat (moist or dry), the condition of the patient and the differences in heat tolerances need to be considered when determining optimum temperatures for applying heat. When the temperature of the skin surpasses approximately 110° F., many individuals are likely to suffer burns.

The temperature of water used for applications is described usually as neutral or warm, hot, very hot. The temperature ranges stated frequently are as follows:

Warm or neutral .... 93° F. to 98° F.
Hot .... 98° F. to 105° F.
Very hot ....105° F. to 115° F.

The common methods for applying heat discussed later in this chapter state the temperature ranges for applications which have been found satisfactory for most persons. However, checking the condition of the patient's skin is still necessary in order to avoid possible tissue damage.

Effects of Very Hot Applications. If very hot applications are applied to the skin for short periods of time, the reaction is similar to that of cold—that is, the cutaneous vessels may contract and decrease the blood supply. This is because the body is protecting itself against excessive loss of internal heat when exposed to an extreme of temperature in the environment. Muscles may fail to relax. Warm applications, on the other hand, lead to relaxation of muscles and increased blood supply. The effects of a warm bath and of a hot shower illustrate this difference in reaction of the body when warmth and heat are used. Contraction of small vessels is a desired reaction when hemorrhage is present, but cold rather than very hot applications are used more commonly to aid in checking bleeding.

There is logic in this when one recalls that cold increases the viscosity of blood. Increased viscosity slows the speed of flow, and blood clotting is facilitated by lower speed of circulation with vasoconstriction resulting from the cold.

Diathermy is the production of heat in body tissue by the use of high-frequency currents. It is used generally for producing heat in deep tissues. Special equipment is used for diathermy; generally, trained technicians are responsible for giving diathermy treatments. The reaction of the deep tissue to the heat produced by diathermy is similar to that of the skin and more superficial tissue when heat is applied locally.

Local Application of Heat

The application of heat to any body area usually requires the order of a physician. Even if heat, such as a hot water bottle, is used as a comfort measure, for warming "cold" feet, many agencies specify that the physician consent to its use. This is not only because of the possibility of burns but also because of the physiologic changes which occur throughout the body when heat is applied locally.

Extreme care should be taken when heating devices are used on children and elderly patients, as well as on irrational and unconscious patients. Such care includes frequent observation of the area to which heat is applied. When patients have known vascular disturbances, there is also a need for close observation as well as extra caution, such as increasing the heat gradually to the desired temperature, avoiding abrupt changes.

Electric Heating Pads. The electric heating pad is a popular means for applying dry heat locally. It is easy to apply, provides constant and even heat and is relatively safe to use. Nevertheless, careless handling can result in injury to the patient or the nurse as well as damage to the pad.

The heating element of an electric pad consists of a web of wires that convert electric current into heat. Crushing or creasing the wires may impair proper functioning, and portions of the pad will overheat. Burns and fire may result. Pins should be avoided for securing a pad, since there is danger of electric shock if a pin touches the wires. Pads with a waterproof covering are preferred, but they should not be operated in a wet or moist condition because of danger of short-circuiting the heating element and consequent shock.

Usually, the selector switch for controlling the heat of an electric pad is within easy reach of the patient. After the heat has been applied and a certain amount of depression of the peripheral nerve endings has taken place, the patient often increases the heat. Many persons have been burned in this manner. In some hospitals, the high heat control is removed by the engineering department before the pad is put into use. As further precaution, electric pads should not be used near oxygen.

Like other devices for applying dry heat, electric pads should be covered with flannel or similar material. This helps to make the heat therapy more comfortable for the patient. The pad can be used repeatedly when the cover is washed after each patient's use. However, it is important not to cover the pad too heavily, for heavy covering over an electric pad prevents adequate heat dissipation.

There also are plastic pads with tubular inner construction which can be filled with water (distilled water is specified by some manufacturers). An attached electric control unit heats the water and keeps it at an even temperature. The temperature is set prior to operation and the patient cannot change it because it requires a key. Such pads are useful on wet dressings when heat must be applied.

Hot Water Bags. When electric heating pads are not available, frequently the hot water bag is used. Hot water bags have disadvantages in that they may leak, and their weight makes them less comfortable than the electric pad.

To help to prevent burning the patient, it is considered essential to test the temperature of the water accurately with a thermometer before pouring it into the bag. A safe temperature range for infants under two years of age is from 105° F. to 115° F.; for children over two years of age and for adults, from 115° F. to 125° F.

In order to keep the bag as light as possible in weight and easy to mold to the body area, it should be filled about two-thirds full. The air remaining in the bag can be expelled in one of two ways: by placing the bag on a flat surface and permitting the water to come to the opening and then screwing in the stopper; or by holding the bag up and twisting the unfilled portion to remove the air and then screwing in the stopper. After the bag has been filled, hold it upside down to test it for leaks. Apply the flannel cover to the bag securely before placing it on the body part. In order that the patient may feel warmth immediately, the cover should be warmed before it is placed on the hot water bag. Otherwise, it will take time for the heat of the bag to be transmitted through the flannel.

The temperature ranges given above will produce the desired local effects if the bag is filled properly and the cover warmed. However, most patients will seem to think that the water is not hot enough. Unless the patient receives an explanation beyond simply telling him that the temperature will not burn him, it is likely that the bag may be filled from the hot water tap when the nurse is not around. If the patient cannot do it, a visitor or another patient may oblige.

Hip or Sitz Baths. As a means of applying tepid or hot water to the pelvic area, patients are often placed in a tub filled with sufficient water to reach the umbilicus. These baths are referred to as hip or sitz baths. When sitz baths are used frequently, as on a gynecologic or a surgical service, special tubs or chairs usually are available. Sitz tubs and chairs are designed so that the patient's buttocks fit into a rather deep seat which is filled with water of the desired temperature and the legs and the feet remain out of water. A regular bathtub is not as satisfactory for a sitz bath because the heat is applied also to the lower extremities, and this alters the effect desired in the pelvic region.

If the purpose of the sitz bath is to apply heat, water at a temperature of 110° F. to 115° F. for 15 minutes will produce relaxation of the parts involved after a short initial period of contraction. Warm water should not be used if considerable congestion is already present.

If the purpose of the sitz bath is to produce relaxation or to help to promote healing in a wound by cleansing it of discharge and slough, then water at a temperature of 94° F. to 98° F. should be used. The temperature of the water should be tested frequently to prevent too great a range from occurring.

Since a large body area is involved when a sitz bath is given, the patient should be observed closely for signs of weakness and faintness. The nature of the procedure also makes it necessary to protect the patient from exposure. Usually, a wash blanket is wrapped around the patient's shoulders and then draped over the tub. After the bath, the patient should be covered adequately and encouraged to remain out of drafts. If a warm sitz bath has been given, it may be best for the patient to go to bed until normal circulation is resumed.

Sitz tubs and chairs are not adjustable to the comfort needs of patients, especially the short patient. After the patient is in the tub or the chair, check to see whether or not there is pressure against the patient's thighs or legs. If the patient's feet do not touch the floor, and the weight of the legs is resting on the edge of the chair, objects such as a stool should be procured to support the feet and relieve the pressure on the vessels in the legs.

In addition to avoiding any pressure areas, it may be necessary to place a towel in the water to support the patient's back in the lumbar region. Fifteen to 20 minutes can seem like a very long time if one's body is not in good alignment and comfortable.

Soaks. The direct immersion of a body area into warm water or a medicated solution is referred to as a soak. The purposes for which soaks are used vary: to increase blood supply to a locally infected area, to aid suppuration, to aid in cleansing large sloughing wounds such as burns, to improve circulation and to apply medication to a locally infected area. A soak has the added advantage of making manipulation of a painful area much easier, since the body part is buoyed up by the weight of water it displaces.

If a soak is prescribed for a large wound, such as might cover an entire arm or lower leg or even an area of the torso, a compromise with sterile technic usually is made. The vessel into which the body area is placed is sterilized before use if possible; if not, the vessel should be cleaned scrupulously. Tap water is used for soaks, since it is accepted generally as being free from pathogens.

During the treatment, which is usually 15 to 20 minutes per soak, the temperature should be kept as constant as possible. This may be done by discarding some of the fluid every five minutes and replacing it, or by adding solution at a higher temperature.

Care must be taken to avoid burning the patient. If hot solution is added and it is not stirred or otherwise agitated, it will not diffuse into the cooler solution quickly enough to prevent discomfort or tissue injury.

Unless the temperature of the soak is prescribed by the physician, a range of 105° F. to 110° F. is considered as being physiologically effective and comfortable for the patient.

The vessel holding the fluid should be placed so that the part to be immersed is comfortable and the patient is in good body alignment. For example, an arm basin placed on top of the bedside stand may cause the patient's shoulders to be thrown out of alignment, and it may also cause pressure on the back of the patient's arm. Or, a hand basin may be so situated as to cause wrist fatigue. Whenever a soak basin is placed in position,

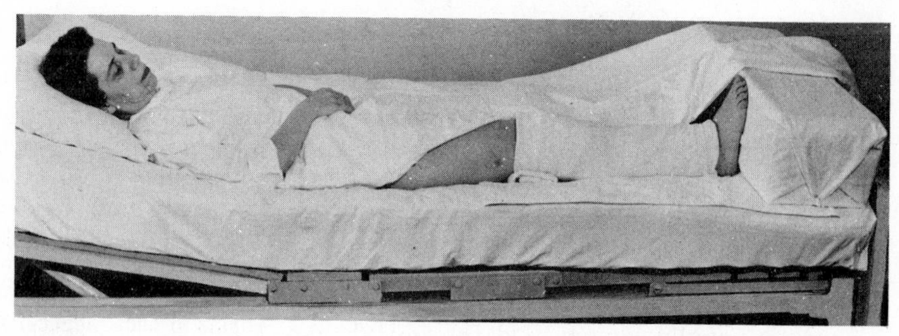

FIG. 31-1. In the application of heat or cold to any large surface area of the body, consideration always must be given to keeping the area in good alignment to prevent fatigue. Here the patient's foot is kept free from the wrapping on the leg so that it may be supported in dorsiflexion. A small support under the knee prevents hyperextension. The weight of a massive pack often restricts motion in the area. This, too, contributes to fatigue.

PRINCIPLES GUIDING ACTION FOR APPLYING HOT MOIST APPLICATIONS TO A BODY AREA

The purpose is to apply heat to an area to produce changes in the blood vessels and the underlying tissues. (Application to the lower leg is used as an example.)

SUGGESTED ACTION	PRINCIPLE
Prepare pieces of woolen or flannel material sufficiently large to cover the area adequately. (Knee to ankle.)	Absorbent and loosely woven fibers hold moisture.
Immerse the packs in hot water.	The woolen or flannel material absorbs the water slowly.
Prepare the patient's body area so that no time will be wasted in applying the pack after it is removed from the hot water. Place a dry pack and a waterproof cover (of plastic or aluminum foil) under the patient's leg so that the dry pack will cover the moist one, and the waterproof cover will be on the outside.	Air will reduce the temperature of the pack. The dry pack and the waterproof cover will act as insulation and will prevent rapid heat and moisture loss from the wet pack.
Lubricate the skin in the area of application with petrolatum.	Petrolatum delays the transmission of the heat from the pack to the skin.
Wring the hot wet packs until water does not drip from them.	Saturated packs will lose water.
Shake once or twice.	Loss of steam helps to reduce temperature.
Place the pack on the skin lightly and, after a few seconds, lift the pack to inspect the patient's skin for degree of redness.	Degree of vasodilatation indicates intensity of heat.
Wrap the pack around the area snugly and mold it to the skin surface.	Air is a poor conductor of heat. Air spaces between the skin and the pack will reduce the effect of the application.
Cover the moist pack with the dry pack and waterproof covering.	Insulation and covering prevent heat and moisture loss.

the nurse should look for pressure areas and observe the patient's degree of comfort.

Hot Moist Packs and Compresses. The application of warm moist flannels to a body area is referred to as a pack; warm moist gauze dressings are referred to as compresses. Packs usually are applied to a more extensive area. Packs and compresses differ from soaks primarily in two ways: the duration of the application of packs and compresses is usually longer, and the initial application of heat is more intense. Packs and compresses are applied as hot as the patient can tolerate them comfortably.

If an area is to be kept warm continuously by means of moist dressings, the frequency of the change of such applications will depend on the thickness of the material used for the application and the amount of protection given to it.

Because of the effect of the moist hot applications on circulation, the patient is likely to feel chilly. Precautionary comfort measures should be taken during and following the treatment to keep the patient, and especially the area which has been treated, warm and free from drafts.

Effects of Local Application of Cold

When cold is applied to the skin, the first visible reaction is vasoconstriction—that is, the caliber of the cutaneous vessels decreases. The skin becomes cool and pale. The skin receptors for cold are stimulated, the impulses are carried to the hypothalamus and the cerebral cortex, and the body reacts to

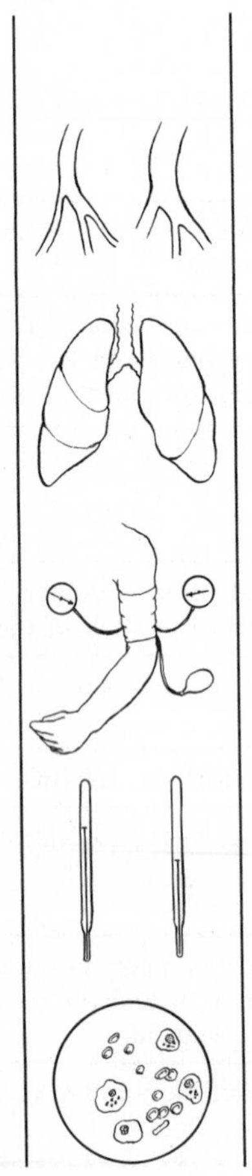

Fig. 31-2. Some major physiologic reactions to applications of heat and cold of short duration.

conserve heat. The constriction of blood vessels reduces circulation in the skin in order that heat may be conserved by preventing loss of heat from the blood to the environment.

In addition to vasoconstriction, there is a decrease in tissue metabolism in the area involved. Less oxygen is used, and fewer wastes accumulate. Cold also has an anesthetic effect on the skin, an important point to remember when applying cold applications, since the patient may become unaware of impulses from the skin which normally serve to warn that tissue damage is occurring.

Cold commonly is used immediately following contusions, sprains and strains in order to prevent the accumulation of fluid in body tissue (edema). If edema is already present, the application of cold will act to retard its relief, since circulating blood in the area is at a minimum, and excess fluid will not be reabsorbed as efficiently. The application of cold will aid in controlling hemorrhage by constricting vessels. Cold has practical uses for its anesthetic value. For example, areas of the body can be frozen and surgery performed without the patient's feeling pain. Lower temperatures are also used for checking inflammation and suppuration by decreasing blood supply, slowing cellular metabolism and inhibiting microbial activity.

Cold also affects remote areas of the body when applied locally. The amount of blood in other parts of the body increases as blood decreases in the part to which cold is applied because blood volume normally remains quite constant. When the body is chilled, it has been observed that vasoconstriction occurs in the nasal passages. This reaction explains the uncomfortable and harmful effects of cold and drafts when one is suffering with an upper respiratory infection.

It was pointed out earlier that, when heat was applied to the leg, underlying tissue temperature increased. The same study was done when an ice bag was placed on the leg and the following results were noted:

Interior of ice bag .... 32° F.
Outside of towel covering ice bag .... 40° F.
Cutaneous temperature declined from .... 84° F. to 43° F. (in 15 minutes)
Subcutaneous temperature declined from .... 94° F. to 70° F. (in about 1 hour)
Intramuscular temperature declined from .... 98° F. to 79° F. (in about 2 hours)

When cold air was blown over the leg, similar local temperature changes were noted, and more remote areas also were cooled.

Cold applied to the forehead demonstrated that the temperature of the interior of the brain, as far as two inches from the forehead, had dropped as much as 1.5° F.

Although the immediate effect of cold application is vasoconstriction, the prolonged effect is vasodilatation, again, a defense measure against excesses, probably largely reflex in nature. Therefore, the effects of prolonged cold and the effects of heat applied for shorter periods are approximately the same. Some authorities believe that prolonged cold causes damage of nerve supply to vessel walls, and that following such damage vasodilatation results.

Temperature for Cold Applications. As is true when heat is being applied, no arbitrary temperature can be stated for cold applications. The selection of temperature depends on such factors as duration of application, method of application, condition of the patient, conditon and sensitivity of the skin, area to be covered and the like. For short periods of time and for small areas, colder temperatures can be tolerated without discomfort or tissue damage. For longer periods of time, usually it is considered dangerous to keep skin temperatures below 40° F. except when ice is used for anesthesia.

The temperature of water used for cold applications usually is described as tepid, cool, cold or very cold. The temperature ranges stated frequently are as follows:

Tepid .... 80° F. to 93° F.
Cool .... 65° F. to 80° F.
Cold .... 55° F. to 65° F.
Very cold .... Below 55° F.

Local Application of Cold

Ice Bags. The device used frequently for applying cold to an area is the ice bag. As mentioned previously, the effect from such application may be either local or reflex in nature.

The ice bag is filled with small pieces of ice, making it easier to mold it to the contour of the body part and also reducing the amount of air spaces which act as insulators. After the bag is approximately two-thirds full, the air should be removed, for air, a poor conductor of heat, will interfere with the removal of heat from the body surface.

A cover should be placed on the ice bag to make it more comfortable for the patient and also to provide for absorption of the moisture which condenses on the outside of the bag.

To be effective as a local application, the ice bag should be applied for one-half to one hour and removed for approximately one hour. In this way the tissues are able to react to the effects of the cold.

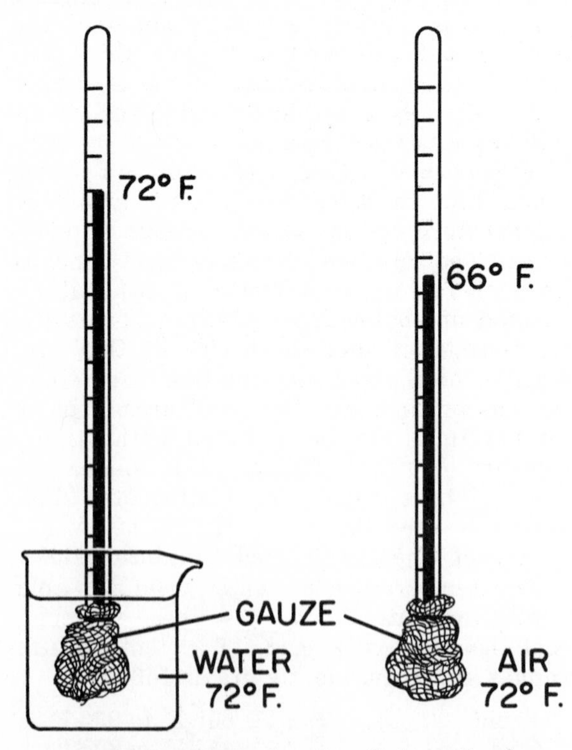

FIG. 31-3. Evidence of cooling effect resulting from evaporation. Gauze on thermometer in air is also saturated with water.

Cold Compresses. Moist, cold, local applications usually are referred to as cold compresses. They might be used for an injured eye, headache, tooth extraction—and, by some physicians, for hemorrhoids. The texture and the thickness of the material used will depend on the area to which it is to be applied. For example, eye compresses could be prepared from surgical gauze compresses which have a small amount of cotton filling. A wash cloth makes an excellent compress for the head or the face.

The material used for the application is immersed in a clean basin, appropriate for the size of the compress, that contains pieces of ice and a small amount of water. The compress should be wrung thoroughly before it is applied to avoid dripping, which is uncomfortable for the patient and may also wet the bed or clothing. The compresses should be changed frequently. Usually, the patient can feel when they have become warm, and many patients like to apply their own compresses. The application should be continued for 15 to 20 minutes and repeated every two to three hours.

Alcohol or Cold Sponge Baths

Occasionally, an alcohol or a cold sponge bath is recommended for reducing a patient's elevated temperature. Alcohol added to tepid water is tolerated more easily than a cold bath by most patients. Alcohol vaporizes at a relatively low temperature and therefore removes heat from the skin surfaces rapidly. Cold water very often produces a strong initial reactionary effect which elevates the temperature further.

When an alcohol or a cold sponge bath is given, it is essential that it be continued until the initial reaction of chilliness, or shivering is overcome and the body has adjusted to the temperature. Therefore, it is best if the procedure lasts for at least 25 to 30 minutes. Each extremity should be bathed for a five-minute period at least, and then the entire back and the buttocks for an additional 5 to 10 minutes.

During the procedure, place moist, cool cloths over large superficial blood vessels, as in the axilla and the groin as a further aid in lowering the temperature. A warm water bottle placed at the feet helps to overcome a sensation of chilliness. To help to prevent congestion and to provide comfort, an ice bag is applied to the head.

An ice mattress, a plastic pad which is filled continuously from a container of melting ice, is used in the care of patients who are in danger of having high temperature elevation or who need to have a high body temperature reduced. An ice mattress is used more commonly with patients having specific clinical problems, such as neurosurgery.

Study Situations

1. Some patients who have heating pads prescribed keep moving the regulator until it is in the "high" position. A patient probably will say that he does this because the pad is not warm enough. Why does he think it is not warm enough?

2. To clarify your understanding of physics principles underlying the correct use of heat and cold, consult a physics textbook and determine whether convection, conduction or evaporation is the primary process involved in each of the following situations:

Feeling chilly on a warm day when the humidity is about 40 per cent and a slight breeze is blowing

Feeling chilly in bed when you have insufficient covering

Feeling warm and uncomfortable when the temperature is 72° F. and the humidity is 85 per cent and there is no air movement

Feeling chilly when only your feet touch a cold floor as you leave a warm bed

If you make the effort to understand the principles in effect in the above situations, it also will increase your understanding of many nursing situations, such as, for example, the effect of air currents on older persons, the need for considering adequate covering for patients who are asleep or inactive, the reaction to being placed on a cold bedpan, the use of electric lamps for supplying heat to an infant's crib or to a patient's legs and the need for considering altering the temperature of bath water during different times of the year and for patients of different age groups.

3. In an attempt to understand more fully some of the effects of heat and cold, consider some of your own experiences and then explain them on the basis of physical or physiologic principles.

For example, why does your entire body feel warm after you have kept only your hands in warm water to wash dishes? Who in your family or among your friends is least able to handle hot objects or cold objects, or requires a higher or lower room temperature to be comfortable?

References

1. Abramson, D. E. *et al*: (Abs.) Comparison of wet and dry heat in raising temperature of tissues.
   AMER. J. NURS., *68*:835-836, April, 1968.
2. Brouha, L.: Heat and the older worker.
   J. AMER. GERIAT. SOC., *10*:35, January, 1962.
3. Gaunt, D.: A small ice bag.
   AMER. J. NURS., *62*:75, April, 1962.
4. Halsell, M.: Moist heat for relief of postoperative pain.
   AMER. J. NURS., *67*:767-770, April, 1967.
5. Hardwick, R. G.: Two cases of accidental hypotherma.
   BRIT. M. J., *5272*:147, January 20, 1962.
6. Licht, S.: Therapeutic Heat and Cold. ed. 2, pp. 126-159.
   New Haven, Conn., Elizabeth Licht, 1965.
7. Sheldon, N. S.: Sterile warm wet compresses.
   AMER. J. NURS., *59*:982, July, 1959.
8. Wise, C. S.: Heat and Cold in Bierman, W., and Licht, S. (eds.): Physical Medicine in General Practice. ed. 3, pp. 1-25, New York, Hoeber, 1955.

Nursing Responsibilities in Relation to Assisting the Physician with Diagnostic and Therapeutic Measures

Unit 6

CHAPTER

32

The Role of the Nurse as Assistant

Introduction

For many diagnostic and therapeutic measures performed by the physician the assistance of the nurse is required. Measures common to most clinical services are discussed in this Unit. Those which are unique to more specific clinical entities are discussed in clinical texts.

When the nurse assists the physician, she is guided by the same three broad principles, first discussed in Chapter 4, of understanding the patient's needs as an individual, maintaining his physiologic functioning and providing for his safety. These principles guide the nurse even though the specific nursing care will vary among patients depending on such factors as his age, health problems, personal problems and the like, or whether the extent of the measure is considered to be simple or radical. The nurse might well ask herself these questions before acting as an assistant to the physician: What does the measure mean to the patient, and what should I understand about the patient in order to put him at ease? Why is the measure necessary, and what should I know about it to understand how it is related to his present state of health? What should be considered for the patient's safety?

Responsibilities of the Nurse

The nurse's responsibilities when she assists the physician fall into several broad categories. Generally, there are responsibilities that she fulfills without the physician's direction or orders for the patient; there are those that she carries out for or with the latter; and there may be agency policies and procedures which she is also obliged to observe.

Understanding the Procedure. The nurse must understand the measure if she is to prepare the patient both mentally and physically and to assist the physician skillfully so that it is carried out with the least distress to the patient. Such knowledge will guide her in her explanation of the treatment and its relationship to the patient's illness and recovery; the amount and the kind of equipment needed; its proper placement for efficiency of performance; the most effective yet most comfortable position for the patient during the treatment; and the kind of aftercare needed by the patient.

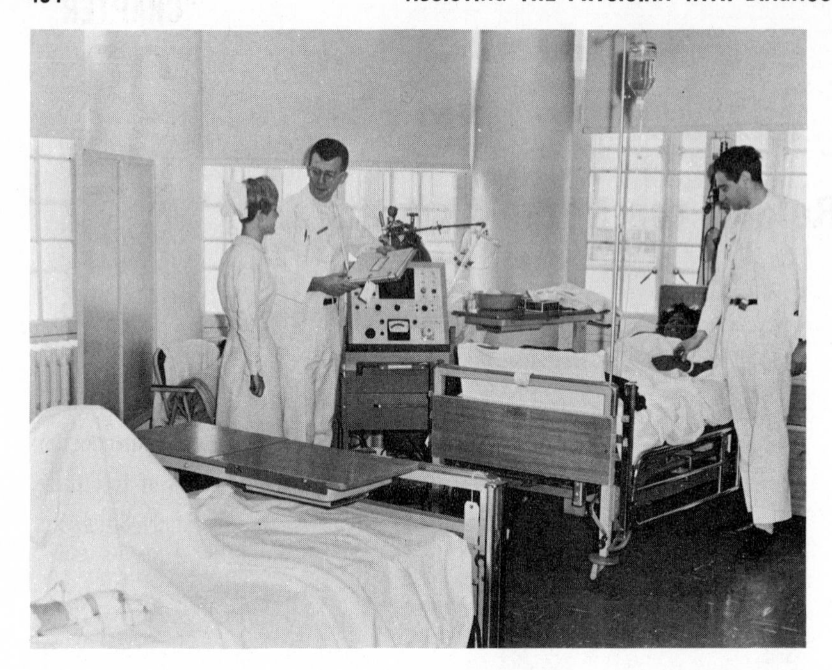

FIG. 32-1. Comprehensive care depends upon the cooperation of many of the health personnel. Here the nurse and physicians are discussing the care of patients in the intensive care unit. (Courtesy of New York Hospital—Cornell Medical Center)

Understanding the Patient, His Illness and His Medical Therapy. In earlier Units, the importance of the nurse's observations was stressed repeatedly. This responsibility is no less important when the nurse assists the physician. Prior to carrying out a treatment and during and following it, the physician depends on the nurse's careful observations as a guide to further decisions concerning the patient's plan of therapy.

In order to observe the patient intelligently, the nurse must be familiar with the following: the patient's diagnosis and the cause of his illness; the physician's plan of therapy for the patient; the patient's response (physical and mental) to his illness and to therapy; the normal physiologic functioning of the body and the manner in which the disease process interferes with normal functioning; the reasons for carrying out the diagnostic or the therapeutic measure; the common effects of it, both desirable and possibly untoward, and symptoms of such; and measures to prevent complications that may occur either during or after treatment.

Preparing the Patient. Although the physician usually is responsible for telling the patient about the procedure which he will perform, the nurse still assumes responsibility in helping the patient to understand it and the reasons for it. No exact rules can be stated as to how to prepare the patient mentally and what to teach him. The same principles apply as have been discussed earlier in relation to teaching the patient and explaining procedures to him. In general, the nurse will be guided by the physician's wishes, the condition of the patient and the individual circumstances that exist.

The physical preparation of the patient depends to a great extent on the nature of the procedure. However, usually the patient will be more comfortable during any procedure if he voids first. A certain amount of anxiety and the excitement associated with the procedure often stimulate the urge to void. Usually, it is inconvenient and sometimes almost impossible to offer a bedpan or a urinal during a treatment measure.

Preparation also may include dressing the patient in garments that will protect him from exposure and free him from concern over soiled linen. In addition, it may be necessary to transport the patient to a location where the treatment can be performed more easily. The advantage of such a move should be explained carefully so that the patient recognizes that it is for his comfort and safety.

Observing Agency Policies. The nurse must acquaint herself with and observe the agency's policies concerning diagnostic and therapeutic measures with which she will assist. For example, a written consent of the patient, the guardian or the responsible family member may be necessary before certain diagnostic or therapeutic measures can be carried out. In some agencies, this is cared for at the time of admission by an admitting officer. In others, the assisting nurse may be responsible for obtaining consent.

In some agencies, policies will govern where and when certain measures may be carried out. In those situations, the nurse, as well as the physician, obliges.

Preparing Equipment for the Procedure. The nurse is responsible for preparing the necessary equipment. Although equipment varies among health agencies, certain basic types are necessary, and the nurse prepares the appropriate equipment accordingly. While assembling and preparing the equipment, the nurse also considers which aspects require medical or surgical asepsis.

Preparing the Working Unit. Many agencies have special rooms for carrying out diagnostic and therapeutic measures which are arranged conveniently and eliminate the necessity of carrying equipment to the patient's unit. If the patient is not able to be moved to such a room, it then becomes necessary for the nurse to prepare a suitable working area in the patient's unit. A blood transfusion is more comfortable and convenient for the patient if he remains in bed, in which case the nurse prepares the patient's unit accordingly.

Whether the procedure is carried out in a special room or at the patient's bedside, the nurse is responsible for seeing that privacy is provided for the patient, that the room is free of drafts and that there is good lighting.

Assisting the Physician. The nurse usually assembles the equipment and the materials in the working unit. She places the patient in the required position so that he is as comfortable as possible but so that it is convenient for the physician. (The position depends on the procedure and will be discussed later in relation to each one.) The patient is draped appropriately and according to local procedure, exposing only the area that is involved.

In some instances, the nurse prepares the skin at the site where the body will be entered. The skin is cleansed thoroughly according to local procedure to minimize the danger of injecting organisms into the tissues. Previous discussions have indicated the necessity of precaution in considering the action of antiseptic solutions on the skin. Since the skin cannot be sterilized, it is of prime importance to cleanse it as thoroughly as possible, remembering that soap and water are very effective for cleansing and that antiseptics at best cannot render the skin sterile.

Items should be placed so that the physician and the nurse will not be required to reach across a sterile field, thus minimizing the danger of contamination. The physician uses gloves where it is necessary for him to handle sterile equipment. He hands necessary pieces to the nurse for connection to containers of solutions, suction equipment, specimen containers and the like. She may hold drugs and anesthesia for the physician to withdraw from vials. If the nurse is asked to handle the drug or a solution for injection, she should not only personally check the label on the container but also provide an opportunity for the physician to read it in order to eliminate the danger of an error or a misunderstanding concerning the nature of the drug or the solution to be injected.

While the physician is working, the nurse has two primary responsibilities: observing the patient and assisting with equipment and materials as necessary.

The nurse observes the patient's reaction to the procedure. She watches for immediate effects, the untoward as well as the desired, and reports them to the physician as indicated. While speaking with the physician during the procedure, the nurse exercises care in her comments and remembers that the patient is usually alert and easily disturbed should the conversation in his opinion suggest some danger or untoward effect.

Caring for the Patient. When the procedure

is completed, the nurse helps return the patient to his unit and to make him comfortable.

The patient should be observed for symptoms, desirable and undesirable, that will indicate the effect of the procedure. These may occur soon afterward, or, in some cases, delayed reactions may occur as late as 24 or 48 hours or longer after the procedure has been completed.

To Record the Procedure. The physician records the treatment on the patient's progress notes. The nurse is responsible for entering it on the Nurses' Notes. Local policy determines the exact manner in which the nurse records the measure and the patient's reaction to it. The following information usually is included: the date and the time; the name of the treatment; if a drug was injected, the name and the amount; if drainage was present, the nature and the amount; if specimens were collected, their number and their nature; the name of the physician and the name of the nurse assisting.

In addition, the patient's reactions are recorded, including those which occur during and immediately following the measure and any delayed reactions.

Caring for the Equipment. In some agencies the nurse takes care of used equipment. If the nurse does not do this, an auxiliary worker may carry out this portion of the procedure. It is important to cleanse the nondisposable equipment as soon as possible, since it is more difficult to remove coagulated substances. This is particularly true when blood has been injected or removed. All persons handling soiled equipment should be aware of the hazards involved, especially from punctures from needles and other sharp instruments which have been in contact with the patient's blood. The patient appreciates having the equipment removed as soon as possible so he does not have to look at it.

Study Situations

1. The role of the nurse as assistant to the physician is not one of being merely another pair of hands. Hopefully, this has been made clear in the text. Rather, the nurse should be an intelligent thinking and functioning teammate of the physician. This may not be the image of the nurse held by many physicians. In some instances, it may not even be the nurse's image of herself. There is much that both can do to foster a relationship that is in harmony with the health team concept. Read the following and consider your own feelings about your relationship with the physicians, your experiences with them and what you think can be done by nurses.

• Macgregor, F. C.: Social Science in Nursing. pp. 265-272.
New York, Russell Sage Foundation, 1960.

2. Although this article focuses on "principles of preparation adapted to a child's way of thinking," they are not without application to the adult who is also the recipient of various kinds of treatments.

• Wu, R.: Explaining treatments to young children.
AMER. J. NURS., *65*:71-73, July, 1965.

CHAPTER 33

Commonly Used Therapeutic and Diagnostic Measures

Since attention has been given in the previous chapter to the nurse's role as assistant, responsibilities common to all measures will not be repeated. What will be stressed are specific nursing points for each situation.

Intravenous Infusion

Intravenous infusions were discussed in Chapter 29, since in some states nurses are taught the principles of injecting a vein. In some health agencies, nurses are permitted to start infusions. However, in many others the physician is still the only one permitted to inject a vein with a drug or to start an infusion.

When the physician performs the treatment, the nurse may assist by preparing all the necessary equipment and the solution and adding the drugs, if ordered. She immobilizes the site of choice, puts the tourniquet in place and removes the air from the tubing. If the set-up so requires, she should also be ready to hand the tubing to the physician after the needle is in the site. The nurse should be ready to adjust the rate of flow as soon as the solution begins to enter the vein;

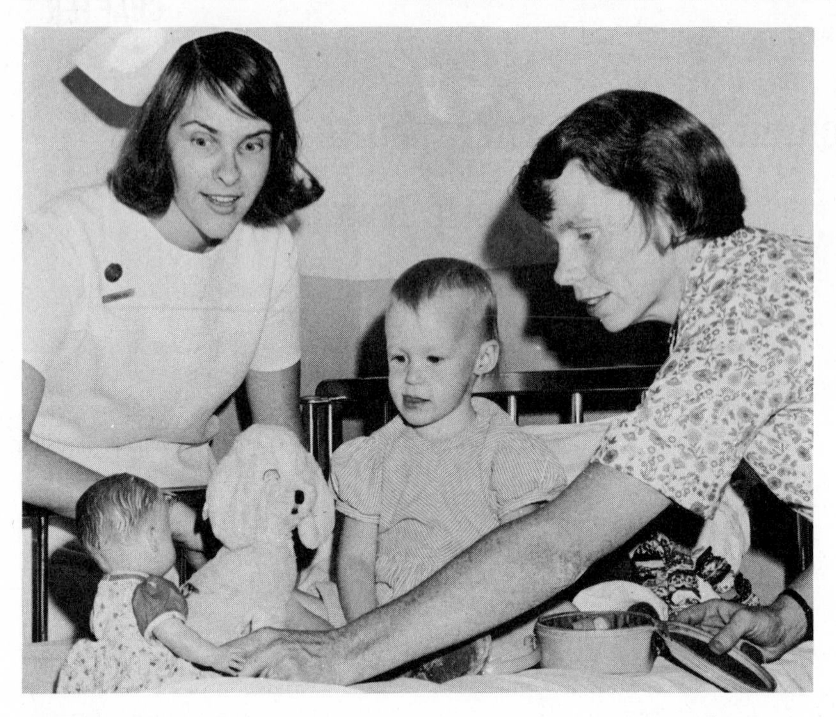

FIG. 33-1. Permitting a parent to assist in the care of a child can be helpful to both parent and child. This is especially so if the child is receiving many treatments or having many diagnostic tests. Here the nurse is instructing a mother in the hospital care of her 18-month-old daughter.

The same applies to older patients. Having a family member remain with the patient following a diagnostic test, or even to feed him, can be helpful. (Courtesy the New York Hospital—Cornell Medical Center)

many times she will be left to anchor the needle also. It is the nurse's responsibility to regulate the flow as needed during the treatment, to add additional solution if ordered and, when all the solution is absorbed, to discontinue the infusion.

Cut-Down to a Vein. When the superficial veins are not readily accessible, it may be necessary to make an incision into the skin over a vein. Cut-down sets, as they are called, usually are obtained from the Central Supply Room. They contain the necessary items for the procedure. This procedure of entering a vein is carried out under surgical asepsis since it constitutes minor surgery. The physician wears sterile gloves, and many agencies specify that the physician and the nurse wear masks. Plastic tubing, (radiopaque) is threaded through the needle and placed into the vein. It is held in place with a suture. When the plastic tubing is removed, a stitch or two is placed in the skin at the site of incision.

Intravenous Injection

Intravenous injection refers to the direct introduction of a drug in solution into a vein. In most health agencies, the physician is responsible for administering intravenous injections. The nurse usually prepares the drug for him and assists him during the procedure if the patient's condition warrants it.

Indications for Intravenous Injection. Drugs are administered intravenously for several reasons. For example, certain ones are so irritating that other routes rarely are used; also, when the quickest possible action of a drug is desired, as in an emergency, the intravenous route is ideal, since no time is lost in absorption. This route is used too when it is particularly desirable to eliminate the variability of absorption.

Dyes are injected intravenously for diagnostic purposes, especially for x-ray studies of the kidneys, the ureters and the bladder. Some anesthetics are administered intravenously, thiopental sodium being an example.

Necessary Equipment for Intravenous Injection. The preparation of a drug for intravenous injection is almost identical with that for an intramuscular or subcutaneous injection. The same precautions are used in selecting and preparing the drug. The size of the syringe will depend on the amount of solution, and the size of the needle will depend on the age and the condition of the patient, the viscosity of the solution and the rapidity with which the physician wishes to inject it. For the average adult patient, a 20- or 22-gauge needle is used most commonly for the injection. When the drug is ready for the physician to inject, the nurse repeats the name of the drug and the dose to him before handing him the syringe. If possible, the container in which the drug was dispensed should be given to him to read. The safest practice is never to prepare drugs for intravenous therapy far in advance of the time to be used and never to leave them unattended or out of sight. A tourniquet, antiseptic and gauze or cotton balls will also be needed by the physician.

Drugs are also injected into intravenous tubing if an infusion is running. The tubing is cleansed before the needle, usually 25 gauge, is inserted. This is done in the area close to the needle.

Blood Transfusion

A blood transfusion is the infusion of whole blood given by a healthy person for injection into a patient's vein. The person giving the blood is referred to as the *donor*, while the patient is called the *recipient*.

Blood may be given by either the *direct* or the *indirect* method. The indirect method is used most commonly. The technic is similar to that for giving an intravenous infusion.

The direct method is used rarely. It involves infusing blood directly from the donor's vein to the recipient's vein and usually is performed only in an operating room.

Selecting Blood Donors. The selection of blood donors must be done with care. It is also important to determine whether or not the donor is free of diseases, as for example, infectious hepatitis. Persons who have allergies usually are not used; nor those with a history of a chronic disease, such as tuberculosis. As a further precaution, some blood banks will not accept blood from a donor who has been immunized recently.

Also, the donor is examined carefully at the time of donation and is permitted to give blood only if his heart and chest sounds, blood count, temperature, pulse and respiratory rate and blood pressure are within normal ranges.

Blood Groupings. Before blood may be given to a patient, it must be determined that the blood of the donor and that of the recipient are compatible. This means not only type and Rh factors, but also crossmatching of the donor's and the recipient's blood.

Table 13. The system of nomenclature for blood groupings in man and their approximate incidence

International Landsteiner	Jansky	Moss	Approximate Per Cent of Incidence
O	I	IV	45
A	II	II	40
B	III	III	10
AB	IV	I	5

Research in this area indicates that an individual's blood is as unique as his fingerprints. In addition to four groups, there are many hundreds of other factors which differentiate one blood from another.

Necessary Equipment for Indirect Blood Transfusion. Because a vein is being entered, sterile technic is employed. The equipment necessary for the procedure is similar to that used for an intravenous infusion by the gravity method. The drip chamber in a transfusion set contains a filter. A slightly larger needle, usually an 18 gauge, is used because of the viscosity of the blood. If the patient is sensitive to the pain of the larger needle as it pierces the skin, the physician may inject a small amount of local anesthetic intradermally at the site of the injection or use a volatile anesthetic spray for numbing the pain receptors.

The blood is dispensed in bottles or in plastic containers by a blood bank or a laboratory and is ready for use. The container is the one used for obtaining the blood from the donor and contains a solution to prevent clotting.

If blood is obtained for a transfusion and then for some reason is not to be used immediately, it should be returned to the place of issue for storage. It is not considered safe to allow blood to stand at room temperature for several hours prior to administration. When the policies of the blood bank or the laboratory governing the management of blood are adhered to, fewer reactions occur, and the patient's safety is assured.

Warming blood prior to infusion is not necessary or even wise. The blood warms sufficiently by the time it has passed the length of the tubing and entered the vein. Furthermore, warming the blood tends to destroy certain blood cells and favors the growth of any organisms that may have entered it accidentally.

Occasionally, when small amounts are being given, as for children, the syringe method is used. The necessary equipment is the same as that used for intravenous injections.

In the management of blood for transfusion, every precaution should be taken. *Check and double check the labels, the numbers, the Rh factors and compatability.* The nurse and the doctor check the blood at the patient's bedside.

Assisting the Physician. The nurse's role in assisting the physician when a transfusion is being started is similar to that for intravenous infusions. Before the transfusion is started, the nurse checks the blood with the physician. The patient's name, his hospital number and the blood group and the Rh factor of the patient and the donor are checked again. Because the dangers of using incorrect blood are so serious, the importance of careful checking cannot be overstressed.

After the transfusion has been started, it is the nurse's responsibility to see that the blood is administered at the rate of flow specified by the physician. However, during the time blood is flowing the nurse should check the rate carefully. Changing the height of the bed and elevating or lowering the patient's head can alter the rate of flow. The chance of injury to the blood cells is minimized when the filter is covered with blood. This avoids having the blood hit the filter as it leaves the container. Repositioning the extremity in which the needle is located may halt or change the rate of flow. In addition, the bottle should be agitated from time to time, since red blood cells settle to the bottom and plasma rises to the top.

The physician may order additional fluids to be given after the blood has been absorbed. Agency policy may determine if a nurse adds these solutions, or if two persons must check the solutions added.

Observing the Patient for Signs of a Reaction. Reactions to transfusion rarely occur when every precaution has been observed in selecting the proper blood and in sterilizing and preparing the equipment. However, because errors sometimes do happen, it is essential that the nurse recognize the signs and the symptoms of untoward effects of a transfusion. While many authors have categorized the reactions most likely to result from incompatible or contaminated blood, the picture is complicated somewhat by the fact that many of the symptoms and signs are common to more than one kind of reaction. No untoward effects or discomfort accompany a blood transfusion if all factors of safety and matching of blood have been observed carefully. Any sign of discomfort or any change in the patient's appearance or expression should be taken into careful consideration if a blood transfusion is being administered or has been recently administered.

The most serious and quickest complication to occur is the hemolytic reaction when incompatible bloods have been mixed. If the patient begins to have symptoms of discomfort, such as headache, sensations of tingling, difficulty in breathing or pain in the lumbar region, stop the transfusion and notify the physician immediately.

Other reactions may occur after the transfusion has been running for a short time, or perhaps many hours later. They are caused by protein substances to which the patient is allergic. The patient may complain of feeling itchy, especially in areas where the skin is warm, as the back and the buttocks. If hives (urticaria) appear near the site of the needle or on other parts of the body, the reaction is easy to recognize. However, the picture may be complicated if the patient also complains of difficulty in breathing and has laryngeal edema. For allergic reactions, the blood is also stopped immediately.

Febrile reactions, which may be due to some contaminant in the blood, usually occur late in the course of the transfusion or after it has been completed. The patient has an elevated temperature and shows signs of a systemic infection. Flushing of the skin and general malaise are typical.

Occasionally, the addition of blood to the existing supply produces circulatory overload, which is noted by increased pulse rate and dyspnea. This may result in pulmonary edema which can be recognized by signs of respiratory distress, moist coughing and possibly expectoration of blood-tinged mucus.

Since blood given by the indirect method contains substances to help prevent clotting, it is not unlikely that some individuals may react to these chemicals. Usually, the reaction is mild and of short duration, but it does produce discomfort for the patient and bears careful watching.

Transfusion of Blood Extracts. Some patients do not need all the constituents of whole blood. For example, one may need red blood cells but not the plasma and its constituents. Red blood cells in concentrated form sometimes are given to these patients. In other situations, only plasma is required. Human serum or plasma is particularly useful in emergencies for immediate restoration of fluids, since serum presents no compatibility problem and time need not be lost matching bloods and seeking donors.

Fractions, such as serum albumin and gamma globulin, have been separated out of plasma and used for the treatment and the prevention of certain diseases.

Hypodermoclysis

A hypodermoclysis is a subcutaneous infusion and is utilized for the purpose of restoring fluids and electrolytes. The fluid is injected slowly into subcutaneous tissue where absorption occurs via the blood capillaries. This route can be used when the oral and the intravenous routes are unsatisfactory.

Indications for Hypodermoclysis. The indications for administering fluids and electrolytes by hypodermoclysis are the same as those for administering them intravenously. Absorption occurs more slowly than when the intravenous route is used; therefore, desired effects cannot be observed as quickly.

The amount and the kind of solution are determined by the physician. The solution usually used is isotonic or occasionally hypotonic. Hypertonic solutions may cause water and salt depletion and damage to the subcutaneous tissue. If a hypertonic solution is indicated and this route must be used, only small amounts of solution are administered because of the associated dangers.

To hasten the rate of absorption, the enzyme (or enzyme complex), hyaluronidase or similar product is used. This drug dissolves cellular protective substances and thus makes it possible for the solution to enter the circulatory system more rapidly. It is effective for this procedure as well as for speeding the absorption of hematomas and certain drugs that ordinarily are absorbed slowly from the tissues.

Necessary Equipment for Hypodermoclysis. Hypodermoclysis usually is administered to adults by the gravity method. For children, the amount of fluid is less and usually is injected slowly at one time, using the syringe method. It is difficult and undesirable to restrain acutely ill children for a prolonged period of time.

Because subcutaneous tissue is being entered, sterile technic is employed for preparing equipment and administering a hypodermocylsis.

The tubing contains a Y connector which makes it possible for the solution to flow through two pieces of tubing. Each of the pieces of tubing to which the needles will be attached has a clamping device. These should be clamped before the tubing is inserted into the container of fluid and hung on the pole. As it is with intravenous infusions, fluid is permitted to flow through the tubing slowly to force out the air. One tube at a time should be released. The tubes are clamped again, and the tips are protected until the needles are attached, to prevent their becoming contaminated. Safest practice is not to attach the needles until the physician is ready to insert them. Some hospitals permit nurses to insert needles in the anterior thighs.

For the adult patient the most common

sites of injection are the anterior thighs. However, for the adult female, the area directly below the breasts can be used. A 19-gauge needle, two and one-half or three inches long, is usually used in these areas. The needles are inserted below the skin into subcutaneous tissue and then moved along horizontally in the tissue.

For children, the sites directly over the scapula are used. An intramuscular needle of 20 or 22 gauge, one and one-half inches long, is usually satisfactory for a child.

To minimize the immediate effect of the needle's penetrating the skin, some physicians may wish to use an application of a local anesthetic to numb the area.

Preparation of the Patient. The patient should be made as comfortable as possible and protected from exposure. His position will depend on the area of the body to be entered. If the thighs are used, it will be necessary to divide the top bedclothes so that the tubing is not disturbed. This necessitates adjusting the bed linen to provide appropriate covering considering the patient's age, physical condition and room temperature. Freedom of movement for the patient is also a consideration. A loin cloth will protect the patient's perineum from exposure.

Since the solution is absorbed slowly and the procedure continues over a period of several hours, the patient should be turned or at least have his position altered somewhat, every half hour. Patients frequently are reluctant to move for fear of dislodging the needles or of creating discomfort for themselves.

Assisting the Physician. After the patient is in the appropriate position for the procedure, the skin is prepared with an antiseptic. Shave the area if necessary. After the physician inserts the needles, each needle is held in place with strips of adhesive placed above the hubs. The physician may wish to place small pieces of sterile gauze under each needle to support them at an angle that permits solution to flow into subcutaneous tissue. Usual practice is to inject the hyaluronidase as soon as the solution begins to flow. A two-cc. syringe and a 25-gauge needle are used to inject the prescribed amount into the rubber inserts in the tubing directly above the needle attachments.

Solutions given by hypodermoclysis must be given slowly enough to allow for absorption. Allowing the solution to enter the subcutaneous tissue too rapidly may damage tissues. The nurse is responsible for adjusting the rate according to the speed of absorption. If absorption occurs slowly, the fluid accumulates in the tissue, the area of injection becomes swollen, and the skin over the area becomes taut. Should this occur, gentle massage over the area helps to speed the absorption of fluid. In addition to keeping check on the rate of flow and the rate of absorption, the nurse observes the patient for signs that indicate the desired effect of the hypodermoclysis. These signs depend to a large extent on the amount and the kind of solution administered. Reactions rarely occur when solutions are given by hypodermoclysis.

If more than one bottle of solution is ordered for the patient, the nurse adds the additional bottles as necessary.

Discontinuing a Hypodermoclysis. When the amount of solution that the physician has ordered has been absorbed, the nurse assumes responsibility for discontinuing the hypodermoclysis. The adhesive strips are removed, and the needles are removed quickly. Some of the solution tends to escape from the subcutaneous tissue where the needles have been inserted. To prevent this from occurring, a small sterile dressing may be applied snugly.

Lumbar Puncture

A lumbar puncture, or spinal tap, is the insertion of a needle into the subarachnoid space in the spinal canal.

Indications for a Lumbar Puncture. Cerebrospinal fluid normally fills the ventricles of the brain, the subarachnoid space and the central canal of the spinal cord. The fluid is clear and transparent. It may be necessary to enter the subarachnoid space for several reasons: to obtain a specimen of the fluid for analysis and for culture, to establish any alterations in the usual pressure of the cerebrospinal fluid, to relieve pressure, to inject drugs or to inject dyes for x-ray visualization.

Necessary Equipment. Because the subarachnoid space is a sterile cavity, surgical asepsis is observed. Normally, the cerebrospinal fluid pressure is greater than atmospheric pressure, and many pathogenic conditions of the central nervous system are characterized by an increase in this normal pressure. Therefore, the lumbar puncture needle contains a carefully and precisely fitted stylet so that fluid will not escape while the needle is in place, except when the physician removes the stylet.

The necessary sterile equipment includes a 20- or 22-gauge lumbar puncture needle, three to five inches long; a small syringe and a 22- or 25-gauge needle for the injection of local anesthesia at the site of injection; a fenestrated drape, gauze and cotton balls and gloves for the physician. Many sets include specimen containers and some a manometer for measuring the pressure of the fluid. If not included, they are added at the appropriate time. If the physician wishes to inject a drug into the spinal canal, another sterile syringe of the appropriate size is necessary. The local anesthetic of the physician's choice is brought to the working unit. One per cent procaine hydrochloride usually is used.

Prior to the procedure, the nurse examines the skin area where the physician will be working. If hair is present, the physician is asked whether he wishes the area to be shaved.

Assisting the Physician. The fourth or the fifth lumbar space is the usual site of entry. The needle enters the subarachnoid space by passing between the vertebrae into the canal. In order to spread the vertebrae and to provide the widest possible space for easier insertion of the needle, the patient is positioned on his side and with his back arched. Figure 33-2 illustrates this position. He is brought near the edge of the bed or the treatment table where the physician will work. The patient is asked to flex his knees and bring his head and shoulders down as close as possible to his knees. A small pillow may be placed under the patient's head and between his knees for comfort. Some patients are unable to assume or maintain this position without assistance. This can be done by facing the patient and grasping him behind his knees with one arm and behind his neck with the other arm so that the back remains arched as much as possible. Other patients may have difficulty in understanding or be disoriented. They will need repeated assurances of what is being done. However, the head should not be pulled down or the knees pressed against the abdomen, since this increases intraspinal fluid pressure, leading to a falsely elevated pressure.

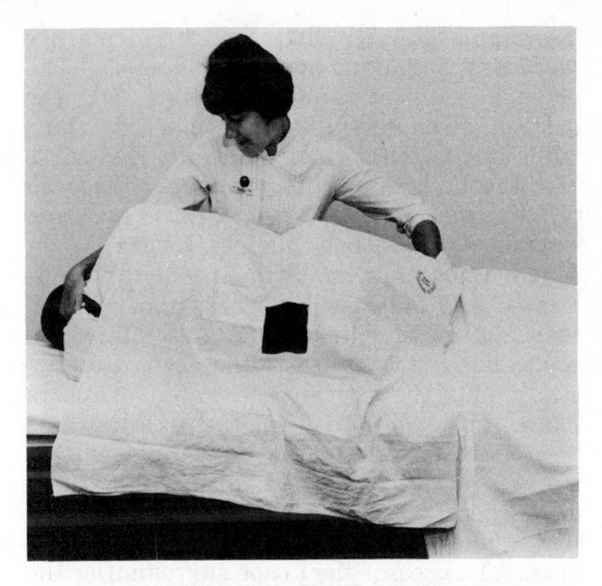

FIG. 33-2. Position of patient for a lumbar puncture. The nurse is helping this patient to assume and maintain the desired position by holding her one arm behind his knees so that they are flexed and bringing his head forward by putting her other arm behind his neck. In this position his back is arched.

The nurse may have to help the patient to maintain the desired position. After helping the physician to get his equipment in order, the nurse returns to the opposite side of the bed to do this. It is important to explain to the patient that he must remain motionless during the procedure. Moving about makes insertion of the needle more difficult and also may cause the needle to break.

Occasionally, the physician may prefer having the patient in the sitting position during the lumbar puncture. The patient sits on the edge of a treatment table, his feet are supported on a chair and his arms are placed over the shoulders of a person who helps to support him in position. Or, the patient straddles a straight-backed chair while facing the back of the chair. He arches his back by bringing his arms over the back of the chair and allowing his head and shoulders to rest over the chair back.

The fourth or the fifth lumbar space is located approximately at the same level on the back as the iliac crest. After an antiseptic has been applied to the area, the physician puts the sterile fenestrated drape in place. The opening is over the area that has been cleansed and where the needle will be inserted. Care should be taken so that the drape does not slip about during the procedure and thereby contaminate the working area. The area of the drape surrounding the working area is kept sterile.

The nurse prepares the bottle of anesthetic that the physician has ordered and holds it so that he can check the label and withdraw some, or the nurse may pour the drug. The physician begins the procedure by anesthetizing the skin and the subcutaneous tissue at the site of injection.

When the anesthesia is effective, the physician inserts the lumbar puncture needle. After the needle is in place, the physician may apply the manometer to the needle to determine the cerebrospinal pressure. The pressure normally is not constant and will be observed to fluctuate somewhat with each pulse beat and each respiration. The normal average range of pressure is about 6 to 12 mm. of mercury or 90 to 150 mm. of water. The physician may ask the nurse to make a notation of the pressure reading. If the lumbar puncture needle is resting freely in the subarachnoid space, pressure usually can be increased when venous compression occurs. The physician may ask the nurse to apply hand pressure to the abdomen. The pressure can also be increased by compressing the jugular vein. This is called the Queckenstedt test and is used if intraspinal lesions are suspected. The most reliable reading can be obtained by the use of the blood pressure cuff wrapped about the neck. This provides for a more even pressure. The mercury column is elevated to 50 mm. Since there is variation in this practice, the nurse should always understand the physician's procedure if she is to assist in this test.

After pressure has been determined, specimens will be collected if desired. If sterile tubes are provided in the set, the physician may collect the specimens himself and hand them to the nurse for proper labeling and handling.

If not included, the physician may ask the nurse to hold the tubes below the opening of the needle while he regulates the flow of cerebrospinal fluid with the stylet. Care should be observed to prevent touching the needle or the hands of the physician with the collecting tubes.

During the procedure, the nurse observes the patient's reaction carefully. His color, pulse rate and respiratory rate are noted and reported to the physician immediately if anything unusual is observed. Care should be exercised to prevent alarming the patient if any report is being given to the physician.

When the procedure is completed, the needle is removed, and compression is applied to the site for a short while. A small sterile piece of gauze may be applied to the site and fastened with adhesive.

Immediately following the procedure, the patient may be placed in the recumbent position, preferably without a pillow. Fluids usually are offered. This is intended to avoid postspinal headache. It generally is believed that the headache is due to the tear in the dura mater made by the needle, which allows for seepage of small amounts of cerebrospinal fluid. Experience has shown that headaches are rare or at least not severe if patients are kept flat immediately following the procedure. If a headache does occur, the patient usually is treated symptomatically.

The patient's general physical reaction to the procedure is observed. This is of particular importance if the procedure was carried out to relieve pressure. Any unusual reactions such as twitching, vomiting, or slow pulse are reported to the physician promptly.

Cisternal Puncture

The subarachnoid space may also be entered by a cisternal puncture. Indications for its use are the same as for a lumbar puncture. The point of entry is in the suboccipital area. The usual site is over the prominent second cervical vertebra. The patient is placed on his side as for a lumbar puncture, but the neck rather than the back is arched. The suboccipital area is shaved prior to the procedure.

The necessary equipment and the procedure are the same as those for a lumbar puncture. The observation of the patient and the charting also are the same. Only rarely do patients complain of headaches following a cisternal puncture.

Thoracentesis

A thoracentesis is the aspiration of fluid from the pleural cavity. The pleural cavity is a potential cavity, since normally it is not distended with fluid or air. Its walls are in approximation, and normal secretions keep them from adhering.

Indications for Thoracentesis. When a thoracentesis is done for diagnostic reasons, the pleural cavity is entered to determine whether fluid is present, if this cannot be established satisfactorily by other means. If fluid is present, specimens usually are obtained and analyzed to assist in diagnosis. If an accumulation of fluid in the pleural cavity causes difficult respiration and discomfort, a thoracentesis may be done for therapeutic reasons to remove the fluid. This, in turn, relieves respiratory embarrassment.

Fluid in the pleural cavity results from inflammation caused by an infection which increases the normal secretions in the pleural cavity. If the fluid is purulent, the condition is called *empyema*. Fluid may accumulate also in the pleural cavity as a result of impaired circulation. This is common when a tumor is present. Air in the pleural cavity is due almost always to accidents when the chest wall has been punctured.

Necessary Equipment. Because the cavity being entered is sterile, surgical technic is used. The basic equipment for entering the pleural cavity includes a small syringe and a 22- or 25-gauge needle for administering a local anesthetic at the site of injection; a blunt 15-gauge needle, two to three inches long, gauze and cotton; sterile rubber gloves for the physician; and a fenestrated drape. A skin antiseptic and a bottle of one per cent procaine hydrochloride are included.

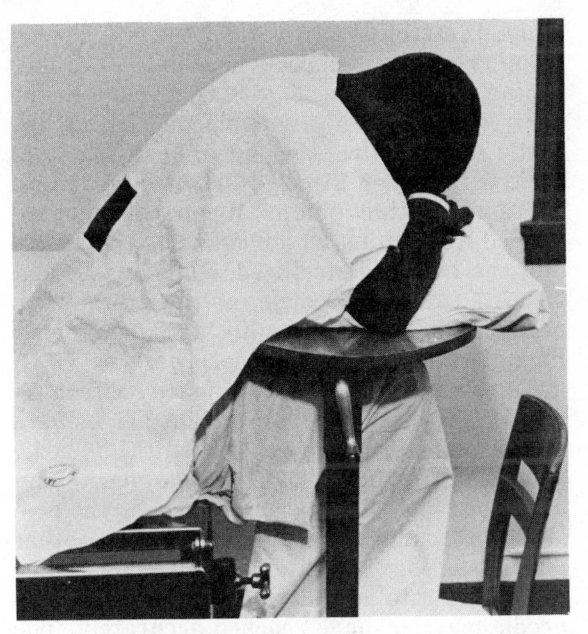

Fig. 33-3. Position of the patient for a thoracentesis.

Normally, the pressure in the pleural cavity is less than atmospheric; therefore, equipment for suction is almost always necessary to remove the fluid. The physician indicates the method that he will use.

One way to remove fluid or air from the pleural cavity is to aspirate it with a syringe. A large syringe—usually 50 cc.—is used. When this method is employed, a sterile syringe with a three-way stopcock attached is added to the sterile equipment. The physician withdraws the fluid into the syringe and adjusts the stopcock so that he may push the fluid into the collecting container. He readjusts the stopcock and reaspirates the pleural cavity.

Another method for removing fluid from the pleural cavity is to drain the fluid into a bottle in which a partial vacuum has been created. The bottle has a stopper on it to which is attached a two-way stopcock. To one opening in the stopcock is attached rubber tubing which connects with the needle in the pleural cavity. Air is removed from the bottle through the other opening in the stopcock with either a motor-driven or a hand-operated suction pump. When this method is used, the tubing which connects the needle and the bottle is sterilized. It is convenient to use a calibrated bottle for the drainage in order to determine readily the amount of fluid that has been removed.

To enhance the safety and the effectiveness of the procedure, physicians are using a plastic catheter to thread through the needle after it is in the site. Then the needle can be withdrawn. The catheter reduces the possibility of puncturing the lung or doing other damage; also, its flexibility makes it possible to feed it into a pocket of fluid which the needle may not have reached accurately. The catheter is also more comfortable for the patient.

Prior to the procedure, the nurse examines the skin area where the physician will be working. If hair is present, the physician is asked whether he wishes the area shaved.

Assisting the Physician. Usually, this procedure is carried out when the patient is in a sitting position on a chair or on the edge of a treatment table or bed with his feet supported on a chair. Figure 33-3 illustrates this position. If the patient cannot sit up, he may lie on his side. Usually, he is placed on the affected side with the hand of that side resting on the opposite shoulder.

The skin is prepared over the area where the physician indicates that he will insert the needle. The exact location will depend on the area where fluid is present and where the physician can best aspirate it. The needle will be inserted between the ribs through the intercostal muscles, the intercostal fascia and into the pleura. After the skin is prepared, the physician places the drape. The nurse may need to help anchor it in front of the patient's shoulders to prevent its slipping about on the field of work. The nurse prepares the bottle of anesthetic drug and holds it so that the physician can read the label before he withdraws some, or she pours some.

The physician begins by anesthetizing the area where the needle is to be inserted. When anesthesia is effective, the physician inserts the needle. After the needle is in place, the nurse is responsible for having the container ready for the physician to empty the syringe if the syringe method is being used. If a bottle is being used to collect the drainage, the nurse assists by operating either the hand- or the motor-driven pump that creates the partial vacuum in the bottle. The nurse usually is asked to assist with the collection of specimens.

During the procedure, the nurse observes the patient for reactions. The patient's color, pulse rate and respiratory rate are observed, and anything unusual is reported to the physician immediately. Fainting, nausea and vomiting may occur.

When the procedure is completed, the needle (or plastic catheter) is removed. The nurse assists with placing a small sterile dressing over the site of entry.

Following the procedure, the patient should be observed for changes in his respirations. If fluid is removed, respirations usually will be eased. If the lung has been punctured accidentally (the use of a blunt needle aids in preventing this accident), respiratory embarrassment becomes acute. If present, sputum should be observed, and if blood appears or if the patient has severe coughing, the physician should be notified promptly.

Abdominal Paracentesis

The withdrawal of fluid from the peritoneal cavity is referred to as an abdominal paracentesis. The word *paracentesis* means the withdrawal of fluid from any body cavity, but it is common practice to use the term when referring to the removal of fluid from the peritoneal cavity. It is used more for diagnostic purposes. There are other therapeutic means for decreasing fluid from this area.

The accumulation of fluid in the peritoneal cavity is called *ascites* and often occurs with certain liver, cardiac and renal diseases.

Indications for a Paracentesis. A paracentesis will help to relieve symptoms caused by the accumulation of fluid in the peritoneal cavity. The symptoms are caused by the pressure of the fluid. For example, respirations may be embarrassed if the fluid causes pressure on the diaphragm, or frequency of voiding may be increased, since the fluid may make it difficult for the urinary bladder to fill to normal capacity.

When used for diagnostic purposes, specimens of the fluid are taken for examination in order to identify certain organisms or cells. For example, the fluid may be analyzed to determine whether or not cells of a malignant tumor are present.

Necessary Equipment. Since the peritoneal cavity is normally a sterile cavity, surgical asepsis is observed for the procedure. Normally, the pressure in the peritoneal cavity is no greater than atmospheric pressure, but, when fluid is present, pressure is greater than atmospheric. Gravity will aid in the removal of fluid; therefore, the fluid will drain of its own accord until pressure is equalized.

A sterile trocar and cannula are used to enter the peritoneal cavity. This instrument is usually four to five inches in length with a bore of approximately one-eighth of an inch. In order to introduce the trocar easily, a very small incision is made in the skin which is sutured following the procedure. The sterile items needed include: a small syringe and a 22- or 25-gauge needle for anesthetizing the skin prior to making the incision; a scalpel for making the incision; suture material, small clamps or forceps, a suture needle and a scissors for closing the incision; sterile tubing to be attached directly to the trocar for drainage; a sterile fenestrated drape or

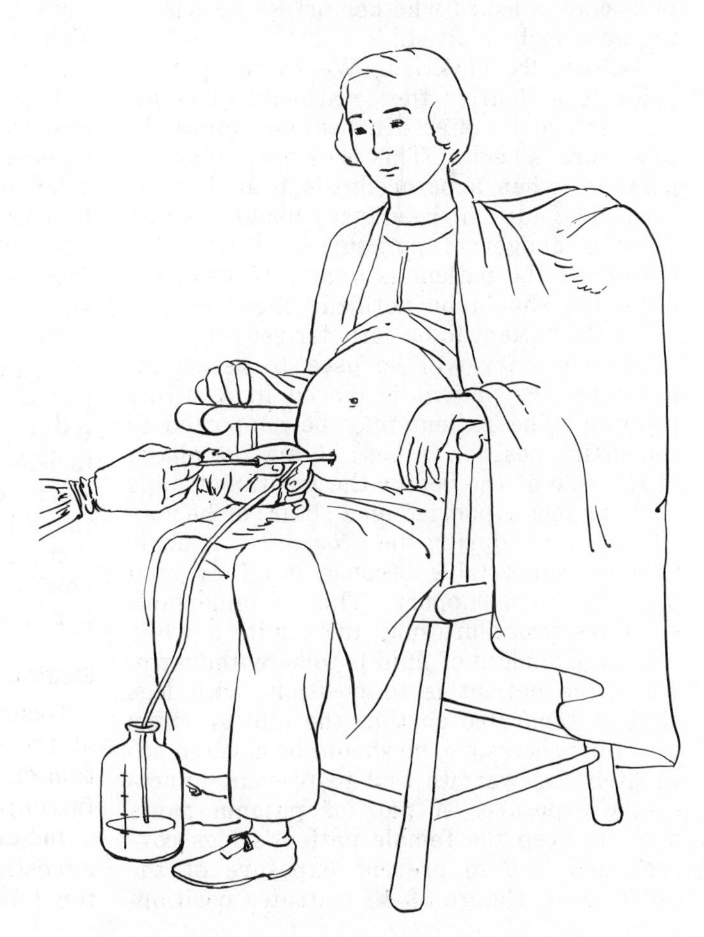

Fig. 33-4. Position of the patient for an abdominal paracentesis.

towels; gauze and cotton balls and gloves. Skin antiseptic and an anesthetic, usually one per cent procaine, will be needed.

A clean container for drainage, preferably a calibrated bottle, is necessary. The use of a plastic catheter threaded through the trocar once it is in place is a method used by some physicians. It provides for greater safety and comfort to the patient. In addition, its small caliber reduces the rate of flow of the fluid. When the plastic catheter is used, both the physician and the nurse may need to consider available equipment for a means of connecting the catheter to drainage tubing. A large-gauge needle inserted into the plastic tubing and then attached to suitable-sized drainage tubing is one means used.

Prior to the procedure, the nurse examines the patient's abdomen. If hair is present, the physician is asked whether or not he wishes the area to be shaved.

Assisting the Physician. Weigh the patient prior to and after the treatment. The patient should be offered a bedpan before the procedure is begun. This is of particular importance when a paracentesis is to be performed because, if the urinary bladder is full, there is danger of puncturing it with the trocar. If the patient is unable to void, the physician should be notified; then he may order the patient to be catheterized.

Since gravity will be used to assist the drainage, the patient is placed in a sitting position. The patient may be supported in the sitting position in bed; he may be placed at the side of the bed or the treatment table with his feet supported on a chair; or he may sit on a chair during the procedure. A chair is most comfortable because it offers good back and arm support. This is important, since the procedure may take quite a while if a large amount of fluid is to be withdrawn. After the patient is in position, with legs slightly separated so that the site of entry is readily accessible, he should be covered adequately for warmth and to prevent unnecessary exposure. A pair of pajama pants helps to keep the female patient's legs covered and also to prevent exposure of the pubic area. Figure 33-4 illustrates positioning and draping. The trocar will be passed through the abdominal wall into the peritoneal cavity near the midline of the abdomen approximately halfway between the umbilicus and the pubis. The skin over this area is cleansed, and the physician places the sterile drape in position. The nurse may need to secure it to prevent its slipping.

The physician then anesthetizes the site of entry, incises the skin and introduces the trocar and the cannula. When the trocar is in place, the physician will pull back on the cannula to see if fluid will drain; if it does, the drainage tube is attached. If a plastic catheter is used it is threaded through at this time. The nurse places the distal end of the tubing in the container for drainage. The greater the vertical distance between the trocar and the container for drainage, the greater will be the pull of gravity. If fluid is draining too rapidly, the container should be elevated on a stool. Rapid drainage may produce symptoms of shock.

During the treatment and after, the nurse observes the patient for untoward reactions associated with electrolyte imbalance. His color and respiratory and pulse rates are noted. Signs of fainting are watched for. The patient may begin to experience relief from the pressure of the fluid, and these signs are observed by the nurse also.

The nurse notes the type and the amount of drainage present and assists with preparing specimens for laboratory examination. After the needle has been withdrawn and the incision sutured, the nurse should place a sterile dressing and a combination pad over the site of incision, since leakage usually occurs. The patient often is more comfortable if an abdominal binder is used for support following the procedure.

Gastric Lavage

Gastric lavage is the mechanical emptying of the contents of the stomach. An irrigation or flushing of the stomach often is done in conjunction with the procedure.

Indications for Gastric Lavage. For some diagnostic purposes, stomach washings are used for laboratory examination. For example, stomach contents may be examined for the presence of *Mycobacterium tuberculosis.*

The procedure also is done to remove contents that have stagnated in the stomach and cannot pass into the small intestine because of the presence of an obstruction or lack of intestinal motility. The obstruction may be due to a tumor, a stenosis at the pyloric valve or adhesions. Gastric lavage relieves symptoms that are distressing to the patient, but it does not remove or treat the cause of the obstruction.

Another indication for a lavage is to empty the stomach of poisonous contents. For example, if a poison has been taken or if an overdose of a drug has been administered orally, the contents are removed, and the stomach is washed in order to prevent the absorption of the drug or the poison, or cool saline is used to remove old blood.

Necessary Equipment. Since the stomach is not a sterile cavity, the equipment need not be sterile, but medical asepsis is observed.

The tube is introduced through one of the nares. It is made of rubber or plastic and is 12 to 24 inches longer than the distance from the patient's mouth to his stomach. The tube commonly used is the Levin tube. Either a bulb-type syringe or a plunger-type syringe is used to aspirate the stomach contents. Usually, a 50-cc. syringe is preferred.

The larger the lumen of the tube, the easier it is to remove thick stomach contents and the more effective is the irrigation of the stomach. Obviously, a large tube is uncomfortable for the patient. Once the stomach contents have been drawn up to fill the tube, the end of the tube may be placed lower than the level of the patient's stomach, and the stomach contents may be removed by siphonage. Lavage tubes may also have a funnel attached so that solutions may be poured easily into the tube for irrigating the stomach. The physician indicates the type of solution to use for irrigating—usually sodium bicarbonate or physiologic saline.

Before the physician inserts the tube, it is helpful to place the tube on cracked ice for 15 or 20 minutes. This cooling of the tube makes it less flexible and therefore easier to handle. In addition, the water from the melting ice serves as lubrication for the tube. Because of the danger of the patient's aspirating a lubricant, water is the safest lubricant to use.

When a small tube is used, it is passed through one of the nares. If a large tube is used, the patient is asked to swallow it through the mouth. If the patient is allowed water, permitting him to take sips while the tube is being passed aids in the ease with which the tube is swallowed.

In addition to the chilled tube, the syringe, the funnel and the solution for irrigation, there should be appropriate containers for specimens and for collecting stomach washings.

Assisting the Physician. In most instances, the patient is placed in the sitting position so that gravity aids the passage of the tube. If the patient is unable to sit up, he may lie either on his back or on his side. The physician introduces and passes the tube, asking the patient to help by swallowing frequently. After the tube is in place, the nurse assists the physician as necessary by helping with collecting specimens and pouring the solution if an irrigation is done.

The tube should be tested to see that it is in place *before any solution is introduced.* This is done by placing the end of the tube in a small amount of water. If the tube has entered a bronchus, air bubbles will appear at regular intervals with each respiration. However, in the conscious adult there usually are other signs of distress, such as coughing, cyanosis and gasping.

Gastric and Duodenal Suction Siphonage

Gastric or duodenal suction siphonage provides for the continuous removal of contents from the stomach or the duodenum or both.

Indications. Continuous siphonage is indicated when it becomes desirable and necessary to keep the stomach and the duodenum empty and at rest. For example, prior to gastric surgery, the surgeon usually wishes to have the area free of gas and undigested food; following surgery performed on the gastrointestinal tract, he will wish to keep the stomach and the duodenum empty and at rest until healing at the site of the operation has begun. The siphonage is effective for removing secretions and air or gas that often accumulate in the gastrointestinal tract following abdominal surgery. This helps to prevent distention. Continuous siphonage is indicated also when there is a paralysis in the gastrointestinal tract and the normal movement of the products of digestion is interrupted, for example, by a paralysis of the ileus which sometimes occurs. Siphonage then is used to prevent distention, discomfort and the dangers associated with the paralysis.

Necessary Equipment. A variety of tubes is available for use for siphoning gastric and duodenal contents. If simple decompression of the stomach is desired, a long plain tube, such as the Levin tube, is used. The disposable tubes are very satisfactory, since they seem to be comfortable for the patient, are less objectionable when secured to the face, and eliminate the difficult problem of thorough cleaning.

If siphonage of the duodenum is desired and to be continued over a period of several hours or days, then one of a variety of other tubes is used. These usually have a device at the end which keeps the tip of the tube in the duodenum.

One type of tube has a double lumen. One lumen connects with a small rubber bag. After the tube is past the pylorus, the bag is inflated with fluid or air. Another type of tube is injected with mercury, usually five cc. The air, the fluid and the mercury tips aid in the forward movement of the tube. These tips also act to keep the tube in situ by preventing the tube from moving back into the stomach. These tubes are chilled on ice and passed through one of the nares in the same manner as other gastric tubes.

Assisting the Physician. The physician is responsible for passing the tube. After it is determined that the tube is in the stomach, peristalsis aids in moving it through the pyloric valve. Usually, it is helpful to have the patient lie on his right side so that gravity will aid the tube in dropping into the duodenum. As a rule every 20 or 30 minutes, a few more inches of the tube are passed until the desired length has entered the gastrointestinal tract. The responsibility of passing a few inches of tube at regular intervals may be delegated to the nurse.

Siphonage either is started as soon as the tube has reached the stomach or is delayed until the tube is in the duodenum, depending on the physician's wishes.

Suction Siphonage. Fluids and gases move from an area of greater pressure to one of lesser pressure. To remove liquids and gases from the gastrointestinal tract, it is necessary to lower the pressure in the tube, thus causing the contents of the gastrointestinal tract to rise in the tube and be drained off.

The manner in which suction is maintained on the drainage tube will depend on each agency's equipment. Some agencies have electric pumps which automatically maintain a partial vacuum in the bottle that collects drainage from the patient; others have wall suction which can be connected to the collecting bottle. A syringe attached to the free end of the tube can be used also to create an area of lesser pressure in the tube by partially evacuating the air from the tube.

To remove gastrointestinal contents with a syringe over a long period of time is not convenient or expedient. Therefore, a mechanical device is used to great advantage. While motor-driven units are used extensively and are highly efficient, a water-created suction apparatus should still be understood by the nurse, because there may be an occasion where she has to set one up, or to improvise a suction device. It is simple to assemble and to operate in the event that other devices are not available.

Study Situations 1 and 2 are concerned with two such set-ups.

Nurse's Responsibilities. The nurse is responsible for seeing that the apparatus is functioning properly at all times. The patient's tube is irrigated at regular intervals, as ordered by the physician. Normal saline or water, usually about 30 cc., is used. When irrigating is done, it is easy to determine whether or not the tube is patent. After the solution has been injected, the suction is started again, and the irrigating fluid should return quickly. Usually, patients having continuous gastrointestinal suction are having intake and output measured. Therefore, the amount injected in the tube and returned should be recorded carefully. Observe for signs of electrolyte imbalance.

The nares require special care while the drainage tube is in place. Regular cleansing and the application of a small amount of lubrication help to keep the mucous membrane in good condition.

The nurse is responsible for noting the type and the amount of drainage present. Most agencies provide a routine for measuring, emptying and cleansing the drainage bottle in every 24-hour period. For esthetic reasons, it is desirable to place a cover around the drainage bottle (if the set-up does not have one) so that the contents are out of view of the patient and the visitors.

Gastric Analysis

Gastric analysis is the mechanical emptying of the stomach for the purpose of examining gastric secretions as an aid in diagnosis. The number of specimens to be taken and the time intervals between them will vary according to the procedure of the laboratories in the various agencies. However, almost all request a fasting specimen and then the administration of a test meal. At intervals following the meal, samples of gas-

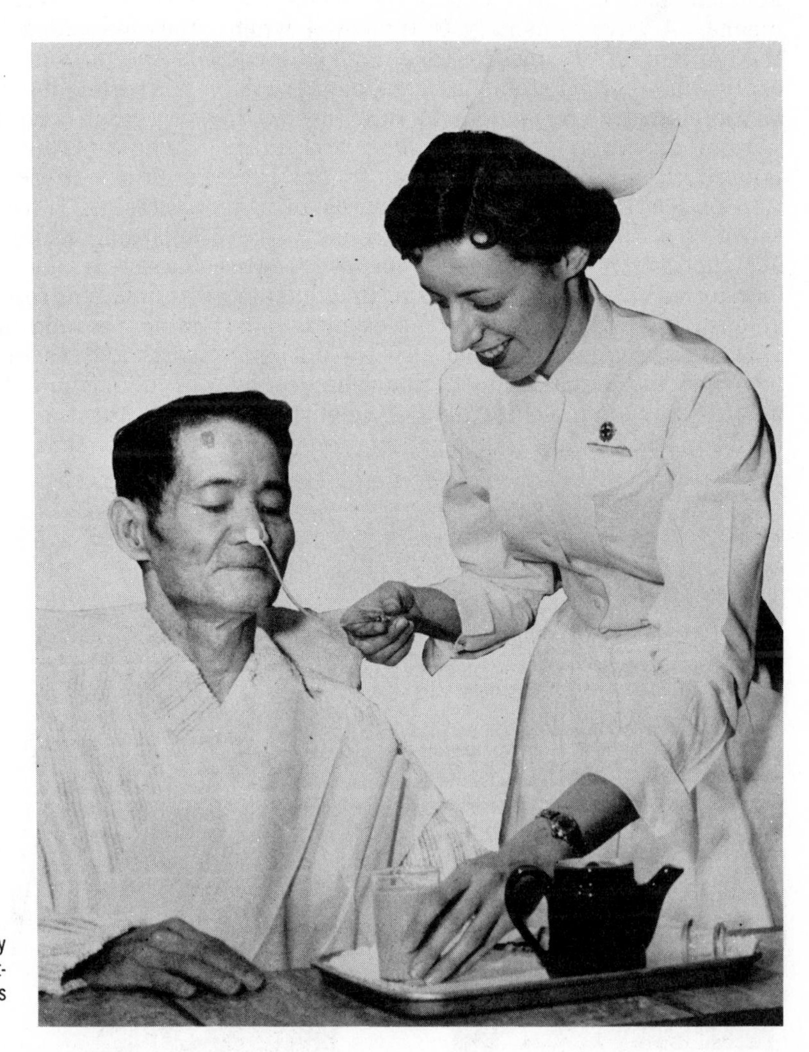

FIG. 33-5. If the patient must be fed by tube, the feeding should be served in an attractive and appetizing manner, so that it is obviously food and not a medication.

tric contents are taken. Gastric analyses are done usually to determine the amount of hydrochloric acid in gastric contents.

Preparation for Gastric Analysis. Preparation for this procedure is similar to all others involving the passing of a tube into the stomach. However, the nurse's role of explaining the procedure to the patient cannot be overemphasized. If the patient does not understand fully the nature of the examination, it is quite possible that fluids and foods might be eaten and the examination necessarily delayed.

Gastric Gavage

Gastric gavage is the introduction of nourishment into the stomach by mechanical means. A gavage usually is indicated when the patient is unable to take nourishment orally but when no stomach or duodenal pathologic changes are present to interfere with normal digestive processes. The procedure is used often when a patient has an obstruction or a stricture in the esophagus or the throat. A tumor may be the cause of an obstruction. A stricture may be congenital or may be caused by scar tissue that has developed following injury to the esophagus.

Gastric gavages are used also for patients who are too weak to take nourishment by mouth. For example, gavages frequently are used for feeding premature infants for whom the physicial effort of sucking is too great. They are also used for patients who are unconscious.

Necessary Equipment. The equipment is similar to that used for a gastric lavage. A tube with a small lumen is passed, usually through the nostril. The nourishment is poured into a funnel attached to the tube leading to the stomach or it may be injected by the syringe method. If continuous nourishment is given, usually to a bed patient, a container of the prescribed feeding is hung at the bedside on a pole and allowed to drip constantly at a slow rate.

The nourishment given by gavage is prepared in liquid form, usually from a blender. Drugs that ordinarily are administered orally may be added to the nourishment according to the physician's order.

Assisting the Physician. The nurse assists the physician and the patient as for a gastric lavage. After the tube is in place, the nurse assumes responsibility for giving the nourishment. If the tube is left in place, it is secured, usually with adhesive or Scotch Tape. If nourishment is to be given continuously, drop by drop, the nurse is responsible for adding to the container as necessary and as ordered. When large amounts of nourishment are given at regular intervals, the food is warmed to room temperature so that the patient does not become

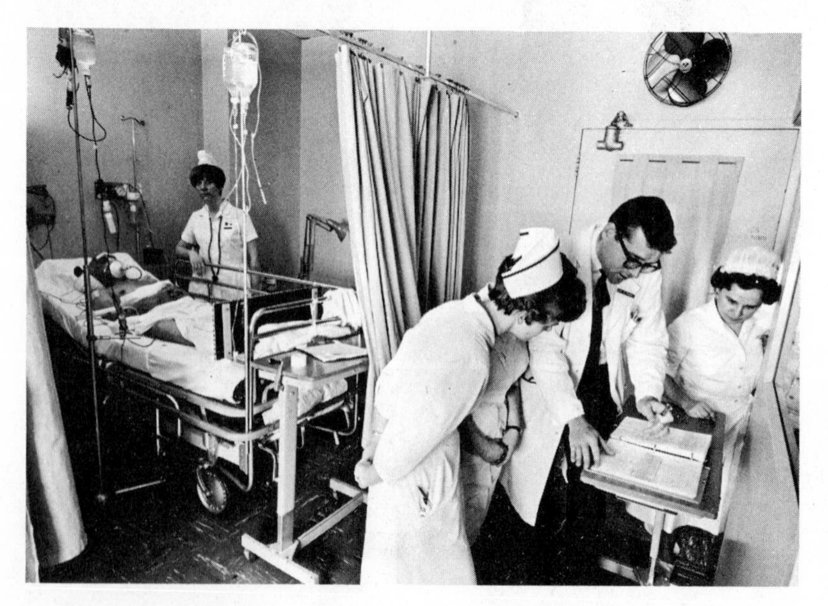

FIG. 33-6. The intensive care unit is an example of an area in which patients have many therapeutic and diagnostic measures performed concurrently. This is a challenge to the nurse, because it requires her to know scientific principles without losing sight of the fact that the person receiving such therapy is an individual. (Photo by Bernard Cole, Hospital Life)

chilled. Food which is given continuously is not warmed, since it will approximate room temperature while it passes through the tubing to the patient's stomach. In addition, warmed milk and cream will sour more quickly during the period of time it takes for a container of nourishment to enter the patient's stomach.

After the feeding is instilled, a small amount of water should be introduced into the tube. This washes the feeding remaining in the tube into the stomach. It also prevents adhered feeding from souring.

The tube is clamped off after the food is instilled. This prevents it from draining back out.

Study Situations

1. The following diagram illustrates an improvised three-bottle set-up. Fluid in the sealed bottle *A* drips into the open-mouth container *C* via tube *B*. *C* must have a means for air to leave as fluid enters; otherwise, an area of greater pressure will be created, and fluid from *A* will not be able to flow into *C*.

As fluid leaves *A*, an area of lesser pressure is created; therefore, "pull" is put on *D*. *D* is able to obtain air from *E*, which is a sealed container. However, soon *E* contains an area of lesser pressure because its contents are moving into *D*. *F*, which is connected to the gastrointestinal tube, then begins to have an area of lesser pressure, and gases and fluids from the patient move into it and collect in *E*.

What would happen if *D* were long enough to reach into the contents at the bottom of *E*?

What would happen if *B* were to become kinked or shut off?

What would happen if *E* were brought to the same level as *A*?

What would happen if air were to leak in *A* at the point where *B* is inserted?

2. The following diagram illustrates an improvised two-bottle set-up. Fluid in the sealed bottle *A* drips into the open-mouth container *C*. An area of lesser pressure is created in *A* and is transmitted into the tube *D*. *D* is attached to the gastrointestinal tube in the patient, and, therefore, gases and liquids in the patient will move toward this area of lesser pressure and be drawn into *A*.

What would happen if the fluid level in *A* were to fall below the inserted tip leading to *B*?

What would happen if *C* were brought to the level of *A*?

3. Check your understanding of why various means are used to *remove* fluids from different body sites. Select from Column 2 the

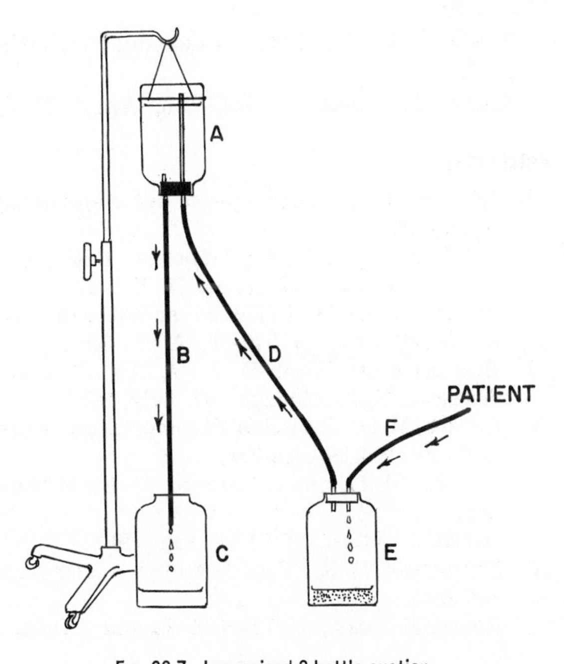

FIG. 33-7. Improvised 3-bottle suction.

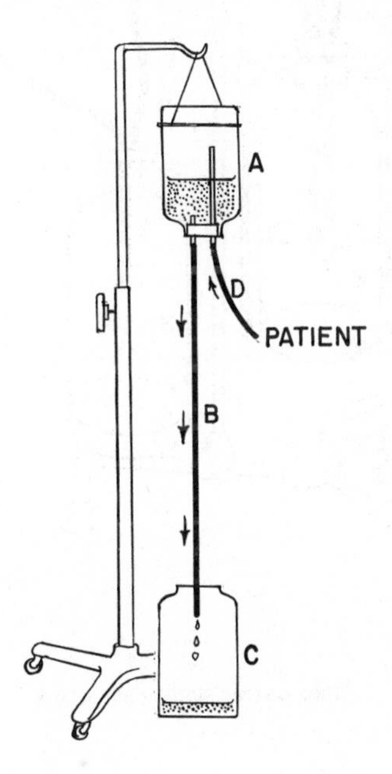

appropriate description of the pressure status of these sites under normal circumstances.

Column 1	Column 2
_____ Venous circulation	1. At atmospheric pressure
_____ Arterial circulation	
_____ Stomach	
_____ Small intestine	2. Below atmospheric pressure
_____ Subarachnoid space	
_____ Peritoneal cavity	
_____ Pleural cavity	3. Above atmospheric pressure

4. In a commercially prepared three-bottle suction, as illustrated below, bottles *1* and *2* are attached to a stand in such a manner

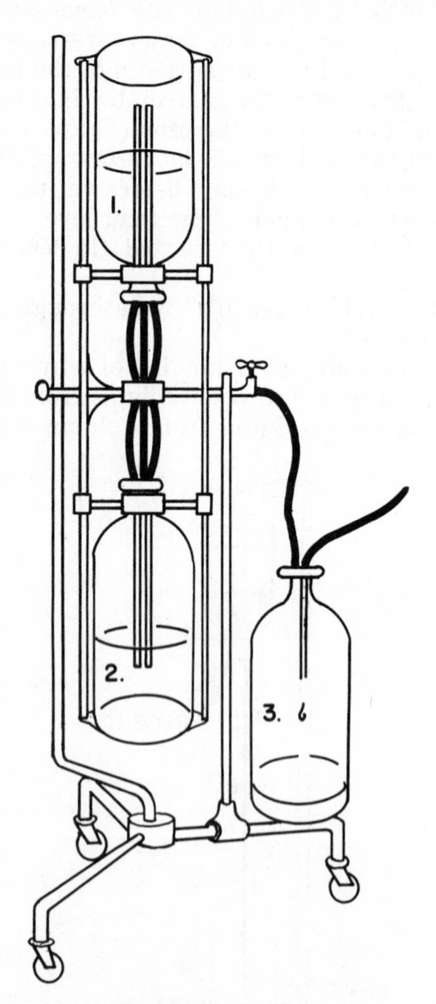

Wangensteen suction apparatus.

that they can be reversed whenever the top bottle is empty. Fluid from the top bottle *1* drips into the lower bottle *2*, creating an area of lesser pressure in bottle *1*. This pressure is transmitted to bottle *3*. Bottle *3* is connected by means of tubing to the patient's gastric tube. The area of lesser pressure in bottle *3* exerts "pull" on the contents in the patient's gastrointestinal tract and drains them into bottle *3*.

How does air get in? What keeps the water in the top bottle from running into the lower one?

5. The importance of explaining to both patient and family whenever a patient is to be removed from his unit for any type of treatment is emphasized in the following article. See how unnecessarily distressed a family may be when explanations are not given.

- Shipp, D. E.: The empty bed.
  AMER. J. NURS., *67*:2129, October, 1967.

6. How would you feel if you could not hear well and therefore had to guess what was going on around you? This is particularly important when patients are not carefully prepared for diagnostic or therapeutic measures. For some valuable hints on how to make it easier for such patients see the following:

- Bender, R. E.: Communicating with the deaf.
  AMER. J. NURS., *66*:757-760, April, 1966.

References

1. Brocker, R. J.: Technique to avoid spinal-tap headache.
   J.A.M.A., *168*:261, September 20, 1958.
2. Brown, B. A., and Jones, O. W., Jr.: Prolonged headache following spinal puncture.
   J. NEUROSURG., *19*:349-50, April, 1962.
3. Buchanan-Davidson, D. J.: A drop of blood.
   AMER. J. NURS., *65*:103-107, July, 1965.
4. Cantor, M. O.: Intestinal decompression tubes.
   G.P., *26*:104, September, 1962.
5. Crouch, M. L., and Gibson, S. T.: Blood therapy.
   AMER. J. NURS., *62*:71, March, 1962.
6. Davenport, R. R.: Tube feeding for long-term patients.
   AMER. J. NURS., *64*:121-123, January, 1964.

7. Drummond, E. E., and Anderson, M. L.: Gastrointestinal suction.
AMER. J. NURS., *63*:109-113, December, 1963.
8. Fason, M. F.: Controlling bacterial growth in tube feedings.
AMER. J. NURS., *67*:1246-1247, June, 1967.
9. Flitter, H. H.: Pressure in Physics and Nursing *in* An Introduction to Physics in Nursing. ed. 4, pp. 93-102.
St. Louis, Missouri, C. V. Mosby, 1962.
10. Jensen, J. T.: Introduction to Medical Physics. pp. 76-80, 87-91, 96-98.
Philadelphia, Lippincott, 1960.
11. McClaughry, R.: Transfusion reactions.
MED. CLIN. N. AMER., *46*:551, March, 1962.
12. Myers, R. S.: One pint transfusions may not be worth the risk.
MOD. HOSP., *95*:106, November, 1960.
13. Nordmark, M. T., and Rohweder, A. W.: *In* Scientific Foundations of Nursing, "Volume and Pressure of Circulating Blood," ed. 2, Chapter 1.
Philadelphia, Lippincott, 1967.
14. Strickler, J. H. *et al*: Diagnostic paracentesis.
ARCH. SURG., *77*:859, December, 1958.
15. Wu, R.: Explaining treatments to young children.
AMER. J. NURS., *65*:71-73, July, 1965.

Nursing in a Home Situation: A Patient Study

Unit 7

CHAPTER 34

Nursing in a Home Situation: A Patient Study

In the basic nursing program almost all—and, in some instances, all—of what is learned about nursing is hospital oriented. This gives the impression that patients with major health problems are in hospitals or other health facilities. However, many persons manage difficult and involved health problems at home, and in some instances even in a one-room apartment. The following describes one home situation. It is about a patient and her family coping with multiple sclerosis. It is an example of what can be done, and hopefully it will give suggestions to nurses who need to help other families. The diagnoses and the problems may vary but there are many families with similar problems.

The patient is Mrs. Ryan. Her history of multiple sclerosis dates back to the time when her youngest daughter, who is now 20 years old, was an infant. Mrs. Ryan has two older children, a son and a daughter, who are married and live far from their parents' home. Her husband teaches and her daughter works in an office. Mrs. Ryan's own parents are dead, as is her mother-in-law. She has no sisters or brothers. So the only other close relative is her father-in-law, who lives reasonably near, visits her, and frequently brings things grown in his garden.

As is often typical of this illness, Mrs. Ryan had been able to manage quite well for several years. There were periods of time when she was "fine," and then there were episodes of remission when her impaired vision and ambulation prevented her from getting about. But her wonderful spirit of hope and good cheer helped her to accept these ups and downs. Eventually she became dependent upon the wheelchair to get about. However, she still retained her hope and her role in the home: planning meals, managing routine household and family problems, and looking after her husband.

The time came when Mrs. Ryan had to remain in bed alone at home. This presented the problem of how to provide for her care and nourishment. Having reached the state of immobility, she could not move her arms voluntarily and was unable to walk. She was, and is, able to sit in a wheelchair for short periods of time.

For a person with many needs for care, one solution is a nursing home. Another is to find a means of providing the care the family cannot give because they must be absent from the home many hours of the day. Being at home and a part of the family means everything to Mrs. Ryan; she mentions this very often. Her family wants her there and are willing to try to give her the care needed, with the help of others to fill the gaps.

The situation developed into a team approach. As in any health team, there is the physician who plans the course of therapy and care needed. Mrs. Ryan's physician, who made the original diagnosis, was able to continue treating her until recently when he moved away. This meant the start of a new medical relationship, but fortunately a pleasant one developed. There is also a visit-

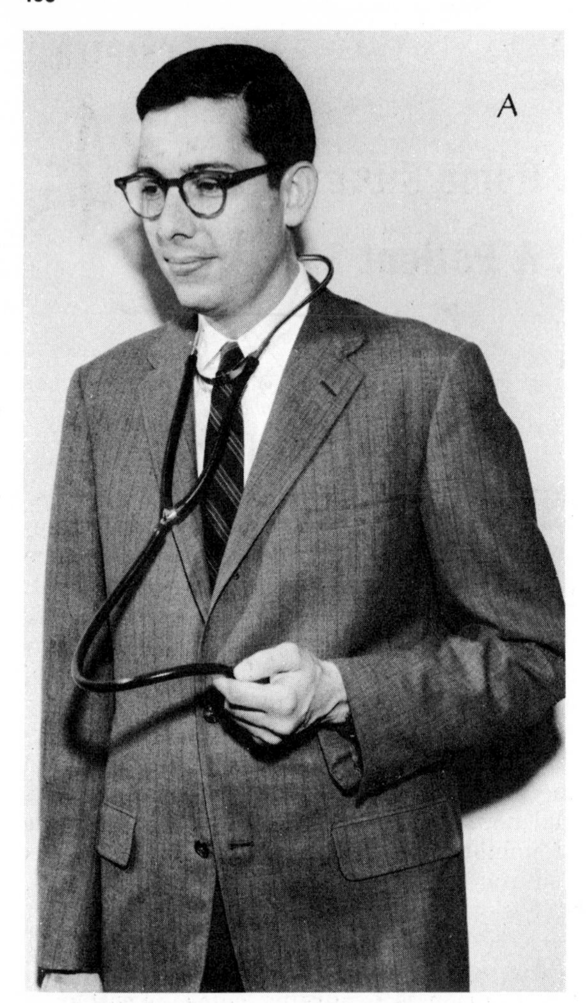

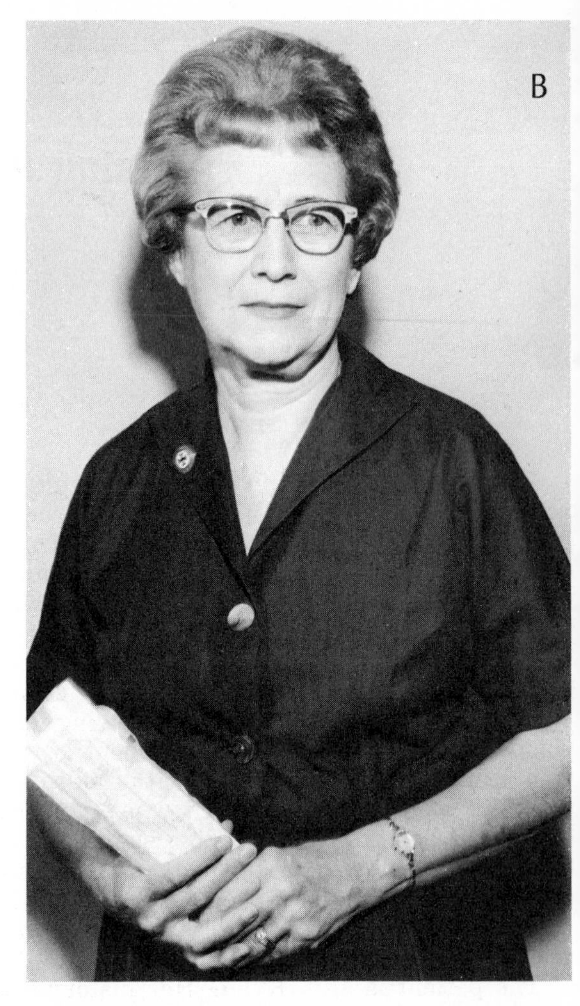

FIG. 34-1A and 1B. The leaders of the home health team. The physician's visits are regular, though not as frequent as in the hospital situation. The visiting nurse determines nursing goals, formulates plans of care, carries out special treatments, and coordinates the activities of the volunteer group.

ing nurse who in the course of her regular visits explained to the family the details of care needed now that bed rest and immobility were to be considered. Mrs. Ryan had several neighbors and friends who knew of her plight and were willing to help, so the visiting nurse taught them how to turn her, care for her back, and exercise her limbs.

Mrs. Ryan was active in her church, so an appeal went out for volunteers so that there would be a sufficient number of persons to carry out the care needed and to have a supply of "reserves" in case of illness, vacations and so forth. Fortunately, one of the neighbors, an R.N., was able to teach others as they joined the team (or "troops" as they came to be called). And so it has been now for several years. Friends bring their friends and teach them as replacements are needed. Some are inactive R.N.s and others are Red Cross Nursing Aide volunteers, so there is plenty of know-how.

Like the time sheet in the hospital, there is a sheet listing the names of the regulars and the substitutes, their days and times and who does what. Even the milkman can be

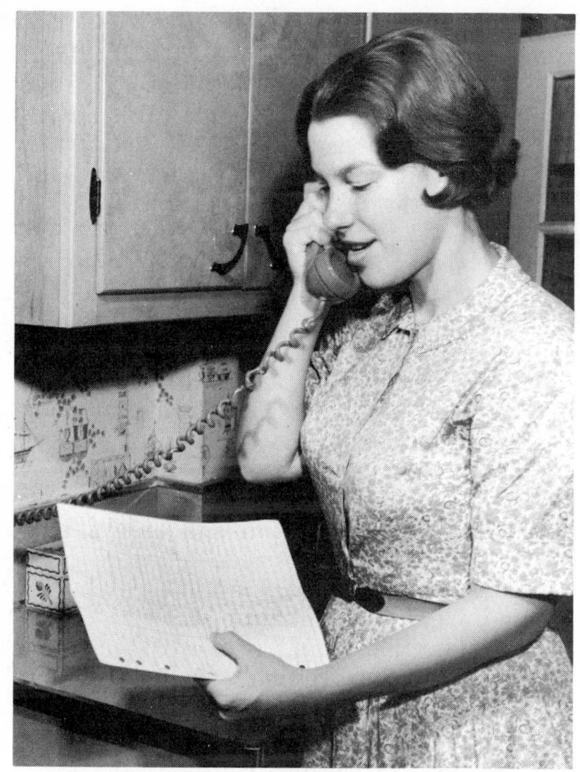

FIG. 34-2. One of the "regulars" has a problem. She is starting to have signs of an upper respiratory infection, so she is calling up a substitute to take her place. The sheet she is holding lists who is where and when, and substitutes who can be called when and for what functions. One thing Mrs. Ryan can do without is an upper respiratory infection.

considered a "dietary" representative on the team. He brings the milk into the house and places it in the refrigerator.

Mrs. Ryan's daily out-of-bed treats are made possible by her husband who is able to lift her out and back into bed by means of a body-mechanics technic of his own design. The patient is in a standard hospital bed which is not adjustable in terms of height. It was obtained through the town's Rescue Squad, which can supply such items.

Mrs. Ryan's care includes irrigation of the retention catheter, which of course means the preparation of the solution and the sterilization of the equipment. It also means the use and care of the collecting bag which is attached when she is out of bed, and the tubing and collecting bottle when she is in bed. There are several medications to be administered at different times of the day, and a vitamin complex injection once a week. There is need for frequent turning and back care to prevent breakdown. There are, of course, her needs for bathing, hair and nail care, and oral hygiene. As mentioned, she cannot move her arms voluntarily, and therefore must be fed.

It is difficult to obtain dental care for a home patient. For dental prophylaxis, or for care of cavities, the person must be transported to the dentist. This can be a major

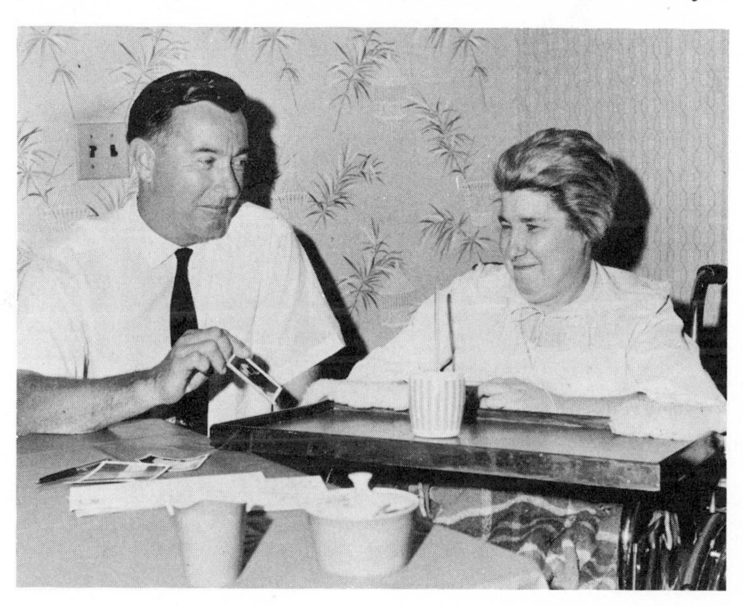

FIG. 34-3. High spots of the day, and especially the weekends, are when Mrs. Ryan can be out of bed in her wheelchair. Her husband made a tray that fits over the arms of the wheelchair so she can rest her arms on it. It is also used for her meals. She has a small sheepskin under each elbow to prevent pressure from the chair. Husband and wife are going through the day's mail containing the latest pictures of their first granddaughter.

undertaking, and such it is each time Mrs. Ryan visits the dentist. Only recently has there been some indication in the literature that dental home services are receiving some attention.

In addition to the physician, the visiting nurse, the daughter, and Mr. Ryan, who carries out the largest share of the care, the volunteer "team" consists of fifteen regulars and fourteen substitutes. Each regular has a fixed day of the week, time and functions. The substitutes are the "back-up" team when a regular cannot keep her appointment.

In mid-morning Mrs. Ryan is given back care and turned. She is given the fluids and the medications due at that time. Some of the persons who volunteered to help are unable to move Mrs. Ryan up in bed or turn her for various reasons; for instance, some have had back injuries, and for others the bed is too high, causing back strain. These members come at mid-day and give Mrs. Ryan her lunch. Often they read to her from books of her choice. They also fix flowers as needed and tend to other needs as they arise.

In the afternoon another member of the team comes to turn the patient again, and give her back care and more fluids and medications. When she is on her left side, she is inclined to have some involuntary movements of her legs, so a bed siderail is always put up. Her television set is located so that she can see it when she is on her left side. A detail of the planning is that the patient decides her "turning pattern" so that she will be on her left side in time for the television programs that she wants to see.

Just as in the hospital, where a patient is in contact with a large number of persons in the course of a week, the major goals of the patient's care must be formulated and made known to all who contribute. In Mrs. Ryan's case, they are:

1. *An adequately nutritious diet:* Because her appetite is good and she enjoys most foods and has no restrictions, there is no problem. However, in recent years she has begun to gain weight. As she was on the "thin" side, the weight gain was acceptable and actually improved her appearance. But, as often happens, there comes a point at which one must call a halt and impose a limit on the caloric intake.

No one likes to deny any person who is physically handicapped anything that he enjoys. But the time comes when it is necessary

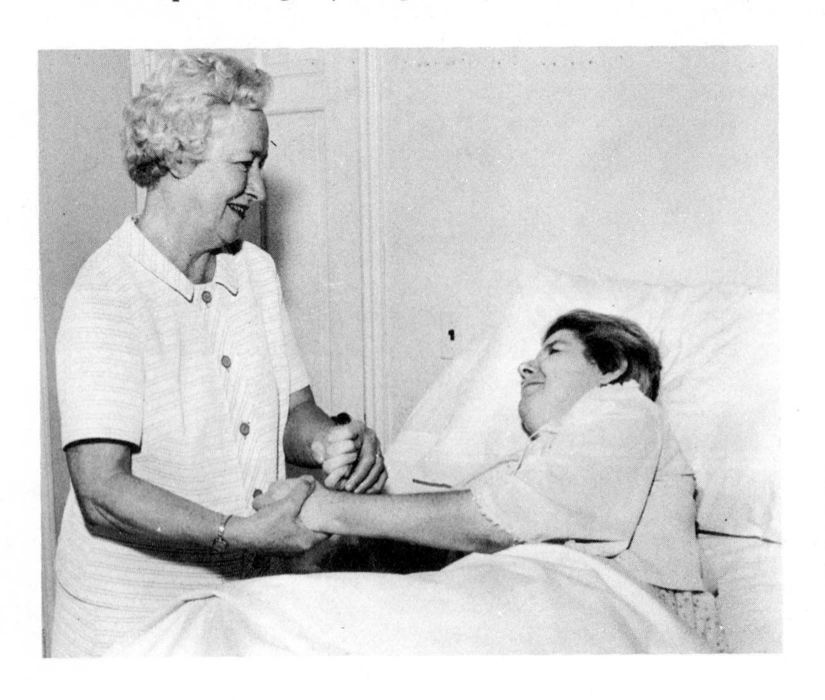

FIG. 34-4. One of the members of the volunteer "team" is starting to put Mrs. Ryan's arm through range of motion. Because she cannot remain on her back unaided, exercises must be done from side-lying positions.

to be "cruel" in order to be kind. Mrs. Ryan admits to having a "sweet tooth." She enjoys rich desserts and candies. The excess adiposity was not any more helpful to her situation than it is to any one else. So more fruit instead of highly caloric desserts, and less candy and other sweets became necessary. Dietetic juices are substituted for the sweetened variety. Butter on toast and other foods is used more sparingly. Mrs. Ryan joins the army of weight watchers.

The diet must not only be nutritious but also promote regularity of bowel evacuation. For the most part the patient is "regular," but occasionally some combination of circumstances may result in temporary constipation. Understandably, this is disturbing to her. One of her medications is a multi-vitamin and mineral combination. Iron preparations can cause constipation for some persons. However, her diet pattern has not made this a chronic problem.

2. *Adequate fluid intake:* Fluid intake is important not only in relation to normal cellular needs and as an aid in bowel elimination, but also for "internal" irrigation. Since Mrs. Ryan has a retention catheter, it is important that she maintain sufficient urinary output to prevent concentration of urine and ascending infection. Sufficient urinary drainage is a form of self-irrigation of the catheter.

Because it is difficult for her to pull up on the drinking tube, it is a mouthful-by-mouthful process. Sometimes the patient jokes about "drink-the-water-it-is-good-for-you" routine by deciding when each kidney has had its drink, and how much went for catheter irrigation.

3. *Prevention of complications of immobility:* The frequent turning, the extremity exercises, and getting the patient up out of bed in the wheelchair all help to improve circulation of blood and lymph, maintain musculoskeletal function to the greatest extent possible, and prevent pressure sores. There is no foot board or block because Mrs. Ryan is never on her back while in bed. She is unable to maintain that position even with the support of pillows. Also, she is not comfortable in that position.

4. *Deep breathing and coughing exercises:* These are done to the extent to which Mrs. Ryan is capable of doing them. However, she does have a choking sensation periodically and this acts almost as a coughing exercise. She is inclined to have such episodes when she is taking fluids. Another very helpful circumstance is that she has a very good sense of humor. She laughs a great deal and this too is a respiratory "assist."

5. *Medications:* In regard to medications, the smallest tablets are the most difficult for her to swallow. Most people find a large capsule a problem, but these she can manage easily. By a bit of experimenting, it was found that it is best for her if the small pills are placed (one at a time) directly in back of her lower teeth at the tip of her tongue. Then when she takes the sip of water, she can move it over her tongue and hopefully on its way down. When a small tablet was placed on her tongue, the water went around it. Inasmuch as it is easier for her to swallow the large capsules, the experiment of obtaining empty capsules and placing the smaller tablets in them is being considered.

In addition to special physical and safety needs, "life as usual" is another goal in planning for Mrs. Ryan's care in her home.

One member of the team added a small bird cage to Mrs. Ryan's room. It is attached to the wall and is filled with artificial flowers and birds and changed with each season of the year. Another member, an artist, brings one of her paintings to hang where Mrs. Ryan can see it, and all may enjoy it. She replaces it with a new one every few weeks. Another member altered her nightgowns so that they open in the back like hospital gowns, facilitating care. There are any number of other "extras" these women do both for the patient and the family.

Mentally, Mrs. Ryan is so alert and has such a good sense of humor and is so accepting of her situation that not infrequently others find themselves telling her about their troubles. Her alertness is not permitted to "go to waste" as it were, as might be the case if she were not living at home. Jokingly she has been credited with having all sorts of information "programmed" into her, such as: where to find various items in the kitchen, like glass drinking straws, the cat's food, clean dish towels, or various foods. She remembers many people's birthdays, dates of past events and telephone numbers. When told what supplies are running low, she reminds her husband to add them to his shopping list.

Recently Mrs. Ryan was ordained a deacon in her church. Although she cannot attend meetings, she contributes her prayers for the church, its members and for others. This helps to give her the feeling that she is still active in the community.

She and her husband discuss meal plans, things that need to be purchased, and the usual problems of maintaining a home. Her daughter provides the usual happiness and tribulations a young adult can bestow upon parents, such as opening up her latest purchases on her mother's bed, or reading to her letters from her male friends in the service, and having discussions as to whether she may or may not accept some invitations. Minor but important experiences such as these are often removed from persons who must become hospitalized. Being at home is therapeutic for all concerned. "Institution-

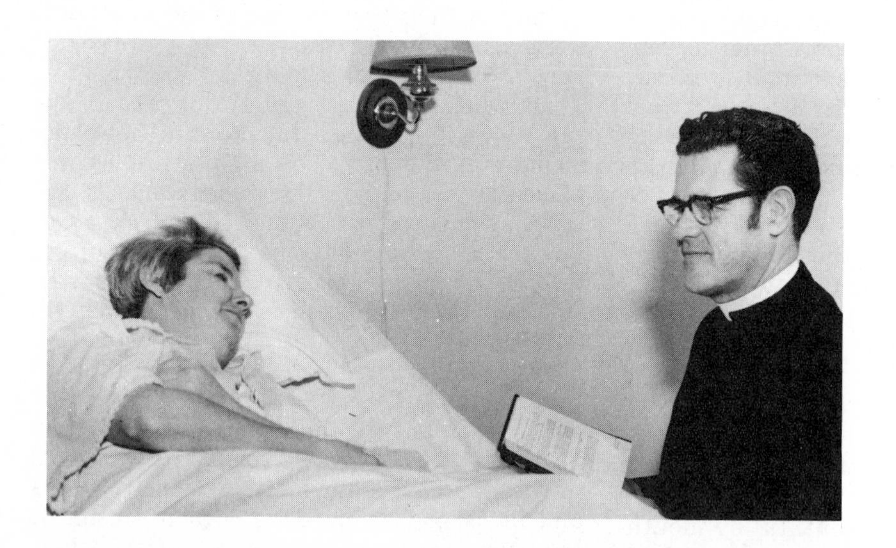

FIG. 34-5. The minister from her church visits frequently, not only because she is a home patient, but because of her position as a deacon. He gives her the sacrament of Communion at the intervals that are customary in their church. A member of the church who assists in Mrs. Ryan's care also is present at these times.

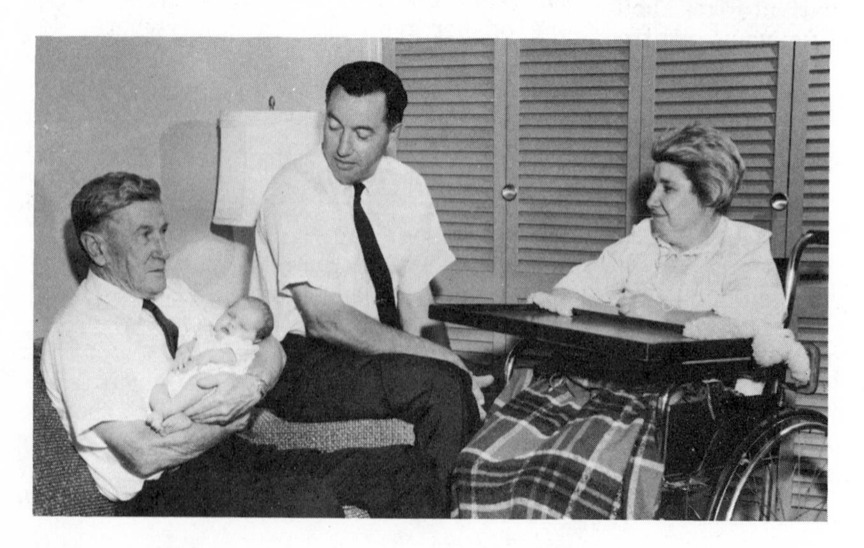

FIG. 34-6. The latest addition to the family pays her first call. Great-grandfather's arms must be mighty comfortable because no amount of pleading can entice her to wake up and smile, but "Grandma" is pleased.

alized" patients are deprived not only of the visual and verbal stimuli of loved ones but also of the loss of 'touch" or contact as well. It is such things as her husband's "hello" and "goodbye" kisses and other affectionate gestures from him and her daughter, her cat jumping up on the bed and cuddling up beside her (and being annoyed at being asked to move when Mrs. Ryan is to be turned), the month-old granddaughter being put in her arms, and the other granddaughter who can now run around, throwing her toys on the bed when she comes to visit. These are some of the things that help to maintain the individuality of the person and are so desperately important when bodily functions become increasingly impaired.

So, with a "team approach," Sally, as she is known by all (including the milkman), is enjoying life as the person she is—wife, mother, grandmother, daughter-in-law, and friend to many. She is thankful for a safe and therapeutic environment and total nursing care in her own home.

Index